Cosmetics for the Skin

Physiological and Pharmaceutical Approach

Cosmetics for the Skin

Physiological and Pharmaceutical Approach

A.K. Mohiuddin
Assistant Professor, Department of Pharmacy,
World University of Bangladesh
Tejgaon, Dhaka

PharmaMed Press
An imprint of BSP Books Pvt. Ltd.
4-4-309/316, Giriraj Lan
Sultan Bazar, Hyderabad - 500 095.

Cosmetics for the Skin: ***Physiological and Pharmaceutical Approach***
by AK Mohiuddin

Published by

PharmaMed Press

An imprint of BSP Books Pvt. Ltd.

4-4-309/316, Giriraj Lane, Sultan Bazar, Hyderabad - 500 095.
Phone: 040-23445688; Fax: 91+40-23445611
E-mail: info@pharmamedpress.com
www.pharmamedpress.com/pharmamedpress.net

ISBN: 978-93-90211-34-0

Preface

Skin is the barrier that segregates the body from the environment. Besides protecting the body from water loss and microbial infections, it plays a significant societal and cosmetic role. Skin health and appearance is often recognized as one of the principal factors representing overall well-being and the perception of "health" in humans and to cater to this notion, the skin care industry bloomed in early 20th century.

Today, skin care is an enormous global industry fostering a business of over 500 billion dollars

In addition to enhancing appearance, cosmetic products are also used extensively to treat various medical problems related to the skin. These products are a complex mixture of chemical compounds that are directly applied to the skin and although they seem harmless when used in small quantities (and their effects poorly advertised) continuous exposure to a mix of these chemicals over long periods has consequences on the health and well-being of people.

This book is a detailed review of the chemical and pharmacological base of these cosmetics, their functions, usage, ingredient details and their impact on our health. Additionally it also delves deeper into the historical facts of skin care products.

This book will empower you to understand cosmeceutical science with methodological reporting of various skin diseases and an insight of next generation technology and new innovative treatments.

-Author

Acknowledgement

I'm thankful to Dr. Mamun Rashid, Assistant Professor of Pharmaceutics, Appalachian College of Pharmacy Oakwood, Virginia for his valuable time to audit my paper and for her thoughtful suggestions. I'm also grateful to the seminar library of Faculty of Pharmacy, University of Dhaka and BANSDOC Library, Bangladesh for providing me books, journal, and newsletters.

-Author

Contents

Chapter 3: Skin Lightening and Management of Hyperpigmentation

Chapter 4: Skin Aging and Modern Age Anti-Aging Strategies

Chapter 5: Sunscreen and Suntan Preparations

CHAPTER 1

COSMETICS IN USE

1.1 BACKGROUND

History of Skin Care - Though cosmetics have likely existed for even longer, the first evidence of cosmetics stems from Ancient Egypt, approximately 6,000 years ago. They used cosmetics for a variety of reasons, the first being for mummification, burial traditions, and honoring their Gods and Goddesses. They also used cosmetics to protect them from the elements — mainly sun rays and insects. Egyptians - like using aloe, myrrh, and frankincense. These products, particularly frankincense, were believed to possess anti-inflammatory properties and were used as anti-wrinkle creams by Ancient Egyptians. Makeup was created using a variety of products including metal ore, copper, water, oil, animal fat, and precious stones. While Ancient Greeks and Romans used the ideas of the Ancient Egyptians, they took their skincare and beauty rituals one step further. Many Greeks and Romans would spend an entire day at the "spa" to focus on their skin. Women commonly used white lead, crocodile dung, and chalk to lighten the appearance of their skin. They also created face masks with starch and eggs, which were believed to tighten the skin, reduce wrinkles, and keep the face looking as youthful as possible. This was even more common in China, particularly under the Shang Dynasty (in 1760 BC). A powdered face with smooth skin was extremely popular and white powders were used to achieve the whitest complexion possible. Taking it another step further, many also used gels and lotions to permanently bleach their skin. As skincare moved to Europe and the Middle East, new ingredients and methods were invented and introduced. The first cold cream was developed using rose oil and water, and melting beeswax into it. They used the mineral alum to treat scabs and used olive lead to fight acne. They combined vinegar and lead to make a whitening foundation and used it to get rid of freckles and whiten their skin. During the Elizabethan Era, many Europeans used this whitening foundation. At the time, it wasn't popular to wash their faces and/or bodies; so typically, they piled on layer after layer of the whitening foundation to achieve a look as pale as possible. Despite the many social strides made in the late 1800s and early 1900s, dark skin was still seen as undesirable. Skin whitening was as popular as ever and products were made nearly exclusively for light-skinned women. By the 1920s, a shift in beauty ideals caused slightly tanned skin to be seen as desirable. Cosmetics, in turn, followed this trend. Tinted face powders and lotions that emulated a tan were introduced.

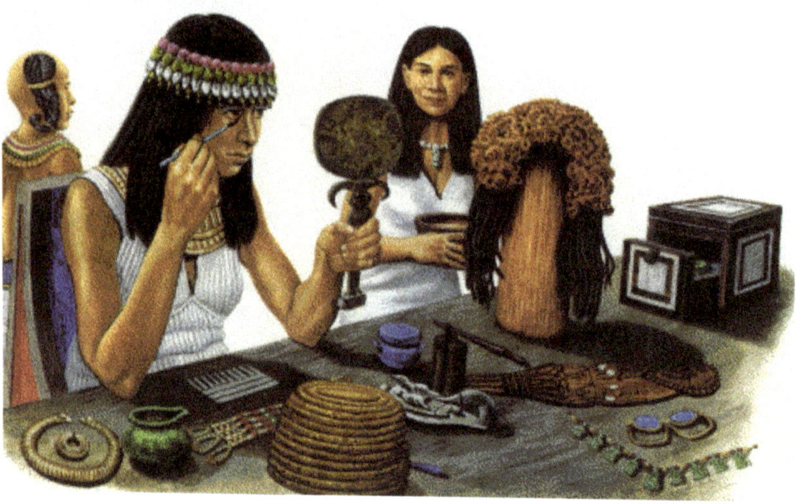

Figure 1.1 The Beauty of Yesterday: Ancient Egypt [183]. Often referred to as the vainest civilization in history, Ancient Egyptians are known to have played a vital role in shaping modern ideals of beauty. For example, these populations used olive oil, honey, and milk to keep their skin wrinkle- free, as well as the pigment from clay to create lip and cheek tints to recreate a healthy glow. Another prime example is their use of a charcoal-like substance called Kohl to create thick black lines around their eyes to enhance their natural shape, believing that by following this technique, it would also protect their eyes from the glare of the sun (*Courtacy:* sarajevograd.space).

1.2 ABSTRACT

The word "cosmetics" actually stems from its use in Ancient Rome. They were typically produced by female slaves known as "*cosmetae*," which is where the word "cosmetics" stemmed from. Cosmetics are used to enhance appearance. Makeup has been around for many centuries. The first known people who used cosmetics to enhance their beauty were the Egyptians. Makeup those days was just simple eye coloring or some material for the body. Nowadays makeup plays an important role for both men and women. In evolutionary psychology, social competition of appearance strengthens women's desires for ideal beauty. According to "The Origin of Species", humans have evolved to transfer genes to future generations through sexual selection that regards the body condition of ideal beauty as excellent fertility. Additionally, since women's beauty has recently been considered a competitive advantage to create social power, a body that meets the social standards of a culture could achieve limited social resources. That's right, even men have become more beauty conscious and are concerned about their looks. Cosmetics can be produced in the organic and hypoallergenic form to meet the demands of users. Makeup is used as a beauty aid to help build up the self-esteem and confidence of an individual. The importance of cosmetics has increased as many people want to stay young and attractive. Cosmetics are readily available today in the form of creams, lipstick, perfumes, eye shadows, nail polishes, hair sprays, etc. Other cosmetics like face powder give a glow to the skin after applying the base cream. Then we have lipsticks, which are applied by many women of all ages. They are made from wax and cocoa butter in the desired amount. Cosmetics like creams, gels, and colognes are used daily by both women and men. Creams act as a cleanser for the face in many circumstances. More recently anti-aging creams have been manufactured which can retain younger looking skin for many years. The best cleansing agents are cleansing cream, soap,s and water. Cosmetic creams serve as a skin food for hard, dry and chapped skin. It mainly lubricates, softens and removes unwanted dirt from the skin. Some popular fat creams that are used include Vaseline and Lanolin. Dry creams are used in the manufacture of soap and gelatin which is used as a base for the skin. Haircare has become one of the fastest developing markets in the beauty industry. Many young men turn to oils and gels to maintain and style their hair. Products like hair gels, oils, and lotions have been introduced in the market to help protect hair fall and dandruff. Some professions, like the show business industry, focus on the importance of the outer appearance. Many personalities and artists have utilized makeup to beat the harsh lights and the glare of camera flashes. They very well know the importance of their looks and maintain them by using a variety of cosmetics. Their appearance is their most valuable asset and they take every endeavor to appear as the fans want them to appear. Recent research has shown that makeup helps in protection from harmful rays of the sun. Many beauty products manufacturers have utilized the needs of people to protect themselves and their skin from the rays of the sun. This is a great achievement because earlier make-up and sun protection could not blend.

Importance of Cosmetics: Today Cosmetics help to enhance our appearance and make us feel more confident. With more cosmetics on the market today than ever before, it becomes obvious to us that they play a great role in our everyday life.

1.3 INTRODUCTION

A cosmetic product is defined as 'a substance or preparation intended for placement in contact with any external part of the human body' (this includes the mouth and teeth). We use cosmetics to cleanse, perfume, protect and change the appearance of our bodies or to alter its odors. Products that claim to 'modify a bodily process or prevent, diagnose, cure or alleviate any disease, ailment or defect' are called therapeutics. Whatever the process one wishes to take, there is one goal in mind: covering up imperfections (**Figure 1.2**). Most cosmetic products are complex mixtures of chemical compounds that are directly applied to the skin. Unlike pharmaceutical products, cosmetics are not intended to cure diseases. However, modern cosmetics are often "functional." Products for whitening, wrinkle care, moisturizing, and treating pores, spots, etc. are produced to meet the needs of today's consumers. Thus, some cosmetic products contain quasi-drugs, although their effects on the body remain mild and gentle. Because cosmetics are freely used by consumers with no daily-exposure limits, the absorption of quasi-drugs (and other ingredients) through the skin needs to be carefully controlled, which makes monitoring transdermal drug absorption one of the important subjects in cosmetic science. Though use and acceptance of the term "cosmeceutical" may largely be confined to the U.S., knowledgeable and increasingly demanding consumers have no national borders – and the onus to live up to these demands is on both brand owners and ingredient suppliers. According to research firm Kline & Company's "Specialty Actives in Personal Care 2011: U.S. Market Analysis and Opportunities," a growing consumer understanding of active ingredients in personal care products, driven by extensive consumer mediacoverage, is pressuring suppliers of active ingredients to produce innovative products ("innovative" and "active" are the hallmarks of cosmeceuticals). When seeking out personal care, consumers want the new and exciting, while their expectations for and of functional and efficacious ingredients and products grow. Also, as a result of global economics, consumer frugality has become the new normal, and this, too, plays a role in what consumers expect from the performance of their products. Consumers will continue to spend on beauty products, but as their spending power decreases, they're ever quicker to move on from a product they deem as not living up to its promises. Consumers set the parameters and will continue to seek out the most effective beauty products for their needs – and value is determined first on efficacy. On the face of it, reaching today's consumers and winning their buy for the long term seems an ever more daunting proposition, but their quest and hunger for ever more efficacious and intriguing products translates to more opportunities to innovate for new unmet needs. Turning innovation into success, though, will truly depend on an open and honest conversation with consumers – listening to their needs and being as clear as possible about claims and the potential for any given product. Brand owners must convey the value of new ingredients, formulas, and products through clear language, with explanations of benefits based on scientific studies or other trials. Backing good ingredients and products by developing smart marketing campaigns that can convey appropriate expectations from the use of products will foster a significant connection with consumers – and that translates to the growth of business.

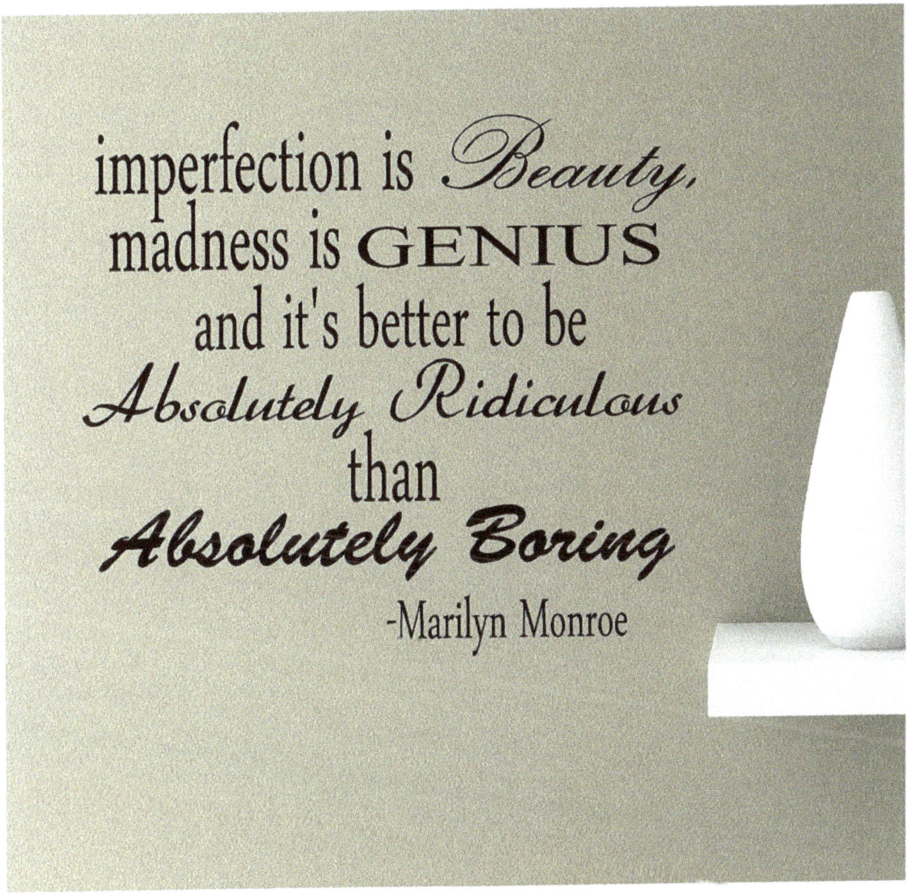

Figure 1.2 Famous Beauty Quote, Marilyn Monroe [66-68]. The "blonde bombshell" had a heavy peach fuzz "beard" but refused to wax it off. But her so- called "imperfection" never left without cosmetics. Monroe used five different lipsticks and glosses to create her pouty look. Between shampoo jobs, she was said to have applied baby powder on the roots of her hair. To get skin glow, Monroe slathered on thick layers of Vaseline or Nivea Cream under her makeup before getting in front of the camera. She was also a huge fan of moisturizers, olive oil, and lanolin. She wasn't always a blonde bombshell—she was born a brunette. She dyed her hair golden blonde when a modeling agency told her it would make her more successful.

1.3.1 GENERAL USE OF COSMETICS

Cosmetic is a Greek word thatmeans to 'adorn' (addition of something decorative to a person or a thing). It may be defined as a substance that comes in contact with various parts of the human body like skin, hair, nail, lips, teeth, and mucous membranes etc. A Cosmetic substances help in improving or changing the outward show of the body and also masks the odor of the body. It protects the skin and keeps it in good condition. In general, cosmetics are external preparations that are applied to the external parts of the body. Even in earlier days, men and women used to decorate their bodies for improvement of appearance. Men used leaves of vegetables and parts of animals whereas women use to wear colored stones and flowers round their neck and wrist. Gradually, they start using colored earth and ointments on their face and body. Even bangles and necklaces made of baked earth materials became very common among the people. Eye shadow was made of copper (colored earth) ore and lampblack (colored earth) while red color was used for dyeing of hair. Nowadays, cosmetics are considered as essential components in life. They not only, attract the people towards it but also impart psychological effects. It has gained popularity in the last 3-4 decades and its use has been increased exponentially both-in males and females (**Figure 1.5**). The most popular cosmetics are hair dyes, powders, and creams.

- Foundation used to smooth out the face and cover spots or uneven skin coloration. Usually a liquid, cream, or powder.
- Powder used to set the foundation, giving a matte finish, and also to conceal small flaws or blemishes.
- Rouge, blush or blusher, cheek coloring used to bring out the color in the cheeks and make the cheekbones appear more defined. This comes in powder, cream, and liquid forms.
- Bronzer used to give skin a bit of color by adding a golden or bronze glow.
- Mascara is used to darken, lengthen, and thicken the eyelashes. It is available in natural colors such as brown and black, but also comes in bolder colors such as blue, pink, or purple. There are many different formulas, including waterproof for those of us prone to allergies or sudden tears.
- Eye liner, eye shadow, eye shimmer, and glitter eye pencils as well as different color pencils used to color and emphasize the eyelids (larger eyes give a more youthful appearance).
- Eyebrow pencils, creams, waxes, gels and powders are used to color and define the brows.
- Nail polish used to color the fingernails and toenails.
- Concealer, makeup used to cover any imperfections of the skin.
- A hair growth tonic contains, as an active ingredient, a filtrate of lactic acid bacterial culture such as Streptococcus lactis, and Lactobacillus bulgaricus. The use of this type of hair growth tonic promotes hair regeneration, hair growth, and hair nourishment. Modern technology is using plant stem cells

to influence the function of certain cells in our skin and hair follicles (**Figure 1.3**).

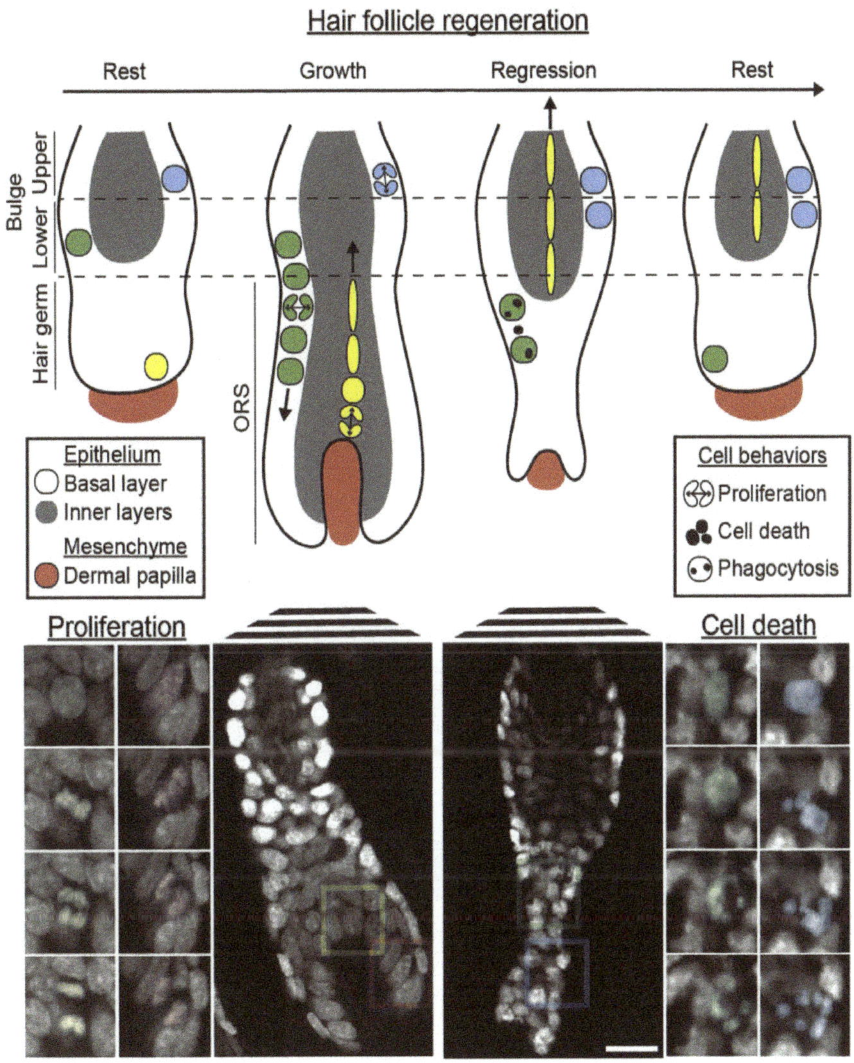

Figure 1.3 How Do Plant Stem Cells Help Hair Growth? [69,70]. Plant stem cells possess similar genetic factors as human stem cells and can be used to influence the function of certain cells in our skin and hair follicles. Active plant stem cells work to increase the lifespan of hair follicles so that hair can remain in the anagen phase of the hair growth cycle for a longer period.. Another hair-growth benefit of Asparagus Stem Cells is their ability to block the most common hair-killing hormone, DHT. High levels of DHT, as well as sensitivity to the hormone, are known for causing most male-pattern baldness and even female alopecia. Asparagus Stem Cells can aid the receptors in the skin to block the intrusion of DHT, and therefore minimizing the hair loss caused by it.

Also included in the general category of cosmetics are skincare products. These include creams and lotions to moisturize the face and body, sunscreens to protect the skin from damaging UV radiation, and treatment products to repair or hide skin imperfections (acne, wrinkles, dark circles under eyes, etc.). Cosmetics can also be described by the form of the product, as well as the area for application. Cosmetics can be liquid or cream emulsions; powders, both pressed and loose; dispersions; and anhydrous creams or sticks [1-5].

Exhibit 1. Interesting facts from history of cosmetics [33-36], [64,65]
Women are susceptible to the societal pressures of using cosmetics to beautifythemselves. One theory behind the origins of the ♀ symbol used to denote "woman" is that it represents the hand mirror used by the Roman goddess Venus or the Greek goddess Aphrodite. In their efforts to look beautiful, both men and women apply cosmetics to hide their flaws and accentuate their features. Cosmetics have been a part of human history as far back as the ancient Egyptians. The ancient Egyptians, Romans, and Greeks used various ingredients to soften, improve, exfoliate, and detoxify skin. The ancient Romans and Greeks used walnut extracts as hair dye, antimony (a known toxic heavy metal) as eye shadow, white lead carbonate as a skin lightener, charcoal crocodile excrement as a skin darkener, and cinnabar as rouge. *Atropa Belladona* is a poisonous plant called deadly nightshade. The name belladonna comes from the Italian, meaning beautiful lady, originating either from its use as a facial cosmetic, or, more probably, from its use to increase pupil size in women because during the Renaissance the herb was used in eye-drops by women to dilate the pupils of the eyes to make them appear seductive (**Figure 1.4**). In Elizabethan England, dyed red hair comes into fashion. Society women wear egg whites over their faces to create the appearance of a paler complexion. Women in Ancient Egypt used kohl, a substance containing powdered galena (lead sulphide—PbS) to darken their eyelids, and Cleopatra is said to have bathed in milk to whiten and soften her skin. By 3000 B.C men and women in China had begun to stain their fingernails with colors according to their social class. The Chinese stained their fingernails with gum arabic, gelatin, beeswax, and egg. Chou dynasty royals wear gold and silver, with subsequent royals wearing black or red. Lower classes were forbidden to wear bright colors on their nails. Greek women used poisonous lead carbonate (PbCO3) to achieve a pale complexion. Clays were ground into pastes for cosmetic use in traditional African societies and indigenous Australians still use a wide range of crushed rocks and minerals to create body paint for ceremonies and initiations.

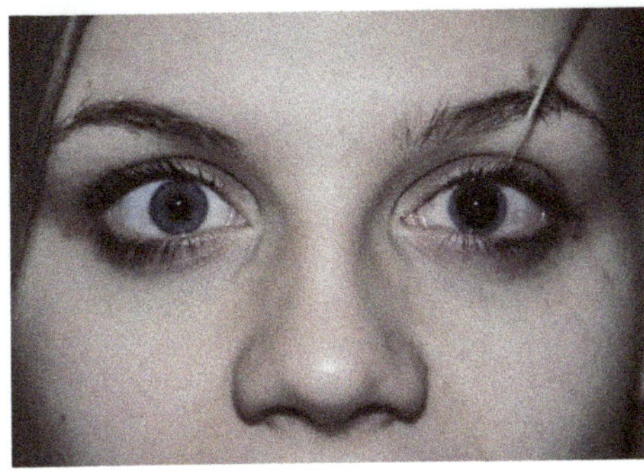

Figure 1.4 Beauty is in the eye of the beholder, and there is nothing better than a pair of gorgeous eyes [184]. Made from an extract of nightshade berries, also called *Atropa belladonna*, the resulting eyedrops dilate the pupils, providing a soft and seductive effect, just like in a romance scene of a novel where someone's eyes 'darken with desire.' In Renaissance Italy, this dusky, lustrous appearance of a lady's eyes was considered to be the height of beauty. One drop per eye would block receptors in the muscles of the eye that constrict pupil size. As one might suspect, this comes at an immediate cost to vision, resulting in blurriness and inability to focus on close objects. Though this would wear off over time, prolonged use of belladonna could cause permanent vision distortion or blindness. It also carried the side effect of increased heart rate because, let's not forget, this tincture was made of poison (*Courtacy:* medpedia.framar.bg).

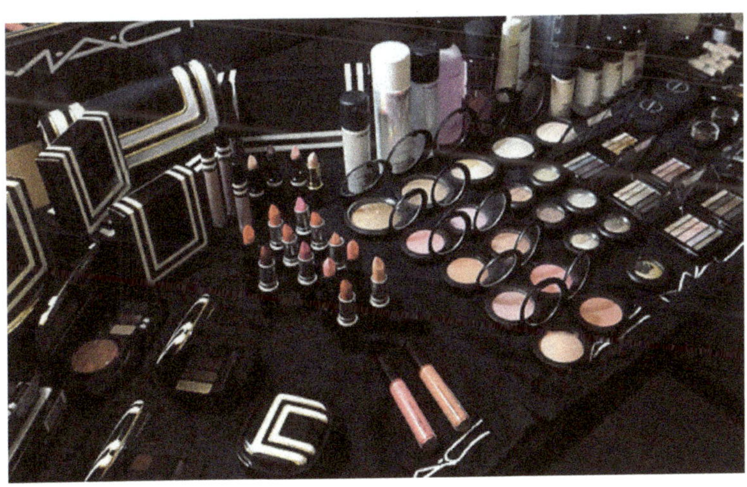

Figure 1.5 Modern Day Cosmetics [71,72]. Professional makeup artists have been perfecting techniques to get ordinary beauty products to multi-task for years. Cosmetics companies are now using advanced technology to develop multi-purpose products that emulate these techniques. Foundations are no longer designed to simply smooth complexions. Many now boast different ingredients to target varying skin needs, such as salicylic acid for acne or jojoba oil for dry skin. Numerous brands have also created multipurpose stains with a creamy consistency and a neutral color that can be used on cheeks, lips, and eyes. Some shades of these creamy all-over-color sticks also offer a little shimmer or gold sparkle, so that it can glide across eyebrow bones, shoulders or cleavage as a highlighter -- Lauren Balukonis, beauty division at 5W Public Relations (*Courtacy:* Odyssey).

1.4 PRODUCTS CLASSIFIED AS COSMETICS

- *Skin Creams* be considered pharmaceutical products as even cosmetic creams are based on techniques developed by pharmacy and un-medicated creams are highly used in a variety of skin conditions in ancient times, creams were simply prepared by mixing two or more ingredients using water as the solvent. With the advancement in technology, newer methods are used for the formulation of creams. These semisolid preparations are elegant to use by the public and society. They show versatility in their functions. Creams can be applied to any part of the body with ease. It is convenient to use the cream by all the age groups of people. Although it may be equally well applied to non-aqueous products such as wax-solvent based mascaras, liquid eye shadows, and ointments. If an emulsion is sufficiently low viscosity to be pourable (flow under influence of gravity alone) is referred to as lotion. Creams are emulsions of oil and water. In the coming future, more advanced technologies and methods will be used for the preparation, formulation, and evaluation of creams. Also, the demand for herbal constituents-based creams is increasing day by day [74-79].

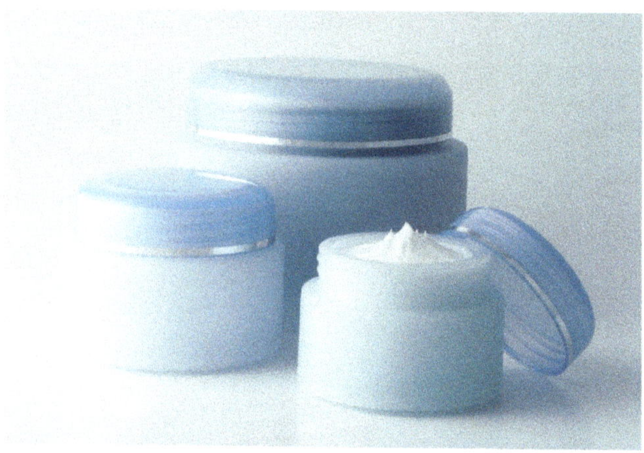

Figure 1.6 Skin Creams [168]. In general, creams for the skin should protect it from the sun and environmental pollutants, while also treating any specific problems. Look for the highest quality ingredients to ensure a cream's ability to live up to its claims. Enhance the circulation of blood flow by massaging creams into your skin several times a day.

- *Lips makeup*-Lipstick, lip gloss, lip liner, lip plumper, lip balm, lip stain, lip conditioner, lip primer, lip boosters, and lip butters. Lipsticks are intended to add color and texture to the lips and often come in a wide range of colors, as well as finishes such as matte, satin, gloss and luster. Lip stains have a water or gel base and may contain alcohol to help the product stay on leaving a matte look. They temporarily saturate the lips with a dye. Usually designed to be waterproof, the product may come with an applicator brush, directly through the applicator, rollerball, or could be applied with a finger. Lip glosses are intended to add shine to the lips and may add a tint of color, as well as being scented or flavored for a pop of fun. Lip balms are most often used to moisturize, tint, and protect the lips. Some brands contain sunscreen. Using a priming lip product such as lip balm or chapstick can prevent chapped lips [6-8], [73].

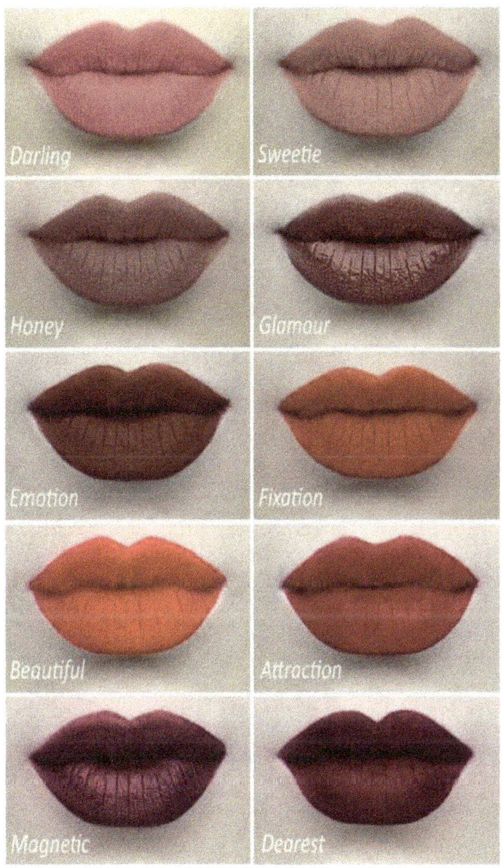

Figure 1.7 Lip Colors [169,170], [181]. Makeup artists and advertisements for cosmetics often claim that lip color can influence facial skin's apparent lightness. Currently, we do not have scientific evidence to either support or deny these claims. The luminance contrast between facial features and facial skin is greater in women than in men, and women's use of make-up enhances this contrast. In black-and-white photographs, increased luminance contrast enhances femininity and attractiveness in women's faces, but reduces masculinity and attractiveness in men's faces. In Caucasians, much of the contrast between the lips and facial skin is in redness. Red lips have been considered attractive in women in geographically and temporally diverse cultures, possibly because they mimic vasodilation associated with eternal desire (*Courtacy:* Bellevous Makeovers).

- *Primers* are so beloved by experts because they can do so much more than just make the foundation go on smoother. Primers are sort of like insurance for makeup. Although they often wear many hats — smoothing, concealing, protecting and prepping — their main roles are to keep makeup on longer and give skin a smooth, flawless finish. This creates another layer between skin to prevent acne and makeup clogging up pores. Primer creates an even tone throughout the skin and makes makeup last longer. Primer is applied throughout the face including eyes, lips, and lashes. This product has a creamy texture and applies smoothly. Many makeup primers are formulated with silicone-based polymers, like dimethicone, because of their ultra-smoothing effects. Photoaged skin is the result from various environmental factors, most importantly chronic sun exposure. Dyschromia and fine lines/wrinkles are common clinical manifestations of photo damaged skin. The facial primer was shown to be effective and well- tolerated for immediate and long-term improvement in the appearance of mild-to-moderate hyperpigmentation and fine lines associated with photodamage when used over a 12-weeks [82-85].
- *Concealer* covers imperfections of the skin. Many people try to manage acne by squeezing pimples, following a thorough skincare routine or wearing foundation. Others hope things will improve if they change their diet or expose their skin to sunlight. Concealer is often used for any extra coverage needed to cover acne/pimple blemishes, undereye circles, and other imperfections. Concealer is often thicker and more solid than foundation, and provides longer-lasting, more detailed coverage as well as creating a fresh clean base for all the rest of the makeup. This product also brightens up the skin and applying under the foundation can remove blemishes and discoloration because of acne scars. In females, in particular, there is a need for cosmetic products that can effectively cover the signs of this highly visible skin condition to reduce the emotional impact of the disease.The use of cosmetics can also increase acne patients' adherence to their medical regimen, which is estimated to be poor in 50% of patients. Perhaps the most important type of concealer is the corrective type, and is most effective in a liquid formula, like La-Roche Posay Toleriane Teint Corrective Pen, which has corrective colors to help tone down ruddiness, fade the appearance of hyperpigmentation, and yes, even cover up any more irritating blemishes [86-90].

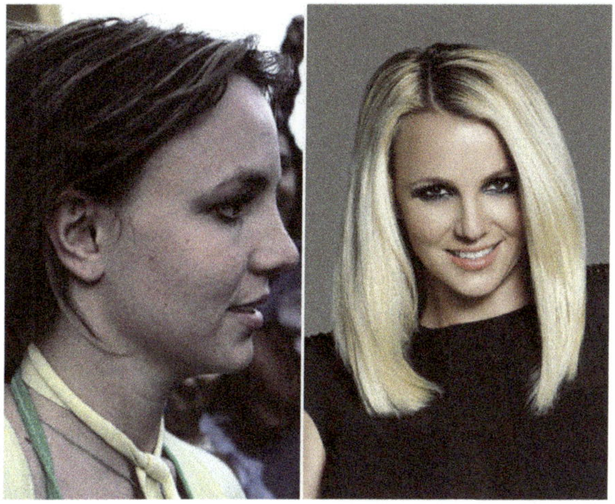

Figure 1.8 Pimpled and no pimpled Britney Spears [185,186]. At glamorous, Hollywood events, the ".... baby one more time" star Britney Spears' skin seems flawless, but in reality, this is far from the truth: redness, pimples, rashes – the singer knows all of these problems too well, first hand. However, Girls and women often use concealer or foundation to cover up their pimples. This makes them feel more comfortable in public. Young men sometimes use subtle foundation, powder, and concealer as well (Courtacy: bestbritneyspearse.blogspot.com).

- *Foundation* is used to smooth out the face by covering spots, acne, blemishes, or uneven skin tone. These are sold in a liquid, cream, or powder, or more recently in a mousse. Foundation provides sheer, matte, dewy or full coverage. Foundation primer is applied before the foundation to fill out pores, create a dewy look or create a smoother finish. They usually come in cream formulas to be applied before foundation as a base. The most classic form of foundation, liquid, offers medium to full coverage for all skin types and is a sure-fire way to achieve a smooth base [2], [91-94].
- *Face powder* sets the foundation and under-eye concealer, giving it a matte finish while also concealing small flaws or blemishes. It can also be used to bake the foundation, so that it stays on longer and create a matte finish. Tinted face powders may be worn alone as a light foundation so that the full face does not look as caked-up as it could. Loose powder comes in a jar, has smaller particles (and therefore a finer consistency), and usually gives lightweight coverage. It's also messy and hard to transport, so this guy is meant to stay at home. The difference between setting powder and finishing powder is a little nebulous. Many companies use these terms interchangeably, so it's partially a matter of marketing [6-8], [95-97].
- *Rouge, blush, or blusher* is cheek coloring to bring out the color in the cheeks and make the cheekbones appear more defined. Blush is having a

major moment, graduating from makeup bag staple to a starring role in almost every red-carpet beauty look. Rouge comes in powder, cream, and liquid forms. Different blush colors are used to complement different skin tones. The ancient Egyptians were the first to incorporate blush into their beauty rituals. The Middle Ages saw a drop in the use of blush, as red cheeks were associated with prostitutes. During the 1500s to the 1700s, blush was made with toxic chemicals. Starting in the 1900s, as America became industrialized; blush began to be mass-produced and became much safer to use [98-100].

- *Highlighter* used to draw attention to the high points of the face such as the cheekbones, below the eyebrows, nose, upper lip, and collar bones. This product also adds a glow; comes in liquid, cream, and powder forms. It often contains a substance to provide shimmer. Alternatively, a lighter-toned foundation/concealer can be used [101].
- *Bronzer* gives skin a bit of color and contours the face for a sharper definition or creates a tan-look. Bronzer is considered to be more of a natural look and can be used for everyday wear. Bronzer enhances the color of the face. It comes in either matte, semi-matte/satin, or shimmer finishes [102-104].

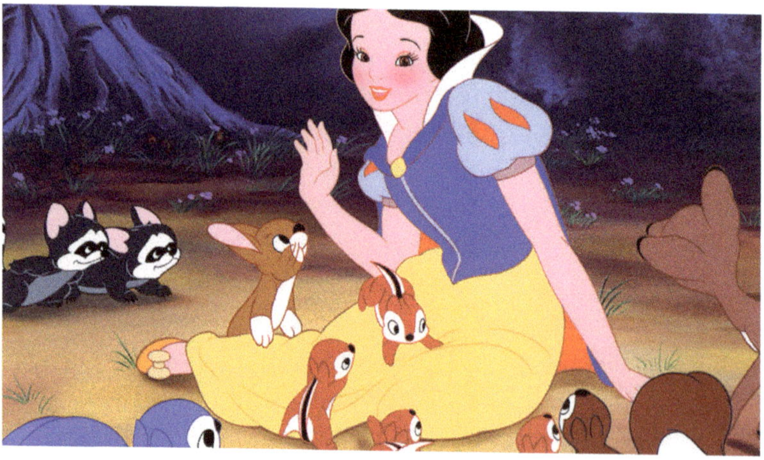

Figure 1.9 Disney princess, Snow White (Fairy Tale) [172,173]. In the time that Snow White was released it was common for the majority of women desired to have blush in their faces like her. Rouge originated as a thick paste and was made from a range of things: from strawberries to red fruits and vegetable juices, to the powder of finely crushed ochre. The difference between blush and rouge is that blush being an act of blushing while rouge is red or pink makeup to add color to the cheeks; blusher. Blushers, those versatile successors to rouge, help light up a complexion and accent face structure and best features (*Courtacy:* DesktopBackground.org).

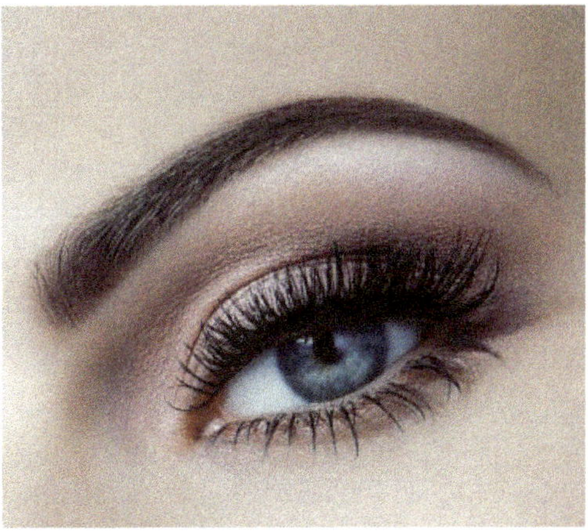

Figure 1.10 Eye Makeup [174-176]. Kohl was a widely used traditional cosmetic. It may be a pervasive source of lead poisoning in those areas and among individuals from those areas who have immigrated to developed nations. Eventhough the cosmetic products undergo rigorous testing to ensure they are safe for human use; some users report mild discomfort following their application. The cutaneous changes, such as allergic dermatitis, are well reported, but the ocular changes associated with eye cosmetic use are less so. Some pigmented cosmetic products may accumulate within the lacrimal system and conjunctivae over many years of use, but immediate reports of eye discomfort after application are most common. Changes to the tear film and its stability may occur shortly after application, and contact lens wearers can also be affected by lens spoliation from cosmetic products. Additionally, creams used in the prevention of skin aging are often applied around the eyes, and retinoids present in these formulations can have negative effects on meibomian gland function and may be a contributing factor to dry eye disease.

- *Mascara* is used to darken, lengthen, thicken, or draw attention to the eyelashes. It is available in various colors. Some mascaras include glitter flecks. There are many formulas, including waterproof versions for those prone to allergies or sudden tears. It is often used after an eyelash curler and mascara primer. Many mascaras have components to help lashes appear longer and thicker [105-107].
- *Eye shadow* is a pigmented powder/cream or substance used to accentuate the eye area, traditionally on, above, and under the eyelids. Many colors may be used at once and blended to create different effects using a blending brush. This is conventionally applied with a range of eye shadow brushes, though it isn't uncommon for alternative methods of application to be used such as fingers. However, it is important to have clean fingers because oils from the skin can result in pimples [108,109].
- *Eyeliner* is used to enhance and elongate the apparent size or depth of the eye. For example, white eyeliner on the waterline and inner corners of the eye makes the eyes look bigger and more awake. It can come in the form of

a pencil, a gel, or a liquid and can be found in almost any color. Conversely, black eyeliner makes eyes look smaller, brightens up the face and draws attention to the eyes [108,109].

- *Eyebrow pencils, creams, waxes, gels, and powders* are used to color, fill in, and define the brows. Popular in recent years, the "Instagram look" is creating fuller eyebrows by filling it, sharper angles, and adding gel to set it [110].
- *Nail polish* is used to color the fingernails and toenails. Transparent, colorless versions may strengthen nails or be used as a top or base coat to protect the nail or polish. This can be found in glossy, matte, and powder [110].
- *Setting spray* is used as the last step in the process of applying makeup. It keeps applied makeup intact for long periods.Inaddition to setting spray is setting powder, which may be either pigmented or translucent. Both of these products claim to keep makeup from absorbing into the skin or melting off [111].
- *False eyelashes* are used when exaggerated eyelashes are desired. Their basic design usually consists of human hair, mink hair, or synthetic materials attached to a thin cloth-like band, which is applied with glue to the lash line. Designs vary in length and color. Rhinestones, gems, and even feathers and lace occur on some false eyelash designs. Eyelashes can be purchased in several drug or beauty supply stores and can be applied with eyelash glue. These eyelashes are not permanent and can be taken off easily by gently taking them off with fingers [108,109].
- *Contouring* is designed to give shape to an area of the face. The aim is to enhance the natural shading on the face to give the illusion of a more defined facial structure which can be altered to preference. Brighter skin-colored makeup products are used to 'highlight' areas which are wanted to draw attention to or to be caught in the light, whereas darker shades are used to create a shadow. These light and dark tones are blended on the skin to create the illusion of a more definite face shape. It can be achieved using a "contour palette" - which can be either cream or powder [102], [112].
- *Cleansers* or foaming washes are used to remove excess dirt, oil, and makeup left on the skin. Different cleansing products are aimed at various types of skin, such as sulfate-free cleansers and spin brushes. Cleansing oil or oil cleanser is an oil-based solution that can contain, but not necessarily, an emulsifier to allow for the oils to gently emulsify on the skin. Cleansing Oils allowing to provide essential fatty acids to the skin [113,114].
- *Toners* are used after cleansing the skin to freshen it up, boost the appearance of one's complexion, and remove any traces of cleanser, mask, or makeup, as well to help restore the skin's natural pH. They are usually applied to a cotton pad and wiped over the skin but can be sprayed onto the

skin from a spray bottle. Toners typically contain alcohol, water, and herbal extracts or other chemicals depending on skin type whether oily, dry, or combination. Toners containing alcohol are quite astringent and usually targeted at oily skins [108], [115].

- *Facial masks* are treatments applied to the skin and then removed. Typically, they are applied to a dry, cleansed face, avoiding the eyes and lips. Clay-based masks use kaolin clay or fuller's earth to transport essential oils and chemicals to the skin and are typically left on until completely dry. As the clay dries, it absorbs excess oil and dirt from the surface of the skin and may help to clear clogged pores or draw comedones to the surface. Because of its drying actions, clay-based masks should only be used on oily skins. Peel masks are typically gel-like in consistency and contain acids or exfoliating agents to help exfoliate the skin, along with other ingredients to hydrate, discourage wrinkles, or treat uneven skin tone. They are left on to dry and then gently peeled off. They should be avoided by people with dry or

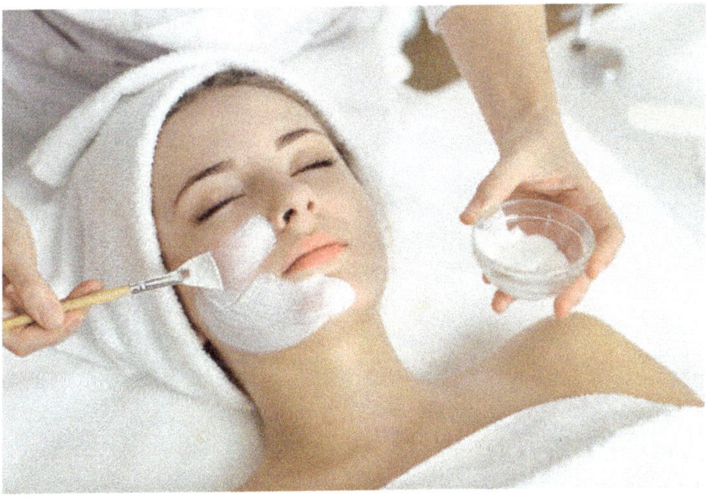

Figure 1.11 Facial Treatment [177-180]. Facial masks are the most prevalent cosmetic products utilized for skin rejuvenation. Facial masks are divided into four groups: (a) sheet masks; (b) peel-off masks; (c) rinse-off masks; and (d) hydrogels. Each of these has some advantages for specific skin types based on the ingredients used. Peel-off facial masks are known for their unique characteristics inherent to the use of film-forming polymers that, after complete drying, create a very cohesive plastic layer allowing for the manual removal of the product without leaving any residue. Most clay-based products on the market consist only of dried clay powder that needs to be moistened before use. After facial application, the product dries naturally, forming a sandy-cracked material due to the low cohesion between the dried particles. The most interesting effects of aloe vera in topical use are anti-inflammatory, antiseptic, antioxidant, and regenerative. It has been demonstrated that the association of green clay and aloe vera exerts a beneficial synergistic effect when it comes to developing a facial mask as a regenerative aid.

sensitive skin, as they tend to be very drying. Sheet masks are a relatively new product that is becoming extremely popular in Asia. Sheet masks consist of a thin cotton or fiber sheet with holes cut out for the eyes and lips and cut to fit the contours of the face, onto which serums and skin treatments are brushed in a thin layer; the sheets may be soaked in the treatment. Masks are available to suit almost all skin types and skin complaints. Sheet masks are quicker, less messy, and require no specialized knowledge or equipment for their use compared to other types of face masks, but they may be difficult to find and purchase outside Asia [116-118].

- *Exfoliants* are products that help slough off dry, dead skin cells to improve the skin's appearance. This is achieved either by using mild acids or other chemicals to loosen old skin cells, or abrasive substances to physically scrub them off. Exfoliation can even out patches of rough skin, improve circulation to the skin, clear blocked pores to discourage acne and improve the appearance and healing of scars. Chemical exfoliants may include citric acid (from citrus fruits), acetic acid (from vinegar), malic acid (from fruit), glycolic acid, lactic acid, or salicylic acid. They may be liquids or gels, and may or may not contain an abrasive to remove old skin cells afterward. Abrasive exfoliants include gels, creams or lotions, as well as physical objects. Loofahs, microfiber cloths, natural sponges, or brushes may be used to exfoliate the skin, simply by rubbing them over the face in a circular motion. Gels, creams, or lotions may contain an acid to encourage dead skin cells to loosen, and an abrasive such as microbeads, sea salt, sugar, ground nut shells, rice bran, or ground apricot kernels to scrub the dead cells off the skin. Salt and sugar scrubs tend to be the harshest, while scrubs containing beads or rice bran are typically very gentle [116], [119].
- *Moisturizers* are creams or lotions that hydrate the skin and help it to retain moisture; they may contain essential oils, herbal extracts, or chemicals to assist with oil control or reducing irritation. Night creams are typically more hydrating than day creams but may be too thick or heavy to wear during the day, hence their name. Tinted moisturizers contain a small amount of foundation, which can provide light coverage for minor blemishes or to even out skin tones. They are usually applied with the fingertips or a cotton pad to the entire face, avoiding the lips and area around the eyes. Eyes require a different kind of moisturizer compared with the rest of the face. The skin around the eyes is extremely thin and sensitive and is often the first area to show signs of aging. Eye creams are typically very light lotions or gels, and are usually very gentle; some may contain ingredients such as caffeine or Vitamin K to reduce puffiness and dark circles under the eyes. Eye creams or gels should be applied over the entire eye area with a finger, using a patting motion. Finding a moisturizer with SPF is beneficial to prevent aging and wrinkles [116], [120].

- *Soaps* composed of long-chain fatty acid alkali salts with a pH of between 9 and 10.The use of soap with high pH causes an increase in skin pH, which in turn causes an increase in dehydrative effect, irritability and alteration in bacterial flora. The majority of soaps and shampoos available in the market do not disclose their pH. Glycerin bars/transparent bars: used rampantly in our country in winter. They contain humectant–glycerin to counter the drying effects of soap. Super-fatted soaps: contain a greater amount of lipids such as triglycerides, lanolin, paraffin, stearic acid, or mineral oils which provide a protective film on the skin. Deodorant soaps/antibacterial soaps: contain antibacterial agents such as triclosan, triclocarban, or carbanile to inhibit the growth of bacteria and thereby odor [80,81].
- *Shampoos* are used primarily to clean the scalp of dirt and other environmental pollutants, sebum, sweat, desquamated corneocytes (scales), and other greasy residues including previously applied hair care products such as oils, lotions, and sprays. It is easy to formulate a shampoo that will remove all of the sebum and dirt from the hair and scalp, but this will leave the hair, frizzy, dry, unmanageable and unattractive. Shampoo now is also supposed to have a secondary function thatserves to condition and beautify

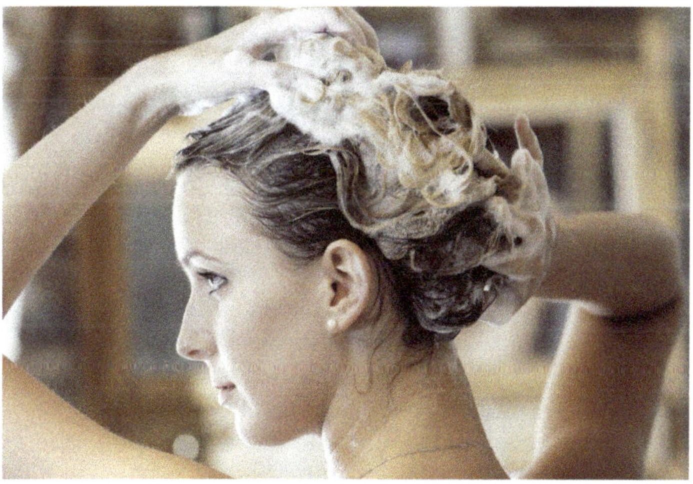

Figure 1.12 Hair Shampoo [187,188]. The main purpose of shampoo is to remove dirt and oil from the surface of the hair fibers and the scalp, while the main purpose of the conditioner is to ensure that the hair is smooth for combing. Shampoos typically contain a primary and secondary surfactant for a thorough cleaning, a viscosity builder, a solvent, conditioning agents, pH adjuster and other non-essential components such as fragrance and color for commercial appeal. Conditioners usually contain silicone polymerS to increase shine and soften hair, cationic polymers such as quaternary nitrogen compounds to reduce static electricity, bridging agents to increase absorption, viscosity builder, pH adjuster and components for commercial appeal (*Courtacy:* Good Housekeeping).

hair and to soothe the irritated scalp skin in conditions like seborrheic dermatitis. The challenge is to remove just enough sebum to allow the hair to appear clean and leave behind enough conditioning agents to leave the hair soft, shiny and manageable. This balancing act between good cleaning and beautifying the hair is an art achieved by mixing various ingredients in the correct proportion in the shampoo preparation. The modern advances in chemistry and technology have made it possible to replace the soap bases with complex formulation which contain cleansing agents, conditioning agents along with functional additives, preservative, aesthetic additives and sometimes even medically active ingredients [121-125].

- *Conditioners* are used to decrease friction, detangle the hair, minimize frizz and improve combability. Conditioners act by neutralizing the electrical negative charge of the hair fiber by adding positive charges and by lubricating the cuticle that reduces fiber hydrophilicity. They contain anti-static and lubricating substances that are divided into 5 main groups: Polymers, oils, waxes, hydrolyzed amino acids, and cationic molecules. The most active and used conditioner agent is a silicone. There are different types of silicones with different deposition, adherence and wash out capacity which will lead to different performances of the conditioner. The ideal conditioner is capable of restoring the hydrophobicity of the fiber and to neutralize the static electricity. Depending on the capacity of entering the fiber, the conditioner may reach the cuticle surface or the inner part of the cortex [122], [125].
- *Deodorant* is one of the most commonly used cosmetic products, with millions of consumers applying these products to their axilla every day. Deodorants are used to mask odor; whereas, antiperspirants are used to reduce the amount of sweat produced. These two activities are often combined into single products. While deodorants are considered cosmetic products because they do not change the function of the skin, antiperspirants are classified as drugs and are therefore subject to rules and regulations set forth by the FDA. The active ingredient in antiperspirants is usually aluminum- based, which reduces sweat by obstructing the eccrine glands. Deodorants work by two different mechanisms—antimicrobial agents decrease the number of bacteria that produce volatile odoriferous substances and fragrances cover any odors that are produced. Recently, naturally occurring zeolite minerals, in the form of potassium alum or ammonium alum crystals, have been marketed as all-natural alternatives to deodorants and antiperspirants. These products are sold in solid crystal form. The consumer is instructed to wet the crystal and apply the product to the underarm area to prevent odor. Although no research has been published evaluating the mechanism of action of these products, the company that markets them, Crystal Body Deodorant (French Transit, Ltd., Burlingame,

California), claims that the mineral salts create an environment in which bacteria cannot survive [126,127].

- *Contouring* is intended to offer shape to a zone of the face. The point is to upgrade the normal shading on the face to give the fantasy of a more characterized facial structure which can be adjusted to inclination. More brilliant skin-colored makeup items are utilized to 'feature' regions which are needed to attract thoughtfulness regarding or to be gotten in the light, while darker shades are utilized to make a shadow. These light and dark tones are mixed on the skin to make the deception of a more unequivocal face shape. It very well may be accomplished utilizing a "shape palette" - which can be either cream or powder [102], [112].

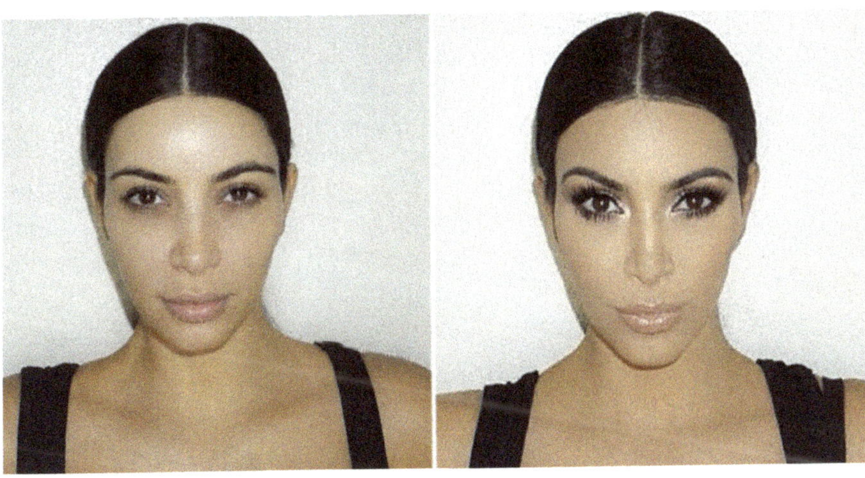

Figure 1.13 Contouring [182]. Contouring is the newest makeup craze that people just can't get enough of! This trend, made famous by none other than the Kardashian sisters, was created to make your face appear slimmer and more sculpted. The basic premise of it is to highlight the areas of the face that someone would like to bring out while shading in the parts she wants to make thinner (Courtacy: Odyssey).

Products classified as therapeutics

- *Antiperspirants* help to reduce the production of sweat. Aluminum salts – the active ingredient found in antiperspirants – dissolve into the moisture on the skin's surface. This forms a gel, which temporarily sits on top of the sweat gland, reducing the amount of sweat released. Antiperspirants that contain alcohol also help the active ingredient to dry faster and create a pleasant, cool feeling. An antiperspirant can also be a deodorant because it can help to control sweat and contain a fragrance at the same time. But deodorants only mask body odor; they don't help to prevent sweating [121], [128, 129].

- *Anti-dandruff shampoo-* Dandruff (pityriasis capitis) is a chronic scalp condition characterized by scaling and sometimes itching and redness. Shampoos containing antifungal agents are used to control the scaling condition. Regular use of anti-fungal shampoos represents a proven therapeutic strategy to improve the most common symptoms of flakes and itch. The therapeutic efficacy of a product based on a complex delivery vehicle such as a shampoo must be considered from a full-product perspective rather than just the active system as the non-active components of the composition will often play a significant role in the overall product pharmacology and resultant efficacy [130-132].

Household products

- *Toothpaste* is a paste or gel to be used with a toothbrush to maintain and improve oral health and aesthetics. Since their introduction several thousand years ago, toothpaste formulations have evolved considerably from suspensions of crushed egg shells or ashes to complex formulations with often more than 20 ingredients. Fluoride is the most important therapeutic substance used in toothpastes, adding to the effect of mechanical toothbrushing on dental caries control. The use of fluoride toothpaste to reduce caries in children and adults is strongly based on evidence and is dependent on the concentration (minimum of 1000 ppm F) and frequency of fluoride toothpaste use (2'/day or higher). The risk of dental fluorosis due to toothpaste ingestion by children has been overestimated, since there is no evidence that: 1) fluoride toothpaste use should be postponed until the age of 3-4 or older, 2) low-fluoride toothpaste avoids fluorosis and 3) fluorosis has a detrimental effect on the quality of life of individuals exposed to fluoridated water and toothpaste. Among other therapeutic substances used in toothpastes, there is evidence that triclosan/copolymer reduces dental biofilm, gingivitis, periodontitis, calculus and halitosis, and that toothpastes containing stannous fluoride reduce biofilm and gingivitis [133-136].
- A *mouthwash* may be defined as a nonsterile aqueous solution used mostly for its deodorant, refreshing, or antiseptic effect. Mouthwashes or rinses, when used as an adjunct to regular oral hygiene methods such as flossing. The first reference to mouth rinse as a formal practice is credited to Chinese medicine, about 2700 B.C.E., to treat the diseases of the gums. Mouthwashes exert adverse effects on teeth, gums and mucous membrane of the oral cavity and their extensive use is being criticized. study revealed that damage to DNA increases many folds when different mouthwashes are combined. Essential oils of six spice plants (black pepper, clove, black seasame, cinnamon, carom seeds and cumin) were evaluated for possessing anti-mutagenic property. These essential oils were found effectively protective against the DNA damaging effect of

mouthwashes but could not inhibit it completely. Black pepper, clove, black seasame, cinnamon, and cumin were stronger protect as compared to carom seeds [79], [137-140].

- *Detergents* - Performing household-cleaning chores involves the use of chemical detergents; these are commonly believed to provide cleaner and safer households. Occupational health studies have associated health risks with detergents, including respiratory and skin problems. Women are the major users of household detergents, as they are in general the primary homemakers. Detergent-handling strategies including storage, use, and precautionary measures affect women's exposure to chemical detergents and thus affect their health. Studies investigating the behavioral component of chemical exposure to detergents at the domestic level are scarce. The different classes of raw materials are surfactants, builders, bleaching agents, enzymes, and minors which remove dirt, stain, and soil from surfaces or textiles gave them pleasant feel and odor. The physicochemical properties of surfactants make them suitable for laundry purposes. Laundry detergent has traditionally been a powdered or granular solid, but the use of liquid laundry detergents has gradually increased over the years, and these days use of liquid detergent equals or even exceeds the use of solid detergent. This review paper describes the history, composition, types, mechanism, consumption, environmental effects and consumption of laundry detergents. Frequent exposure to antimicrobial household products has been hypothesized to lead to allergic diseases in children [141-145].
- *Baby Products* - Although the U.S. pediatric skincare market is a $1.7 billion industry, little is known regarding the usage pattern of skincare products in very young children. The natural baby skin-care products were well tolerated by infants and toddlers when used alone or as part of a skin-care regimen. Immediately after birth, the skin barrier of healthy, full-term neonates is competent, yet skin-barrier function continues to develop through at least the first year of life. This developing state of infant skin results in infant skin being susceptible to dryness and irritation from external factors, such as cold weather and wind, as well as harsh topical skin-care products. Therefore, it is critical that infant cleansers and moisturizers be well tolerated and not disrupts the stratum corneum. Infant skin is also exposed to other factors, such as saliva, nasal secretions, urine, feces (including fecal enzymes), and dirt, which can be irritants and result in disruption of the skin barrier. Lower-income households reported a higher frequency of product use and were less likely to purchase fragrance-free products or ones that were made for sensitive skin. As a result of normal daily exposure to these external factors, proper skin cleansing and protection of the infant skin-barrier are essential to the maintenance of skin-barrier function. Recent studies

suggest that some phthalates can alter human male reproductive development, the association was strongest in young infants, who may be more vulnerable to developmental and reproductive toxicity of phthalates given their immature metabolic system capability and increased dosage per unit body surface area. There was some evidence to suggest that daily use of full-body emollient therapy may help to reduce the risk of atopic eczema in high-risk babies with a genetic predisposition to eczema; however, the use of olive oil or sunflower oil for baby dry skin may adversely affect skin barrier function [146-152].

- *Toiletries* - Greater emphasis on cleanliness has led to widening the use of disinfectants and other cleaning agents in the home.The real picture is, an estimated 2.3 billion people lacked access to improved sanitation facilities, worldwide found in a 2017 study. Inadequate access to sanitation and hygiene facilities is known to be a leading cause of morbidity and mortality, particularly in low-income countries. Approximately 10% of the global burden of disease is thought to be attributed to inadequate Water, Sanitation, And Hygiene (WASH), which is largely driven by increased exposure to human pathogens transmitted via the fecal-oral route. An undesirable effect (UE) of a cosmetic product is a harmful reaction attributable to its normal or reasonably foreseeable use. However, the knowledge of UEs, at the population level, is limited by the absence of formal and reliable cosmetovigilance systems, which nevertheless are characterized by underreporting. Triclosan is a widely used antimicrobial pesticide; in fact it's so widely used that there is concern that triclosan could be contributing to making bacteria resistant to antibiotics. Triclosan not only irritates the skin; it may also promote cancer and disrupt the endocrine system. Toluene is a toxic chemical commonly found in nail products and hair dyes. It is also listed on labels as benzene, toluene, phenylmethane, or methylbenzene. Toluene can affect the respiratory and central nervous systems, damage the liver and kidneys, and cause birth defects and spontaneous abortion. Most cosmetics and toiletries products contain scents, which are typically labeled as 'fragrances,' and do not include the list of chemicals they are comprised of. Fragrances can contribute to air pollution and health issues such as hormone disruption, asthma, allergies, and migraines. Parabens are oestrogen-mimicking preservatives found in many cosmetics and other body-care products. A study by the Centers for Disease Control and Prevention showed that most of the participants tested for paraben exposure came up positive. Studies have shown a potential link between paraben exposure and the proliferation of breast cancer cells. The European Union deemed butylated hydroxyanisole (BHA) unsafe for use in fragrance, but BHA can still be found in cosmetics and other personal care products in the United States. The National Toxicology Program considers BHA a carcinogen, and animal studies have indicated it damages the reproductive system. Found in hundreds of personal care products and other merchandise, from shower curtains to wood finishes. Most Americans tested by the Centers for Disease Control and Prevention in the National Health and Nutrition Examination Survey from 2003 to 2004 showed the metabolites of several phthalates in their urine. Phthalates are considered toxic to normal development and the reproductive system, and can potentially cause endocrine disruption and cancer. Much of the market is dominated by big brand owners. The type of products in the household sectors often directs the packaging material choice with some more aggressive bleach-based products having to use HDPE. Plastic waste is also generated as a non-biodegradable waste, which can cause environmental pollution from unsanitary disposal and toxic leachates and gases, especially carbon monoxide and black smoke produced from open burning [153-165].

1.5 SAFETY ISSUES OF COSMETICS

Cosmetic products are frequently applied to the skin by a large number of people, but some contain potentially toxic compounds if absorption through the skin is sufficient. Makeup, shampoo, skin lotion, nail polish, and other personal care products contain chemical ingredients that lack safety data. Moreover, some of these chemicals have been linked in animal studies to male genital birth defects, decreased sperm counts, and altered pregnancy outcomes. There is no definitive evidence for the same effects in humans, but widespread exposure, primarily to phthalates, has been shown to occur. Phthalates, as key components in plastics, appear in many consumer products. The main phthalates in cosmetics and personal care products are dibutyl phthalate in nail polish, diethyl phthalate in perfumes and lotions, and dimethyl phthalate in hair spray. Often, their presence is not noted on labels [9]. For serious health problems to arise, exposure to these rapidly-clearing compounds must daily . Two such classes of compounds are the phthalate plasticizers and parabens, both of which are used in many personal care products, some medications, and even foods and food preservation. The phthalates are commonly found in foods and household dust. Even though they have relatively short half-lives in humans, phthalates have been associated with several serious health problems, including infertility, testicular dysgenesis, obesity, asthma, and allergies, as well as leiomyomas and breast cancer. Parabens, which can be dermally absorbed, are present in many cosmetic products, including antiperspirants. Their estrogenicity and tissue presence are a cause for concern regarding breast cancer. Fortunately, these compounds are relatively easy to avoid and such steps can result in dramatic reductions of urinary levels of these compounds [23]. An extensive number of cosmetic products are applied topically on and around the human breast on a daily basis, often multiple times a day, including not only underarm antiperspirant/deodorant products but also body lotions, body sprays, moisturizing creams, breast firming/enhancing creams and sun care products. These products are not rinsed off but left on the skin, allowing for continuous dermal exposure, absorption and deposition into underlying tissues, which may be further increased by abrasions in the skin created by shaving. Clinical studies dating back decades report a disproportionately high number of female breast cancers originating in the upper outer quadrant of the breast, and although this is attributed to a greater amount of epithelial tissue in that region, it is also the area to which underarm cosmetic products are applied. Early studies reported 31% of cancers in the upper outer quadrant, but later studies in the 1990s report up to 61%. On the basis, the antiperspirant formulations are designed to block underarm sweat ducts and breast cysts arise from blocked breast ducts in the adjacent region of the body [29]. The percutaneous absorption of N-nitrosodiethanolamine (NDELA), an impurity in many cosmetic products, has been evaluated in diffusion cells using excised human skin [39]. The Cosmetic Ingredient Review (CIR) program was established in 1976 by the Cosmetics, Toiletry, and Fragrance Association, with the support of the Food and Drug Administration (FDA) and the Consumer Federation of America (CFA). CIR performs independent, expert reviews to determine if ingredients used in cosmetics are safe. CIR staff prepares summaries of available data and the CIR Expert Panel reviews the data in open, public meetings. If more data are needed, requests are made. Unpublished studies may be provided, but become public and available for review once summarized in CIR safety assessments. Tentative conclusions are supported with a rationale and public comment is sought. Considering any input, a final safety assessment monograph is issued. These monographs are submitted for publication in the peer-reviewed International Journal of Toxicology. Hair dyes represent an important product category reviewed by CIR. In considering hair dyes, the CIR Expert Panel reviews experimental and clinical data specific to the particular chemical structure of each hair dye and reviews epidemiologic studies that address hair dye use that are less specific. CIR Expert Panel concluded that the available epidemiologic studies are insufficient to conclude there is a causal relationship between hair dye use and cancer and other end points. New information will inevitably become available concerning ingredients for which safety assessments were completed in the early days of the program. To consider new data, the CIR Expert Panel has instituted a re-review program. Sodium lauryl sulfate (SLS), formaldehyde, and parabens are discussed as examples. Safety assessments currently underway are listed, along with high-priority ingredients from which new work will be chosen. Although supported by the cosmetics industry, the CIR program has remained independent in its decision making, based on its open, public process; the integrity of the expert panel members; the participation of the FDA and the CFA; and the cooperation of the cosmetics industry [10]. Over the years, some activist groups have targeted cosmetics as possible human health threats, claiming that cosmetic ingredients are not adequately tested for safety and may pose risks to consumers. The groups allege that industry practices related to safety testing are flawed, that there is little government oversight, and that cosmetics contain cancer-causing chemicals and other toxicants. A critical review of the scientific data related to these claims indicates:

(a) Industry has the primary responsibility to ensure that all ingredients, preservatives, and co-formulants used in products are safe for their intended uses.

(b) The US FDA has regulatory oversight of the cosmetic industry. Its authority includes the banning or restriction of ingredients for safety reasons.

(c) The Cosmetic Ingredient Review (CIR), an independent, scientific review board, critically evaluates chemical ingredients used in cosmetics and publishes the results of its findings in the peer-reviewed literature.

(d) Health-related allegations about cosmetic ingredients are generally based on the results of high-dose laboratory testing in animals and have little relevance for humans. As true now as when Paracelsus said it in the 16th century, "It is the dosc that makes the poison."

(e) Chemicals such as phthalates, parabens, bisphenol A (BPA) and triclosan (TCS), used in a wide variety of consumer products, are suspected endocrine disrupters although their level of toxicity is thought to below. Combined exposure may occur through ingestion, inhalation and dermal exposure, and their toxic, as well as combined effects are poorly understood.

(f) Animal and human physiology differs in crucial ways, further invalidating simplistic attempts to extrapolate rodent testing to human health risks.

The cosmetic industry should be encouraged to publish more of its toxicity studies and safety evaluations, which would aid in dispelling the uncertainty that some consumers have about cosmetic safety [21, 22]. Since the FDA does not specify acceptable levels, the cosmetic industry generally follows the guidelines of the Personal Care Products Council (PCPC) (formerly the Cosmetic, Toiletry, and Fragrance Association (CTFA)) regarding the level of microbial contamination and the absence of pathogens [52].

Exhibit 2. FDA in Action [44-51]

- Under a structure originally established in 1938 that places regulation of cosmetics under the Food and Drug Administration (FDA), cosmetics manufacturers in the United States are not required to register their products or forward consumer complaints to the FDA, leading to broad under-reporting of adverse events. The FDA has limited authority to mandate product recalls.
- In July 2018, Johnson & Johnson was ordered to pay a $4.96 billion settlement to 22 women who found asbestos in talc in baby powder caused their ovarian cancer.
- Guthy-Renker, the manufacturer of WEN hair products, settled a class-action lawsuit for $26 million after consumers said it caused rashes and hair loss.
- After decades of use in soaps, the FDA finally banned triclosan from soap in 2016 over concerns about its long-term safety and contribution to antibiotic-resistant bacteria. Unfortunately, it is still used in many products like toothpaste, mascara, and foundation.

1.6 SKIN AND OTHER SENSITIVITY ISSUES OF COSMETICS

Human skin is the front line of defenses against external infectious or toxic substances and is an environmental habitat that various microorganisms, including bacteria, fungi, yeasts, and viruses, can colonize. Human skin is a complex ecosystem with various microenvironmental conditions, and thus, skin microbial communities are very diverse and complex. Skin structures such as hair follicles, sebaceous glands, eccrine and apocrine sweat glands as well as subepidermal skin compartments, provide distinct biological niches that are colonized by their unique skin microbiota. The current understanding is that most of these skin microbes are harmless or commensal organisms that play essential roles in inhibiting colonization by pathogenic microbes or modulating innate and adaptive immune systems [11]. Skin sensitivity is not the only issue with cosmetics. Beauty salon workers and consumers suffered such injuries as eye and nervous system disorders, respiratory tract problems, chest pain, vomiting, and rash as a result of using the straightener but it remains on the market because the FDA is not authorized to recall cosmetics [12]. Sensitive skin is less tolerant to frequent and prolonged use of cosmetics and toiletries. It is self-diagnosed and typically unaccompanied by any obvious physical signs of irritation. With the change in lifestyle and also with increased opportunity to use many new brands of cosmetics and toiletries, there has been an increase in females complaining of unique sensations in their facial skin. Sensitive skin presents as smarting, burning, stinging, itching, and/or tight sensation in their facial skin. The condition is found in more than 50% of women and 40% of men, creating a sizable demand for products designed to minimize skin sensitivity. Good numbers of invasive and non-invasive tests are designed to evaluate and predict the sensitive skin. Management includes guidelines for selecting suitable cosmetics and toiletries in sensitive skin individuals [13]. In Europe, 1% of the population is estimated to be allergic to fragrances and 2-3% to ingredients of cosmetics; 10% of outpatients patch-tested for cosmetics allergy were found to be positive. Allergenic ingredients of cosmetics can be fragrances, hair dye, preservatives, antioxidants, emollients, surfactants, UV absorbers, pigments or resins used in nail cosmetics. Among standard allergen series, eight substances are related to cosmetics; in Japan in 2003, p-phenylenediamine (hair dyes) induced allergic reactions with the highest rate of 7.9% in outpatients patch-tested. Cosmetic allergy symptoms tend to be mild except those caused by hair dye [42].

1.7 NATURAL PRODUCTS FOR COSMETIC USES

Some natural products have been shown to benefit the skin, especially for the restoration of the skin barrier. Dead Sea mud and water, balneotherapeutic water preparations, deep- sea sponges, milk, and pearl, for example, have been used in ancient to modern formulations for topical application to provide healthy ageless skin. Results were not always well documented, but the effects have been observed and triggered many investigations. The Dead Sea, the deepest and most salinc lake on earth, has been known from biblical times for its healing properties. The systematic review aimed to present critically the level of evidence for the claims of therapeutic effects of Dead Sea treatments in several rheumatologic diseases and psoriasis as well as to review these treatments' safety [14]. Among many components within these materials, calcium is one notable ingredient in common. Plants and natural products with skin-whitening effects are gaining interest among consumers and researchers because they are perceived to be milder, safer, and healthier than synthetic alternatives [15]. Biological activities of plants and natural extracts are therefore available for cosmetic formulators and dermatologists interested in naturally derived ingredients for skin hyperpigmentation treatment as per the consumers' preferences and expectations upon natural cosmetic products. Photoaging is a leading concern for patients and many of these patients will express a desire to utilize natural ingredients as treatment. Mushrooms, feverfew, green tea, licorice, olive oil, soy, and coffee berry have been shown to have antioxidant properties and may play a role in the treatment and prevention of photoaging [16]. Botanical compounds for which dermatologic and cosmetic applications have emerged include olive oil, chamomile, colloidal oatmeal, oat kernel extract, feverfew, acai berry, coffee berry, curcumin, green tea, pomegranate, licorice, paper mulberry, arbutin, and soy. Many of these botanical sources offer biologically active components that require further in vitro and in vivo investigation regarding over-the-counter products based on these ingredients

[17]. The natural baby skin-care products were well tolerated by infants and toddlers when used alone or as part of a skin-care regimen. Although traditional skin-cleansing, lotion, and shampoo products still comprise a large share of the personal care market, increasing numbers of consumers and health care professionals have begun scrutinizing products and product labels, which has created a sizeable market for products that contain natural ingredients. Immediately after birth, the skin barrier of healthy, full-term neonates is competent, yet skin-barrier function continues to develop through at least the first year of life. This developing state of infant skin results in infant skin being susceptible to dryness and irritation from external factors, such as cold weather and wind, as well as harsh topical skin-care products. Therefore, it is critical that infant cleansers and moisturizers be well tolerated and not disrupts the stratum corneum. Infant skin is also exposed to other factors, such as saliva, nasal secretions, urine, feces (including fecal enzymes), and dirt, which can be irritants and result in disruption of the skin barrier. As a result of normal daily exposure to these external factors, proper skin cleansing and protection of the infant skin barrier are essential to the maintenance of skin-barrier function [18]. Nutraceuticals represent a promising strategy for preventing, delaying, or minimizing premature ageing of the skin and also to alleviate certain skin disorders. Among them, bioactive peptides and oligosaccharides, plant polyphenols, carotenoids, vitamins, and polyunsaturated fatty acids are the most widely used ingredients. Supplementation with these products has shown evidence of affecting the signs of ageing and protection against UV radiation ageing in several human trials [19]. Traditional formulation techniques have focused on creating the best performing products at the lowest cost. Little regard has been given to the source of the starting raw materials. However, issues of sustainability, consumer desires, and regulatory pressures have led to the need for the development of cosmetics using primarily plant-based, renewable resourced raw materials. This presents a special challenge to formulators as the starting materials often do not work as well as traditional synthetic ingredients. Since the cosmetics and personal care industry is not regulated, various organizations have offered conflicting positions on standardized guidelines for natural and organic claims. To improve communication on this topic, it will therefore, become important to dissociate claims regarding the naturalness of ingredients from the perception of safety. Safety is inherent in the raw materials used for formulating, regardless of their origin and in the synergies among ingredients—for more than 50 years, the industry has worked hard to monitor the safety of products on the market, supported by the US Food and Drug Administration (FDA). And recently, more governmental agencies such as the FDA, the US Department of Agriculture (USDA) and the Council of Europe's Committee of Experts on Cosmetic Products have taken a proactive role in sorting out the meanings of natural and organic for the cosmetics and personal care industry. Such organizations act as a

clearer scientific focal point in deciding what ingredients are safe for use in cosmetic products.Besides this,, several organizations currently are monitoring the safety of cosmetics and personal care ingredients, such as the Cosmetic Ingredient Review (CIR) panel [53].

1.8 TARGETED COSMETICS

Skin compartments traditionally targeted by cosmetic actives - epidermis and dermis - are anchored and nourished by the underlying hypodermis, which therefore should be a key target for skin-rejuvenating formulations. Given the difficulty to reach even the superficial layers of the skin, and to its 'unglamorous' fatty composition, the regenerative potential of hypodermis remains largely untapped. Nutraceutical grade cosmetics have the potential to induce signal transduction pathways in facial hypodermis, resulting in anti-aging effects throughout all skin compartments, including dermal and epidermal layers [20]. Skin whitening products are commercially available for cosmetic purposes to obtain a lighter skin appearance. They are also utilized for clinical treatment of pigmentary disorders such as melasma or post-inflammatory hyperpigmentation. Whitening agents act at various levels of melanin production in the skin. Many of them are known as competitive inhibitors of tyrosinase, the key enzyme in melanogenesis. Others inhibit the maturation of this enzyme or the transport of pigment granules (melanosomes) from melanocytes to surrounding keratinocytes. In Western culture it is still considered desirable to obtain a (bronze) tan. Despite warnings about the consequences of excessive sun or UV exposure, the artificial tanning business has expanded strongly in the last decades. In the Eastern world, however, a centuries- long tradition exists whereby a light complexion is regarded as equivalent to youth and beauty. Development of preparations for bleaching hyperpigmented lesions or to safely achieve overall whitening is one of the challenges for the cosmetic industry. In recent years, the interest in skin whitening has grown tremendously [24]. It is estimated approximately 15% of the world population invest in skin whitening agents with Asia is being dominated. Global industry analysts (GIA) have predicted that the universal market for skin lighteners will reach $23 billion by 2020, driven by new markets in Asia, particularly India, Japan, and China. According to the SIRONA biochem (a biotechnology company, Vancouver, British Columbia) report, approximately $13 billion spent on skin care products and cosmetics in Asia Pacific's. In India alone, it is estimated that $432 million was spent in 2010 on skin lightening creams and skin care agents. A recent survey showed that 80% of Indian men use fairness creams and the number of consumers are growing 18% annually. The molecular mechanism of these skin lightening agents is to reduce the melanin, which is the main source of skin color [25,26]. The number of patients that visit dermatologists with pigmentary disorders is significant. Patients are often overwhelmed with numerous over-the-counter skin lightening agents, many without clinical evidence of efficacy. Botanical and natural ingredients have become popular as depigmenting products and provide an alternative to the current gold standard, hydroquinone. Despite the need for more long-term, well-designed, randomized, controlled studies, several botanical and natural ingredients do show initial promise in treating disorders of hyperpigmentation based on the results of clinical trials. These ingredients are AA, soy, lignin peroxidase, ascorbic acid iontophoresis, arbutin, ellagic acid, licorice extracts, niacinamide, and mulberry. In addition to showing promise in treating hyperpigmentation, these agents also provide greater insight into the pathogenesis of dyschromia, thus enhancing our understanding of the many complexities of pigment disorders [27]. Cellulite is a serious cosmetic concern for most of the 90% of women affected by it. The phenomenon is most commonly seen on the hips, buttocks, and thighs but can also touch other areas, including the abdomen. Up to 90% of women, over 20 years of age, are affected at various degrees, against only 2% of men. Cellulite is seen as a normal condition by the medical community, but it is a serious cosmetic concern for most women affected by it. It is a complex phenomenon that requires a complex approach, and no single ingredient is solely responsible for the benefits reported. Some disorders have also been associated with cellulite, such as venous insufficiency, kidney problems, metabolic perturbations, and gastrointestinal alterations [28]. Many cosmetic products are available in spray form. Even though the principal targets of these products are the skin and hair, spraying leads to the partitioning of the product between the target and the surrounding air [30]. Aluminium chlorohydrate and aluminium zirkonium tetrachlorohydrate glycine complex are the most frequently used active ingredients in commercial antitranspirants today. Aluminium chloride and propantheline bromide, the anticholinergic substance, are important alternatives although less common. Active ingredients of deodorants are mainly perfuming or bactericidal/bacteriostatic substances, such as triclosan. Also, there are substances that are meant to bind offending smells (e.g. zinc ricinoleate) or to influence the skin surface pH (e.g. triethyl citrate) [31]. A shampoo not only provides the cleaning of the scalp skin and hair as its primary function, but in addition also serves to condition and beautify hair and acts as an adjunct in the management of various scalp disorders. To achieve this, various ingredients in the correct proportion are mixed to provide a shampoo which is suitable for individuals having different hair types and hair need. Among the ingredients that go into the making of a shampoo are detergents, conditioners, thickeners, sequestering agents, pH adjusters, preservatives and specialty additives. Hair conditioners are designed to improve hair manageability, decrease hair static electricity and add luster. They are used in several ways depending upon the state of hair and requirement of the individual [32]. In the 2000s, nail polish manufacturers started promoting "3-Free" products, phasing out three widely publicized toxic chemicals: toluene, formaldehyde, and dibutyl phthalate (DnBP). However, DnBP was sometimes replaced by another endocrine-disrupting plasticizer, triphenyl phosphate (TPHP). Many new "n-Free" labels have since appeared, without any standardization on which n chemicals are excluded. This study aimed to compare measured plasticizer content against nail polish labels. The limited regulation of ingredients in nail polish may leave nail polish users and nail salon workers vulnerable. Consumers that use nail polish mostly consist of women, often of child-bearing age, and even children. Market research suggests that consumers apply nail polish two to six times per month on average, or as much as once per day [33]. Lipsticks may not only increase the contrast between lips and facial skin but may also influence the perceived lightness of skin. Therefore, it would be both scientifically interesting and beneficial for practical purposes to test the effect of lip color on facial skin's perceived lightness. Kobayashi et. al., 2017 reviewed that lip color was assimilated into facial skin's perceived color. For example, they found that orange lip color makes facial skin appear yellowish, and reddish lip color makes facial skin appear reddish and lighter [37]. Acceptable lipstick for the consumers should have a suitable texture and spreadability. Descriptive sensory profiling is an essential tool in this process as it allows an experienced panel to assess the qualitative and quantitative characteristics of a product [38].

1.9 COSMETICS VEHICLES

Consumers will pay a premium for high-performance skin and hair care products. The demand exists, and in return for the high cost, consumers expect the product to perform as claimed and to meet aesthetic standards beyond many products found in the mass market. To be successful in this highly competitive market, products must function as claimed or consumers will not repurchase. Effective contemporary high-end products must be properly formulated in nonirritating vehicles that consumers will perceive as elegant [40]. Cosmetic products mean any substance or mixture intended to be placed in contact with the external parts of the human body (eg, epidermis, lips) and should not pass to the lower parts and penetrate to the skin [41]. In cosmetics, the term "active ingredient" is a marketing term for an ingredient that people believe has some effect but is not legally allowed to. For example, some marketers say Vitamin C is an active ingredient for skin lightening. While there may be some lab studies to show this ingredient may have an effect it is not an approved ingredient for skin lighting, so it's not an active ingredient. If it had affected skin like that it would be a mislabeled drug. Basically, there is no such thing as an active ingredient in cosmetics. If a product has an active ingredient, it is a drug. Functional cosmetic ingredients are those whose main purpose in the formula is to deliver a benefit to a consumer. They may have some secondary effect of improving the feel of the product when it's applied or stabilizing the formula but the primary reason, they are added is for the effect they have on skin or hair [43]. Cosmetic surfactant performs detergency, wetting, emulsifying, solubilizing, dispersing and foaming effects. Adverse reactions of chemical synthesis surfactants affect the environment and humans, particularly severe in the long term. Biodegradability, low toxicity and ecological acceptability which are the benefits of naturally derived surfactant that promises cosmetic safety are, therefore, highly on demand. Biosurfactant producible from microorganisms exhibiting potential surface properties suitable for cosmetic applications especially incorporate with their biological activities. Sophorolipids, rhamnolipids and mannosylerythritol lipids are the most widely used glycolipids biosurfactant in cosmetics. Indeed, many of these biosurfactants could exhibit a "prebiotic" character [54,55]. In addition to their surfactant capacity, many biosurfactants can act as good emulsifiers, which is an extra advantage in the preparation of green cosmetic products. In this work, a biosurfactant obtained from *Lactobacillus paracasei* was used as a stabilizing agent in oil-in-water emulsions containing essential oils and natural antioxidant extract [56]. Surface-active polysaccharides typically have to be used at relatively high levels to produce small droplets, but the droplets formed are highly resistant to environmental changes. Conversely, surface-active proteins are typically utilized at low levels, but the droplets formed are highly sensitive to changes in pH, ionic strength, and temperature. Certain phospholipids are capable of producing small oil droplets during homogenization, but again the droplets formed are highly sensitive to changes in environmental conditions. Biosurfactants (saponins) can be utilized at low levels to form fine oil droplets that remain stable over a range of environmental conditions. Some nature-derived nanoparticles (e.g., cellulose, chitosan, and starch) are effective at stabilizing emulsions containing relatively large oil droplets. Future research is encouraged to identify, isolate, purify, and characterize new types of natural emulsifier, and to test their efficacy in food, cosmetic, detergent, personal care, and other products [57].

1.10 CAUTIONS WITH SENSITIVE SKIN IN USING REGULAR SKIN CARE COSMETICS

Sensitive skin is generally defined as skin that is reactive to external aggressors both in the environment and skincare. When this barrier is weakened due to exposure to environmental aggressors, harsh products or because the body is worn down through stress, for example, it is unable to function properly and the sensitive nerve endings just under the skin become irritated and subsequently react [189]. Therefore, sensitive skin can be a result of either nerve ending becoming more prone to irritation, or the skin barrier function breaking down. Sensitive skin presents as smarting, burning, stinging, itching, and/or tight sensation in their skin. These symptoms may occur minutes to hours after contact with a cosmetic product/ environmental stimulant or even after several episodes of use of a topic product, triggering the conduction by cumulative effect [190]. Sensitive skin: often feels tight and uncomfortable; is sometimes sore or sensitive to touch; needs extra hydration in winter; dries out during flights; can be oily in summer; flushes easily after a spicy meal or drinking alcohol; has patches of redness that may or may not fade; has areas of uneven texture, with dryness and flakiness; reacts to skincare; becomes itchy or develops a rash after contact with irritants; can feel itchy after wearing coarse, synthetic fabrics; turns red and dries out after a hot shower or bath; becomes irritable after continued washing with hard water. common causes of sensitive skin can include: (i) sun exposure (ii) exposure to air pollution (iii) frequent changes in temperature (iv) cold, harsh weather (v) hard water (water with higher mineral content) (v) very hot water (vi) lack of sleep (vii) hormonal changes during your menstrual cycle or pregnancy (viii) stress and late nights (ix) chlorine in swimming pools (x) dry skin (xi) dehydration [191]. Sensitive skin is less tolerant of frequent and prolonged use of cosmetics and toiletries. With the change in lifestyle and also with increased opportunity to use many new brands of cosmetics and toiletries, there has been an increase in females complaining of unique sensations in their facial skin. The condition is found in more than 50% of women and 40% of men, creating a sizable demand for products designed to minimize skin sensitivity. Good numbers of invasive and non-invasive tests are designed to evaluate and predict the sensitive skin. Management includes guidelines for selecting suitable cosmetics and toiletries in sensitive skin individuals [192].

1.11 COSMETICS REGULATIONS

The regulatory framework, compliance requirement, efficacy, safety, and marketing of cosmetic products are considered the most important factors for the growth of the cosmetic industry. The two most important laws aboutcosmetics marketed in the United States are the Federal Food, Drug, and Cosmetic Act (FD&C Act) and the Fair Packaging and Labeling Act (FPLA). FDA regulates cosmetics under the authority of these laws. In the United States, federal laws are enacted by Congress. To make the laws work on a day-to-day level, Congress authorizes certain government agencies. such as the FDA, to create regulations. A change in FDA's legal authority over cosmetics would require Congress to change the law [58]. Different regulatory bodies across the globe have their own insights for regulation; moreover, governments such as the United States, European Union, and Japan follow a stringent regulatory framework, whereas cosmetics are not so much strictly regulated in countries such as India, Brazil, and China [59]. The alignment of a regulatory framework will play a significant role in the removal of barriers to trade, growth of the market at an international level, innovation in the development and presentation of new products, and most importantly safety and efficacy of the marketed products. Unfortunately, despite the efforts of European Authorities, the current legislation is still stratified and several criticisms remain because of the lack of well-established scientific knowledge on nanomaterials. Although the regulatory framework for cosmetic products is almost complete, the efficacy and/or safety assessment of nanomaterials in medicinal products and medical devices is still based on case-by-case evaluation because of the complexity of such systems [60]. The United States (U.S.) and European Union (EU) share a common goal of ensuring the safety of cosmetics for consumers through rigorous science-based regulation. The manner by which each regulates the safety of cosmetics is quite similar. The present contribution gives insight into the important cosmetic regulations in areas of premarket approval, ingredient control, and labeling and warnings, with a special focus on the cosmetic regulatory environments in the United States, European Union, Japan, and India. The European Union's framework of chemical and cosmetics regulations are binding on all Member States Regulations and are enforced at the national level. Under the EU Commission, Regulation (EC) No. 1223/2009 is the key European legislation governing finished cosmetics products in the EU Each country in the EU has a competent authority that is responsible for upholding compliance [59], [61]. In India, cosmetics are regulated as per the Drugs and Cosmetics Act 1940 and Rules 1945. Part-XIII (regulates import and registration of cosmetics), part-XIV (manufacture of cosmetic for sale or distribution) and part-XV (regulates labeling, packing and standards of cosmetics) [62]. In Japan, cosmetics are regulated by the Ministry of Health, Labor, and Welfare (MHLW) under the Pharmaceutical Affairs Law (PAL). For legal reasons, cosmetics are divided into quasi-drugs and cosmetics [63]. In Australia, the importation, manufacture, and use of chemicals—including those used in cosmetics—are regulated by the Australian Government's National Industrial Chemicals Notification and Assessment Scheme (NICNAS). NICNAS works to ensure that chemicals used in consumer products do not cause significant harm to users or the environment [65].

EPILOGUE

Civilizations have used cosmetics – though not always recognizable compared to today's advanced products – for centuries in religious rituals, to enhance beauty, and to promote good health. Cosmetics usage throughout history can be indicative of a civilization's practical concerns, such as protection from the sun, an indication of class, or conventions of beauty. People use cosmetics to keep clean and enhance their beauty. These products range from lipstick and nail polish to deodorant, perfume, hairspray, shampoo, shower gel, tattoos, hair adhesives, hair removal products, hair dyes, most soaps, some tooth whiteners, and some cleansing wipes. Physical appearance is an integral component of self-presentation in all social situations, including that of applying for a job. Cosmetics contain a vast number of chemicals, most of which are not under the regulatory purview of the Food and Drug Administration. Only a few of these chemicals have been evaluated for potential deleterious health impact: parabens, phthalates, polycyclic aromatic hydrocarbons, and siloxanes. While the current scientific thinking on many of these chemicals is that they are safe to use, it is up to each consumer to make their own decision as to whether they purchase and use a product containing certain ingredients or not. Consumers should also try to purchase reputable brands from established sellers—cheap imports or copies bought online may not have been through the proper testing and assessment process and may not contain what they claim to.

SUMMARY

Cosmetology incorporates the most advanced scientific knowledge and technology including chemistry, pharmacology, molecular biology, genetic/new materials engineering, immunology, and neurology, etc. Cosmetics are readily available today in the form of creams, lipstick, perfumes, eye shadows, nail polishes, hair sprays etc. Other cosmetics like face powder give a glow to the skin after applying the base cream. Cosmetic ingredients/excipients are incorporated to obtain detergency, wetting, emulsifying, staining and soothing effects. Adverse reactions of chemicals have effects on the environment and humans, particularly severe in the long term. Many cosmetics have therapeutic effects in use. Again, different populations have a different profile of cosmetics use. As a consequence of this increasing application of science to beauty, the line between cosmetic and medical research is becoming blurred; the laboratories of major cosmetic companies perform cutting-edge research in areas such as matrix biology, antioxidants and aging processes. Proper rules and regulations should be imposed on their manufacturing, marketing and distributions along with pricing.

ABBREVIATIONS

The Cosmetic Ingredient Review (CIR); Consumer Federation of America (CFA); Sodium lauryl sulfate (SLS); Global industry analysts (GIA); dibutyl phthalate (DnBP); triphenyl phosphate (TPHP); N-nitrosodiethanolamine (NDELA); Ministry of Health, Labor, and Welfare (MHLW); Pharmaceutical Affairs Law (PAL); National Industrial Chemicals Notification and Assessment Scheme (NICNAS), Water, Sanitation, And Hygiene (WASH), High Density Polyethylene (HDPE)

BIBLIOGRAPHY AND WEBLIOGRAPHY

1. Chapter 2. The body with limits. In: The Future of Post-Human Performing Arts: A Preface to a New Theory of the Body and its Presence by Peter Baofu, Published by Cambridge Scholars Publishing, 2013, ISBN 1443844853, 9781443844857
2. Unit 1. Cosmetics. In: Cosmetic Chemistry: An Instant Approach by Ayaz Mahmood Dar, Published by Educreation Publishing
3. International Modeling Guide -5th Edition by Regina Niallah, published by FTC Publications, Inc., 2007 ISBN 0977477126, 9780977477128
4. Web L'Oréal Paris USA. Bronzer vs. Contour: What's the Difference? Available From: https://www.lorealparisusa.com/beauty-magazine/makeup/face-makeup/ bronzer -vs-contour-difference.aspx
5. Tolentino G. In What Order Do I Apply My Skin Care Products? Web DermStore.com (Skin Care Blogs), August 9, 2018. Available From: https://www.dermstore.com/blog/in-what-order-do-i-apply-my-skin-care-products-infographic/
6. Web narscosmetics. LIPS TO STYLE. Available From: https://www.narscosmetics.com/USA/lips
7. Dionisio KL, Phillips K, Price PS, Grulke CM, Williams A, Biryol D, Hong T, Isaacs KK. The Chemical and Products Database, a resource for exposure-relevant data on chemicals in consumer products. Sci Data. 2018 Jul 10;5:180125. doi: 10.1038/sdata.2018.125.
8. EWG's Skin Deep® Cosmetic Database. Available From: https://www.ewg.org/skindeep/site/about.php
9. Barrett JR. The ugly side of beauty products. Environ Health Perspect. 2005 Jan;113(1):A24.
10. Bergfeld WF, Belsito DV, Marks JG Jr, Andersen FA. Safety of ingredients used in cosmetics. J Am Acad Dermatol. 2005 Jan;52(1):125-32. Erratum in: J Am Acad Dermatol. 2005 Jul;53(1):137.
11. Lee HJ, Jeong SE, Lee S, Kim S, Han H, Jeon CO. Effects of cosmetics on the skin microbiome of facial cheeks with different hydration levels. Microbiologyopen. 2018 Apr;7(2):e00557. doi: 10.1002/mbo3.557. Epub 2017 Nov 29.
12. Vogel L. US legislators propose crackdown on toxic cosmetics. CMAJ. 2011 Nov 8;183(16):E1169-70. doi: 10.1503/cmaj.109-4019. Epub 2011 Oct 11.
13. Inamadar AC, Palit A. Sensitive skin: an overview. Indian J Dermatol VenereolLeprol. 2013 Jan-Feb;79(1):9-16. doi: 10.4103/0378-6323.104664.
14. Katz U, Shoenfeld Y, Zakin V, Sherer Y, Sukenik S. Scientific evidence of the therapeutic effects of dead sea treatments: a systematic review. SeminArthritis Rheum. 2012 Oct;42(2):186-200. doi: 10.1016/j.semarthrit.2012.02.006.
15. Handbook of Cosmetic Science and Technology, 4th Edition by André O. Barel, Marc Paye, Howard I. Maibach, published by CRC Press, 2014 ISBN 1842145649, 9781842145647

16. Kanlayavattanakul M, Lourith N. Plants and Natural Products for the Treatment of Skin Hyperpigmentation - A Review. Planta Med. 2018 Sep;84(14):988-1006. doi: 10.1055/a-0583-0410.
17. Baumann L, Woolery-Lloyd H, Friedman A. "Natural" ingredients in cosmetic dermatology. J Drugs Dermatol. 2009 Jun;8(6 Suppl):s5-9.
18. Coret CD, Suero MB, Tierney NK. Tolerance of natural baby skin-care products on healthy, full-term infants and toddlers. Clin CosmetInvestig Dermatol. 2014 Feb 5;7:51-8. doi: 10.2147/CCID.S56939.
19. Pérez-Sánchez A, Barrajón-Catalán E, Herranz-López M, Micol V. Nutraceuticals for Skin Care: A Comprehensive Review of Human Clinical Studies. Nutrients. 2018 Mar 24;10(4). pii: E403. doi: 10.3390/nu10040403.
20. Bojanowski K. Hypodermal delivery of cosmetic actives for improved facial skin morphology and functionality. Int J Cosmet Sci. 2013 Dec;35(6):562-7. doi: 10.1111/ics.12077.
21. Ross G. A perspective on the safety of cosmetic products: a position paper of the American Council on Science and Health. Int J Toxicol. 2006 Jul-Aug;25(4): 269-77.
22. Larsson K, Ljung Björklund K, Palm B, Wennberg M, Kaj L, Lindh CH, Jönsson BA, Berglund M. Exposure determinants of phthalates, parabens, bisphenol A and triclosan in Swedish mothers and their children. Environ Int. 2014 Dec;73:323-33. doi: 10.1016/j.envint.2014.08.014.
23. Crinnion WJ. Toxic effects of the easily avoidable phthalates and parabens. Altern Med Rev. 2010 Sep;15(3):190-6.
24. Smit N, Vicanova J, Pavel S. The hunt for natural skin whitening agents. Int J Mol Sci. 2009 Dec 10;10(12):5326-49. doi: 10.3390/ijms10125326.
25. Pillaiyar T, Manickam M, Namasivayam V. Skin whitening agents: medicinal chemistry perspective of tyrosinase inhibitors. J Enzyme Inhib Med Chem. 2017 Dec;32(1):403-425. doi: 10.1080/14756366.2016.1256882.
26. Desmedt B, Courselle P, De Beer JO, Rogiers V, Grosber M, Deconinck E, De Paepe K. Overview of skin whitening agents with an insight into the illegal cosmetic market in Europe. J Eur Acad Dermatol Venereol. 2016 Jun;30(6):943-50. doi: 10.1111/jdv.13595.
27. Hollinger JC, Angra K, Halder RM. Are Natural Ingredients Effective in the Management of Hyperpigmentation? A Systematic Review. J Clin Aesthet Dermatol. 2018 Feb;11(2):28-37. Epub 2018 Feb 1.
28. Dupont E, Journet M, Oula ML, Gomez J, Léveillé C, Loing E, Bilodeau D. An integral topical gel for cellulite reduction: results from a double-blind, randomized, placebo-controlled evaluation of efficacy. Clin CosmetInvestig Dermatol. 2014 Feb 20;7:73-88. doi: 10.2147/CCID.S53580.
29. Darbre PD. Underarm antiperspirants/deodorants and breast cancer. Breast Cancer Res. 2009;11 Suppl 3:S5. doi: 10.1186/bcr2424.
30. Steiling W, Buttgereit P, Hall B, O'Keeffe L, Safford B, Tozer S, Coroama M. Skin exposure to deodorants/antiperspirants in aerosol form. Food Chem Toxicol. 2012 Jun;50(6):2206-15. doi: 10.1016/j.fct.2012.03.058.

31. Lukacs VA, Korting HC. [Antiperspirants and deodorants--ingredients and evaluation]. DermBeruf Umwelt. 1989 Mar-Apr;37(2):53-7.
32. Young AS, Allen JG, Kim UJ, Seller S, Webster TF, Kannan K, Ceballos DM. Phthalate and Organophosphate Plasticizers in Nail Polish: Evaluation of Labels and Ingredients. Environ Sci Technol. 2018 Oct 10. doi: 10.1021/acs.est.8b04495
33. Chow ET, Mahalingaiah S. Cosmetics use and age at menopause: is there a connection? FertilSteril. 2016 Sep 15;106(4):978-90. doi: 10.1016/ j.fertnstert.2016.08.020
34. Berdai MA, Labib S, Chetouani K, Harandou M. Atropa belladonna intoxication: a case report. Pan Afr Med J. 2012;11:72.
35. Richard Evans Schultes, Albert Hofmann. Plants of the Gods: Origins of Hallucinogenic Use (pp 88), published by Hutchinson, 1980 ISBN 0091416000, 9780091416003.
36. Tombs, S., & Silverman, I. (2004). Pupillometry: A sexual selection approach. Evolution and Human Behavior, 25(4), 221-228. http://dx.doi.org/10.1016/j.evolhumbehav.2004.05.001
37. Kobayashi Y, Matsushita S, Morikawa K. Effects of Lip Color on Perceived Lightness of Human Facial Skin. Iperception. 2017 Jul 11;8(4):204 1669517717500. doi: 10.1177/2041669517717500. eCollection 2017 Jul-Aug.
38. Kasparaviciene G, Savickas A, Kalveniene Z, Velziene S, Kubiliene L, Bernatoniene J. Evaluation of Beeswax Influence on Physical Properties of Lipstick Using Instrumental and Sensory Methods. Evid Based Complement Alternat Med. 2016;2016:3816460.
39. Bronaugh RL, Congdon ER, Scheuplein RJ. The effect of cosmetic vehicles on the penetration of N-nitrosodiethanolamine through excised human skin. J Invest Dermatol. 1981 Feb;76(2):94-6.
40. Epstein H. Cosmeceutical vehicles. Clin Dermatol. 2009 Sep-Oct;27(5):453-60. doi: 10.1016/j.clindermatol.2009.05.007.
41. Pavlačková J, Egner P, Polašková J, Hojerová J, Pinďáková L, Mokrejš P, Varaďová V. Transdermal absorption of active substances from cosmetic vehicles. J Cosmet Dermatol. 2019 Jan 30. doi: 10.1111/jocd.12873.
42. Minamoto K. [Skin sensitizers in cosmetics and skin care products]. Nihon EiseigakuZasshi. 2010 Jan;65(1):20-9.
43. Romanowski P (2017). What is an active ingredient in cosmetics? Web chemistscorner.com
44. Cornell EM, Janetos TM, Xu S. Time for a makeover-cosmetics regulation in the United States. J Cosmet Dermatol. 2019 Apr 4. doi: 10.1111/jocd.12886.
45. Hsu T. Johnson & Johnson Told to Pay $4.7 Billion in Baby Powder Lawsuit (Business Article). The New York Times July 12, 2018
46. Bellon T. Jury orders J&J to pay $4.7 billion in Missouri asbestos cancer case ((Business Article). Web euters.com, July 13, 2018
47. Narayan P. The cosmetics industry has avoided strict regulation for over a century. Now rising health concerns has FDA inquiring. CNBC News Thu, Aug 2 2018.

48. Edgar J. WEN Case Spurs Call for Beauty Product Regs. WebMD Health News, February 7, 2018.
49. McMillen M. Banned From Soap, Is Triclosan Still a Concern? - Medscape - Jul 09, 2018.
50. Louis CS. Why a Chemical Banned From Soap Is Still in Your Toothpaste? The New York Times Sept. 7, 2016.
51. Helmenstine AM. Toxic Chemicals in Cosmetics. Web ThoughtCo, February 11, 2019.
52. Halla N, Fernandes IP, Heleno SA, Costa P, Boucherit-Otmani Z, Boucherit K, Rodrigues AE, Ferreira ICFR, Barreiro MF. Cosmetics Preservation: A Review on Present Strategies. Molecules. 2018 Jun 28;23(7). pii: E1571. doi: 10.3390/molecules23071571.
53. Eric S. Abrutyn. Chapter 1. Building Natural Products. In: Primer on Formulating NATURAL Products, edited by Angela C. Kozlowski, published by Marian Raney, 2012. ISBN: 978-1-937235-07-9
54. Lourith N, Kanlayavattanakul M. Natural surfactants used in cosmetics: glycolipids. Int J Cosmet Sci. 2009 Aug;31(4):255-61. doi: 10.1111/j.1468-2494.2009.00493.x.
55. Vecino X, Cruz JM, Moldes AB, Rodrigues LR. Biosurfactants in cosmetic formulations: trends and challenges. Crit Rev Biotechnol. 2017 Nov;37(7):911-923. doi: 10.1080/07388551.2016.1269053.
56. Ferreira A, Vecino X, Ferreira D, Cruz JM, Moldes AB, Rodrigues LR. Novel cosmetic formulations containing a biosurfactant from Lactobacillus paracasei. Colloids Surf B Biointerfaces. 2017 Jul 1;155:522-529. doi: 10.1016/j.colsurfb.2017.04.026.
57. McClements DJ, Gumus CE. Natural emulsifiers - Biosurfactants, phospholipids, biopolymers, and colloidal particles: Molecular and physicochemical basis of functional performance. Adv Colloid Interface Sci. 2016 Aug;234:3-26. doi: 10.1016/j.cis.2016.03.002.
58. Suhag J, Dureja H. Cosmetic Regulations: A Comparative Study. Skinmed. 2015 May-Jun;13(3):191-4.
59. Web US FDA. FDA Authority Over Cosmetics: How Cosmetics Are Not FDA-Approved, but Are FDA-Regulated. Available From: https://www.fda.gov/Cosmetics/GuidanceRegulation/ucm074162.htm
60. Musazzi UM, Marini V, Casiraghi A, Minghetti P. Is the European regulatory framework sufficient to assure the safety of citizens using health products containing nanomaterials? Drug Discov Today. 2017 Jun;22(6):870-882. doi: 10.1016/j.drudis.2017.01.016.
61. Web cosmeticinfo.org. U.S. and EU Cosmetics Regulation. Available From: https://www.cosmeticsinfo.org/cosmetics-regulation
62. Sarma P, Kumar H, Medhi B. Cosmetovigilance in India: Need of the day. Indian JPharmacol. 2017 Sep-Oct;49(5):341-343. doi: 10.4103/ijp.IJP_45_18.
63. Pharmacopeia T.J. The Japanese Pharmacopeia. 64th ed. Japan Ministry of Health, Labour and Welfare; Tokyo, Japan: 2016. pp. 2486–2489.

64. Web cosmeticsinfo.org. A History Of Cosmetics From Ancient Times. Available From: https://cosmeticsinfo.org/Ancient-history-cosmetics
65. Jones O, Selinger B. The chemistry of cosmetics. Web Australian Academy of Science November 20, 2018.
66. Laliberte M. 10 Beauty Secrets to Steal from Marilyn Monroe. Web Reader's Digest. Available from: https://www.rd.com/health/beauty/marilyn-monroe-makeup/
67. Forster A. Marilyn Monroe's beauty secrets: The most surprising tips from Hollywood's ultimate icon. Fashion Magazine, June 1, 2016.
68. Marilyn Monroe Quotes Pinterest. Blog I'm Still a woman, October 27, 2012.
69. REVEALED: Asparagus Stem Cells Are The Answer To Hair Loss! Available From: https://www.cel.md/blogs/news/revealed-plant-stem-cells-are-the-answer-to-hair-loss
70. Trehan S, Michniak-Kohn B, Beri K. Plant stem cells in cosmetics: current trends and future directions. Future Sci OA. 2017 Jul 12;3(4):FSO226. doi: 10.4155/fsoa-2017-0026.
71. MAC-Makeup-Collection-Holiday-2013. Web chicprofile.com, October 15, 2013
72. Balukonis L. Cosmetics A Look into the Past, Present and Future. Available From: https://www.dermascope.com/resources/cosmetics-a-look-into-the-past-present-and-future
73. Anna Savina. Permanent Lip Makeup, published by Anna Savina LLC, Dec 28, 2013.
74. Donna Maria. Making Aromatherapy Creams & Lotions: 101 Natural Formulas to Revitalize & Nourish Your Skin, published by Storey Publishing, LLC, 2018 ISBN 161212240X, 9781612122403
75. Sandi Brenner. Beauty and the Budget, published by Sandi Brenner, 2006, ISBN 1589399269, 9781589399266
76. Stephen M. Schleicher. Skin Sense! A Dermatologist's Guide to Skin and Facial Care; Third Edition, published by iUniverse, 2009, ISBN1440174288, 9781440174285
77. Nelson Lee Novick. Super Skin: A Leading Dermatologist's Guide to the Latest Breakthrough in Skin Care, published by iUniverse, 2000 ISBN 1475922132, 9781475922134
78. Brandith Irwin, Mark McPherson. Your Best Face Without Surgery: Looking Your Best Without Plastic Surgery, published by Hay House Inc., September 2002., ASIN: B004C03L1E
79. John Toedt, Darrell Koza, Kathleen Van Cleef-Toedt. Chemical Composition of Everyday Products, ABC-Clio ebook Gale virtual reference library, published by Greenwood Publishing Group, 2005, ISBN 0313325790, 9780313325793
80. Tarun J, Susan J, Suria J, Susan VJ, Criton S. Evaluation of pH of Bathing Soaps and Shampoos for Skin and Hair Care. Indian J Dermatol. 2014 Sep;59(5):442-4. doi: 10.4103/0019-5154.139861.
81. Mukhopadhyay P. Cleansers and their role in various dermatological disorders. Indian J Dermatol. 2011 Jan;56(1):2-6. doi: 10.4103/0019-5154.77542.

82. Oliver D. What Is Makeup Primer, And Do You Need It? The Huffington Post, December 21, 2017.
83. How to Use Primer Like a Pro – Superdrug. Available From: https://www.superdrug.com › Home › Beauty Manuals › How to Use Primer Like a Pro
84. Roberts WE, Jiang LI, Herndon JH Jr. Facial primer provides immediate and long-term improvements in mild-to-moderate facial hyperpigmentation and fine lines associated with photoaging. Clin CosmetInvestig Dermatol. 2015 Sep 2;8:471-7. doi: 10.2147/CCID.S88443.
85. Denton-Hurst. T. How to Pick the Best Makeup Primer for You and Apply it Like a Pro. Web makeup.com Tutorial, September 7, 2018.
86. Rayner VL. Camouflage therapy. Dermatol Clin. 1995 Apr;13(2):467-72. PubMed PMID: 7600717.
87. Monfrecola G, Cacciapuoti S, Capasso C, Delfino M, Fabbrocini G. Tolerability and camouflaging effect of corrective makeup for acne: results of a clinical study of a novel face compact cream. Clin CosmetInvestig Dermatol. 2016 Oct 11;9:307-313
88. Levy LL, Emer JJ. Emotional benefit of cosmetic camouflage in the treatment of facial skin conditions: personal experience and review. Clin CosmetInvestig Dermatol. 2012;5:173-82. doi: 10.2147/CCID.S33860.
89. Sarveswari KN. Cosmetic camouflage in vitiligo. Indian J Dermatol. 2010 Jul-Sep;55(3):211-4. doi: 10.4103/0019-5154.70663.
90. Concealer for Skin Imperfections. Available From: https://www.carobels.com/en/makeup/makeup/face/concealer-for-skin-imperfections/287
91. Draelos ZD. Active agents in common skin care products. PlastReconstr Surg. 2010 Feb;125(2):719-24. doi: 10.1097/PRS.0b013e3181c83192.
92. Moore A. The biochemistry of beauty. The science and pseudo-science of beautiful skin. EMBO Rep. 2002 Aug;3(8):714-7.
93. Tagai K, Shimakura H, Isobe H, Nittono H. The light-makeup advantage in facial processing: Evidence from event-related potentials. PLoS One. 2017 Feb 24;12(2):e0172489. doi: 10.1371/journal.pone.0172489.
94. Kilkeary AM. What Comes First — Foundation or Concealer? Here's What You Need To Know. Web makeup.com Tutorial, January 2, 2019.
95. Under Eye Concealer Setting Powder: Top Selected Products and Reviews. Available From: https://www.amazon.com/slp/under-eye-concealer-setting-powder/pg46h58wak4t3hg
96. ATKINS F. Analysis of face powder. Manuf Chem Aerosol News. 1948 Dec;19(12):565.
97. Everything you need to know about face powders. Available From: https://hellogiggles.com/beauty/everything-to-know-about-face-powders/
98. Lubitz R. The gruesome and lengthy history of why we use blush. Web .businessinsider.com, June 1, 2017.
99. These are the best blushes for making your dewy skin dreams come true (including a £10 steal). Glamour Magazine, Friday 8 March 2019.

100. Carole Jackson. Color Me Beautiful Makeup Book, published by Ballantine Books, 1988, ISBN 0345348427, 9780345348425
101. Janet Simms. A Practical Guide to Beauty Therapy for NVQ Level 2, publisher Nelson Thornes, 2003, ISBN 0748771506, 9780748771509
102. Bronzer vs. Contour: What's the Difference? Available From: https://www.lorealparisusa.com/beauty-magazine/makeup/face-makeup/bronzer-vs-contour-difference.aspx
103. Sandra Morris. The beauty manual: how to look your best ever, published by Lowell House, 1999, ISBN0737305053, 9780737305050
104. Should I Use Shimmer Bronzer, Matte Bronzer, or Sheer Bronzer? Available From: https://www.adorebeauty.com.au/bronzer/guide/bronzer-types
105. Writeup: Cosmetics/Makeup. Available From: https://rayorconcept.blogspot.com /2016/10/writeup-cosmeticsmakeup.html
106. Sinks T. Everything You Need to Know About Mascara. Web lifehacker.com, January 5, 2017.
107. Michelle Phan. Make Up: Your Life Guide to Beauty, Style, and Success--Online and Off, published by Potter/Ten Speed/Harmony/Rodale, 2014, ISBN 1101903074, 9781101903070
108. Sharon Parsons. The Chemistry of Cosmetics, published by Cengage Learning Australia, 2013, ISBN0170229513, 9780170229517
109. Eye makeup. Available From: http://www.gulabifashion.com/eye-makeup/
110. Marjorie Grimm. Permanent Cosmetics: The Foundation of Fundamental Applications, Independent Publisher, 2018, ISBN 1532368526, 9781532368523
111. What Is Makeup Setting Spray and How Does It Help Keep Your Makeup in Place. Available From: https://www.lorealparisusa.com/beauty-magazine/makeup/ face-makeup/makeup-setting-spray.aspx
112. Stan Place, Bobbi Ray Madry. The Art and Science of Professional Makeup Skin Series, published by Cengage Learning, 1989, ISBN 0873503619, 9780873503617
113. Face Wash vs. Cleanser vs. Scrub: What's the Difference? Available From:
114. Villette M. How to Choose the Best Cleanser for Your Skin? Villette M. Web theskincareedit.com February 3, 2016.
115. Charlotte Cho. The Little Book of Skin Care: Korean Beauty Secrets for Healthy, Glowing Skin, published by HarperCollins, 2015 ISBN 0062416383, 9780062416384
116. General skincare programs. Available From: https://cosmeticsproduct.org/general-skincare-programs
117. Julie Gabriel. The Green Beauty Guide: Your Essential Resource to Organic and Natural Skin Care, Hair Care, Makeup, and Fragrances, published by Health Communications, Inc., 2008 ISBN 0757307477, 9780757307478
118. Shahnaz Husain. Shahnaz Husain's Beauty Book, published by Orient Paperbacks, 1998 ISBN 8122200605, 9788122200607
119. Krieger L. 10 Important Things You Need to Know Before Exfoliating Your Face. Web cosmopolitan.com, October 18, 2018.

120. Mark Lees. Skin Care: Beyond the Basics, published by Cengage Learning, Jun 25, 2013, ISBN 1133708390, 9781133708391

121. S.D. Williams. Chemistry and Technology of the Cosmetics and Toiletries Industry, edited by D. F. Williams, W.H. Schmitt, published by Springer Science & Business Media, 1996 ISBN 0751403342, 9780751403343

122. D'Souza P, Rathi SK. Shampoo and Conditioners: What a Dermatologist Should Know? Indian J Dermatol. 2015 May-Jun;60(3):248-54. doi: 10.4103/0019-5154.156355.

123. Trüeb RM. Shampoos: ingredients, efficacy and adverse effects. J Dtsch Dermatol Ges. 2007 May;5(5):356-65.

124. Draelos ZD. Essentials of Hair Care often Neglected: Hair Cleansing. Int J Trichology. 2010 Jan;2(1):24-9. doi: 10.4103/0974-7753.66909.

125. Gavazzoni Dias MF. Hair cosmetics: an overview. Int J Trichology. 2015 Jan-Mar;7(1):2-15. doi: 10.4103/0974-7753.153450.

126. Benohanian A. Antiperspirants and deodorants. Clin Dermatol. 2001 Jul-Aug;19(4):398-405.

127. Zirwas MJ, Moennich J. Antiperspirant and deodorant allergy: diagnosis and management. J Clin Aesthet Dermatol. 2008 Sep;1(3):38-43.

128. Burry JS, Evans RL, Rawlings AV, Shiu J. Effect of antiperspirants on whole body sweat rate and thermoregulation. Int J Cosmet Sci. 2003 Aug;25(4):189-92. doi: 10.1046/j.1467-2494.2003.00184.x.

129. Callewaert C, Hutapea P, Van de Wiele T, Boon N. Deodorants and antiperspirants affect the axillary bacterial community. Arch Dermatol Res. 2014 Oct;306(8):701-10. doi: 10.1007/s00403-014-1487-1. Epub 2014 Jul 31. PubMed PMID: 25077920.

130. Lodén M, Wessman C. The antidandruff efficacy of a shampoo containing piroctone olamine and salicylic acid in comparison to that of a zinc pyrithione shampoo. Int J Cosmet Sci. 2000 Aug;22(4):285-9. doi: 10.1046/j.1467-2494.2000.00024.x.

131. Schwartz JR, Bacon RA, Shah R, Mizoguchi H, Tosti A. Therapeutic efficacy of anti-dandruff shampoos: a randomized clinical trial comparing products based on potentiated zinc pyrithione and zinc pyrithione/climbazole. Int J Cosmet Sci. 2013 Aug;35(4):381-7. doi: 10.1111/ics.12055

132. Victor R. Preedy. Handbook of Hair in Health and Disease, Issue 1 of Human health handbooks, ISSN 2212-375X, published by Springer Science & Business Media, 2012 ISBN 9086867286, 9789086867288

133. Cury JA, Tenuta LM. Evidence-based recommendation on toothpaste use. Braz Oral Res. 2014;28 Spec No:1-7. doi: 10.1590/S1806-83242014.50000001.

134. Lippert F. An introduction to toothpaste - its purpose, history and ingredients. Monogr Oral Sci. 2013;23:1-14. doi: 10.1159/000350456. Epub 2013 Jun 28. PubMed PMID: 23817056.

135. C. van Loveren. Toothpastes Volume 23 of Monographs in oral science, published by Karger Medical and Scientific Publishers, 2013 ISBN 3318022063, 9783318022063

136. Davies RM, Ellwood RP, Davies GM. The rational use of fluoride toothpaste. Int J Dent Hyg. 2003 Feb;1(1):3-8.
137. Jahangir GZ, Ashraf DS, Nasir IA, Sadiq M, Shahzad S, Naz F, Iqbal M, Saeed A. The myth of oral hygiene using synthetic mouthwash products. Springerplus. 2016 Sep 2;5(1):1481. doi: 10.1186/s40064-016-3158-5.
138. Ciancio SG. Mouthwashes: Rationale for use. Am J Dent. 2015 Sep;28 Spec No A:4A-8A.
139. Alshehri FA. The use of mouthwash containing essential oils (LISTERINE®) to improve oral health: A systematic review. Saudi Dent J. 2018 Jan;30(1):2-6. doi: 10.1016/j.sdentj.2017.12.004.
140. Pereira EM, da Silva JL, Silva FF, De Luca MP, Ferreira EF, Lorentz TC, Santos VR. Clinical Evidence of the Efficacy of a Mouthwash Containing Propolis for the Control of Plaque and Gingivitis: A Phase II Study. Evid Based Complement Alternat Med. 2011;2011:750249. doi: 10.1155/2011/750249.
141. Bajpai D, Tyagi VK. Laundry detergents: an overview. J Oleo Sci. 2007;56(7):327-40.
142. Habib RR, El-Masri A, Heath RL. Women's strategies for handling household detergents. Environ Res. 2006 Jun;101(2):184-94.
143. Liu X, Lao XQ, Wong CC, Tan L, Zhang Z, Wong TW, Tse LA, Lau APS, Yu ITS. Frequent use of household cleaning products is associated with rhinitis in Chinese children. J Allergy Clin Immunol. 2016 Sep;138(3):754-760.e6. doi: 10.1016/j.jaci.2016.03.038.
144. Hong S, Kwon HJ, Choi WJ, Lim WR, Kim J, Kim K. Association between exposure to antimicrobial household products and allergic symptoms. Environ Health Toxicol. 2014 Nov 21;29:e2014017. doi: 10.5620/eht.e2014017.
145. Sherriff A, Farrow A, Golding J, Henderson J. Frequent use of chemical household products is associated with persistent wheezing in pre-school age children. Thorax. 2005 Jan;60(1):45-9.
146. Coret CD, Suero MB, Tierney NK. Tolerance of natural baby skin-care products on healthy, full-term infants and toddlers. Clin CosmetInvestig Dermatol. 2014 Feb 5;7:51-8. doi: 10.2147/CCID.S56939.
147. Sathyanarayana S, Karr CJ, Lozano P, Brown E, Calafat AM, Liu F, Swan SH. Baby care products: possible sources of infant phthalate exposure. Pediatrics. 2008 Feb;121(2):e260-8. doi: 10.1542/peds.2006-3766.
148. Kuller JM. Infant Skin Care Products: What Are the Issues? Adv Neonatal Care. 2016 Oct;16 Suppl 5S:S3-S12.
149. Gao X, Simpson EL. Market trends in baby skin care products and implications for clinical practice. Pediatr Dermatol. 2014 Nov-Dec;31(6):734-8. doi: 10.1111/pde.12424.
150. Cooke A, Bedwell C, Campbell M, McGowan L, Ersser SJ, Lavender T. Skin care for healthy babies at term: A systematic review of the evidence. Midwifery. 2018 Jan;56:29-43. doi: 10.1016/j.midw.2017.10.001.
151. The Choice Guide to Baby Product: The Buying Guide for Parents, published by ReadHowYouWant.com, 2010, ISBN 1459603427, 9781459603424

152. Lawrence F. Eichenfield, Ilona J. Frieden, Erin Mathes, Andrea Zaenglein, Nancy B. Esterly, Neonatal Dermatology E-Book, 2nd Edition, published by Elsevier Health Sciences, 2007 ISBN 1437720773, 9781437720778

153. Dennis Laba. Rheological Properties of Cosmetics and Toiletries Cosmetic Science and Technology, CRC Press, 1993 ISBN 0824790901, 9780824790905

154. Groot AC, Nater JP, Lender R, Rijcken B. Adverse effects of cosmetics and toiletries: a retrospective study in the general population. Int J Cosmet Sci. 1987 Dec;9(6):255-9. doi: 10.1111/j.1467-2494.1987.tb00481.x.

155. Sportiello L, Cammarota S, de Portu S, Sautebin L. Notification of undesirable effects of cosmetics and toiletries. Pharmacol Res. 2009 Feb;59(2):101-6. doi: 10.1016/j.phrs.2008.10.008.

156. Household, Toiletries and Personal Care. Available From: http://www.esterform.com/market-sectors/household-toiletries-and-personal-care/

157. Poonyakan A, Rachakornkij M, Wecharatana M, Smittakorn W. Potential Use of Plastic Wastes for Low Thermal Conductivity Concrete. Materials (Basel). 2018 Oct 11;11(10). pii: E1938. doi: 10.3390/ma11101938.

158. Weatherly LM, Gosse JA. Triclosan exposure, transformation, and human health effects. J Toxicol Environ Health B Crit Rev. 2017;20(8):447-469. doi: 10.1080/10937404.2017.1399306.

159. Proma AM. Zero chemicals; hero toiletries!. The Daily Star, February 25, 2019.

160. McNary JE, Jackson EM. Inhalation exposure to formaldehyde and toluene in the same occupational and consumer setting. InhalToxicol. 2007 May;19(6-7):573-6.

161. Kim S, Lee S, Shin C, Lee J, Kim S, Lee A, Park J, Kho Y, Moos RK, Koch HM, Kim S, Choi K. Urinary parabens and triclosan concentrations and associated exposure characteristics in a Korean population-A comparison between night-time and first-morning urine. Int J Hyg Environ Health. 2018 May;221(4):632-641. doi: 10.1016/j.ijheh.2018.03.009.

162. Nowak K, Ratajczak-Wrona W, Górska M, Jabłońska E. Parabens and their effects on the endocrine system. Mol Cell Endocrinol. 2018 Oct 15;474:238-251. doi: 10.1016/j.mce.2018.03.014.

163. Koniecki D, Wang R, Moody RP, Zhu J. Phthalates in cosmetic and personal care products: concentrations and possible dermal exposure. Environ Res. 2011 Apr;111(3):329-36. doi: 10.1016/j.envres.2011.01.013. Epub 2011 Feb 18. PubMed PMID: 21315328.

164. Kim YM, Kim J, Cheong HK, Jeon BH, Ahn K. Exposure to phthalates aggravates pulmonary function and airway inflammation in asthmatic children. PLoS One. 2018 Dec 17;13(12):e0208553. doi: 10.1371/journal.pone.0208553.

165. Johansen JD, Rastogi SC, Andersen KE, Menné T. Content and reactivity to product perfumes in fragrance mix positive and negative eczema patients. A study of perfumes used in toiletries and skin-care products. Contact Dermatitis. 1997 Jun;36(6):291-6.

166. Zhou J, Tierney NK, McCarthy TJ, Black KG, Hernandez M, Weisel CP. Estimating infants' and toddlers' inhalation exposure to fragrance ingredients in baby personal care products. Int J Occup Environ Health. 2017 Oct;23(4):291-298. doi: 10.1080/10773525.2018.1475446.

167. Steinemann A. Fragranced consumer products: exposures and effects from emissions. Air Qual Atmos Health. 2016;9(8):861-866.
168. Patrick M. Skin Creams, Web skincare.lovetoknow.com
169. Cosmetic tattoo Sydney specialist Lana Shine. Available From: http://lanashine.com/#!/pageLips
170. Why the Mineral Primer is the Best Friend of Your Makeup? Available From: https://stuffweblog.com/why-the-mineral-primer-is-the-best-friend-of-your-makeup/
171. Kobayashi Y, Matsushita S, Morikawa K. Effects of Lip Color on Perceived Lightness of Human Facial Skin. Iperception. 2017 Jul 11;8(4):2041669517717500. doi: 10.1177/2041669517717500.
172. Seikali A. Disney Unveils Seven Dwarfs Mine Train Footage (VIDEO). Web Variety.com, February 24, 2014.
173. Ruth Drake. Redbook's complete guide to beauty, published by Grosset& Dunlap, 1973 ISBN044801291X, 9780448012919
174. Natural eye makeup for blue eyes. Web lakesidersrochester.com, November 11, 2018.
175. Parry C, Eaton J. Kohl: a lead-hazardous eye makeup from the Third World to the First World. Environ Health Perspect. 1991 Aug;94:121-3.
176. Ng A, Evans K, North RV, Jones L, Purslow C. Impact of Eye Cosmetics on the Eye, Adnexa, and Ocular Surface. Eye Contact Lens. 2016 Jul;42(4):211-20. doi: 10.1097/ICL.0000000000000181.
177. Top Facial Treatment Stock Photos. Web istockphoto.com.
178. Nilforoushzadeh MA, Amirkhani MA, Zarrintaj P, Salehi Moghaddam A, MehrabiT, Alavi S, MollapourSisakht M. Skin care and rejuvenation by cosmeceutical facial mask. J Cosmet Dermatol. 2018 Oct;17(5):693-702. doi: 10.1111/jocd.12730. Epub 2018 Aug 21.
179. O'Reilly Beringhs A, Rosa JM, Stulzer HK, Budal RM, Sonaglio D. Green clay and aloe vera peel-off facial masks: response surface methodology applied to the formulation design. AAPS PharmSciTech. 2013 Mar;14(1):445-55. doi: 10.1208/s12249-013-9930-8.
180. Abu-Jdayil B, Mohameed HA. A facial mask comprising Dead Sea mud. J Cosmet Sci. 2006 Nov-Dec;57(6):441-54
181. Stephen ID, McKeegan AM. Lip colour affects perceived sex typicality and attractiveness of human faces. Perception. 2010;39(8):1104-10.
182. How to Contour Your Face Like a Celebrity? Glam and Gowns by FAVIANA, October 20, 2018
183. Ancient Egypt, Skin Scanners & Algorithmic beauty... what we've been reading this week at Brand Genetics. Brand genetics (Human Experience), August 30, 2018.
184. Masterson M. Bad Decisions in History: featuring Belladonna. Blog Meghan Masterson, February 6, 2017.
185. Health Candy. Celebrities With Acne Prone Skin - Only Human! Available From: https://healthkandy.com/blogs/news/only-human-10-stars-who-have-acne-prone-skin

186. InformedHealth.org [Internet]. Cologne, Germany: Institute for Quality and Efficiency in Health Care (IQWiG); 2006-. Skin care for acne-prone skin. 2013 Jan 16 [Updated 2016 Jul 28]. Available from: https://www.ncbi.nlm.nih.gov/books/NBK279208/

187. Corinne M. Tips for Growing out your Hair. Daily MOM, March 26, 2014.

188. Zhang Y, Alsop RJ, Soomro A, Yang FC, Rheinstädter MC. Effect of shampoo, conditioner and permanent waving on the molecular structure of human hair. PeerJ. 2015 Oct 1;3:e1296. doi: 10.7717/peerj.1296.

189. Understanding Sensitive & Reactive Skin. SkinCeuticals, February 27th 2017.

190. Duarte I, Silveira JEPS, Hafner MFS, Toyota R, Pedroso DMM. Sensitive skin: review of an ascending concept. An Bras Dermatol. 2017 Jul-Aug;92(4):521-525. doi: 10.1590/abd1806-4841.201756111. Review. PubMed PMID: 28954102; PubMed Central PMCID: PMC5595600.

191. What Is Sensitive Skin & What Are The Causes? La Roche-Posay, March 06th 2017.

192. Inamadar AC, Palit A. Sensitive skin: an overview. Indian J Dermatol VenereolLeprol. 2013 Jan-Feb;79(1):9-16. doi: 10.4103/0378-6323.104664.

CHAPTER 2

SKIN CREAMS

2.1 BACKGROUND

Until the beginning of the 1900s, no clear difference existed between active and inactive components in dermatological and cosmetic preparations. Later, it became possible to assign specific therapeutic effects to certain chemical

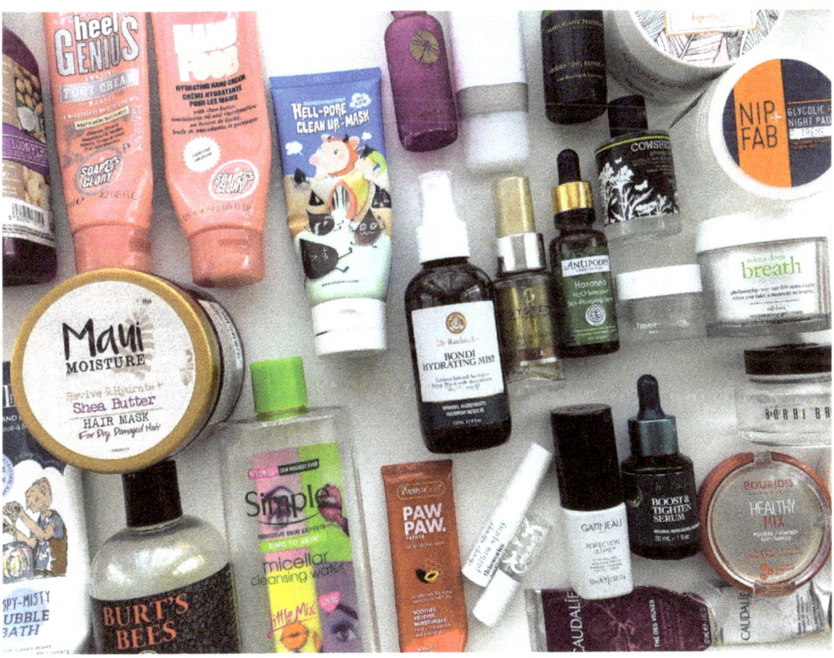

Beauty Secrets. Cosmetics insiders share little-known secrets behind the products applied to the face and other skin surfaces. Some manufacturers make both high-end and drugstore products using similar formulas! This is what the symbols on the back of beauty products mean (Courtacy: ummbabybeauty.com).

substances, and the concept of vehicle, i.e., a rather inactive carrier substance, started to be developed. Nowadays, formulations are mixtures of components that include one or more vehicles and one or more active principles. The efficacy of dermatological and cosmetic products is influenced by the type of vehicle and active principles. In general, formulations will work if the active ingredients penetrate the epidermis. Hence, the correct selection of a suitable vehicle plays an important role during the development of a product. Pharmaceutical preparations are aimed at obtaining a curative effect. In these cases, the role of the vehicle is primarily to allow the delivery of the active principles to the site of application. Cosmetic formulations do not contain strictly curative drugs, but their purpose is rather to help skin homeostasis and prevent degenerative processes. As we have seen, a clear boundary between the medical and cosmetic fields cannot be easily traced, while the marked tendency of cosmetic industries to develop products containing pharmaceutically active principles has led to the introduction of the concept of cosmeceuticals. This term indicates cosmetic-pharmaceutical hybrids aimed at enhancing the beauty of the skin using ingredients that modify skin functionality or provide additional health-related function or benefit.

2.2 ABSTRACT

Skin reflects origin, lifestyle, age, and state of health. Skin color, tone and evenness, pigmentation, as well as skin surface characteristics are signs of skin's health. The cosmetic and pharmaceutical industry offers a vast armamentarium of skin care products and procedures to clean, soothe, restore, reinforce, protect and t treat our skin and hence to keep it in "good condition". Skin care products are readily available in daily life and they play a major role in health and nursing care. The promotion of skin care products including their claims are often based on an effect (e.g., moisturizing, antioxidant), evoked by an active (e.g., urea, tocopherol) that is delivered through a vehicle (e.g., lotion) that relies on a specific technology (e.g., nanotechnology). In addition, "without" claims (e.g., without parabens) often accompany nowadays promotions. Today, modern skin care includes cleansing, soothing, restoring, reinforcing and protecting. With increasing age, the emphasis on skin care is changing. The importance of soothing, restoring, reinforcing increases and cleansing should be executed with particular care. The character of skin care shifts from more cosmetic objectives e smooth, healthy looking skin e to more therapeutic and preventive objectives e soothing, restoring, reinforcing and protecting stressed skin. Even though skin care and skin protection play an important role throughout lifetime the skin areas in primary need of care and protection also change. In younger years, environmental factors (e.g., UV radiation) are of primary importance whereas, in advanced years, age-related factors (e.g., prolonged exposure to various sources of moisture, including urine or feces, perspiration, wound exudate, and their contents) become more important. Subsequently, the skin areas in need of care and protection also change e initially skin areas (e.g., face, arms, legs) exposed to the external environment and later enclosed skin areas (e.g., skin folds, perianal, perigenital skin, groin, feet) become the vulnerable zones (hot spots). Aging per se changes the skin structure and function across the life course increasing its susceptibility to numerous clinically relevant skin problems (e.g. xerosis cutis). Skin diseases (e.g., bacterial/fungal infections), accumulating effects of systemic diseases (e.g., diabetes mellitus, renal insufficiency) or pharmacotherapies (e.g., cancer therapies) also necessitate special skin care.

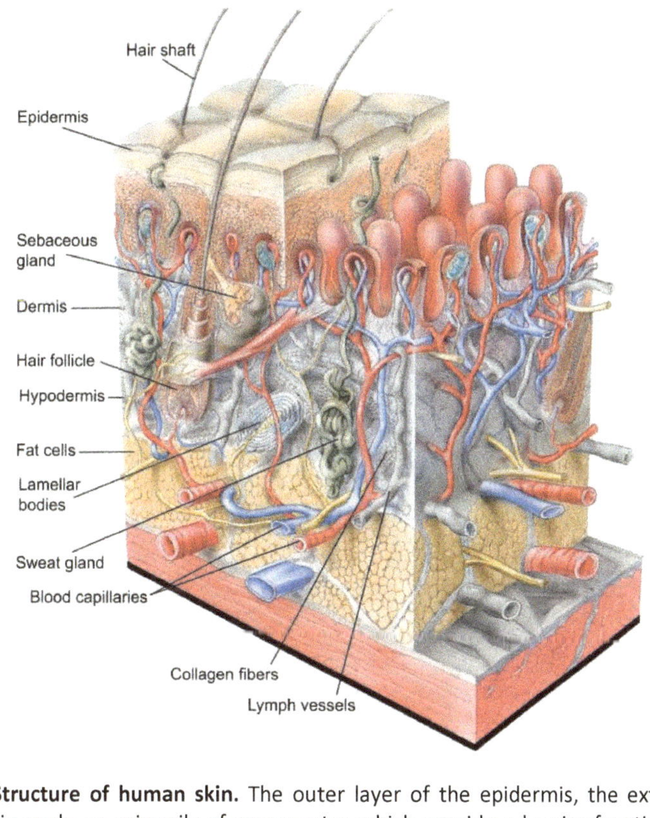

Figure 2.1 Structure of human skin. The outer layer of the epidermis, the external layer of human skin, is made up primarily of corneocytes which provide a barrier function. Underlying the corneocytes are viable keratinocytes, which migrate outward and terminally differentiate to become corneocytes. The epidermis is organized into extensions called rete ridges that project between dermal papillae (pink) into the underlying connective tissue. Underlying the epidermis is the dermis, which is primarily made up of collagen, elastin fibers, and other extracellular matrix components. Collagen and elastin fibers are synthesized by fibroblasts to provide tensile strength, firmness, and elasticity to the skin. The innermost layer of the skin, the hypodermis, is composed largely of fat cells, which helps provide structure to the skin. Blood capillaries, lymph vessels, sweat glands, sebaceous glands, hair follicles, and lamellar bodies lie within the dermis and hypodermis.

2.3 INTRODUCTION

Now, a variety of skincare products are available for almost any beauty concern one can have, including body washes, gels, lotions, exfoliants, moisturizers, toners, and sun protection. There is mainly a focus on helping skin from the inside out. The existence of the FDA keeps known toxic ingredients from being used, though many skincare products still do unfortunately have side effects. From time immemorial creams as topical preparations are considered an important part of cosmetic products. Creams may be considered pharmaceutical products as even cosmetic creams are based on techniques developed by pharmacy and un-medicated creams are highly used in a variety of skin conditions in ancient times, creams were simply prepared by mixing two or more ingredients using water as the solvent. With the advancement in technology, newer methods are used for the formulation of creams. These semisolid preparations are elegant to use by the public and society. They show versatility in their functions. Creams can be applied to any part of the body with ease. It is convenient to use the cream by all the age groups of people. Also it may be equally well applied to non-aqueous products such as wax-solvent based mascaras, liquid eye shadows, and ointments. If an emulsion is sufficiently low viscosity to be pourable (flow under influence of gravity alone) is referred to as lotion. Creams are emulsions of oil and water. In the coming future, more advanced technologies and methods will be used for the preparation, formulation and evaluation of creams. Also, the demand for herbal constituents-based creams is increasing day by day.

2.3.1 SKIN CARE PROCEDURES AND SKIN CARE PRODUCTS

The information on skin care procedures is plentiful but little scientifically documented and the number of products available for cleansing, soothing, restoring, reinforcing and protecting is of an almost infinite variety. Nonetheless, their functionalities may be described as

- Removal of dirt, sebum, microorganisms, exfoliated corneocytes and other non-wanted substances from the skin
- Reduction of unpleasant skin symptoms (e.g., pruritus, burning, odor)
- Restoration of (sub-clinically) damaged skin (e.g., dry and inflamed skin)
- Reinforcement of undamaged but vulnerable skin (e.g., skin surface pH balance, germ reduction)
- Protection of damaged, undamaged and vulnerable skin from various noxious factors.
- Providing a pleasant skin feel (well-being) [1].

2.3.2 MAINTAINING THE FUNCTIONAL INTEGRITY OF THE STRATUM CORNEUM

It has been recognized for approximately 7 decades that the stratum corneum exhibits biological properties that contribute directly to maintaining and sustaining healthy skin. Continued basic science and clinical research coupled with keen clinical observation has led to more recent recognition and general acceptance that the stratum corneum completes many vital "barrier" tasks, including but not limited to regulating epidermal water content and the magnitude of water loss; mitigating exogenous oxidants that can damage components of skin via an innate antioxidant system; preventing or limiting cutaneous infection via multiple antimicrobial peptides; responding via innate immune mechanisms to "cutaneous invaders" of many origins, including microbes, true allergens, and other antigens; and protecting its neighboring cutaneous cells and structures that lie beneath from damaging effects of ultraviolet radiation. Additionally, specific abnormalities of the stratum corneum (**Figure 2.2**) are associated with the clinical expression of certain disease states [2].

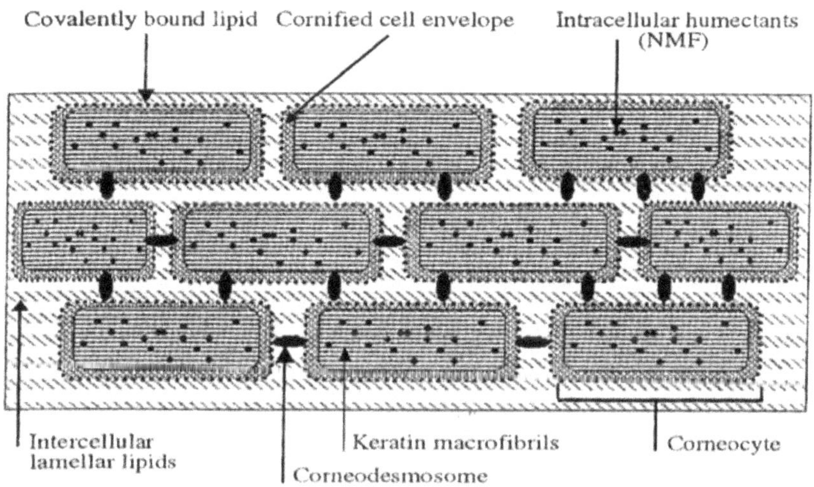

Figure 2.2 This figure depicts the "bricks and mortar" structure of the stratum corneum [2]. The corneocytes represent the bricks and the intercellular lamellar lipid membrane represents the mortar. Corneocytes comprise primarily keratin macrofibrils, are protected externally by a cornified cell envelope, and are held together by corneodesmosomes. The intercellular lamellar lipid membrane is primarily composed of ceramides, cholesterol, and fatty acids. A mixture of multiple small hygroscopic compounds presents within corneocytes, referred to collectively as a natural moisturizing factor (NMF), plays a vital role in the physiological maintenance of stratum corneum hydration.

The functionality of the skin care products ranges from mono-functional, e.g., protecting barrier creams to poly-functional, e.g., soothing and restoring cleansers. They unfold their functionality as leave-on products (e.g., moisturizing or skin barrier products), or as rinse-off products (e.g., cleansers). Skin care procedures like washing/drying and the application of leave-on products- should be as benign as possible. The unduly removal of natural skin components (e.g., lipids), prolonged exposure to water (e.g., long-term immersion in full-baths), a (repeated) disruption of the physiological skin surface pH, and excessive and/or prolonged occlusion of the skin should be avoided. However, epidermal acidification is known to be fragile and it is commonly accepted that cosmetic products, especially soaps and skin cleansing products, can induce significant changes in skin surface pH. The skin pH recovery needs time up to several hours before it can reach the physiological level. Skin care delivered to improve, e.g., the outcome of an eczema therapy or to reduce, e.g., the adverse effects of cancer therapy are often termed as adjuvant skin care. Nonetheless, adjuvant or the above described classic preventive skin care pursues similar goals. Moisturizing prevents and alleviates skin irritation, soothing the skin by slowing the evaporation of water. Many liquid face cleansers also moisturize, which may be all that is needed for a patient with oily skin. Protection from sun and environmental damage is important for all patients. While sunscreens are often irritants, the best options for young, oily, acne-prone skin tend to have a water or light liquid base. Moisturizing sunscreens are appropriate for patients with dry, sun-damaged skin, as well as those who wear makeup, have other skin diseases, or are easily irritated by- products [3-6].

2.4 TYPES OF SKIN CREAMS

They are divided into two types: oil-in-water (O/W) creams which are composed of small droplets of oil dispersed in a continuous phase, and water-in-oil (W/O) creams which are composed of small droplets of water dispersed in a continuous oily phase. Whether the aqueous or the oil phase becomes the dispersed phase depends primarily on the emulsifying agent used and the relative amounts of the two liquid phases. Hence, an emulsion in which the oil is dispersed as droplets throughout the aqueous phase is termed an oil-in-water (O/W) emulsion. When water is the dispersed phase and oil the dispersion medium, the emulsion is of the water-in-oil (W/O) type. Oil-in-water creams are more comfortable and cosmetically acceptable as they are less greasy and more easily washed off using water. Water-in-oil creams are more difficult to handle but many drugs that are incorporated into creams are hydrophobic and will be released more readily from a water-in-oil cream than an oil-in-water cream.

Water-in-oil creams are also more moisturizing as they provide an oily barrier which reduces water loss from the stratum corneum, the outermost layer of the skin. Pharmacists need to know the type of emulsion they have prepared or are dealing with because this can affect its properties and performance. Unfortunately, the several methods available can give incorrect results, so the type of emulsion determined by one method should always be confirmed by usinga second method [7,8].

Table 2.1 Characteristics of Skin Creams [9]

Functional	Physicochemical	Subjective
Cleansing Creams Cold Creams Massage Creams Night Creams	Medium to High oil content O/W or W/O Low Slip Point oil phase Neutral pH May contain surfactant that improve penetration	Oily Difficult to 'Rub in' May be stiff and rich Also popular as lotions
Moisturizing Creams Foundation Creams Vanishing Creams	Low oil content Usually O/W Low slip-point oil phase Neutral to slightly acidic pH May contain emollients & special moisturizing ingredients	Easily spreadable and 'Rub in' quality Available as creams and lotions
Hand & Body Protective	Low to medium oil content Usually O/W Medium slip point oil phase Slightly alkaline or acidic pH May containing protective factors, especially silicon and lanolin	Easily spreadable but do not 'Rub in' with the ease of vanishing creams Very popular in lotion form
All- Purpose Creams	Medium oil content O/W or W/O	Very often slightly oily but should be easy to spread

2.4.1 CLEANSING CREAMS

In the earliest times, cleansing was done by using a piece of bone or stone to scrape the skin. Later civilizations used materials of plant origin along with water for cleansing. Many different civilizations can be given credit for discovering soap. The earliest mention of the soap making process can be found in Sumerian clay tablets dating to ca. 2000 BC. By 600 BC, tree ash and animal fat had been used by the Phoenicians to prepare soap. The first cosmetic cleansing cream to be manufactured on an industrial scale was cold cream, an emulsion made with mineral or almond oil along with beeswax, borax, and water. A second type of cleanser was introduced around 1920. It was made solely from oils and waxes, so it was water-free (anhydrous) and was not an emulsion. Cleansers of this type were designed to melt or liquefy when applied to the skin – they were thixotropic – which is why they were referred to as liquefying cleansing creams. Skin permeability was found to depend very strongly on temperature and less strongly on the duration of heating. The pores of the skin are like little thermostats; they expand with heat and contract with cold. Now when a cream containing a high percentage of water is applied to the skin it is obvious that the pores will at once contract and prevent the deep penetration which is essential if the skin is to be thoroughly cleansed. Some chemists who favor cold cream type cleansers argue that such a reaction is momentary and that with continued rubbing the skin warms up and the pores open again. But they overlook the simple fact that water begins to evaporate immediately upon exposure and in evaporating it abstracts heat from the skin, which causes the pores to contract again. Many of the environmental impurities and cosmetic products are not water-soluble and so washing the skin with simple water would not be sufficient to remove them. Substances capable of emulsifying them into finer particles are to be used for making these fat-soluble impurities water soluble. Herein, cleansers fit into the picture. Skin cleansers are surfaceactive substances (i.e. emulsifiers/detergents/surfactants/soaps) that lower the surface tension on the skin and remove dirt, sebum, oil from cosmetic products, microorganisms, and exfoliated corneum cells in an emulsified form. Careful face washing helps to improve and prevent acne; however, intensive washing has a risk of inducing skin barrier impairment and dry skin, especially in sensitive skin. An ideal cleanser should do all these without damaging or irritating the skin, on the contrary, it should try to keep the skin surface moist. With the advent of advanced technologies, newer cleansers are now being manufactured which are mild, provide moisturizing benefits and can be easily washed off. The combined use of a facial skin cleanser and moisturizers is safe and effective for the care of acne in post-adolescent women with sensitive skin. The key ingredients in cleansing creams, which are also known as cold creams, are usually petrolatum, mineral oil, waxes, and water. Many cleansing creams also contain emulsifiers, which prevent the ingredients of the cream from separating into layers. It can moisturize the skin and remove dirt, sweat, make-up at the same time. The layers of make-up, dust, and sweat remain as a layer on the face and prevent the skin from breathing this may eventually lead to wrinkles and dullness. With their mild and effective action, cleansing creams now days have become a beneficial approach to healthy skincare [10-16].

Table 2.2 Typical Formulation: Cleansing Creams

Ingredient	Formulation 1 (%)	Formulation 2 (%)	Justification of Use
Stearic Acid	10	12.5	A key component of corneum lipids, an antioxidant and also potent anti-inflammatory lipid, non-toxic and non-irritant [17,18].
Mineral Oil	5	-	Mineral oil has been shown to improve skin softness and barrier function better than some other emollients. Benefits skin through hydration and occlusion [19].
Petrolatum	2	-	Emollient- base; it is poorly absorbed by the skin [24].
Cetostearyl Alcohol	1.5	2	It is used as an emulsion stabilizer, opacifying agent, and foam boosting surfactant, as well as an aqueous and non-aqueous viscosity-increasing agent [23].
Isopropyl Myristate	3	5	Emollient; oleaginous vehicle; skin penetrant; solvent, thickening agent, or lubricant [18], [27].
Sorbitan Monolaureate	2	-	Lubricants, processing aids, specific to petroleum production. Solvents (for cleaning and degreasing), surface active agents [28].
Glycerin	6.5	-	Humectant/Emollient
Na-Lauryl SO4	5	-	Anionic surfactant; detergent; emulsifying agent; skin penetrant; wetting agent [33].
Triethanolamine	1.5	-	A surfactant or pH adjuster [35], alkalizing agent; emulsifying agent
Polyoxyethylene Sorbitan Mono Laurate	2	-	Preventing surface adsorption and as stabilizers [37].
Water	61.5	68.5	
Lanolin	-	0.4	Emulsifying agent
Coco-Na Isothionate	-	12	Surface active agents; Cleansing Agent
Perfume, Preservative	q.s.	q.s.	

There is strong evidence that mineral oil hydrocarbons are the greatest contaminant of the human body, amounting to approximately 1 g per person. Possible routes of contamination include air inhalation, food intake, and dermal absorption. The present study aims to identify the most relevant sources of mineral oil contamination [20]. Petrolatum is thought to be occlusive, thereby blocking transcutaneous water loss and trapping water under the skin's surface [21]. Petrolatum is a common moisturizer (Discussed in detail is often used in the prevention of skin infections after ambulatory surgeries and as a maintenance therapy of atopic dermatitis (AD) [22]. Common ingredients in emollients include petroleum products, glycerin, fatty acids, and plant oils. An ideal emollient should contain a combination of occlusive agents to slow down water loss, humectants to increase the capacity to withhold moisture and lubricants to reduce friction against skin [25]. The exotic fats used in skin care are known to exhibit their effects through the restoration of a sufficient layer of skin lipids and skin elasticity, boost natural skin regeneration and increased skin hydration by forming an inert, epicutaneous occlusive membrane. Besides these facts, mango butter which is one of several exotic fats is viewed as an ingenious replacement for cocoa butter, mineral, and petroleum-based emollients because of its appreciable contents which are very important as a source of skin active ingredients [26]. Isopropyl myristate is a non-greasy emollient that is absorbed readily by the skin. It is used as a component of semisolid bases and as a solvent for many substances applied topically [18]. IPM, the isopropyl ester of myristic acid, is used in cosmetics as a substitute for natural oils because it has excellent spreading properties and is absorbed easily into the skin. In many topical and transdermal preparations, IPM is also used as a co-solvent with skin penetration enhancement properties of active ingredients [27]. Polysorbate20 is a nonionic surfactant and emulsifier derived from sorbitan monolaurate and is distinguished from the other members in the polysorbate range by the length of the polyoxyethylene chain and the fatty acid ester moiety. Due to non-toxic nature, it is used as a wetting agent in flavored mouth drops such as Ice Drops, helping to provide a spreading feeling to other ingredients like SD alcohol and mint flavor [29,30]. Glycerin is widely used in cosmetics and well as in pharmaceutical formulations, mainly as a humectant. In vitro studies have shown glycerin to prevent crystallization of stratum corneum model lipid mixture at low room humidity (**Figure 2.3**). Ten days treatment of normal skin with 20% glycerin significantly increased skin corneometer values, indicating an increased hydration [31].

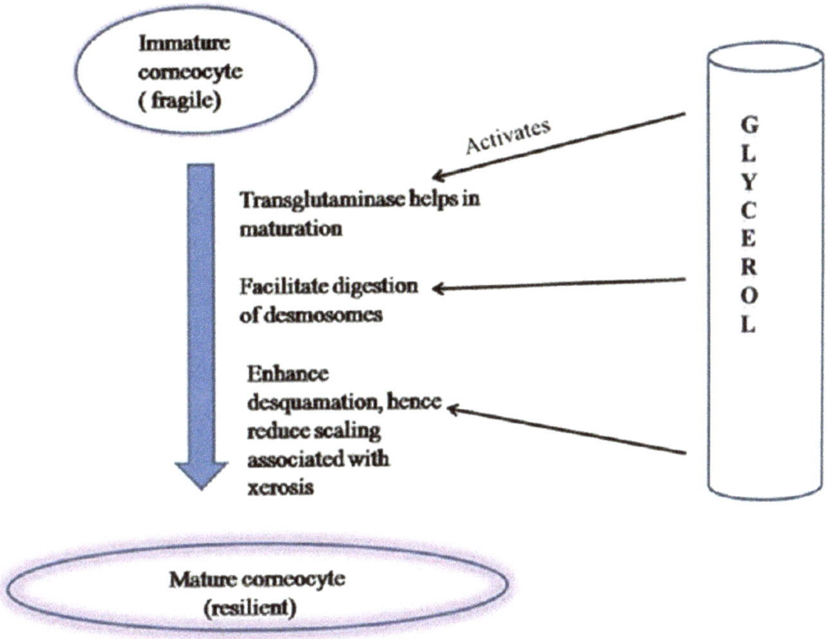

Figure 2.3 The mechanism of action of glycerol [32], [81]. A humectant attracts and retains the moisture in the air nearby via absorption, drawing the water vapor into or beneath the organism's or object's surface. Much more is now known about the epidermis, and in particular, the stratum corneum. The "bricks and mortar" model suggests that its role is as an active membrane. Loss of intercellular lipids, i.e., the ceramides, cholesterol and fatty acids that form the bilayers, damages the water-barrier function. The stratum corneum then calls into action repair mechanisms. Scientifically, the moisturizing treatment involves a 4-step process: (a) Repairing the skin barrier (b) Increasing water content (c) Reducing TEWL (d) Restoring the lipid barriers' ability to attract, hold and redistribute water

The intended application of detergents and cleaners should not result in direct contact with product ingredients; however, misuse of the product could potentially cause dermal (skin and ocular) or inhalation exposure. Sodium Lauryl Sulfate (SLS) enters and maintains residual levels in the heart, the liver, the lungs and the brain from skin contact. SLS is cited as causing severe eye damage and blindness. A second erroneous ocular health claim made about SLS is its link to cataract formation [32], [34]. For cleaning and industrial uses, it is monitored by the Environmental Protection Agency (EPA). Sodium cocosulfate, made from coconut oil, can be used as a replacement for SLS in your beauty product recipes [35]. Recent studies suggest that coconut oil can be a useful surfactant when combined with Yucca schidigera extract [36]. The polysorbates are amphipathic, nonionic surfactants composed of fatty acid esters of polyoxyethylene sorbitan being polyoxyethylene sorbitan monolaurate for polysorbate 20 and polyoxyethylene sorbitan monooleate for polysorbate 80. The polysorbates used in the formulation of biopharmaceuticals are mixtures of different fatty acid esters with the monolaurate fraction of polysorbate 20 making up only 40-60% of the mixture and the monooleate fraction of polysorbate 80 making up >58% of the mixture [37]. The Cosmetic Ingredient Review (CIR) Expert Panel assessed the safety of 39 polyether lanolin ingredients as used in cosmetics. The Panel concluded that these polyether lanolin ingredients are safe in the practices of use and concentration as given in this safety assessment [38]. Nasrollahi et.al 2018 revealed that Linoleic acid (LA) containing w/o emulsion exhibited erythema-reducing effects [39]. Sodium cocoyl isethionate (SCI) is an important surfactant ingredient in mild, syndet (synthetic detergent) cleansing bars. In vitro and in vivo studies have demonstrated that SCI is mild and less damaging to the skin barrier than soaps and surfactants such as sodium dodecyl sulfate (SDS) [40]. The Cosmetic Ingredient Review Expert Panel assessed the safety of triethanolamine (TEA) and 31 related TEA-containing ingredients as used in cosmetics. The TEA is reported to function as a surfactant or pH adjuster; the related TEA-containing ingredients included in this safety assessment are reported to function as surfactants and hair- or skin-conditioning agents. The exception is TEA-sorbate, which is reported to function as a preservative. The panel concluded that TEA and related TEA-containing ingredients named in this report are safe as used when formulated to be nonirritating. These ingredients should not be used in cosmetic products in which N-nitroso compounds can be formed [41]. A cleansing cream or lotion is spread onto the skin, using the fingertips, and massaged onto the surface. This action serves to loosen and suspend the grime and soil in the emulsion. A subsequent wipe with a tissue or cotton wool pad removes the majority of the applied cleansing emulsion and with it the skin soil, grime or makeup. The cream should have a medium-to-high percentage oil phase and be easily spreadable, should not "rub in" and should not irritate the skin. In addition, if it can leave a residual emollient film on the skin, so much the better [99]. Surfactants in skin cleansers interact with the skin in several manners. In addition to the desired benefit of providing skin hygiene, surfactants also extract skin components during cleansing and remain in the SC after rinsing. These side effects disrupt SC structure and degrade its barrier properties. Hydrophobically modified polymers (HMPs) have been introduced to create skin compatible cleansing systems. At the presence of HMP, surfactants assemble into larger, more stable structures. These structures are less likely to penetrate the skin, thereby resulting in less aggressive cleansers and the integrity of the skin barrier is maintained. By creating these large polymer/surfactant complexes, the cleanser becomes less aggressive. In these HMP/surfactant systems, because less surfactant enters the SC, there is less inflammation, and therefore the skin barrier is less disturbed [146].

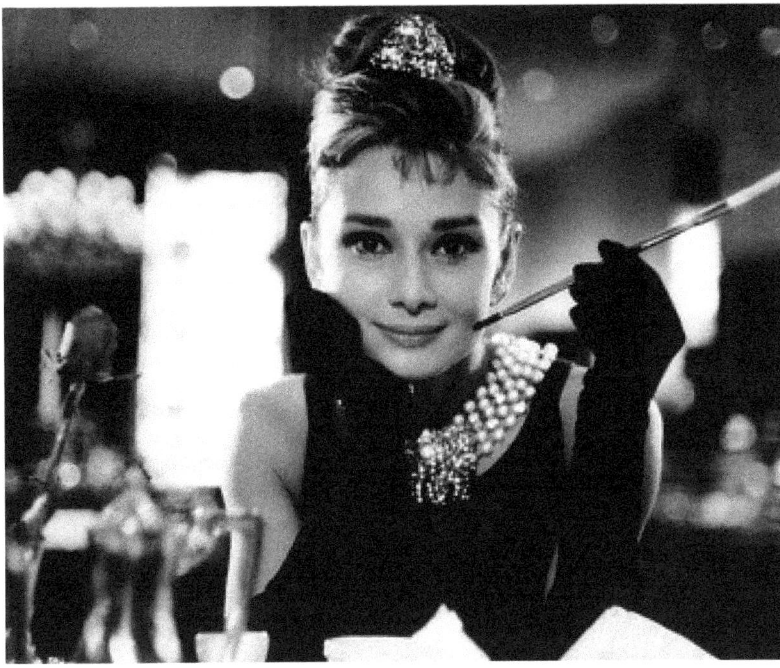

Figure 2.4 Audrey Hepburn [141-143]. The legendary Roman Holiday actress once famously said, "I owe 50% of my beauty to my mother and the other 50% to Erno Laszlo." Erno Laszlo, a pioneer in 20th Century skin care, believed beautiful skin was no miracle. He analyzed women's (and men's) skin giving them precise techniques for their cleansing and prescribed the exact products for their particular skin type and concern. The backbone of any cosmeceutical skin care regimen is facial cleansing and moisturizing. Moisturizers create the illusion of smooth, soft skin by placing a temporary film over the skin surface or by imparting a transient hydration benefit that does not clinically improve the quality or appearance of skin. Cleansing, aggressive exfoliation, and sebum reduction in the absence of a traditional moisturizer safely and effectively improved multiple clinical endpoints of photoaged skin.

2.4.2 COLD CREAM

The invention of cold cream is credited to Galen, a physician in the second century from Greece. This cold cream is thick and softens when it touches the skin. It is perfect for dry skin on elbow, feet, and knees and also perfect for natural ways of removing makeup and to avoid eczema in dry parts of your body. The combination of fats and water in this product helps moisturize – the cream gets its name because it's cold to the touch – with people using it to soften their skin, soothe sunburns, and protect faces from wintry weather, too. The emulsion is of a "water in oil" type unlike the "oil in water" type emulsion of vanishing cream, so-called because it seems to disappear when applied on the skin. Lubricating creams, night creams, or massage creams are a type of cold cream with the addition of lanolin (wool fat) and its derivatives. The name "cold cream" derives from the cooling feeling that the cream leaves on the skin. Cold creams were usually made as water-in-oil (W/O) emulsions. After the creams are applied to the skin much of the water evaporates leaving the remaining oil to act as a solvent that cleanses the skin of cosmetics and other grime. There may also be some surfactant activity. Some chemists suggested that as the water evaporated it cooled the skin which is why the creams are called 'cold cream'. An alternative explanation is that in the days before mineral oil or petrolatum was used, the creams needed to be stored in a cool place to stop them going rancid. This made them cold to the touch and so gave them their name. The first cold cream has been attributed to the Roman physician Galen (C.E. 150) who reputedly made a primitive emulsion by mixing water with molten beeswax and olive oil. It was laborious to make – requiring a great deal of mixing – and tended to separate on standing. However, the formulation persisted – generally using rose-water and/or oil of roses as a perfume – and was included in the first edition of the 'Pharmacopœa Londinensis' in 1618. Vegetable oils like almond oil are liable to deteriorate when they are mixed with water, so early forms were not long-lasting. Their short shelf- life meant that cold creams were usually made up at home or purchased in small quantities, freshly made up by a local pharmacist, chemist or druggist. Borax-beeswax cold creams were white, opaque, had a high luster and spread easily on the skin, but the use of almond oil still limited the shelf life of the cream. When borax-beeswax cold creams were made with petrolatum and mineral oil rather than almond oil, cold creams were produced that were stable, cheap to produce and had a long shelf life. This made borax-beeswax cold creams ideal preparations for industrial manufacture and distribution. Cold creams that contained a high percentage of mineral oil (liquid paraffin) or petrolatum were regarded primarily as cleansers, to be spread on thickly, then removed with a cloth or tissues. However, depending on the formulation, they could be used for a variety of purposes and were often advertised as beauty creams or night creams. City air in most large western cities was a good deal grimier than it is today. Dust, soot and other particulate matter collected on the face, making it an enduring problem. Early advertisements for cold cream stressed the need to "cleanse your skin of all the dirt which lodges in the pores through the day, and which, more than anything else, injures the skin". It was also suggested that the cream be used at night to give it additional time to act. Cold creams were widely used in the theatrical trades to remove greasepaint with several suppliers producing products labelled as Theatrical Cold Cream. As the use of street make-up increased, cold creams were also promoted as a way to remove face powder, lipstick, rouge, foundation and other forms of personal make-up. Cold creams formed the basis of early beauty regimes developed by Pond's, Elizabeth Arden, Helena Rubinstein, and others. By establishing a daily regime, cosmetic companies hoped they would increase the usage of their creams and widen consumer consumption to entire product lines. Guidance from beauty authorities saw many women adopt the practice of applying cold cream before sleep to remove the dirt, grime and cosmetics of the day. It cleansed the skin and, if not removed with soap and water, leave a thin film with moisturizing properties. One wonders, for example, how many women discovered that leaving it liberally on their face when they retired, helped them avoid the 'ministrations' of their husbands, enabling them to get a night of uninterrupted sleep. The all-purpose nature of cold cream, which had been its strength, proved to be its weakness. The recognition of different skin types and skin conditions along with the proliferation of skin creams containing 'beneficial additives' saw the need for an all-purpose skin cream decline. This fracturing of the commercial skin-care market which began with the introduction of stearate (vanishing) creams in 1892, picked up pace in the 1920s and 1930s and eroded the prestige of cold creams and pushed them increasingly into the low-end of the skin-care market. Although the use of cold creams has declined, they are still available. However, when more recent products are compared to original formulations marked differences are evident, primarily in the replacement of borax with modern surfactants [42-50].

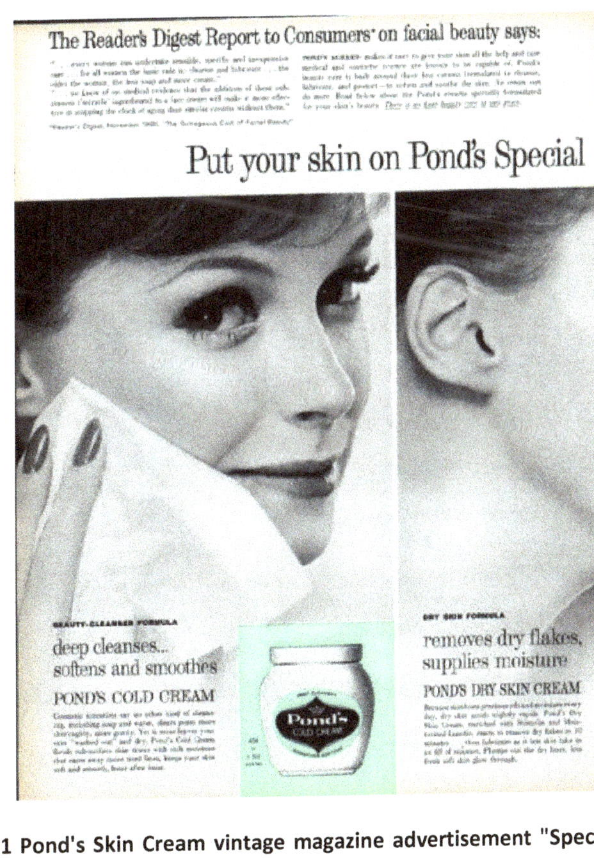

Figure 2.5 1961 Pond's Skin Cream vintage magazine advertisement "Special Formula Care" claims about soft and smooth skin [140].

Cold cream is an emulsion of water and certain fats, usually including beeswax and various scent agents, designed to smooth skin and remove makeup. Beeswax itself suffers from 2 disadvantages as an ingredient in skin creams. The first of this is that it has a distinctive smell which usually has to be masked in the final product; the odor is not unpleasant but not found that compatible with the products of modern days' sophisticated image. And the quality and price also vary with season. The original cold cream recipe or the basic cold cream formula contains Borax. Borax was added to the basic combination of ingredients at the end of the nineteenth century. It reacts with fatty acids in the beeswax to form an emulsion and makes the cream stable. Borax plays many different roles in cold creams in that; it promotes emulsification and reduces surface tension of water. Borax is used in various household laundry and cleaning products but to its highly alkaline nature, it might cause skin irritation. There are also reports of adverse reproductive and developmental impact on the fetus. Its use in the long term is not recommended as there is a possibility of causing renal dysfunction as the borax accumulates in the body. It can also cause fatigue or vomiting due to toxicity. Some research suggests it could also cause genetic damage and be toxic to lymphocytes, the building block of the body's immune system [51-56].

INGREDIENT	FORMULA (WT. %)			
	G	E	F	H
Mineral Oil	35.2	46.0	48.2	49.0
Sodium Behenoyl Lactylate	6.0	6.0	4.0	5.0
Beeswax	3.5	2.0	1.0	2.0
Ceresin Wax	2.0	1.5	0.9	2.0
Carbopol 934 (2% Aqueous)	5.0	5.0	5.0	5.0
Butylene Glycol	3.0	4.0	4.0	4.5
PEG-100 Stearate	1.5	1.5	1.8	1.8
Petrolatum (2.5 Soft)	1.0	1.0	1.0	1.0
Glycerin	0.9	1.3	1.0	1.0
Sorbitan Sesquioleate	0.9	0.8	1.0	0.9
Glyceral Stearate	0.5	0.7	1.0	0.5
Cetyl Alcohol	0.3	0.3	0.3	0.3
Stearic Acid	0.3	0.3	0.3	0.3
Fragrance	0.2	0.2	0.2	0.2
Dimethicone	0.1	0.1	0.1	0.1
Triethanolamine	0.1	0.1	0.1	0.1
Glydant Plus®	0.1	0.1	0.1	0.1
Glycolic Acid	0.02	0.02	0.02	0.02
Vitamin E Acetate	0.01	0.01	0.01	0.01
Ascorbyl Palmitate	0.01	0.01	0.01	0.01
Hydroxycaprylic Acid	0.01	0.01	0.01	0.01
Water	to 100	to 100	to 100	to 100

Figure 2.6 A borax-free cold cream [57,58]. Since borax is a naturally occurring mineral and is so useful in producing skincare and cleaning products, it is somewhat puzzling why there is so much fuss about its use. It's important to remember that "natural" doesn't always equal safe, nor does it guarantee we are protected from adverse effects.

Sodium Behenoyl Lactylate can be used as an emulsifying agent, humectants and conditioner in skin and hair care. Sodium Behenoyl Lactylate is vegetable-derived and can be used in creams, lotions, facial cleansers, and bath products such as bath butters and scrubs [59,60]. White beeswax is a chemically bleached form of yellow wax and is used in similar applications: for example, to increase the consistency of creams and ointments, and to stabilize water-in-oil emulsions. White wax is used to polish sugar-coated tablets and to adjust the melting point of suppositories. Beeswax has been used since ancient times for its antimicrobial properties in European and Asian traditional medicines. Preservative effects are possibly at the basis of its use in embalming and mummification practices by old Egyptians and Persian, or to model death masks by ancient Romans. A total of about 50 aroma components has also been reported. The ester/acid ratio is important for beeswax characterization by different Pharmacopeias, being generally lower (3–4) in European, and higher (8–9) in Asian beeswax [61,62]. Ceresin is often used as a substitute for ozokerite wax due to its similar properties, and also as a substitute for beeswax and paraffin wax. It acts as a rheological modifier at low concentrations (2–3%) and can create very small crystallites, which crosslink and establish a network structure that does not allow flow in practical conditions. Ceresin produces stable mixtures with oils and prevents bleeding or sweating of oil, and it produces a lighter cream that is less greasy [18], [63]. Carbopol® 934 polymer is a white powder, cross-linked polyacrylic acid polymer. It exhibits short flow properties and a creamy sensory profile, and is therefore well suited for use as a rheology modifier in lotions and creams [64]. Butylene glycol is an antimicrobial preservative; humectant; solvent; water-miscible cosolvent. It is used in topical ointments, creams, and lotions, and it is also used as a vehicle in transdermal patches. Cottage cheese whey was unsatisfactory, but B. polymyxa produced large amounts of the glycol in sweet whey, about 60 mmol of glycol per 100 mmol of lactose utilized [18], [65]. It is widely used in cosmetics, including low-irritant skin care products and topical medicaments, as an excellent and low-irritation humectant [66]. Polyethylene glycols (PEGs) are products of condensed ethylene oxide and water that can have various derivatives and functions. PEG-100 STEARATE (a polyethylene glycol ester of stearic acid, commercially available as HallStar® PEG 4400 MS; Jeemate 4400 DPS; Sabowax SE 100) is a non-ionic emulsifier (o/w) from petrochemical and vegetal sources. PEG-100 stearate is an off-white, solid ester of polyethylene glycol (a binder and a softener) and stearic acid. The surfactant qualities of glyceryl stearate and PEG-100 stearate allow oil and water to mix. Used in after sun skin care, antiperspirants, beachwear sun care, cleansing wipes. When it comes to evaluating skin care chemicals to find the best ingredients for skin care, PEG 100 Stearate can be one of those cases where it's difficult to make a clear-cut assessment. On the one hand, this ingredient has many positive properties, such as the ability to moisturize and cleanse the skin.

However, some studies point to a potential link between PEG 100 Stearate and development of toxicity within the body. Some skin care experts even suggest that this ingredient has been linked to problems with reproductive health and even cancer. When looking at PEG 100 Stearate as an emollient, there are other ingredients, like shea and cocoa butter that can also do the job very well. Glycerin is another well-known emollient that can increase skin hydration and softness. When it comes to emulsification properties of PEG 100 Stearate, alternative chemicals that are sometimes used include ceteareth 20, glycol stearate, or laureth 3 [67-70]. Sorbitol-based emulsifiers such as sorbitan sesquioleate (SSO) is used in a variety of products including skin care products, skin cleansing products, moisturizers, eye makeup and other makeup, primarily as an emollient. It is added to formulas as a skin soother and moisturizer and is derived from sorbitol, a humectant. They are commonly used in topical corticosteroids, topical antibiotics, topical antifungals, moisturizing creams and lotions, and topical retinoids. Contact dermatitis from sorbitol derivatives appears to be increasingly prevalent. Patch-testing with SSO can be useful in the work-up of patients with presumptive cosmetic allergic contact dermatitis. Those sensitized to SSO can be counseled to avoid sorbitol-containing products, especially topical corticosteroids [71-73]. Glyceryl Stearate acts as emollient; emulsifying agent; solubilizing agent; stabilizing agent; sustained-release agent; tablet and capsule lubricant. As a lubricant on the skin's surface, it gives the skin a soft and smooth appearance. It also slows the loss of water from the skin by forming a barrier on the skin's surface. Glyceryl Stearate, and Glyceryl Stearate SE help to form emulsions by reducing the surface tension of the substances to be emulsified. In cosmetics and personal care products, Glyceryl Stearate is widely used and can be found in lotions, creams, powders, skin cleansing products, makeup bases and foundations, mascara, eye shadow, eyeliner, hair conditioners and rinses, and suntan and sunscreen products [18], [74,75]. Cetyl Alcohol is a synthetic, solid, fatty alcohol and nonionic surfactant. Cetyl alcohol is used as an emulsifying agent in pharmaceutical preparations. Often confused with the bad alcohols, such as denatured alcohol, fatty alcohols include, among others, cetyl alcohol and stearyl alcohol. Typically, fatty alcohols are used as emollients and thickeners in skin-care products. Fatty alcohols are not irritating and can be beneficial for dry skin [76-80]. Dimethicone is an antifoaming agent; emollient; water-repelling agent. Dimethicones of various viscosities are widely used in cosmetic and pharmaceutical formulations. In topical oil-in-water emulsions, dimethicone is added to the oil phase as an antifoaming agent. It is hydrophobic and is also widely used in topical barrier preparations. Also called polydimethylsiloxane, is a type of silicone oil with distinctive properties that make it a useful ingredient in many skin care products. The combination of silicone with methyl groups tends to make it extremely resistant to water yet it keeps them flexible and moving free, ideal properties for a lubricant. Dimethicone is viscoelastic meaning that, at high temperature, acts like a viscous liquid and, at low temperature, acts like elastic solid, similar to rubber. According to USFDA, dimethicone at concentrations between 1 and 30% is considered as a safe skin protectant. Besides being water and UV resistant, dimethicone is not greasy and is not expensive [82]. Glydant Plus™ is a unique and cost-effective preservative featuring a high level of antimicrobial activity in a wide variety of cosmetic and personal care formulations. Glydant Plus is also highly effective in inhibiting the growth of gram- positive and gram-negative bacteria, yeasts and molds without the need of additional auxiliary preservatives. This water-soluble preservative has a low odor and is stable for extended periods over wide pH and temperature ranges [83]. Alpha-hydroxy acids (AHA) such as glycolic acid has been used extensively in cosmetic and dermatological formulas. In low concentration (2-5%) glycolic acid is believed to facilitate progressive weakening of cohesion of the intercellular material of the stratum corneum (SC), resulting in uniform exfoliation of its outermost layers (the stratum disjunctum) [84]. Exposure to UVB radiation induces inflammation and free radical-mediated oxidative stress through reactive oxygen species (ROS) that play a crucial role in the induction of skin cancer. Clinically chronic photoaging may result in fine wrinkles, texture abnormalities, pigment dyschromia, and actinic keratoses [151]. Glycolic acid (GA) chemical peels are a popular treatment for photoaged skin rejuvenation although retinaldehyde (RAL)-based cosmetic creams are potentially better tolerated than chemical peels [85]. Short-term topical application of glycolic acid in a cosmetic formulation increased the sensitivity of human skin to solar simulated radiation (SSR), while a comparable treatment with salicylic acid did not [86]. Glycolic acid also stimulates the growth of new skin. Although the exact mechanism of action of glycolic acid is still unknown, alpha-hydroxy acids decrease corneocyte cohesion and it has been suggested that this occurs by interference with the formation of ionic bonds. They dissolve adhesions between cells in the upper layers of the skin, inducing shedding of dry scales from the skin's surface, commonly referred to as exfoliation [87]. AHAs have been used as superficial peeling agents as well as to ameliorate the appearance of keratoses and acne in dermatology. However, caution should be exercised about certain adverse reactions among patients using products with AHAs, including swelling, burning, and pruritus [88]. GA suppressed the mRNA expression levels of NLRC4 and AIM2 among the inflammasome complexes. GA also blocked interleukin (IL)-1β by reducing the activity of caspase-1 in the NHEKs. Treatment with GA (2%) inhibited UVB-induced inflammation marker NLRC4 protein levels in mouse dorsal skin. The photoprotective activity of GA was ascribed to the inhibition of ROS formation and DNA damage, as well as a reduction in the activities of inflammasome complexes and IL-1β. GA has anti-inflammatory and photoprotective effects against UVB irradiation (**Figure 2.7**).

GA is potentially beneficial to the protection of human skin from UV damage [89].

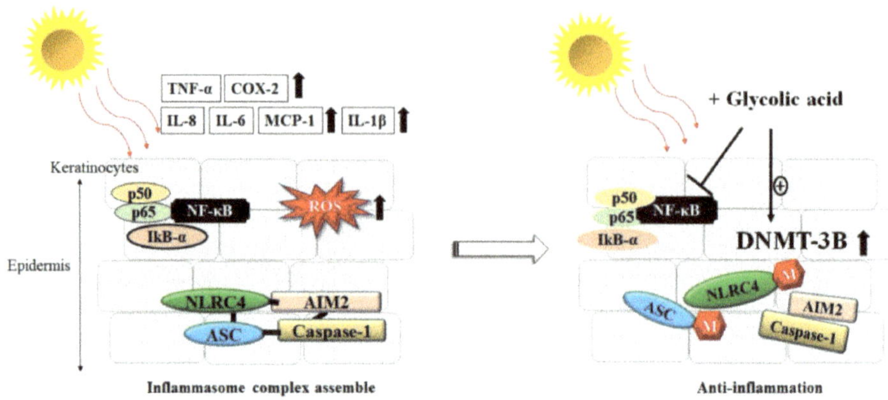

Figure 2.7 Glycolic acid (GA) had anti-inflammatory and photoprotective effects against UVB-irradiation in keratinocytes [88]. (Left) UVB-irradiation activated the nuclear factor-kappa B (NF-kB) pathway and promoted the inflammasome complex assembly, which in ROS accumulation and the release of several proinflammatory cytokines (e.g., interleukin (IL)-6, IL-8, monocyte chemoattractant protein (MCP)-1, IL-Iβ, COX-2, and IL-1β; (Right) Pretreatment with GA could activate DNMT-3B activity and induce the hypermethylation of promoters of NLRC4 and ASC genes, which subsequently hinder of the assembly of the inflammasome complex. GA also inhibited the UVB-induced promoter activity of NF-kB in keratinocyte cells.

A natural tocopherol and one of the most potent antioxidant tocopherols. It exhibits antioxidant activity because of the phenolic hydrogen on the 2H-1-benzopyran-6-ol nucleus [90]. The stability of vitamin E depends on its form, dl-α-Toc acetate being the most stable. It protects the skin from various deleterious effects due to solar radiation by acting as a free-radical scavenger. Experimental studies suggest that vitamin E has antitumorigenic and photoprotective properties [91]. Although many cosmeceuticals contain vitamins C and E, very few are effective in topical application because the stability is compromised as soon as the product is opened and exposed to air and light. However, when a stable formulation delivers a high concentration of non-esterified, optimal isomer of the antioxidant, vitamins C and E inhibit the acute UV damage as well as chronic UV photoaging and skin cancer [92]. The solubility of ascorbyl palmitate in alcohol permits it to be used in nonaqueous and aqueous systems and emulsions. It is an antimutagenic agent; antioxidant [93]. Ascorbic acid-6-palmitate reduced cellular levels of reactive oxygen species following ultraviolet B irradiation. Ascorbic acid-6-palmitate strongly promoted ultraviolet-B-induced lipid peroxidation, c-Jun N-terminal kinase activation, and cytotoxicity, however. Despite its antioxidant properties, ascorbic acid-6-palmitate may intensify skin damage following physiologic doses of ultraviolet radiation [94]. Vitamin C also improves the elasticity of the skin and reduces wrinkles by stimulating collagen synthesis. Since it suppresses pigmentation and decomposes melanin, it is used as a skin-whitening agent. However, applied ascorbic acid is extremely reactive and therefore unstable in dispersions due to the fast oxidation and further irreversible chemical transformation. Therefore, the use of less reactive derivatives like ascorbyl phosphate salts (pro-antioxidant) or lipophilic ascorbyl esters is an attempt to prolong their stability [95]. Ascorbyl palmitate widely used in cosmetic and pharmaceutical preparations. Light accelerated the degradation of ascorbyl palmitate. In contrast, sodium ascorbyl phosphate was stable in both types of microemulsions. Sodium ascorbyl phosphate is shown to be convenient as an active ingredient in topical preparations [96]. The most common AHAs in cosmetic products are glycolic acid and lactic acid. Among others are citric acid, hydroxycaprylic acid, and hydroxycapric acid [97].

2.4.3 NIGHT CREAMS

Night and massage creams are designed to be left on the skin for several hours or to remain mobile on the skin even after vigorous rubbing [98]. Therefore, they are composed of a substantial oil phase that will spread easily without disappearing but also without rubbing off on to clothing or bed linen in use. Such creams tend to be high-oil-content, water-in-oil, soft solid or viscous liquid creams. A moisturizing effect is resulted due to the formation of the occlusive layer on the skin surface thereby reducing the rate of trans-epidermal water loss. Hence, the skin surface feels smooth by lubricating action and allowing any "saw tooth" cells in the outer layer of the stratum corneum to be smoothed down. The occlusive layer prevents epidermal moisture loss and also gives lubrication. Massage has a valuable part to play in skin care since it is well known that vigorous rubbing of the skin prevents dead surface cells and keeps epidermal blood supply in good condition. The term "moisturizing" has also been applied to water-in-oil creams of this type. The recent research has broadened the concept of moisturizing from the simple occlusive skin barrier principle. Many night moisturizing creams are comparatively light and easy to rub in comparison with those of the overnight and massage types, although there still remains a market for the heavier moisturizing creams [99]. Recently, day and night creams containing Melatonin, vehiculated in lipospheres (Melatosphere™), have been developed (Nutriage day cream and Nutriage night cream; Cantabria Labs, Difa Cooper, Caronno Pertusella, VA, Italy). Melatonin is considered as a strong antioxidant molecule, and it is one of the most potent ·OH radical scavenger in nature. The liposphere carrier system could further improve the penetration of the Mel molecules through the skin layers. In women with skin aging, Melatonin-based creams improved significantly skin tonicity and skin hydration with a significant reduction in skin roughness, supporting the skin antiaging effect of this molecule applied topically [100].

Table 2.3 Lightening Night Cream Formulation [110]

Phase				
A	**Product**	**INCI**	**Supplier**	**%**
	Deionized Water	Water	-----	62.10
	Glycerin	Glycerin	Interchimie	4.00
	Dermosoft® GMCY	Glyceryl Caprylate	Dr Straetmans*	0.50
	Satiaxane™ CX 911	Xanthan Gum	Cargill	0.50
	Biophilic™ H	Hydrogenated Lecithin (and) C12-16 Alcohols (and) Palmitic Acid	Lucas Meyer Cosmetics	4.00
	Product	INCI	Supplier	%
B	Sunflower Oil	Helianthus Annuus (Sunflower) Seed Oil	Emile Noel	5.00
	Hazelnut Oil	Corylus Avellana (Hazel) Seed Oil	Emile Noel	5.00
	Cerabeil Blanche Selection	Beeswax	Baerlocher	4.00
	Vitapherole® E1000	Tocopherol (and) *Helianthus Annuus* (Sunflower) Seed Oil	VitaeNaturals	0.20
	Lipex® 102	*Butyrospermum Parkii* (Shea) Butter	AAK	3.00
C	Deionized Water	Water	-----	5.00
	Whitessence™	*Artocarpus Heterophyllus* Seed Extract (and) Maltodextrin (and) Disodium Phosphate (and) Sodium Phosphate	Lucas Meyer Cosmetics	2.00
	Mamaku Vital Essence Nature PF	Water (and) Glycerin (and) Cyathea Medullaris Leaf Extract	Lucas Meyer Cosmetics	2.00
	Exo-T™	Butylene Glycol (and) *Vibrio Alginolyticus* Ferment Filtrate	Lucas Meyer Cosmetics	1.00
	Tyrostat™ 09	Water (and) Glycerin (and) Rumex Occidentalis Extract	Lucas Meyer Cosmetics	1.00
	Product	**INCI**	**Supplier**	**%**
D	Potassium Sorbate	Potassium Sorbate	-----	0.30
	Product	**INCI**	**Supplier**	**%**
E	Relax 2020/2	Fragrance	Vanessence	0.40

* International Nomenclature of Cosmetic Ingredients (INCI)

Deionized (DI) water is water that has been treated to remove all ions – typically, that means all of the dissolved mineral salts [111]. Glycerin is used as humectant/emollient. Dermosoft® GMCY (Glyceryl Caprylate) is a skin-conditioning agent - emollient; surfactant - emulsifying agent [112,113]. synergistic effects of isopropyl myristate and glyceryl monocaprylate (GEFA-C8) enhanced transdermal permeation of PTZ by disrupting SC lipids [114]. There is a considerable interest in the development of preservative-free or self-preserving cosmetics. Lonicera caprifoleum and Lonicera japonica in combination with glyceryl caprylate and/or levulinic acid, p-anisic acid, and ethanol (5%) gave an important assistance to boost the self-preserving system and to produce stable and safe cosmetic products [115]. Glyceryl Caprylate is a preferred ingredient in many natural care products (claimed safe for baby products). It is derived from plants, and a valuable resource because of its many properties. Glyceryl Caprylate moisturizes and balances the pH of the skin. Its antimicrobial and antifungal properties keep bacteria-causing germs at bay. It also contains a natural preservative that prevents mold from forming. It is very compatible with known organic ingredients but can also interact with extra iron [116]. It's moisturizing and re-fatting properties assist with improving and maintaining the moisture and balanced environment of the skin. It can also help to combat impurities due to its strong activity against Propionibacterium acnes [117]. Xanthan gum (XG) is a complex exopolysaccharide produced by the plant-pathogenic bacterium *Xanthomonas campestris* pv. (Xanthomonas bacteria, a Gram-negative bacteria genus that exhibits several different species) and is widely used as a thickener (gelling agent) or viscosity modifier [118]. It is also used as a stabilizing agent; suspending agent; sustained-release agent [18]. The use of bioadhesive hydrogels for skin care presents important advantages such as long residence times on the application site and reduced product administration frequency. Hydrogel formulations showed a prevalently elastic rheological behaviour. Complex viscosity of carbomer homopolymer type C hydrogels was higher than that of the kappa carrageenan hydrogels. Formulations that combined carbomer homopolymer type C with xanthan gum or with carbomer copolymer type B were the most promising for bioadhesive skin products [119]. It has widely been used as an additive in various industrial and biomedical applications such as food and food packaging, cosmetics, water-based paints, toiletries, petroleum, oil-recovery, construction and building materials, and drug delivery. Recently, it has shown great potential in issue engineering applications and a variety of modification methods have been employed to modify xanthan gum as polysaccharide for this purpose [120]. Biophilic™ H is a patented phospholipid-based O/W lamellar emulsifier designed to create elegant and very comfortable formulas. Its lamellar structure has a particular affinity to the skin, resulting in a second skin effect for maximum biocompatibility and tolerance [121]. Hydrogenated Lecithin is the product of the controlled hydrogenation of Lecithin. Bilayers of these phospholipids in water may form liposomes, a spherical structure in which the acyl chains are inside and not exposed to the aqueous phase. Lecithin and Hydrogenated Lecithin are used in a large number of cosmetic formulations as skin conditioning agents-miscellaneous and as surfactant-emulsifying agents. Hydrogenated Lecithin is also used as a suspending agent-non-surfactant. Based on the available data, Lecithin and Hydrogenated Lecithin are safe as used in rinse-off cosmetic products; they may be safely used in leave-on products at concentrations up to 15%, the highest concentration tested in clinical irritation and sensitization studies; but the safety of use could not be substantiated in cosmetic products likely to be inhaled. Because of the possibility of the formation of nitrosamines, these ingredients should not be used in cosmetic products in which N-nitroso compounds may be formed [122]. Functionally sunflower oil is a diluent; emollient; emulsifying agent; solvent; tablet binder. Skin care influences skin barrier function during the first postnatal weeks. Sunflower oil did not harm skin barrier function adaptation in healthy term neonates during the first five weeks of life [123]. Natural oils are applied topically as part of a traditional oil massage to neonates in many developing countries. Topical application of linoleate-enriched oil such as sunflower seed oil might enhance skin barrier function and improve the outcome in neonates with compromised barrier function. Mustard oil, used routinely in newborn care throughout South Asia, has toxic effects on the epidermal barrier that warrant further investigation [124,125]. The topical application of olive oil for 4 weeks caused a significant reduction in stratum corneum integrity and induced mild erythema in volunteers with and without a history of atopic dermatitis. Sunflower seed oil preserved stratum corneum integrity, did not cause erythema, and improved hydration in the same volunteers. In contrast to sunflower seed oil, topical treatment with olive oil significantly damages the skin barrier and therefore has the potential to promote the development of and exacerbate existing, atopic dermatitis [126]. Several studies have shown significant differences between the moisturizing effects and skin tolerances of virgin and refined vegetable oils when incorporated in cosmetic emulsions. The phospholipid content of Hazelnut oil decreased from 286 ppm in virgin oil to traces in refined oil. Still, the moisturizing effect obtained with the emulsion containing the enriched refined oil was shown to be the same as that obtained with the virgin oil emulsion [127]. Hazelnut oil contains 66-85% oleic acid, 7-25% linoleic acid, 4-9% palmitic acid and 1-6% stearic acid. When used in cosmetics and personal care products, hazelnut oil and Hydrogenated Hazelnut

Oil function as skin-conditioning agents - emollient and skin-conditioning agents – occlusive. It's loaded with skin-nourishing vitamins and essential fatty acids that help protect skin against sun damage, boost collagen production, and more. Hazelnut is non-greasy and is best used for those who have oily skin but still want to enjoy the many benefits of carrier oils [128]. Vitapherole E1000 (Tocopherol and *Helianthus Annuus* Seed Oil combination); Vitapherole® is a line of IP natural-source vitamin E or tocopherols including α-tocopherols, mixed tocopherols, and acetates. They protect the skin from environmental stressors like pollution and UV. Tocopherols also help tighten and firm the look of skin which makes vitamin E the perfect addition to any anti-aging formula [129]. Shea butter is a vegetable fat obtained from the fruit of a tree native to Africa, *Butyrospermum parkii*. Shea butter is primarily composed of fatty acids such as stearic and oleic acids. This product can be used in formulations from 1% to 100%. It is a natural emollient that will add moisture back into the skin while also reducing swelling. Shea tree is abundantly found in the wide belt of savannah including West African countries like Nigeria, and further east in Uganda. Nowadays, shea butter, mainly the traditional one (called BIO-shea butter) interests cosmetic and pharmaceutical firms, contained nutritional elements like essential fatty acids (oleic and linoleic acids), minerals (calcium, iron, copper, magnesium, sodium, potassium and zinc), vitamins (A and E) and carotene, which would present them as available, cheap and accessible nutritive edible fats [130,131]. Whitessence ™ is a strong natural lightening agent extracted from Asian nangka seeds. The specific proteins of Whitessence ™ inhibit the transfer of melanin from melanocytes to keratinocytes. The decrease in the melanin quantity at the surface of the skin results in a clear and unified complexion [132,133]. Exo-T™, exopolysaccharide from Kopara (microorganisms mat) living in unique ecosystem in the rims of French Polynesian atolls, acts as an anti-wrinkle agent, anti-aging agent and regenerating/revitalizing (manufacturer's claim) [134]. Also, Tyrostat™ 9 is claimed as a potent strong inhibitor of tyrosinase enzymatic activity, one of the main enzymes involved in the pigmentation process [135]. Potassium sorbate is a potassium salt having sorbate as the counterion. Potassium Sorbate is a mild preservative being used in cosmetic and skin care formulas as a paraben alternative to prevent or retard the growth of microorganisms and protect products from spoiling. Phenoxyethanol, citric acid, sodium benzoate, and potassium sorbate were very common in all the cosmetic product categories, found in a study where 2300 products commercially available in Spain were collected and examined to identify the frequency of a wide variety of preservatives in different product categories [136].

Exhibit 1. Benefits of day and night creams [144,145]	
Why Day Cream?	A day cream is designed to primarily protect and support skin during the day against damaging UV rays, pollution and environmental stress. They contain SPF to prevent burning and photoaging, antioxidants to fight free radicals, and ingredients like caffeine to make skin look energized and firm. Day creams are usually designed to be worn under cosmetics, so they have light, non-greasy formulas that are absorbed quickly and allow pores to breathe.
Why Night Cream?	Night cream works differently as it repairs and moisturizes your skin to make it look supple and wrinkle-free. Good night creams contain antioxidants and anti-wrinkle ingredients which help to slow down our natural process of ageing. For night cream, there's also the whitening night cream available. Most common ingredients to be found in a night cream are AHA, BHA*, Retinol, Vitamin A and so forth. A topical cream containing retinol 0.5% in combination with niacinamide, resveratrol, and hexylresorcinol is efficacious and tolerable for skin brightening/anti-aging when used with a complimentary skin care regimen including SPF 30 sun protection (**Figure 2.8**).

* Unlike AHAs, BHAs can get deeper into the pores to remove dead skin cells and excess sebum.

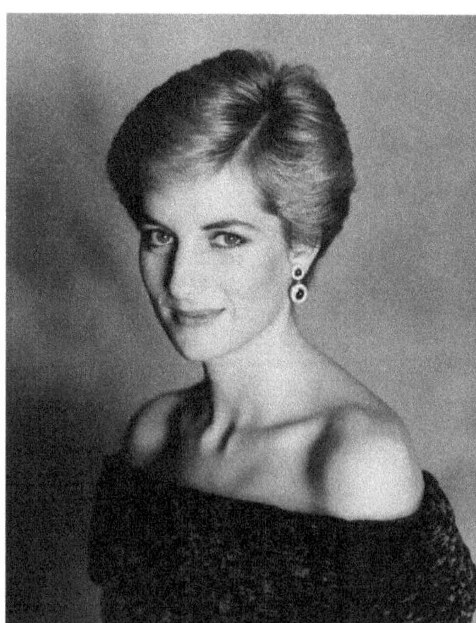

Figure 2.8 Diana, Princess of Wales, 1986 [154-156]. According to the magazine Longevity, Princess Diana was "scrupulous about using an SPF-8 sunblock." While the American Academy of Dermatology recommends applying at least SPF 30, protection against UV rays can prevent both sunburn and dangerous skin cancers (*Courtacy:* Britannica).

2.4.4 MASSAGE CREAMS

A beauty massage cream that promotes resilience and firmness while helping prevent sagging and other signs of aging. The great interest in eternal youth has developed a large market for skin care products claiming anti-wrinkle effects. Facial massage is an extremely popular form of beauty treatment and is thought to rejuvenate the skin. It may refresh the subjects by reducing their psychological distress and activating the sympathetic nervous system [152]. Performing short-term facial massage with a roller increases SkBF, and long-term use improves the vascular dilatation response [150]. Facial beauty treatment generally consists of three steps: vigorous massaging of the face with creams, steaming (using a hot towel or a steaming gadget), and application of a face mask containing adsorbents and astringents. Combining massage with moisturizer application is a popular technique in beauty spa sessions. The subjective positive psychological effects of massage with moisturizer application in hand and face beauty treatment are documented by many people attending spa sessions. Interestingly, the daily performance of massage after moisturizer application was not an effective external intervention for enhancing moisturizer efficacy [147]. The action of rubbing a cream or emollient into the skin is a form of massage, and this simple action will go a very long way towards the recovery of skin integrity and in the prevention of harm and infection [148]. Anecdotally, the addition of aromatherapy oils to massage cream may have a positive effect on symptom relief in people with cancer, although evidence is again lacking [149]. Although there are several subjective benefits with a facial beauty treatment, there may be immediate side-effects, such as erythema and edema, as well as delayed problems, such as dermatitis and acneiform eruption (follicular eruptions characterized by papules and pustules resembling acne), in about one-third of patients [101]. Gentle massage is often facilitated using a cream to reduce friction on the skin. However, there is also the possibility of massage causing harm - massage or rubbing of vulnerable skin may exert shear stresses which may themselves potentially cause damage. Also, it is also possible that the use of a cream or emollient as part of the massage regimen may increase epidermal hydration and prevent dermal stripping and the subsequent exposure of fragile dermal tissue [102]. Cellulite has been treated with massage which decreases tissue edema but it is also likely to have its effects at the cellular level by stimulating fibroblast (and keratinocyte) activity while decreasing adipocyte activity. In addition to massage, effective topical creams with a variety of agents were used to ameliorate the condition [103]. Slimming Cream Containing 3.5% Water-Soluble Caffeine and Xanthenes appears to be effective for the treatment of cellulitis without serious adverse effects. Moreover, massage is also used to remove interstitial fluid and accelerate lymphatic drainage, which leads to the reduction of cellulite [157]. Client-preferred massage creams are ideal for all modalities and offer a unique combination of medium glide, friction, and typically absorb completely into the skin. Massage Warehouse carries a wide range of organic massage cream brands including TheraPro, Massage FX, Lotus Touch, Soothing Touch, Bon Vital and much more! [104]. Massage therapy has been shown to have beneficial effects on varying conditions including prenatal depression, preterm infants, full-term infants, autism, skin conditions, pain syndromes including arthritis and fibromyalgia, hypertension, autoimmune conditions including asthma and multiple sclerosis, immune conditions including HIV and breast cancer and aging problems including Parkinson's and dementia [105]. Thai foot massage may be one of the alternative therapies to improve balance performance for diabetic patients as a result of increasing range of motion (ROM) and sensation of the foot [106]. Massage in infancy improves growth and post-massage sleep. However, only sesame oil showed significant benefit [107]. Swedish Massage Therapy (SMT) is a complementary treatment that is believed to provide relaxation and therefore able to reduce blood pressure caused by stress [108]. Massage creams and lotions are well-suited to deep tissue and other high-friction massages. They tend to provide medium glide, and while they can be nourishing to the skin, they are typically absorbed fairly slowly. Lotion and cream are often similar products, but tend to have a different consistency. Creams are generally quite a bit thicker, while lotions are more liquid. Lotions tend to give more bang for the buck, as they are more spreadable. Creams do better for topical treatments on tough areas of skin. Some creams and lotions, particularly water-based ones, can leave the skin feeling dried out. Creams generally come in jars or tubs which don't fit into holsters, which can be a hassle during treatments. Creams and lotions are often cold when first applied to the skin and can be difficult to heat. Many are also scented, which will bother some clients [109].

Table 2.4 Massage Cream Formulation [158]

Ingredient	% of total	500 g	2 cups	Function
Part A				
Distilled Water	38.10	190.50	3/4 cup + 1 TBS	Diluent
Glycerin	2.00	10.00	2 tsp	Humectant
Part B				
Cetyl Alcohol	4.25	21.25	4 1/4 tsp	Thickener
Ethylhexyl Palmitate	23.00	115.00	1/2 cup	Occlusive oil for slip
Grapeseed Oil	8.50	42.50	3 TBS	Vegetable oil for moisturizing
Cetearyl Alcohol (and) Ceteareth-20	3.55	17.75	3 1/2 tsp	Emulsifier blend
Caprylic/ Capric Triglycerides	10.00	50.00	1/4 cup	Occlusive oil for slip

Table 2.4 ***Contd...***

Ingredient	% of total	500 g	2 cups	Function
Sweet Almond Oil	3.50	17.50	3 1/2 tsp	Vegetable oil for moisturizing
Glyceryl Stearate (and) PEG-100 Stearate	6.10	30.5	2 TBS	Emulsifier blend
Part C				
Germaben II	1.00	5.00	1 tsp	Preservative
Total	**100 %**	**500g**	**2 cups**	

Ethylhexyl palmitate is an ingredient that functions as an emollient, solvent, pigment wetting agent, and fragrance fixative in cosmetics and personal care products. As an emollient, ethylhexyl palmitate helps to keep the skin moist and supple by reducing water loss from the epidermis (the outer layer of skin). Emollients also act as lubricants by reducing friction when anything rubs against the skin. Ethylhexyl palmitate is considered to be a non-occlusive emollient, which means it does not form a film on the surface of the skin. It is often used as an organic replacement to silicones in a cosmetic formulation because it provides a dry-slip, silky feel that is very similar to how a silicone would feel. While all skin types can benefit from emollients like ethylhexyl palmitate, emollients are very beneficial for those who have dry, rough and/or flaky skin. Emollients can treat these symptoms, leaving the skin looking and feeling soft and smooth. Also, emollients can benefit those that suffer from conditions such as eczema, psoriasis, or other inflammatory skin condition [159]. Instruments that have been used for assessing epidermal hydration are based on measurements of conductance, capacitance and impedance of the skin. Most of the commercial moisturizer contains *Aloe barbadensis* (Aloe vera) as a moisturizing agent. Ingestion of Aloe preparations is associated with diarrhea, hypokalemia, pseudomelanosis coli (a disorder of pigmentation of the wall of the colon), kidney failure, as well as phototoxicity and hypersensitive reactions [160]. However, there so many other herb's extract/juices/oils like grape seed, cucumber, basil, jojoba oil, almond oil, olive oil, etc. present in the commercial moisturizer section claiming for restoring skin hydration and viscoelasticity [161]. Many of grapeseed oil's beauty benefits may be due to its omega-6 fatty acid content and vitamin E, an antioxidant that helps to build tissue, and linoleic acid, a fatty acid which promotes hair and skin growth. Nonionic emulsifiers depend chiefly upon hydroxyl groups and ether linkages (from polyhydric alcohol anhydrides and polyoxyethylene chains) for their hydrophobic effects [164]. Nonionic emulsifiers are usually less irritating than their ionic counterparts. Examples of nonionic emulsifiers include cholesterol, a natural component of the lipid bilayer, polyethylene glycol, cetearyl alcohol, ceteareth-20, and stearyl alcohol [162]. This non-ionic emulsifier blend, INCI Cetearyl

Alcohol and Ceteareth 20, is a waxy pastille and creates a thicker, waxier end product. It is derived from coconut fatty acid. It is excellent for foot and elbow creams, which are slightly heavier.It rovides good emollience and feel. It forms highly stable emulsions with excellent appearance and feel, compatible with a wide range of ingredients and pH [163]. Chemically, caprylic /capric triglyceride contains a high concentration of fatty acids, which allows it to provide an occlusive layer to help increase moisture-retention at the skin's surface. As a result, caprylic /capric triglyceride can have emollient properties that may boost skin-hydration levels [166]. Application of the o/w emulsion formulation containing either HP or capric/caprylic triglyceride significantly elevated skin moisture content and thus reduced transepidermal water loss (TEWL) by a maximal approximately 33% against the control formulation within 3 h and maintained this up to 6h [167]. Germaben II-E can be used in problem formulations, without the need for additional co-preservatives. It is compatible with almost all cosmetic ingredients, including surfactants and proteins. Germaben II-E is a clear viscous liquid preservative system with a characteristic mild odor. It is readily soluble at a level of 1.0% in both water/oil and oil/water emulsions, but not in water alone. Germaben II contains propylene glycol, propylparaben, methylparaben, and diazolidinyl urea. There are some studies which have raised concerns that paraben substances may be carcinogenic owing to their effect of mimicking the body's hormone estrogen" [168-170].

2.4.5 VITAMINS USED IN SKIN CREAMS

The number of cosmetic products which include vitamins as a constituent has increased three-fold since 1991. Vitamins are commonly used as ingredients of products designed to improve the appearance and health of the skin; for this reason, the cutaneous benefits of such products are actively researched by dermatologists and chemists. It has been claimed that fat-soluble, as well as water-soluble vitamins are capable of being taken up through the skin. The use of stabilized vitamins in cosmetic preparations for external application is justified [171]. Pantothenic acid is a part of the water-soluble vitamin B complex. Its precursor and the related materials – panthenol, pantethine and pangamic acid have all been quoted as having a beneficial action on the skin and being useful in skin and/or hair preparations. Skin softening ability of pantothenic acid-based topical products have also been demonstrated in a few recent clinical trials [172]. Although there is no certain proof that they penetrate the skin and reach the location where they might exert an influence, vitamin B complex, panthenol and vitamin B6 (pyridoxine) are used in some cosmetics. Vitamin D, like vitamin A, is oil-soluble and is essential for skin health, but deficiencies are best corrected by oral administration to achieve a systemic effect. However, vitamins D2 and D3 (calciferol) are used, sometimes in conjunction with vitamin A. A mixture of vitamins A, E and D3 has been claimed to be synergistic. Vitamin E is said to enhance percutaneous resorption, and vitamin H is claimed to help fat and cholesterol synthesis. Other vitamins having some using topical preparations include the so-called vitamin F, now known as essential (unsaturated) fatty acids (EFA) [173].

2.4.6 MOISTURIZER

This term was developed by marketers, promoting its function to moisten the skin. Moisturizer and emollient are often regarded as synonymous, even when occlusives and humectants are also part of it. Emollients are mostly made up of lipids and their components, which fill intercorneocyte cluster gaps to enhance skin hydration, smoothness, softness, flexibility. Occlusives are another type of moisturizer which is mostly oil-based and serve the function of maintaining skin water content by creating a hydrophobic barrier over the skin and blocking trans-epidermal water loss. The last type of moisturizers are humectants, that consist of hygroscopic substances that help the stratum corneum to absorb water by attracting water from dermis and a humid environment into the epidermis. The efficacy of moisturizers depends largely on proper selection and compliance to continuously use it [199]. Moisturizers, among all other skin creams are most widely used. If water is lost more rapidly from stratum corneum than it is received from the lower layer of the epidermis, the skin becomes dehydrated and loses its flexibility. Water alone will not restore the flexibility [174,175]. There are two basic types of dry skin. The first is due to prolonged exposure to low humidity and air movement. The second is due to ageing related physicochemical changes. Again, Dry skin or xeroderma is an extremely common problem which can be induced by complex interactions between environmental and individual factors including, but not limited to: low environmental temperature, low humidity, exposure to chemicals, microorganisms, aging, psychological stress, atopic dermatitis and eczema. Eczema is common among young children. Other conditions, such as psoriasis and type 2 diabetes, can also cause skin to dry out [32], [184]. Xerosis is abnormal dryness of the skin (**Figure 2.9**), mucous membranes, or conjunctiva (xerophthalmia). There are many causes of xerosis, and treatment depends on the particular cause [198]. Dry skin conditions are often not considered important by health professionals, and as a consequence treatment are frequently under-prescribed. As a result of this, problems with untreated dry skin can lead to a variety of issues. Conditions such as pruritus and ichthyosis vulgaris can be distressing, while ezcema and psoriasis can lead to more serious consequences such as fissures and infections and can result in a reduced quality of life and social isolation [200]. Moisturizers are topical products designed to improve and maintain the skin barrier function and to help prevent dry skin. It is common to think that a moisturizer adds water to the skin; however, this is a misunderstanding. Rather, a moisturizer works by preventing or reducing water evaporation from the skin.8 This action allows the skin to rehydrate from within. There are three classes of chemical ingredients that regularly serve as moisturizers: occlusives, humectants, and emollients. Often these chemicals are either the same as or similar to natural components in the SC. They are often used in combination, with some ingredients providing the overlap of characteristics [176,177].

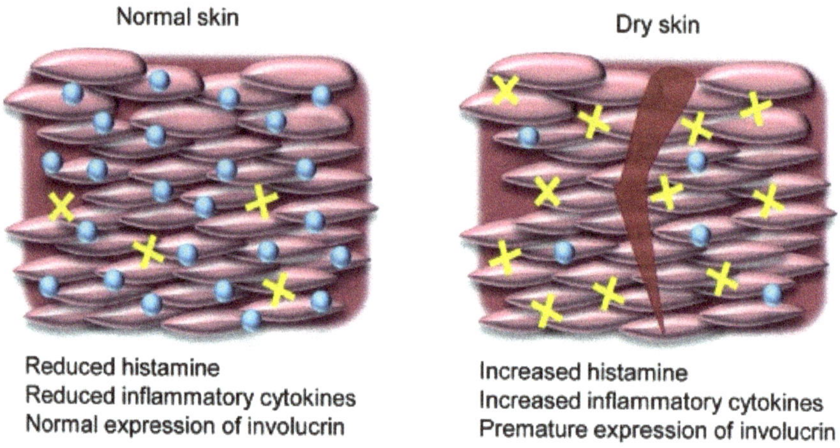

Figure 2.9 Mechanisms of xerosis [196]. Normal skin contains lower levels of histamine and inflammatory cytokines compared to dry skin. Premature expression of involucrin, a protein that forms a protective envelope around corneocytes, has been implicated in the pathophysiology of dry skin. In addition, xerotic skin has been shown to contain higher levels of keratin 5 and 14 and lower levels of keratin 1 and 10 compared to normal skin. The schematic on the right shows the cracked stratum corneum that is characteristic of dry skin and associated with decreased water content (blue spheres) and increased involucrin cross-linking (yellow crosses).

Occlusion (by lanolin, petroleum, silicones, mineral and vegetable oil) prevents water loss from healthy normal skin causing the stratum corneum to be more hydrated, making it softer and supple. Examples of occlusive are mineral and vegetable oils, lanolin and silicones. Their effect is increased by the use of mixtures of lipids and other fatty chemicals which have been designed to imitate the composition of the skin's natural oily secretions. More recently, skin substantive barrier materials (mainly based on quaternary ammonium complexes) have become available which seem to be able to influence the rate of trans-epidermal water loss without putting an inclusive or greasy barrier on the skin surface. These materials can be shown to be substantive to skin (and hair) and act not only as moisturizers, but as emollients and skin conditioning agents. Examples are quaternium, a hydroxyethyl-cellulose derivative [178]. Humectants (Glycerol, Ethylene Glycol, PG, sorbitol alone or in admixture at various levels) attract water from the atmosphere, so supplementing the skin water content. They can be used alone or in a mixture at various levels. Whether or not they penetrate the skin surface is a moot point, but at least they will attract moisture to the skin. [179,180]. The third and most valuable approach to miniaturization to supplementing Natural Moisturizing Factors (NMF) from the skin that are removed by polar solvents and detergent solutions. The NMF contains a combination of several naturally occurring free amino acids, urocanic acid, inorganic salts, sugars, lactic acid, and urea. Many of these are highly efficient at attracting and binding water from the atmosphere, allowing adequate hydration of corneocytes even in low humidity environment. Once applied to the skin, the ingredients can stay on the surface, be absorbed into the skin, be metabolized, or disappear from the surface by evaporation, sloughing off, or by contact with other materials. In addition to substances considered as actives, e.g. fats and humectants, moisturizers contain substances conventionally considered as excipients (e.g. emulsifiers, antioxidants, preservatives). Partitioning of antioxidants, hydrogen bonding, interphase transport, surface accessibility, and interaction of emulsifiers with antioxidants are considered to be important parameters that determine antioxidant activity in lipid-containing systems. Some formulations may deteriorate the skin condition, whereas others improve the clinical appearance and skin barrier function. For example, emulsifiers may weaken the barrier. On the other hand, petrolatum has an immediate barrier-repairing effect in delipidized stratum corneum. Moreover, one ceramide-dominant lipid mixture improved atopic dermatitis and decreased TEWL in an open-label study in children [181-183]. A typical moisturizing formulation is detailed in **Table 2.5.**

Table 2.5 Moisturizer Formulation [185-195]

No.	Ingredient	%	Justification
1	Isopropyl Linoleate	2	Lubricant
2	Glyceryl Stearate	3	Emollient; emulsifying agent
3	Diisopropyl adipate	2	Plasticizer, moisturizer, cleaning agent
4	Myristyle myristate	1	Emollient
5	PEG 40 Stearate	1	Surfactant; cleansing agent
6	Cetyl alcohol	1.5	Emollient; emulsifying agent; stiffening agent
7	Ceteareath-20	0.5	Emulsifying agent
8	Quaternium-22	2	Antistatic
9	Hydroxyethyl cellulose (2% aq)	25	Emulsifying, bubble-forming agent, viscosity-increasing agent.
10	PG	3	Preservative; disinfectant; humectant
11	Water	59	
12	Prfume, preservative	q.s.	

Isopropyl Linoleate the ester of isopropyl alcohol, it is a pale yellow, oily liquid. In cosmetics and personal care products, Isopropyl Linoleate may be used in the formulation of face and skin care products, hair care products, and eye and facial makeup. It acts as a lubricant on the skin's surface, which gives the skin a soft and smooth appearance [185]. The structure of a stable O/W cream is characterized by a more or less pronounced mixed crystal bilayer. The addition of co-emulsifiers in order to achieve a soft formulation often leads to a mixed crystal bilayer network of high viscosity and even leads to phase separation. In order to avoid this component of different chemical identities are used which often are not inert or harmless if they are absorbed. The amount of co-emulsifier used should not be too high, as it would crystallize increasingly during storage which gives the preparation an optical in homogeneity and a lack in softness which is needed for a suitable cosmetic acceptance. A slightly higher concentration than is necessary for the mixed emulsifier system can be advantageous, as the formation of a separate crystalline lipophilic network in the preparation increases its viscosity which will lead to a higher physico-chemical stability of the formulation. These results were obtained with the co-emulsifiers glyceryl monostearate (Imwitor 900), cetylstearyl alcohol (Lanette O), and PEG-20-glycerolstearate (Tagat S2) as O/W emulsifier [186]. Glyceryl Monostearate Emollient; emulsifying agent; solubilizing agent; stabilizing agent [18]. Diisopropyl adipate (DIPA) is a fatty acid ester and an isopropyl ester; clear, colorless to light yellow viscous liquids. It is used for a variety of applications, such as the production of moisturizers, shaving lotions and cleaning agents. DIPA acts as a lubricant on the skin surface which gives the skin a soft and smooth appearance. Its solvent properties allow its use as a carrier for other cosmetic ingredients and also to soften synthetic compounds by reducing brittleness and cracking [187]. Myristyl Myristate is a 100% natural vegetable- derived ester utilizing only the Myristic fatty acids. Non-greasy solid emollient, enhances esthetic properties of skin care products, gives more body & spreadability, results in superior whitening to the product and improved benefits to the skin [188]. About PEG-40 STEARATE: PEG-40 stearate is a synthetic polymer composed of PEG (polyethylene glycol) and stearic acid, a naturally occurring fatty acid. Products and formulas containing PEG 40 Stearate should not be used on broken or irritated skin. Although PEGs are considered safe for use topically on healthy skin, studies showed that patients suffering from severe burns were treated with PEG-based antimicrobial cream; this treatment resulted in kidney toxicity. Due to the presence of PEG, this ingredient may contain potentially toxic manufacturing impurities such as 1,4-dioxane [189]. Cetyl alcohol is a common choice of emollient. It forms a layer on the skin, which traps the water on the skin and prevents it from escaping, thereby inhibiting skin dehydration [190]. Ceteareth-20 functions as an emollient and emulsifier. It's usually used in conjunction with other alcohols and fatty acids, working to thicken a solution and help other ingredients dissolve in a solvent. It also functions as a nonionic stabilizer in oil in water emulsions. Ceteareth-20 is the polyethylene glycol ether of cetearyl alcohol; may contain potentially toxic impurities such as 1,4-dioxane [191]. Quaternium-22 is a light amber-colored liquid, a quaternary ammonium salt. The unreacted monomer content of these ingredients was considered low and of no toxicological concern. Limited data showed no skin irritation/sensitization. Although these ingredients were nongenotoxic in bacterial assays, mammalian genotoxicity, carcinogenicity, and reproductive and developmental toxicity data were not available [192]. However, its toxicity is due to its ability to act as a nitrosating agent, releasing potentially carcinogenic nitrosamines [193]. Hydroxyethyl cellulose is a polysaccharide derivative with gel thickening, emulsifying, bubble-forming, water-retaining and stabilizing properties. It is used as a key ingredient in many household cleaning products, lubricants and cosmetics due to its non-ionic and water-soluble nature [194]. Propylene glycol is a synthetic liquid substance that absorbs water. It is a clear, colorless, viscous, practically odorless liquid, with a sweet, slightly acrid taste resembling that of glycerin. It is a propanediol that exists as a clear, colorless and hygroscopic liquid and consists of propane where the hydrogens at positions 1 and 2 are substituted by hydroxyl groups. It acts as Antimicrobial preservative; disinfectant; humectant; plasticizer; solvent; stabilizing agent; water-miscible cosolvent. Propylene glycol is used as an organic solvent and diluent in pharmaceuticals and many other industrial applications [195].

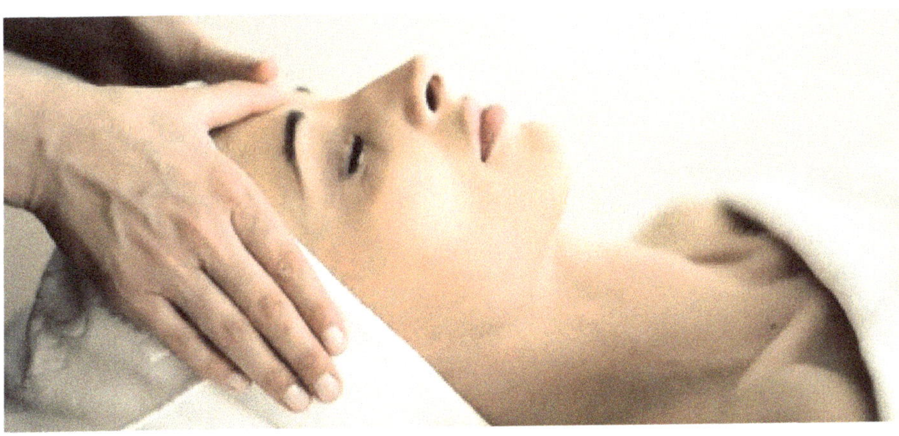

Figure 2.10 Winter treatments [137-139]. In the winter season when the air is crisp and chilly, special skin care is necessary. Dry skin in the winter has been reported to involve scaling, defects in water-holding and barrier functions, and decreased ceramide levels in the stratum corneum (SC). Indicators of dry skin conditions (conductance, dryness, roughness, and scaliness) strongly correlated with the level of ceramide. Daily application of a moisturizing cream is effective in improving mild subclinical inflammation that is induced on the facial skin by the winter environment.

Exhibit 2. Types of Moisturizers [196], [199]

	Emollients	Humectants	Occlusives	Protein Rejuvenators
Mechanism of action	Saturated & unsaturated hydrocarbons with variable length which improves skin barrier function, membrane fluidity and cell signaling, resulting in overall improvement of skin texture and appearance. Often combined with an emulsifier	Low molecular substances in majority, with the capability to attract water into stratum corneum. Frequently used with other compounds which may retain the water content	Consist of oils and waxes, forming an inactive layer on the skin surface to physically block water evaporation from the skin (transepidermal water loss)	Small molecular weight proteins, believed to aid skin rejuvenation by replenishing skin's essential proteins
Indication	Routine skin care, dry and rough skin, papulosquamous skin disease	Xerosis, ichthyosis	Prevention of contact dermatitis, xerosis, atopic dermatitis	Photodamaged skin, skin rejuvenation
Adverse effect	Contact irritation (seldom)	Irritation (lactic acid, urea)	Oily application, cosmetically disagreeable, folliculitis (mineral oil), contact dermatitis (lanolin), acneiform eruption	Contact dermatitis
Substance	Fatty acids, fatty alcohols, cholesterol, squalene, pseudoceramides	Urea, sorbitol, panthenol, glycerol, propylene glycol, hyaluronic acid, alpha hydroxy acids	Mineral oil, petroleum jelly, beeswax, silicones, zinc oxide	Collagen, elastin, keratin

Exhibit 3. Emollients used in skin creams [196-205]
"Emollience" is another ill-defined term often used in connection with skin creams. Emollient means imparting a smoothness and general sense of well-being to the skin, as determined by touch. In a sense, therefore, water is an emollient. Emollients may also cause flattening of the skin surface, pluming of each corneocyte, and general smoothing and diminishing of facial lines. Every liquid, semi-solid or low-melting-point solid of a bland nature and cosmetic quality has been used as an emollient. Among the most popular water-soluble emollients are glycerine, sorbitol, propylene glycol, and various ethoxylated derivatives of lipids. Oil-soluble emollients include hydrocarbon oils and waxes, silicone gels, vegetable oils and fats, alkyl esters, fatty acids and alcohols, together with ethers of fatty alcohols (including polyhydric alcohols). The choice is determined by personal preference, data on potential skin irritation, the degree of "greasiness" and apparent residual film on the skin, cost, and availability. Mineral oils and silicone oils do not "disappear" from the skin very readily when used in any quantity and are therefore useful in cleansing and night creams. Propylene glycol is an efficient preservative against certain micro-organisms at concentrations of more than 8%, but it is a potential sensitizer. The alkyl esters represent a range of interesting emollients ranging, as they do, through lactates, oleates, myristates, adipates, linoleates with the possibility of straight-chained, branch-chained, unsaturated, or saturated precursors. Some are almost water-thin liquids that rub quickly into the skin (decal and isodecyl oleates, isopropyl myristate), and others are waxy solids that melt near body temperature and give "body" to creams. Lanolin was once considered to be an extremely desirable emollient and the claim "contains lanolin" was felt to be a product "plus". Caution: Some emollients, particular those containing white soft paraffin or petroleum jelly can catch fire if used near a naked flame. One should keep children away from candlelight if applied emollients to them, near an open fire or while smoking a cigarette. Once the emollients have been applied to the child's skin, he or she should also avoid naked flames, such as candles or open fires. Emollients should be stored in a cool, dry place away from any naked flames or heat sources such as radiators. The moisturizing effect of emollients can make the bath or shower tray very slippery. One should use a non-slip bath mat and clean it and the bath thoroughly after each use.

Exhibit 4. Comparison between moisturizers and cold creams [209-2013]		
	Moisturizer	**Cold Cream**
General description	Moisturizer is a complex mixture of chemical agents specially designed to make the external layers of the skin (epidermis) softer and more pliable.	Cold cream is an emulsion of fats and water that can be used to clean and soften the skin.

Contd...

Nature	It is thinner	It is thicker
Time of usage	Used in the day and in all seasons.	Used at night and generally in winter.
Functions	Moisturizers are strictly for moisturizing.	Cold creams are typically a cleanser or a very rich moisturizer
Common Examples	Olay Moisturizing Lotion, Himalaya Intensive Moisturizing Body Lotion, Lakme Peach Milk Moisturizers, etc.	Ponds Moisturising Cold Cream, Garnier Nourishing Cold Cream, Aromamagic Aloe Vera Cold Cream, etc.

2.4.7 VANISHING AND FOUNDATION CREAM

The majority of the products are moisturizers with added ingredients to support marketing claims. Whether the product is a facial foundation, an antiaging night cream, a sunscreen, a topical antioxidant, or a skin-lightening serum, the formulation is a moisturizer. Skin care products are numerous and perplexing, yet there is a certain commonality among 80% of the formulations [208]. To achieve rapid 'Rub in' effect, vanishing creams are composed of emollient esters in oil phase which leave little apparent film over skin. For this reason, a low percentage oil phase usually chosen. The presence of the humectant glycerin was also used to claim that they helped reduce moisture loss from dry skin. Vanishing Cream is made especially for the outer skin. It is greaseless. It contains a marvelous substance that prevents loss of skin moisture replaces lost moisture [209]. Major difference with cold cream is that cold cream is an emulsion of water and certain fats, usually including beeswax and various scent agents, designed to smooth skin and remove makeup. The emulsion is of a "water in oil" type unlike the "oil in water" type emulsion of vanishing cream, so-called because it seems to disappear when applied on the skin [210]. The history of foundation use can be traced back as far as 200 B.C. It was considered fashionable to have a pale complexion, so Greek women applied white lead powder and chalk to lighten their skin. Roman women and men also lightened their skins using white lead, chalk, and tin oxide-based creams. This fashion continued during the middle ages up to the early 19th century when consumers used numerous toxic concoctions to lighten their skin [217]. Foundation creams possess many of the same properties of vanishing creams. Foundation creams process many of the same properties. These creams are for daytime use to protect and "condition" the cleansed skin. It is important to know whether a foundation provides sun protection and whether it meets the standards set for other sunscreen products. Sunscreen agents help to protect the consumer's skin from the harmful, aging effects of shortwave solar radiation.

Foundation cream comes in several forms: the original cream, a lighter mousse version, a heavier stick version, and a "pancake" version, a powder that turns creamy after spraying it with water. There's also a relatively new hybrid called cream to powder foundation (also called dual-finish foundation), which looks like a powder and applies like a cream if it is wet, and then dries to a powder finish. Protection which is imbalanced for either UV-B or UV-A radiation is potentially harmful for users believing themselves adequately protected. Foundations proved to be much more interesting because they possess a non-negligible SPF as well as good photostability making these products safe in terms of their mode of application (applied once daily in a study) [214]. They must therefore leave the skin non-greasy and preferably matte so that other makeup can easily be applied over it. Modern foundation creams are of excellent appearance and stability. They contain emollients and moisturizers. In terms of spreadability, coverage, and adhesion, the results of the group who used the 'oscillation applicator' were significantly twice as high as the other group who applied by hand [215].

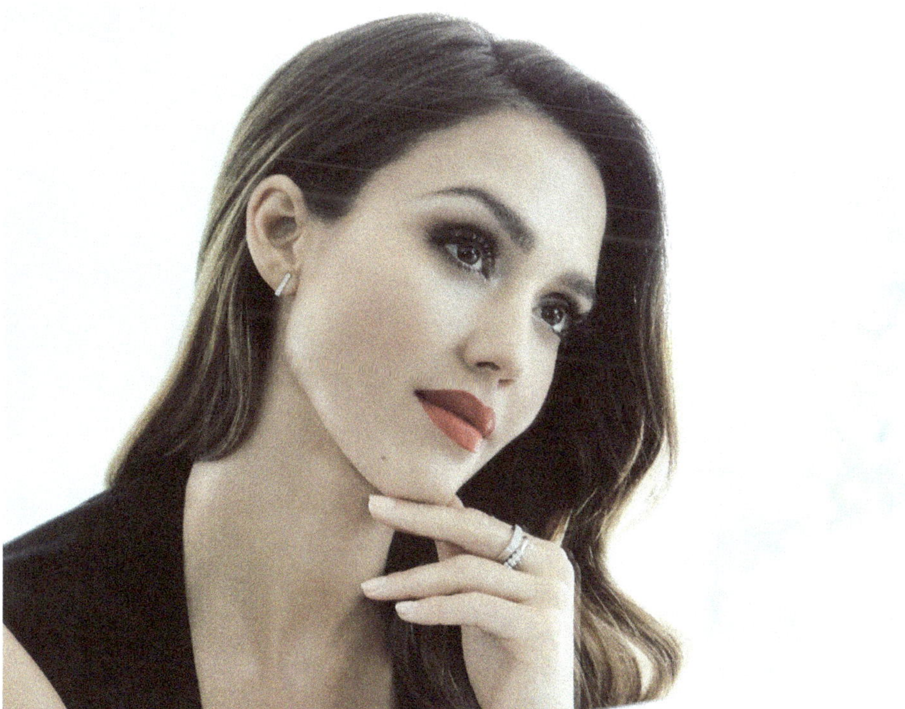

Figure 2.11 Jessica Alba [221,222]. The Dark Angel (TV series by James Cameron, premiered in Y2K) superstar uses an all-natural, organic foundation, according to Glamour magazine, UK. "Vapour's foundation makes my complexion flawless without having to use powder," she told in an interview (*Courtacy:* InStyle).

The right foundation helps to create an illusion of flawless skin. Foundation is arguably the most important part of our makeup routine. It covers blemishes, evens out skin tone and mattifes or illuminates depending on needs (**Figure 2.11**).[221]. Clients with pigmented skin are often coerced into purchasing a foundation that has too much white pigment [216]. Pigmented foundation creams can contain from 3 – 25% of pigments. Those with between 3 and 10% form a suitable substrate for the use for the subsequent use of powder, whereas those with higher pigment concentrations can be used as complete makeup and are often termed powder creams. They can be water-continuous or oil-continuous systems in liquid or solid form. The difficulties encountered in the preparations are: (a). The preferential absorption of emulsifier in the high surface of the pigment may sometimes cause inversion of the emulsion; (b). The inadequate dispersion of the pigment for reproducible colors. Pigments can be suspended by the use of cellulose derivatives or inorganic silicates such as bentonite or hydrated magnesium silicate [99]. According to dermatologists, it has been researched that the foundation cream covers the skin pores to produce a radiant look causing pore congestion and disrupt the skin from breathing. Not only that, after a long time it has been observed that the cream becomes oily which might result into blemishes and peeling especially dry skin. It is therefore advisable that after using foundation cream the layer should be thoroughly washed in the evening or else face the consequences of inflammation, acnes, rashes, and pimples as the skin might be stuck with this. Women with status cosmetics cannot tolerate makeup and complain of a continuous burning sensation after any application [219].

Table 2.6 Typical Vanishing Cream Formulation [206]

Stearic Acid Based Vanishing Cream		Palm Oil Based Vanishing Cream	
Ingredients	**(%)**	**Ingredients**	**(%)**
Stearic Acid	12.5	Natural palm oil base	12.5
Cetyl alcohol	1	Triethanolamine	1
Glycerol	6	Glycerol	6
Potassium hydroxide	1	Citric acid	0.2
Propyl Paraben	0.025	Propyl Paraben	0.025
Methyl Paraben	0.05	Methyl Paraben	0.05
Rose oil	Qs	Rose oil	Qs
Purified water	29.34	Purified water	30.1

2.4.8 HAND AND BODY CREAMS (ALL PURPOSE CREAMS)

True to its name, all-purpose cream is a flexible and versatile type of cream that can be used for both your savory and sweet creations [207]. They act nourishing or night cream when applied excessively, they function as hand creams when applied sparingly, thus they are called all-purpose cream [220]. All-purpose creams are typified by a W/O emulsion or by high oil content O/W emulsions. These products are for general face and body usage and generally have a heavy consistency and significant drag on rub-out [42]. The cream is pourable at room temperature but is also able to be easily whipped when chilled. Preparations should comply following requirements: (a) As a foundation cream for general use it must provide a satisfactory foundation base for make-up without being too greasy (b) As a cleansing cream it should be liquified quickly, be of oily nature but should be free from 'Drag'. It should not be readily absorbed by the skin (c) As a hand cream it should be emollient yet not leave a greasy or sticky film on the skin (d) As a protective and emollient cream, it should leave a continuous but non-occlusive oil film on the skin. There appears to be a market for all-purpose cream because: (i) Unsophisticated user who are unwilling to pay money therefore buys one cream to do as much as possible (ii) Slightly more sophisticated user who buys a specialty cream for one particular function and uses it as a specialty cream (iii) User who finds the cream ideally suited to their particular skin (iv) The user who particularly fragments their skin creams but resorts to an all-purpose cream when travelling or on holiday (v) For general family use and protection against the elements [48].

EPILOGUE

The skin plays many roles ranging from barrier function to highly complex biochemical and photobiochemical processes. If we follow the definition above then skin care products are inherently not simply cosmetics to beautify the appearance of the skin. Many cosmetic formulations have complex mixtures of actives the interactions of which are not all well-defined. They then affect either the structure or the function (or both) of the skin. Unlike drugs, cosmetics typically are very safe and have few significant serious adverse events. However, like drugs, these active agents can impact many diverse functions of the skin and we do not fully comprehend the implications of these actions in many cases. Skin care products are readily available and their promotions with fanciful claims are omnipresent. The promotions are based on effects, evoked by actives that are delivered through vehicles that rely on specific technologies. Due to the fact, that these products are in direct contact to the target tissue, their vehicle and ingredients can profoundly modulate the characteristics of the skin and some of its functions. This makes products for the skin absolutly unique and versatile delivery systems. Currently the majority of skin care products are cosmetics. In cosmetic products claims often describe their functionalities and may be as simple as "soothe signs of dry skin" but may also be more fanciful like "Multi-ingredient anti-aging moisturizer designed to improve the appearance of facial skin". Skin care products are characterized by effects, evoked by actives that are delivered through vehicles that rely on specific technologies. The regulatory situation is unknown to most of the consumers and healthcare professionals. They have to trust the current regulations on cosmetic products and quality standards used by the manufacturer. This means that professional healthcare practitioners have a substantial responsibility for skin health while delivering skin care

SUMMARY

Skin care provides almost any possible kind of vehicle, including emulsifiers, surfactants, oils and butters, waxes, and hydrophilic solutions. These substances combine the properties of drug delivery to the skin, typical of vehicles, with the ability to produce specific actions on the skin, such as occlusive, moisturizing, smoothing, firming, soothing, and conditioning effects. This term "Cosmetics" indicates cosmetic-pharmaceutical hybrids aimed at enhancing the beauty of the skin using ingredients that modify skin functionality or provide additional health-related function or benefit. As well as giving beauty to a person via the skin, the cosmetic industry has now strongly linked its products medicinally to the subject of anti-ageing of the skin. The industry has also coined such terms as actives, cosmeceuticals, nutricosmetics, etc., and the legislation associated with cosmetology and dermatology has become similar.

ABBREVIATIONS

Isopropyl Myristate (IPM); Atopic Dermatitis (AD); Sodium Lauryl Sulfate (SLS); Environmental Protection Agency (EPA); Triethanolamine (TEA); Cosmetic Ingredient Review (CIR); Linoleic acid (LA); Sodium Cocoyl Isethionate (SCI); Sodium Dodecyl Sulfate (SDS); Polyethylene glycols (PEGs); Sorbitan Sesquioleate (SSO); Glycolic acid (GA); Retinaldehyde (RAL); solar simulated radiation (SSR); Alpha-hydroxy acids (AHA); BHA (Beta hydroxy acid) reactive oxygen species (ROS); range of motion (ROM); International Nomenclature of Cosmetic Ingredients (INCI); Sun Protection Factor (SPF); Hydrophobically Modified Polymers (HMPs); Nucleotide binding domain and leucine rich repeat containing proteins (NLRs); NLRC4 (NLR Family CARD Domain Containing 4); absent in melanoma 2 (AIM2); Normal Human Epidermal Keratinocytes (NHEK); Skin blood flow (SkBF); transepidermal water loss (TEWL); Natural Moisturizing Factors (NMF)

BIBLIOGRAPHY AND WEBLIOGRAPHY

1. Surber C, Dragicevic N, Kottner J. Skin Care Products for Healthy and Diseased Skin. CurrProbl Dermatol. 2018;54:183-200. doi: 10.1159/000489532. Epub 2018 Aug 21. Review. PubMed PMID: 30130786.

2. Del Rosso JQ, Levin J. The clinical relevance of maintaining the functional integrity of the stratum corneum in both healthy and disease-affected skin. J Clin Aesthet Dermatol. 2011 Sep;4(9):22-42. PubMed PMID: 21938268; PubMed Central PMCID: PMC3175800.
3. Goodman G. Cleansing and moisturizing in acne patients. Am J Clin Dermatol. 2009;10 Suppl 1:1-6. doi: 10.2165/0128071-200910001-00001. Review. PubMed PMID: 19209947.
4. Johnson AW. Overview: fundamental skin care--protecting the barrier. Dermatol Ther. 2004;17 Suppl 1:1-5. PubMed PMID: 14728693.
5. Simion FA, Abrutyn ES, Draelos ZD. Ability of moisturizers to reduce dry skin and irritation and to prevent their return. J Cosmet Sci. 2005 Nov-Dec;56(6):427-44. PubMed PMID: 16538297.
6. Blaak J, Staib P. The Relation of pH and Skin Cleansing. CurrProbl Dermatol. 2018;54:132-142. doi: 10.1159/000489527. Epub 2018 Aug 21. Review. PubMed PMID: 30130782.
7. Chapter 11. Semi-solid dosage forms. In: Alekha Dash, Somnath Singh, Justin Tolman. Pharmaceutics: Basic Principles and Application to Pharmacy Practice, published by Academic Press, 2013 ISBN 0123868912, 9780123868916
8. Swarbrick J, Rubino JT, Rubino OP. Chapter 22. Coarse Dispersions. In: Remington: The Science and Practice of Pharmacy Volume 1, edited by David B. Troy, Paul Beringer, published by Lippincott Williams & Wilkins, 2006 ISBN 0781746736, 9780781746731
9. Chapter 4. Skin Creams. In: Harry's Cosmeticology 7th edition, edited by John Bernard Wilkinson, Raymond Jack Moore, published by Chemical Pub., 1982, ISBN 0820602957, 9780820602950
10. Chapter 6. Creams and Liquid Emulsions for facial Cleansing. In: Handbook of Cosmetic Skin Care, 2nd Ed, Informa Health Care, 2009, edited by Avi Shai, Howard I. Maibach, Robert Baran, published by CRC Press, September 21, 2009 ISBN 9780415467186
11. Ertel K. Modern skin cleansers. Dermatol Clin. 2000 Oct;18(4):561-75. Review. PubMed PMID: 11059364.
12. Kuehl BL, Fyfe KS, Shear NH. Cutaneous cleansers. Skin Therapy Lett. 2003 Mar;8(3):1-4. Review. PubMed PMID: 12858234.
13. Park JH, Lee JW, Kim YC, Prausnitz MR. The effect of heat on skin permeability. Int J Pharm. 2008 Jul 9;359(1-2):94-103. doi: 10.1016/j.ijpharm.2008.03.032. Epub 2008 Mar 29. PubMed PMID: 18455889; PubMed Central PMCID: PMC2464624.
14. Liquefying Cleansing Creams. Available From: https://www.cosmetics andskin.com/ded/liquefying-cleansers.php
15. Corazza M, Lauriola MM, Zappaterra M, Bianchi A, Virgili A. Surfactants, skin cleansing protagonists. J Eur Acad Dermatol Venereol. 2010 Jan;24(1):1-6. doi: 10.1111/j.1468-3083.2009.03349.x.Epub 2009 Jul 14. Review. PubMed PMID: 19614860.
16. Isoda K, Seki T, Inoue Y, Umeda K, Nishizaka T, Tanabe H, Takagi Y, Ishida K, Mizutani H. Efficacy of the combined use of a facial cleanser and moisturizers for

the care of mild acne patients with sensitive skin. J Dermatol. 2015 Feb;42(2):181-8. doi: 10.1111/1346-8138.12720. Epub 2014 Dec 6. PubMed PMID: 25483138.

17. National Center for Biotechnology Information. PubChem Database. Stearic acid, CID=5281, https://pubchem.ncbi.nlm.nih.gov/compound/5281 (accessed on Apr. 17, 2019)
18. Raymond C. Rowe, Paul J. Sheskey, Marian E. Quinn. Handbook of Pharmaceutical Excipients 6th edition, Pharmaceutical Press, 2009, ISBN 1582121354, 9781582121352
19. Rawlings AV, Lombard KJ. A review on the extensive skin benefits of mineral oil. Int J Cosmet Sci. 2012 Dec;34(6):511-8. doi: 10.1111/j.1468-2494.2012.00752.x.Epub 2012 Sep 21. Review. PubMed PMID: 22994201.
20. Concin N, Hofstetter G, Plattner B, Tomovski C, Fiselier K, Gerritzen K, Semsroth S, Zeimet AG, Marth C, Siegl H, Rieger K, Ulmer H, Concin H, Grob K. Evidence for cosmetics as a source of mineral oil contamination in women. J Womens Health (Larchmt). 2011 Nov;20(11):1713-9. doi: 10.1089/jwh.2011.2829. Epub 2011 Oct 4. PubMed PMID: 21970597.
21. Ghadially R, Halkier-Sorensen L, Elias PM. Effects of petrolatum on stratum corneum structure and function. J Am Acad Dermatol. 1992 Mar;26(3 Pt 2):387-96. PubMed PMID: 1564142.
22. Czarnowicki T, Malajian D, Khattri S, Correa da Rosa J, Dutt R, Finney R, Dhingra N, Xiangyu P, Xu H, Estrada YD, Zheng X, Gilleaudeau P, Sullivan-Whalen M, Suaréz-Fariñas M, Shemer A, Krueger JG, Guttman-Yassky E. Petrolatum: Barrier repair and antimicrobial responses underlying this "inert" moisturizer. J Allergy Clin Immunol. 2016 Apr;137(4):1091-1102.e7. doi: 10.1016/j.jaci.2015.08.013. Epub 2015 Oct 1. PubMed PMID: 26431582.
23. Zondlo Fiume M. Final report on the safety assessment of Acrylates Copolymer and 33 related cosmetic ingredients. Int J Toxicol. 2002;21 Suppl 3:1-50. Review. PubMed PMID: 12537929.
24. Wheeler T. Petroleum, oats, shea butter: are 'natural' emollients best? Br J Nurs. 2011 Jan 27-Feb 9;20(2):70. PubMed PMID: 21278652.
25. Hon KL, Kung JSC, Ng WGG, Leung TF. Emollient treatment of atopic dermatitis: latest evidence and clinical considerations. Drugs Context. 2018 Apr 17;7:212530. doi: 10.7573/dic.212530. eCollection 2018. Review. PubMed PMID: 29692852; PubMed Central PMCID: PMC5908267.
26. Mandawgade SD, Patravale VB. Formulation and evaluation of exotic fat based cosmeceuticals for skin repair. Indian J Pharm Sci. 2008 Jul-Aug;70(4):539-42. doi: 10.4103/0250-474X.44615. PubMed PMID: 20046792; PubMed Central PMCID: PMC2792546.
27. Vadgama RN, Odaneth AA, Lali AM. Green synthesis of isopropyl myristate in novel single phase medium Part I: Batch optimization studies. Biotechnol Rep (Amst). 2015 Oct 24;8:133-137. doi: 10.1016/j.btre.2015.10.006. eCollection2015 Dec. PubMed PMID: 28352582; PubMed Central PMCID: PMC4980752.

28. National Center for Biotechnology Information. PubChem Database. Sorbitan monolaurate, CID=11046239, https://pubchem.ncbi.nlm.nih.gov/compound /11046239 (accessed on Apr. 17, 2019)
29. Kima C, Hsieh YL. Wetting and absorbency of nonionic surfactant solutions on cotton fabrics. Colloids and Surfaces A: Physicochemical and Engineering Aspects Volumes 187–188, 31 August 2001, Pages 385-397. https://doi.org/10.1016/S0927-7757(01)00653-7
30. D.R. Karsa, P.J. Donnelly, J.M. Goode. Surfactants Applications Directory, published by Springer Science & Business Media, 2012, ISBN 9401130388, 9789401130387
31. Lodén M, Wessman W. The influence of a cream containing 20% glycerin and its vehicle on skin barrier properties. Int J Cosmet Sci. 2001 Apr;23(2):115-9. doi: 10.1046/j.1467-2494.2001.00060.x. PubMed PMID: 18498456.
32. Sethi A, Kaur T, Malhotra SK, Gambhir ML. Moisturizers: The Slippery Road. Indian J Dermatol. 2016 May-Jun;61(3):279-87. doi: 10.4103/0019-5154.182427. Review. PubMed PMID: 27293248; PubMed Central PMCID: PMC4885180.
33. National Center for Biotechnology Information. PubChem Database. Sodium lauryl sulfate, CID=3423265, https://pubchem.ncbi.nlm.nih.gov/ compound/3423265 (accessed on Apr. 17, 2019)
34. Bondi CA, Marks JL, Wroblewski LB, Raatikainen HS, Lenox SR, Gebhardt KE. Human and Environmental Toxicity of Sodium Lauryl Sulfate (SLS): Evidence for Safe Use in Household Cleaning Products. Environ Health Insights. 2015 Nov 17;9:27-32. doi: 10.4137/EHI.S31765. eCollection 2015. Review. PubMed PMID: 26617461; PubMed Central PMCID: PMC4651417.
35. Anderson S. How to Replace Sodium Lauryl Sulfate? Available From: https://www.livestrong.com/article/334607-how-to-replace-sodium-lauryl-sulfate/
36. Leland A. Sodium Lauryl Sulfate: What it is and How to Avoid it? Available From: https://bettersheabutter.com/sodium-lauryl-sulfate-what-it-is-and-how-to-avoid-it/
37. Kerwin BA. Polysorbates 20 and 80 used in the formulation of protein biotherapeutics: structure and degradation pathways. J Pharm Sci. 2008 Aug;97(8):2924-35. Review. PubMed PMID: 17973307.
38. Becker LC, Bergfeld WF, Belsito DV, Hill RA, Klaassen CD, Liebler DC, Marks JG Jr, Shank RC, Slaga TJ, Snyder PW, Andersen FA, Heldreth B. Safety Assessment of PolyetherLanolins as Used in Cosmetics. Int J Toxicol. 2018 May/Jun;37(1_suppl):19S-27S. doi: 10.1177/1091581817740120. PubMed PMID: 29761732.
39. Nasrollahi SA, Ayatollahi A, Yazdanparast T, Samadi A, Hosseini H, Shamsipour M, Akhlaghi AA, Yadangi S, Abels C, Firooz A. Comparison of linoleic acid-containing water-in-oil emulsion with urea-containing water-in-oil emulsion in the treatment of atopic dermatitis: a randomized clinical trial. Clin CosmetInvestig Dermatol. 2018 Jan 5;11:21-28. doi: 10.2147/CCID.S145561. eCollection 2018. PubMed PMID: 29379309; PubMed Central PMCID: PMC5759849.
40. Ghosh S, Blankschtein D. Why is sodium cocoyl isethionate (SCI) mild to the skin barrier? - An in vitro investigation based on the relative sizes of the SCI micelles

and the skin aqueous pores. J Cosmet Sci. 2007 May-Jun;58(3):229-44. PubMed PMID: 17598025.

41. Fiume MM, Heldreth B, Bergfeld WF, Belsito DV, Hill RA, Klaassen CD, Liebler D, Marks JG Jr, Shank RC, Slaga TJ, Snyder PW, Andersen FA. Safety assessment of triethanolamine and triethanolamine-containing ingredients as used in cosmetics. Int J Toxicol. 2013 May-Jun;32(3 Suppl):59S-83S. doi: 10.1177/1091581813488804. Review. PubMed PMID: 23696578.
42. Schmitt WH. Chapter 3. Skin Care Products. S.D. In: Williams, W.H. Schmitt. Chemistry and Technology of the Cosmetics and Toiletries Industry, published by Springer Science & Business Media, 2012 ISBN 9400915551, 9789400915558, Page 104-120
43. Halevi S, Shai A. Chapter 3. Principles in the Preparation of Medical and Cosmetic Products. In: handbook of Cosmetic Skin Care, 2nd Ed, Informa Health Care, 2009: Cosmetic Skin Care, 2009 Volume 1 of handbook of Cosmetic Skin Care, published by Bukupedia, Page 20
44. Cold Creams. Available From: https://cosmeticsandskin.com/aba/cold-cream.php
45. Marquez R, Forgiarini AM, Langevin D, Salager J-L. Instability of Emulsions Made with Surfactant–Oil–Water Systems at Optimum Formulation with Ultralow Interfacial Tension. Langmuir 2018 34 (31), 9252-9263. DOI: 10.1021/acs.langmuir.8b01376
46. Baloch MK, Hameed G. Emulsification of oil in water as affected by different parameters. J Colloid Interface Sci. 2005 May 15;285(2):804-13. PubMed PMID: 15837500.
47. Draelos ZD. Cosmetics and skin care products. A historical perspective. Dermatol Clin. 2000 Oct;18(4):557-9. PubMed PMID: 11059363.
48. Harry Ralph G. Chapter 4. Skin Creams. In: Wilkison JB, Moore RJ, editors. Harry's Cosmeticology. 7th edition. London, UK: George Godwin; 1982. pp. 50-73.
49. Jones ER. Greasy Cold Creams. The Journal of the American Pharmaceutical Association (1912) Volume 4, Issue 6, June 1915, Pages 708-714. https://doi.org/10.1002/jps.3080040613
50. Galen (Author), Peter N. Singer (Translator). Selected Works (Oxford World's Classics), published by Oxford University Press; New edition edition (June 20, 2002). ISBN-10: 0192839373 ISBN-13: 978-0192839374
51. Hubbard SA. Comparative toxicology of borates. Biol Trace Elem Res. 1998 Winter;66(1-3):343-57. Review. PubMed PMID: 10050929.
52. Benefits of Borax And Its Side Effects. Available From: https://www.lybrate.com/topic/borax-benefits-and-side-effects
53. Pongsavee M. Effect of borax on immune cell proliferation and sister chromatid exchange in human chromosomes. J Occup Med Toxicol. 2009 Oct 30;4:27. doi: 10.1186/1745-6673-4-27. PubMed PMID: 19878537; PubMed Central PMCID: PMC2776007.
54. Fort, D.J., Propst, T.L., Stover, E.L. et al. Adverse reproductive and developmental effects inXenopus from insufficient boron. Biol Trace Elem Res (1998) 66: 237. https://doi.org/10.1007/BF02783141

55. Lanoue, L., Taubeneck, M.W., Muniz, J. et al. Assessing the effects of low boron diets on embryonic and fetal development in rodents using in vitro and in vivo model systems. Biol Trace Elem Res (1998) 66: 271. https://doi.org/10.1007/BF02783143
56. Douglas J. Fort, Troy D. Fort, Michael B. Mathis, R. Wayne Ball, Boric Acid Is Reproductively Toxic to Adult Xenopus laevis, but Not Endocrine Active, Toxicological Sciences, Volume 154, Issue 1, November 2016, Pages 16–26, https://doi.org/10.1093/toxsci/kfw138
57. Cold creams containing acyl lactylates. Available From: https://patentimages.storage.googleapis.com/bd/29/9d/4c6acecb4b2b08/imgb0003.png
58. The Truth About Borax In Skincare. Available From: https://www.scratchmommy.com/the-truth-about-borax-in-skincare/
59. Sodium Behenoyl Lactylate. Available From: https://www.theherbarie.com/Sodium-Behenoyl-Lactylate.html
60. Sodium Behenoyl Lactylate. Available From: https://cosmetics.specialchem.com/product/i-the-herbarie-sodium-behenoyl-lactylate
61. Cornara L, Biagi M, Xiao J, Burlando B. Therapeutic Properties of Bioactive Compounds from Different Honeybee Products. Front Pharmacol. 2017 Jun 28;8:412. doi: 10.3389/fphar.2017.00412. eCollection 2017. Review. PubMed PMID: 28701955; PubMed Central PMCID: PMC5487425.
62. Kameda T. Molecular structure of crude beeswax studied by solid-state 13C NMR. J Insect Sci. 2004;4:29. Epub 2004 Aug 30. PubMed PMID: 15861244; PubMed Central PMCID: PMC1081567.
63. CERESIN WAX Basic information. Available From: https://www.chemicalbook.com/ProductChemicalPropertiesCB1303742_EN.htm
64. Carbopol® 934 polymer – Lubrizol. Available From: https://www.lubrizol.com/Personal-Care/Products/Product-Finder/Products-Data/95
65. Speckman RA, Collins EB. Microbial production of 2,3-butylene glycol from cheese whey. Appl Environ Microbiol. 1982 May;43(5):1216-8. PubMed PMID: 16346020; PubMed Central PMCID: PMC244211.
66. Aizawa A, Ito A, Masui Y, Ito M. Case of allergic contact dermatitis due to 1,3-butylene glycol. J Dermatol. 2014 Sep;41(9):815-6. doi: 10.1111/1346-8138.12603. PubMed PMID: 25182293.
67. Jang HJ, Shin CY, Kim KB. Safety Evaluation of Polyethylene Glycol (PEG) Compounds for Cosmetic Use. Toxicol Res. 2015 Jun;31(2):105-36. doi: 10.5487/TR.2015.31.2.105. Review. PubMed PMID: 26191379; PubMed Central PMCID: PMC4505343.
68. PEG-100 STEARATE. Available from: https://www.ewg.org/skindeep/ingredient/721388/PEG-100_STEARATE/
69. PEG 100 Stearate. Available From: https://thedermreview.com/peg-100-stearate/
70. Glyceryl Stearate & PEG-100 Stearate. Available From: https://uk.lush.com/ingredients/glyceryl-stearate-peg-100-stearate
71. Asarch A, Scheinman PL. Sorbitansesquioleate: an emerging contact allergen. Dermatitis. 2008 Nov-Dec;19(6):339-41. PubMed PMID: 19134439.

72. National Center for Biotechnology Information. PubChem Database. Sorbitansesquioleate, CID=71308589, https://pubchem.ncbi.nlm.nih.gov /compound/71308589 (accessed on Apr. 17, 2019)
73. SorbitanSesquioleate* An emollient. Available From: https://www.truthin-aging.com/ingredients/sorbitan-sesquioleate
74. Glyceryl Stearate. Available From: https://cosmeticsinfo.org/ingredient/glyceryl-stearate
75. National Center for Biotechnology Information. PubChem Database. Glyceryl monostearate, CID=24699, https://pubchem.ncbi.nlm.nih.gov/compound/24699 (accessed on Apr. 17, 2019)
76. National Center for Biotechnology Information. PubChem Database. 1-Hexadecanol, CID=2682, https://pubchem.ncbi.nlm.nih.gov/compound/2682 (accessed on Apr. 17, 2019)
77. Alcohol In Skincare: The Facts. Available From: https://www.paulaschoice-eu.com/alcohol-in-skincare-the-facts
78. Michael Ash. Handbook of Green Chemicals, published by Synapse Info Resources, 2004 ISBN 1890595799, 9781890595791, Page 665
79. Martin Rieger, Linda D. Rhein. Surfactants in Cosmetics, Second Edition,
80. Volume 68 of Surfactant Science, published by CRC Press, 1997 ISBN 0824798058, 9780824798055
81. Lynde CW. Moisturizers: What They Are And How They Work, Web SkinTherapyLetter, Volume 6 Number 13, December 1, 2001.
82. Pellicoro C, Marsella R, Ahrens K. Pilot study to evaluate the effect of topical dimethicone on clinical signs and skin barrier function in dogs with naturally occurring atopic dermatitis. Vet Med Int. 2013;2013:239186. doi: 10.1155/2013/239186. Epub 2013 Apr 17. PubMed PMID: 23710417; PubMed Central PMCID: PMC3654275.
83. Glydant Plus™. Available From: https://dewolfchem.com/shop/glydant-plus/
84. Fartasch M, Teal J, Menon GK. Mode of action of glycolic acid on human stratum corneum: ultrastructural and functional evaluation of the epidermal barrier. Arch Dermatol Res. 1997 Jun;289(7):404-9. PubMed PMID: 9248619.
85. Rouvrais C, Baspeyras M, Mengeaud V, Rossi AB. Antiaging efficacy of a retinaldehyde-based cream compared with glycolic acid peel sessions: A randomized controlled study. J Cosmet Dermatol. 2018 Dec;17(6):1136-1143. doi: 10.1111/jocd.12511. Epub 2018 Jul 19. PubMed PMID: 30027612.
86. Kornhauser A, Wei RR, Yamaguchi Y, Coelho SG, Kaidbey K, Barton C, Takahashi K, Beer JZ, Miller SA, Hearing VJ. The effects of topically applied glycolic acid and salicylic acid on ultraviolet radiation-induced erythema, DNA damage and sunburn cell formation in human skin. J Dermatol Sci. 2009 Jul;55(1):10-7. doi: 10.1016/j.jdermsci.2009.03.011. Epub 2009 May 2. PubMed PMID: 19411163; PubMed Central PMCID: PMC2791365.
87. Maia Campos PM, Gaspar LR, Gonçalves GM, Pereira LH, Semprini M, Lopes RA. Comparative effects of retinoic acid or glycolic acid vehiculated in different topical formulations. Biomed Res Int. 2015;2015:650316. doi: 10.1155/2015

/650316. Epub 2015 Jan 6. PubMed PMID: 25632398; PubMed Central PMCID: PMC4302967.

88. Tang SC, Yang JH. Dual Effects of Alpha-Hydroxy Acids on the Skin. Molecules. 2018 Apr 10;23(4). pii: E863. doi: 10.3390/molecules23040863. Review. PubMed PMID: 29642579; PubMed Central PMCID: PMC6017965.
89. Hung SJ, Tang SC, Liao PY, Ge JS, Hsiao YP, Yang JH. Photoprotective Potential of Glycolic Acid by Reducing NLRC4 and AIM2 Inflammasome Complex Proteins in UVB Radiation-Induced Normal Human Epidermal Keratinocytes and Mice. DNA Cell Biol. 2017 Feb;36(2):177-187. doi: 10.1089/dna.2016.3471. PubMed PMID: 28112987.
90. National Center for Biotechnology Information. PubChem Database. Vitamin E acetate, CID=86472, https://pubchem.ncbi.nlm.nih.gov/compound/86472 (accessed on Apr. 18, 2019)
91. Keen MA, Hassan I. Vitamin E in dermatology. Indian Dermatol Online J. 2016 Jul-Aug;7(4):311-5. doi: 10.4103/2229-5178.185494. PubMed PMID: 27559512; PubMed Central PMCID: PMC4976416.
92. Burke KE, Clive J, Combs GF Jr, Commisso J, Keen CL, Nakamura RM. Effects of topical and oral vitamin E on pigmentation and skin cancer induced by ultraviolet irradiation in Skh:2 hairless mice. Nutr Cancer. 2000;38(1):87-97. PubMed PMID: 11341050.
93. National Center for Biotechnology Information. PubChem Database. Ascorbyl palmitate, CID=54680660, https://pubchem.ncbi.nlm.nih.gov/compound/54680660 (accessed on Apr. 18, 2019)
94. Meves A, Stock SN, Beyerle A, Pittelkow MR, Peus D. Vitamin C derivative ascorbyl palmitate promotes ultraviolet-B-induced lipid peroxidation and cytotoxicity in keratinocytes. J Invest Dermatol. 2002 Nov;119(5):1103-8. PubMed PMID: 12445199.
95. Gosenca M, Obreza A, Pečar S, Gašperlin M. A new approach for increasing ascorbyl palmitate stability by addition of non-irritant co-antioxidant. AAPS PharmSciTech. 2010 Sep;11(3):1485-92. doi: 10.1208/s12249-010-9507-8. Epub 2010 Sep 16. PubMed PMID: 20845090; PubMed Central PMCID: PMC2974129.
96. Spiclin P, Gasperlin M, Kmetec V. Stability of ascorbyl palmitate in topical microemulsions. Int J Pharm. 2001 Jul 17;222(2):271-9. PubMed PMID: 11427357.
97. Alpha Hydroxy Acids. Available From: https://www.fda.gov/Cosmetics /ProductsIngredients/ucm107940.htm
98. Dr. P. V. Kasture, Dr. A. R. Paradkar. Pharmaceutics – Ii, published by Pragati Books Pvt. Ltd., 2015 ISBN 8185790221, 9788185790220, Page 159
99. Making Cosmetics & Makeup. Available From: http://www.australab.com/blog/ making-cosmetics-makeup/
100. Milani M, Sparavigna A. Antiaging efficacy of melatonin-based day and night creams: a randomized, split-face, assessor-blinded proof-of-concept trial. Clin CosmetInvestig Dermatol. 2018 Jan 24;11:51-57. doi: 10.2147/CCID.S153905. eCollection 2018. PubMed PMID: 29416368; PubMed Central PMCID: PMC5788993.

101. Khanna N, Datta Gupta S. Rejuvenating facial massage--a bane or boon? Int J Dermatol. 2002 Jul;41(7):407-10. PubMed PMID: 12121555.
102. National Clinical Guideline Centre (UK). The Prevention and Management of Pressure Ulcers in Primary and Secondary Care. London: National Institute for Health and Care Excellence (UK); 2014 Apr. (NICE Clinical Guidelines, No. 179.) 10, Skin massage. Available from: https://www.ncbi.nlm.nih.gov /books/NBK333138/
103. Rawlings AV. Cellulite and its treatment. Int J Cosmet Sci. 2006 Jun;28(3):175-90. doi: 10.1111/j.1467-2494.2006.00318.x. PubMed PMID: 18489274.
104. Facial & Body Massage Creams. Available From: https://www.massageware house.com/shop-by-department/oils-creams-and-lotions/massage-creams/
105. Field T. Massage therapy research review. Complement Ther Clin Pract. 2016 Aug;24:19-31. doi: 10.1016/j.ctcp.2016.04.005. Epub 2016 Apr 23. Review. PubMed PMID: 27502797; PubMed Central PMCID: PMC5564319.
106. Chatchawan U, Eungpinichpong W, Plandee P, Yamauchi J. Effects of thai foot massage on balance performance in diabetic patients with peripheral neuropathy: a randomized parallel-controlled trial. Med Sci Monit Basic Res. 2015 Apr 20;21:68-75. doi: 10.12659/MSMBR.894163. PubMed PMID: 25892354; PubMed Central PMCID: PMC4416467.
107. Agarwal KN, Gupta A, Pushkarna R, Bhargava SK, Faridi MM, Prabhu MK. Effects of massage & use of oil on growth, blood flow & sleep pattern in infants. Indian J Med Res. 2000 Dec;112:212-7. PubMed PMID: 11247199.
108. Supa'at I, Zakaria Z, Maskon O, Aminuddin A, Nordin NA. Effects of Swedish massage therapy on blood pressure, heart rate, and inflammatory markers in hypertensive women. Evid Based Complement Alternat Med. 2013;2013:171852. doi: 10.1155/2013/171852. Epub 2013 Aug 18. PubMed PMID: 24023571; PubMed Central PMCID: PMC3759268.
109. Rose L. Should I Use Massage Oils, Creams, Lotions or Waxes? Massage Warehouse Blog, September 24, 2016.
110. Personal Care Magazine (UK). Lightening Night Cream. Available From: https://www.personalcaremagazine.com/formulation-details/2171/lightening-night-cream?companyid=1325
111. Deionized Water Vs Distilled Water - US Water Systems. Available From: https://www.uswatersystems.com/deionized-water-vs-distilled-water
112. GLYCERYL CAPRYLATE. Available From: https://www.ewg.org/skindeep /ingredient/702630/GLYCERYL_CAPRYLATE/
113. Glyceryl Caprylate. Available From: https://cosmeticsinfo.org/ingredient/glyceryl-caprylate
114. Furuishi T, Fukami T, Suzuki T, Takayama K, Tomono K. Synergistic effect of isopropyl myristate and glyceryl monocaprylate on the skin permeation of pentazocine. Biol Pharm Bull. 2010;33(2):294-300. PubMed PMID: 20118556.
115. Papageorgiou S, Varvaresou A, Tsirivas E, Demetzos C. New alternatives to cosmetics preservation. J Cosmet Sci. 2010 Mar-Apr;61(2):107-23. PubMed PMID: 20447363.

116. Is Glyceryl Caprylate Safe For Baby? Available From: https://madeof.com/blog/is-glyceryl-caprylate-safe-for-baby
117. Artificial Preservatives in Skincare: Why They Are Not Worth the Risk. Web FEY Cosmetics, March 25, 2019.
118. Takeuchi A, Kamiryou Y, Yamada H, Eto M, Shibata K, Haruna K, Naito S, Yoshikai Y. Oral administration of xanthan gum enhances antitumor activity through Toll-like receptor 4. Int Immunopharmacol. 2009 Dec;9(13-14):1562-7. doi: 10.1016/j.intimp.2009.09.012. Epub 2009 Sep 27. PubMed PMID: 19788935.
119. Parente ME, Ochoa Andrade A, Ares G, Russo F, Jiménez-Kairuz Á. Bioadhesive hydrogels for cosmetic applications. Int J Cosmet Sci. 2015 Oct;37(5):511-8. doi: 10.1111/ics.12227. Epub 2015 May 14. PubMed PMID: 25854849.
120. Kumar A, Rao KM, Han SS. Application of xanthan gum as polysaccharide in tissue engineering: A review. CarbohydrPolym. 2018 Jan 15;180:128-144. doi: 10.1016/j.carbpol.2017.10.009. Epub 2017 Oct 5. Review. PubMed PMID: 29103488.
121. Web Lucas Meyer Cosmetics. Biophilic™ H. The biomimetic emulsifier with a cashmere touch. Available From: http://lucasmeyercosmetics.com/en/products /product.php?id=66
122. Fiume Z. Final report on the safety assessment of Lecithin and Hydrogenated Lecithin. Int J Toxicol. 2001;20 Suppl 1:21-45. Review. PubMed PMID: 11358109.
123. Kanti V, Günther M, Stroux A, Sawatzky S, Henrich W, Abou-Dakn M, Blume-Peytavi U, Garcia Bartels N. Influence of sunflower seed oil or baby lotion on the skin barrier function of newborns: A pilot study. J Cosmet Dermatol. 2017 Dec;16(4):500-507. doi: 10.1111/jocd.12302. Epub 2017 Jan 10. PubMed PMID: 28070970.
124. Darmstadt GL, Mao-Qiang M, Chi E, Saha SK, Ziboh VA, Black RE, Santosham M, Elias PM. Impact of topical oils on the skin barrier: possible implications for neonatal health in developing countries. Acta Paediatr. 2002;91(5):546-54. PubMed PMID: 12113324.
125. Kanti V, Grande C, Stroux A, Buhrer C, Blume-Peytavi U, Garcia Bartels N. Influence of sunflower seed oil on the skin barrier function of preterm infants: a randomized controlled trial. Dermatology. 2014;229(3):230-9. doi: 10.1159/000363380. Epub 2014 Oct 15. PubMed PMID: 25323538.
126. Danby SG, AlEnezi T, Sultan A, Lavender T, Chittock J, Brown K, Cork MJ. Effect of olive and sunflower seed oil on the adult skin barrier: implications for neonatal skin care. Pediatr Dermatol. 2013 Jan-Feb;30(1):42-50. doi: 10.1111/j.1525-1470.2012.01865.x.Epub 2012 Sep 20. PubMed PMID: 22995032.
127. Masson P, Merot F, Bardot J. Influence of hazelnut oil phospholipids on the skin moisturizing effect of a cosmetic emulsion. Int J Cosmet Sci. 1990 Dec;12(6):243-51. doi: 10.1111/j.1467-2494.1990.tb00539.x. PubMed PMID: 19291034.
128. M. VariniaMichalun, Joseph C. DiNardo. Skin Care and Cosmetic Ingredients Dictionary, published by Cengage Learning, 2014 ISBN 1285060792, 9781285060798

129. Annmarie Skin Care. Vitamin E (Tocopherol) for Skin, the Classic Antioxidant. Available From: https://www.annmariegianni.com/vitamin-e-for-skin-tocopherol-the-classic-antioxidant/
130. Megnanou RM, Niamke S. Improving the optimized shea butter quality: a great potential of utilization for common consumers and industrials. Springerplus. 2015 Nov 4;4:667. doi: 10.1186/s40064-015-1454-0. eCollection 2015. PubMed PMID: 26558170; PubMed Central PMCID: PMC4631807.
131. Ajala EO, Aberuagba F, Olaniyan AM, Onifade KR. Optimization of solvent extraction of shea butter (Vitellaria paradoxa) using response surface methodology and its characterization. J Food Sci Technol. 2016 Jan;53(1):730-8. doi: 10.1007/s13197-015-2033-7. Epub 2015 Sep 24. PubMed PMID: 26787993; PubMed Central PMCID: PMC4711458.
132. WHITESSENCE™. Available From: https://asia.in-cosmetics.com/__nova documents/17685?v=634874761651870000
133. Anti-ageing range - Infinity Ingredients. Available From: https://infinity-ingredients.co.uk/assets/uploads/.../Infinity-Anti-ageing-Range-21.pdf
134. Exo-T™. Available From: https://cosmetics.specialchem.com/product/i-lucas-meyer-cosmetics-exo-t
135. Tyrostat™ 9 by Lucas Meyer Cosmetics - Personal Care & Cosmetics. Available From: https://www.ulprospector.com/en/eu/PersonalCare/Detail/4499/125064/Tyrostat-9
136. Pastor-Nieto MA, Alcántara-Nicolás F, Melgar-Molero V, Pérez-Mesonero R, Vergara-Sánchez A, Martín-Fuentes A, González-Muñoz P, de Eusebio-Murillo E. Preservatives in Personal Hygiene and Cosmetic Products, Topical Medications, and Household Cleaners in Spain. ActasDermosifiliogr. 2017 Oct;108(8):758-770. doi: 10.1016/j.ad.2017.04.003. Epub 2017 Jun 30. English, Spanish. PubMed PMID: 28673419.
137. Ishikawa J, Yoshida H, Ito S, Naoe A, Fujimura T, Kitahara T, Takema Y, Zerweck C, Grove GL. Dry skin in the winter is related to the ceramide profile in the stratum corneum and can be improved by treatment with a Eucalyptus extract. J Cosmet Dermatol. 2013 Mar;12(1):3-11. doi: 10.1111/jocd.12019. PubMed PMID: 23438136.
138. Kikuchi K, Kobayashi H, Hirao T, Ito A, Takahashi H, Tagami H. Improvement of mild inflammatory changes of the facial skin induced by winter environment with daily applications of a moisturizing cream. A half-side test of biophysical skin parameters, cytokine expression pattern and the formation of cornified envelope. Dermatology. 2003;207(3):269-75. PubMed PMID: 14571069.
139. Winter treatments - Source Marine Facial and Cold Cream Marine Facial. Available From: https://totalbodyconcept.co.nz/blog/2018/06/winter-treatments-source-marine-facial-and-cold-cr
140. Web Vintage Adventures. 1961 POND'S SKIN CREAM vintage magazine advertisement. Available From: https://www.vintage-adventures.com/vintage-cosmetics-beauty-shaving-ads/2667-1961-pond-s-skin-cream-ad-special-formula-care.html

141. The Laszlo Glow. Imagine telling the most beautiful women in the world, "You need to wash your face." Elements Beauty Blog, Posted on July 10, 2017.
142. Draelos ZD. Cosmeceuticals: What's Real, What's Not. Dermatol Clin. 2019 Jan;37(1):107-115. doi: 10.1016/j.det.2018.07.001. Epub 2018 Nov 1. Review. PubMed PMID: 30466682.
143. Draelos ZD. A Novel Approach to Enhancing the Quality and Appearance of Photoaged Skin. J Drugs Dermatol. 2019 Jan 1;18(1):28-31. PubMed PMID: 30681790.
144. Lam C. Benefits of Day and Night Creams. Blog Let's Roll With Carol
145. Farris P, Zeichner J, Berson D. Efficacy and Tolerability of a Skin Brightening/Anti-Aging Cosmeceutical Containing Retinol 0.5%, Niacinamide, Hexylresorcinol, and Resveratrol. J Drugs Dermatol. 2016 Jul 1;15(7):863-8. PubMed PMID: 27391637.
146. Walters RM, Mao G, Gunn ET, Hornby S. Cleansing formulations that respect skin barrier integrity. Dermatol Res Pract. 2012;2012:495917. doi: 10.1155/2012/495917. Epub 2012 Aug 13. PubMed PMID: 22927835; PubMed Central PMCID: PMC3425021.
147. Hamed SH, Assakir I, Almalty AM, Bweir S. Does massage postapplication improve moisturizer's efficacy? A 2-week regression study. J Cosmet Dermatol. 2012 Sep;11(3):239-44. doi: 10.1111/j.1473-2165.2012.00626.x. PubMed PMID: 22938011.
148. Pyke C. Massage: a helping hand for people with chronic oedema and lymphoedema. Br J Community Nurs. 2010 Apr;15(4):S28-30. PubMed PMID: 20559174.
149. Barclay J, Vestey J, Lambert A, Balmer C. Reducing the symptoms of lymphoedema: is there a role for aromatherapy? Eur J Oncol Nurs. 2006 Apr;10(2):140-9. Epub 2006 Mar 23. PubMed PMID: 16563861.
150. Miyaji A, Sugimori K, Hayashi N. Short- and long-term effects of using a facial massage roller on facial skin blood flow and vascular reactivity. Complement Ther Med. 2018 Dec;41:271-276. doi: 10.1016/j.ctim.2018.09.009. Epub 2018 Sep 14. PubMed PMID: 30477852.
151. Holck DE, Ng JD. Facial skin rejuvenation. CurrOpinOphthalmol. 2003 Oct;14(5):246-52. Review. PubMed PMID: 14502051.
152. Hatayama T, Kitamura S, Tamura C, Nagano M, Ohnuki K. The facial massage reduced anxiety and negative mood status, and increased sympathetic nervous activity. Biomed Res. 2008 Dec;29(6):317-20. PubMed PMID: 19129675.
153. Aldag C, Nogueira Teixeira D, Leventhal PS. Skin rejuvenation using cosmetic products containing growth factors, cytokines, and matrikines: a review of the literature. Clin CosmetInvestig Dermatol. 2016 Nov 9;9:411-419. eCollection 2016. Review. PubMed PMID: 27877059; PubMed Central PMCID: PMC5108505.
154. Diana, Princess of Wales. Given by the photographer's widow, Diana Donovan, 1998. Web National Portrait Gallery, UK.
155. Picard C. 25 Beauty Secrets to Steal From Princess Diana. Web GoodHousekeeping.com, Mar 7, 2017

156. Nahar VK, Wilkerson AH, Ghafari G, Martin B, Black WH, Boyas JF, Savoy M, Bawa G, Stafford FC Jr, Scott M, Grigsby TB, Gromley Z, Grant-Kels JM, Brodell RT. Skin cancer knowledge, attitudes, beliefs, and prevention practices among medical students: A systematic search and literature review. Int J Womens Dermatol. 2018 Mar 14;4(3):139-149. doi: 10.1016/j.ijwd.2017.10.002. eCollection 2018 Sep. Review. PubMed PMID: 30175215; PubMed Central PMCID: PMC6116816.
157. Byun SY, Kwon SH, Heo SH, Shim JS, Du MH, Na JI. Efficacy of Slimming Cream Containing 3.5% Water-Soluble Caffeine and Xanthenes for the Treatment of Cellulite: Clinical Study and Literature Review. Ann Dermatol. 2015 Jun;27(3):243-9. doi: 10.5021/ad.2015.27.3.243. Epub 2015 May 29. PubMed PMID: 26082579; PubMed Central PMCID: PMC4466275.
158. Massage Cream Formulation - The Personal Formulator. Available From: www.thepersonalformulator.com/formulations/friendly/massagecream.htm
159. Ethylhexyl Palmitate. Available From: https://thedermreview.com/ethylhexyl-palmitate/
160. Guo X, Mei N. Aloe vera: A review of toxicity and adverse clinical effects. J Environ Sci Health C Environ CarcinogEcotoxicol Rev. 2016 Apr 2;34(2):77-96. doi: 10.1080/10590501.2016.1166826. Review. PubMed PMID: 26986231; PubMed Central PMCID: PMC6349368.
161. Kapoor S, Saraf S. Assessment of viscoelasticity and hydration effect of herbal moisturizers using bioengineering techniques. Pharmacogn Mag. 2010 Oct;6(24):298-304. doi: 10.4103/0973-1296.71797. PubMed PMID: 21120032; PubMed Central PMCID: PMC2992143.
162. Levin J, Miller R. A Guide to the Ingredients and Potential Benefits of Over-the-Counter Cleansers and Moisturizers for Rosacea Patients. J Clin Aesthet Dermatol. 2011 Aug;4(8):31-49. PubMed PMID: 21909456; PubMed Central PMCID: PMC3168246.
163. ChemConx Creamblend-20 4 Oz. Available From: https://www.saveoncitric.com/cealandce208.html
164. Summer A. Benefits of Grapeseed Oil for Hair. Available From: https://www.livestrong.com/article/265547-how-to-get-elmers-glue-out-of-hair/
165. Bail S, Stuebiger G, Krist S, Unterweger H, Buchbauer G. Characterisation of various grape seed oils by volatile compounds, triacylglycerol composition, total phenols and antioxidant capacity. Food Chem. 2008 Jun 1;108(3):1122-32. doi: 10.1016/j.foodchem.2007.11.063. Epub 2007 Dec 3. PubMed PMID: 26065780.
166. Web L'Oréal Paris USA. Caprylic. Available From: https://www.lorealparisusa.com /ingredient-library/caprylic.aspx
167. Dayan N, Sivalenka R, Chase J. Skin moisturization by hydrogenated polyisobutene--quantitative and visual evaluation. J Cosmet Sci. 2009 Jan-Feb;60(1):15-24. PubMed PMID: 19296892.
168. Personal Care Product Preservatives, And The Truth (Part II). Web Nature's Complement.
169. Germaben II-E. Available From: https://www.chemistrystore.com/Preservatives-Germaben_II-E.html

170. Germaben. Available From: https://www.revolvy.com/page/Germaben
171. Grammaticopoulos GT, Furtunopoulos DG, Zisova LG. Topically applied vitamins and their cutaneous effects. Folia Med (Plovdiv). 2004;46(2):18-24. Review. PubMed PMID: 15506546.
172. Yang M, Moclair B, Hatcher V, Kaminetsky J, Mekas M, Chapas A, Capodice J. A randomized, double-blind, placebo-controlled study of a novel pantothenic Acid-based dietary supplement in subjects with mild to moderate facial acne. Dermatol Ther (Heidelb). 2014 Jun;4(1):93-101. doi: 10.1007/s13555-014-0052-3. Epub 2014 May 16. PubMed PMID: 24831048; PubMed Central PMCID: PMC4065280.
173. Schagen SK, Zampeli VA, Makrantonaki E, Zouboulis CC. Discovering the link between nutrition and skin aging. Dermatoendocrinol. 2012 Jul 1;4(3):298-307. doi: 10.4161/derm.22876. PubMed PMID: 23467449; PubMed Central PMCID: PMC3583891.
174. Tanaka M, Okada M, Zhen YX, Inamura N, Kitano T, Shirai S, Sakamoto K, Inamura T, Tagami H. Decreased hydration state of the stratum corneum and reduced amino acid content of the skin surface in patients with seasonal allergic rhinitis. Br J Dermatol. 1998 Oct;139(4):618-21. PubMed PMID: 9892905.
175. van Logtestijn MD, Domínguez-Hüttinger E, Stamatas GN, Tanaka RJ. Resistance to water diffusion in the stratum corneum is depth-dependent. PLoS One. 2015 Feb 11;10(2):e0117292. doi: 10.1371/journal.pone.0117292. eCollection 2015. PubMed PMID: 25671323; PubMed Central PMCID: PMC4324936.
176. Spada F, Barnes TM, Greive KA. Skin hydration is significantly increased by a cream formulated to mimic the skin's own natural moisturizing systems. Clin CosmetInvestig Dermatol. 2018 Oct 15;11:491-497. doi: 10.2147/CCID.S177697. eCollection 2018. PubMed PMID: 30410378; PubMed Central PMCID: PMC6197824.
177. Greive K. Cleansers and moisturisers: The basics. Wound Pract Res. 2015;23(2):78–81.
178. Levin J, Miller R. A Guide to the Ingredients and Potential Benefits of Over-the-Counter Cleansers and Moisturizers for Rosacea Patients. J Clin Aesthet Dermatol. 2011 Aug;4(8):31-49. PubMed PMID: 21909456; PubMed Central PMCID: PMC3168246.
179. Lee T, Friedman A. Skin Barrier Health: Regulation and Repair of the Stratum Corneum and the Role of Over-the-Counter Skin Care. J Drugs Dermatol. 2016 Sep 1;15(9):1047-51. Review. PubMed PMID: 27602965.
180. Towey JJ, Dougan L. Structural examination of the impact of glycerol on water structure. J Phys Chem B. 2012 Feb 9;116(5):1633-41. doi: 10.1021/jp2093862. Epub 2011 Dec 13. PubMed PMID: 22126327.
181. Jownie JB. Understanding moisturizers and their clinical benefits. Pract Dermatol Pediatr. 2010:19–22.
182. Lodén M. Role of topical emollients and moisturizers in the treatment of dry skin barrier disorders. Am J Clin Dermatol. 2003;4(11):771-88. Review. PubMed PMID: 14572299.

183. Schwarz K, Huang SW, German JB, Tiersch B, Hartmann J, Frankel EN. Activities of antioxidants are affected by colloidal properties of oil-in-water and water-in-oil emulsions and bulk oils. J Agric Food Chem. 2000 Oct;48(10):4874-82. PubMed PMID: 11052748.
184. Moore K. What Causes Dry Skin and How to Treat It. Medically reviewed by Cynthia Cobb, DNP, APRN. Healthline, May 10, 2018.
185. Isopropyl Linoleate. Available From: https://cosmeticsinfo.org/ingredient/isopropyl-linoleate-0
186. Ballmann C, Mueller BW. Stabilizing effect of cetostearyl alcohol and glyceryl monostearate as co-emulsifiers on hydrocarbon-free O/W glyceride creams. Pharm Dev Technol. 2008;13(5):433-45. doi: 10.1080/10837450802247952 . PubMed PMID: 18728995.
187. Kurohane K, Kimura A, Terasawa R, Sahara Y, Kobayashi K, Suzuki W, Matsuoka T, Watanabe T, Imai Y. Adjuvant Effect of an Alternative Plasticizer, Diisopropyl Adipate, on a Contact Hypersensitivity Mouse Model: Link with Sensory Ion Channel TRPA1 Activation. Biol Pharm Bull. 2015;38(7):1054-62. doi: 10.1248/bpb.b15-00199. Epub 2015 May 9. PubMed PMID: 25959058.
188. What is Diisopropyl Adipate? Available From: https://www.chemoxy.com/products-and-applications/products/chemoxycare-range/diisopropyl-adipate/
189. PEG 40 Stearate. Available From: https://www.truthinaging.com/ingredients/peg-40-stearate
190. Alcohol in Skincare Products. Available From: https://blackpaint.sg/alcohol-in-skincare/
191. Ceteareth-20 - Truth In Aging. Available From: https://www.truthinaging.com/ingredients/ceteareth-20
192. Johnson W Jr, Heldreth B, Bergfeld WF, Belsito DV, Hill RA, Klaassen CD, Liebler DC, Marks JG Jr, Shank RC, Slaga TJ, Snyder PW, Andersen FA. Safety Assessment of Polyquaternium-22 and Polyquarternium-39 as Used in Cosmetics. Int JToxicol. 2016 Nov;35(3 suppl):47S-53S. PubMed PMID: 27913787.
193. Quaternium-22. The Toxin and Toxin Target Database (T3DB).Available From:http://www.t3db.ca/toxins/T3D3633
194. National Center for Biotechnology Information. PubChem Database. Hydroxyethylcellulose, CID=4327536, https://pubchem.ncbi.nlm.nih.gov/compound/4327536 (accessed on Apr. 20, 2019)
195. National Center for Biotechnology Information. PubChem Database. Propylene glycol, CID=1030, https://pubchem.ncbi.nlm.nih.gov/compound/1030 (accessed on Apr. 20, 2019)
196. Wan DC, Wong VW, Longaker MT, Yang GP, Wei FC. Moisturizing different racial skin types. J Clin Aesthet Dermatol. 2014 Jun;7(6):25-32. Review. PubMed PMID: 25013536; PubMed Central PMCID: PMC4086530.
197. Allergic Skin Disorders. Available From: https://www.medicinenet.com/image-collection/xerosis_picture/picture.htm

198. The Influence of Emollients on Dermal and Transdermal Drug Delivery. Available From: https://plasticsurgerykey.com/the-influence-of-emollients-on-dermal-and-transdermal-drug-delivery/
199. Purnamawati S, Indrastuti N, Danarti R, Saefudin T. The Role of Moisturizers in Addressing Various Kinds of Dermatitis: A Review. Clin Med Res. 2017 Dec;15(3-4):75-87. doi: 10.3121/cmr.2017.1363. Epub 2017 Dec 11. Review. PubMed PMID: 29229630; PubMed Central PMCID: PMC5849435.
200. Dyble T, Ashton J. Use of emollients in the treatment of dry skin conditions. Br J Community Nurs. 2011 May;16(5):214, 216, 218 passim. Review. PubMed PMID: 21642925.
201. Lodén M. The clinical benefit of moisturizers. J Eur Acad Dermatol Venereol. 2005 Nov;19(6):672-88; quiz 686-7. Review. PubMed PMID: 16268870.
202. Lazar AP, Lazar P. Dry skin, water, and lubrication. Dermatol Clin. 1991 Jan;9(1):45-51. Review. PubMed PMID: 2022097.
203. Nalawade TM, Bhat K, Sogi SH. Bactericidal activity of propylene glycol, glycerine, polyethylene glycol 400, and polyethylene glycol 1000 against selected microorganisms. J Int Soc Prev Community Dent. 2015 Mar-Apr;5(2):114-9. doi: 10.4103/2231-0762.155736. PubMed PMID: 25992336; PubMed Central PMCID: PMC4415329.
204. Shokrollahi K. Paraffin-based ointments and fire hazard: understanding the problem, navigating the media and currently available downloadable patient information. Scars Burn Heal. 2017 Apr 12;3:2059513117704932. doi: 10.1177/2059513117704932. eCollection 2017 Jan-Dec. PubMed PMID: 29799576; PubMed Central PMCID: PMC5965335.
205. Nola I, Kostović K, Kotrulja L, Lugović L. The use of emollients as sophisticated therapy in dermatology. Acta Dermatovenerol Croat. 2003;11(2):80-7. Review. PubMed PMID: 12773264.
206. Ugandar RE, Deivi KS. Formulation And Evaluation Of Natural Palm Oil Based Vanishing Cream. IJPSR, 2013; Vol. 4(9): 3375-3380. DOI :http://dx.doi.org/10.13040/IJPSR.0975-8232.4(9).3375-80
207. Know Your Cream. Available From: https://www.createwithcream.ph /knowyourcream/types-of-cream
208. Draelos ZD. Active agents in common skin care products. PlastReconstr Surg. 2010 Feb;125(2):719-24. doi: 10.1097/PRS.0b013e3181c83192. Review. PubMed PMID: 20124857.
209. Zoe Diana Draelos. Cosmetics and Dermatologic Problems and Solutions, published by CRC Press, 2011 ISBN 1841847410, 9781841847412
210. Susan West Kurz, Tom Monte. Awakening Beauty: The Dr. Hauschka Way, published by CLAIRVIEW BOOKS, 2006, ISBN 1905570031, 9781905570034
211. John L. Pfenninger, Grant C. Fowler. Pfenninger and Fowler's Procedures for Primary Care, Elsevier Health Sciences, 2010 ISBN 1455700924, 9781455700929
212. H. Butler. Poucher's Perfumes, Cosmetics and Soaps, published by Springer Science & Business Media, 2013 ISBN 9401727341, 9789401727341

213. Difference between Moisturizer and Cold Cream. Available From: http://www.differencebetween.info/difference-between-moisturizer-and-cold-cream
214. Choquenet B, Couteau C, Paparis E, Coiffard LJ. Foundations and self-tanning products: Do they provide any protection from the sun? J Dermatol. 2009 Nov;36(11):587-91. doi: 10.1111/j.1346-8138.2009.00714.x. PubMed PMID: 19878391.
215. Lee SY, Baek JH, Shin MK, Koh JS. The quantitative analysis of spreadability, coverage, and adhesion effect after application of the base make-up product. Skin Res Technol. 2014 Aug;20(3):341-6. doi: 10.1111/srt.12124. Epub 2013 Dec 12. PubMed PMID: 24329816.
216. Aliesh Pierce. Milady's Aesthetician Series: Treating Diverse Pigmentation, published by Cengage Learning, 2012 ISBN 1133712193, 9781133712190
217. From the Bottom Up: Contemporary Foundation Formulations. Available From: https://knowledge.ulprospector.com/7389/pcc-contemporary-foundation-formulations/
218. Shocking side effect of foundation cream. Available From: http://www.naijapr.com/shocking-side-effect-of-foundation-cream/
219. Abraham A, Roga G. Topical steroid-damaged skin. Indian J Dermatol. 2014 Sep;59(5):456-9. doi: 10.4103/0019-5154.139872. PubMed PMID: 25284849; PubMed Central PMCID: PMC4171912.
220. Singh A. Pharmaceutical creams. Web slideshare.net
221. Brotherton H. These are the foundations celebrities swear by From Kim Kardashian to Gigi Hadid... Glamour Magazine, UK 28 March 2018.
222. Blackstone T. Jessica Alba's Reinvention. redbook, March 15, 2018.

CHAPTER 3

SKIN LIGHTENING AND MANAGEMENT OF HYPERPIGMENTATION

3.1 BACKGROUND

Skin bleaching, a practice to chemically lighten the skin, has become increasingly more common around the world in the past 40-60 years. Historically, skin bleaching actually starts in the Victorian era with the age of powder and paint, the precursor to us wearing foundation. Queen Elizabeth (1st) was known to take arsenic complexion wafers, which were essentially little bits of poison to give her that ghostly look. Her early and meticulous efforts to appear ghostly white and nearly transparent during her 16th century rule soon became known as the "Elizabethan ideal of beauty". To great surprise, the history of skin whitening practice began within the white community itself. European women were painting their faces with lead paint. Even fair look women were involved in whiteness because it was their way of communicating purity. And at that time, the race was being solidified as a concept and whiteness was being defined as pure. The 1920s were the heyday of the French colonial empire. At that time France controlled more land in Africa than any other European country. During the colonization process, they imported their language, norms and traditions to Africa, where they imposed on local populations. Colonized populations sought to imitate the light skin of their colonizers to enhance their quality of life and improve their self-image. Black women in the Western Cape Province, in particular, were more likely to find employment as domestic workers and cooks if they appeared to have a lighter complexion. European colonization practices from Asia to Africa to India during the later half of the second millennium rapidly began to spread these beliefs to all corners of the globe. Among such ideologies were associations of darkness and blackness with primitiveness, unrestrained sexuality, and pollution, while whiteness was associated with purity, power, and beauty. Throughout medieval and modern history, the Indian subcontinent has been on the radar of various European settlers and traders, including, from the 15th to 17th centuries, the Portuguese, Dutch and French. The subcontinent was invaded and partly ruled by the Mughals in the 16th century, and colonized by the British from the 17th century onwards until independence in 1947. All these foreign "visitors" were of relatively fair complexion, and many claimed to be superior. According to a study we conducted from 2013 to 2016, 70% of the 300 women and men we interviewed reported wanting a date or partner with someone who had light skin. This colorism is what pushes so many Indians to lighten their skin, creating a phenomenon termed "bleaching syndrome". "Let's scrub out that tan" is a common refrain in beauty parlors in the Indian subcontinent, where girls grow up with constant reminders that only fair skin is beautiful. Even sentiments like, "She got lucky that he married her despite her [dark] complexion" are still whispered around. Skin fairness products include whitening and skin-lightening creams, face washes, deodorants, and lotions. This industry is one of the fastest growing segments of the global beauty industry, particularly in Asia and Africa, with marketing forecasters predicting it will be worth an estimated $US 31.2 billion by 2024.

3.2 ABSTRACT

Skin color, along with hair and eye color, is genetically determined by the amount of melanin found in the top layers of skin. Its varied presence – which accounts for different skin colors – is linked to a population's historic levels of sun exposure. Skin-lightening is just one of the multiple options for augmenting the skin's surface appearance, including but not limited to tanning, scarification, makeup, tattooing, face lifts, nose jobs, botox, lip extensions, and piercings. Skin-bleaching practices, such as using skin creams and soaps to achieve a lighter skin tone, are common throughout the world and are triggered by cosmetic reasons that oftentimes have deep historical, economic, sociocultural, and psychosocial roots. The cosmetics industry has traditionally relied on convincing people that they are incomplete without a particular product. Yet, unlike makeup or fake tan, skin-whitening creams base beauty on a racial hierarchy, fueling intolerance and causing serious social harm. Lighter and fairer skin is something that everyone craves for, and celebrities play a massive part in paving the way. Just like ladies, men also aspire to get immaculate, glowing and healthy-looking skin to accentuate their personality and overall looks. It's for everyone to understand that men feel shy to discuss the skincare routines as they feel it's all-girl stuff. But there is no denying that even boys need to uplift and improve their skin texture to feel good. Studies have documented the use of skin fairness products, sometimes referred to as "skin whitening products," "skin bleaching products," "depigmenting agents," in

Africa, Europe, North America, and Asia, with prevalence of use ranging from 30 to 80% among various community samples. Skin fairness products include whitening and skin-lightening creams, face washes, deodorants, and lotions. These agents act in different ways to lighten skin, but generally work by suppressing the production of melanin, the pigment which gives human skin its color. While traditionally a female practice, use has also become more popular among men in recent years. These agents selectively target hyperplastic melanocytes and inhibit key regulatory steps in melanin synthesis. Historically marketed to women, companies have recently expanded their offerings to include products designed and marketed specifically for men. Advertisements and packaging overtly claim that products will make consumers' skin fairer and more even-toned, while product names and the use of well-known models and actors in advertisements imply that they will enhance consumers' cultural capital via improvements in attractiveness, youthfulness, confidence, and success. The relevance of skin fairness products to public health is highlighted by the scope of the industry, the widespread use of these products, and the potential health risks associated with their use. Skin-whitening cosmetics are a multi-billion-dollar industry pushing the idea that beauty equates with white skin and that lightening dark skin is both achievable and preferable.

Key Terms: skin bleaching; whiteners; hyperpigmentation; fairness creams; melasma; tyrosinase inhibitors; dark skin; melanosomes

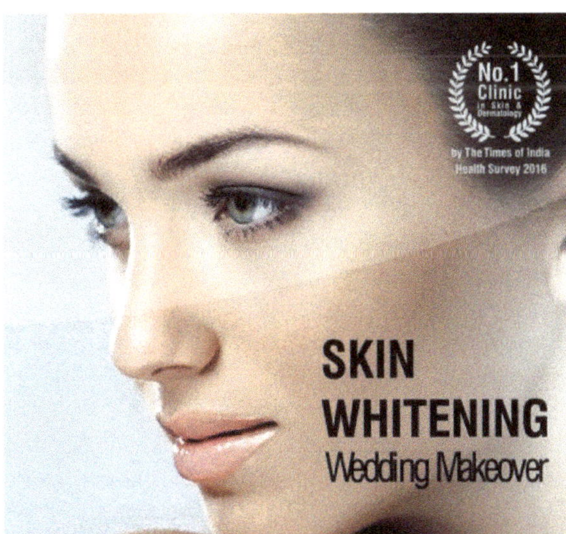

A typical advertisement pointing at a sensitive issue of Indian unwed women. But recently, researchers have found that skin whitening or fairness cream advertisements are playing a major role in creating skin-based discrimination in society and disgracing womanhood. The manufacturers broadcast enticing advertisements to attract customers. Most of the time, advertisers make false and misleading promises (Courtacy: Justdial).

3.3. INTRODUCTION

Global aesthetic regimes continue to emphasize on, and preference for, lighter shades of brown. Consumer choice now fashions lightening as a form of human agency, where the surface of the skin can be manipulated to conform to, or resist global and local beauty standards. Capitalism is thus implicated in the process of commoditization identity politics. The belief and practice to have lighter skin has been rooted from ancient times. For instance, the Chinese myth believes that pearls can lighten one's complexion by taking a small amount of pearl powder together with hot water every day. Children are grown up with stories like "Snow White" a princess skin as white as snow and lips red as blood and hair black as ebony. Sure, for a little girl who wants to be a fairy princess the idea of ethereal, magical, mystical and winged creatures all come to mind. TV, movies, radio, and general culture give us the tools to draw these pictures, however, they also give us, directly or indirectly, a standard by which to live, think, and believe. Every time we turn on the TV, listen to the radio, read a magazine, or simply go out somewhere, we get our daily dose. Women are going to extremes to enhance their body image. Curvier, lighter-skinned women are considered more beautiful, more successful and more likely to get married. Skin color bias affects people psychologically. It affects how a child performs in school because their confidence level goes down: they feel they are not good enough. And when it comes to marriage, we again find skin color plays such a vital role. Women are now embracing anything thrown at them to increase the size of their breasts, hips and change their complexion to suit the community 'standard of beauty'. However, skin lightening products are readily available from major cosmetics companies, from local convenience stores, and widely over the internet. Although both men and women engage in the skin lightening practice, of various sorts, women generally have higher rates of practice than men. Hyperpigmentation-related diseases include melasma, lentigines, nevus, ephelis, freckles, post-inflammatory hyperpigmentation, and age spots. Post-inflammatory hyperpigmentation appears in many skin conditions, including acne, eczema, and contact dermatitis. Multiple agents are available for the treatment of hyperpigmentation, a cosmetically important condition seen most often in middle-aged and elderly individuals and resulting from exposure to ultraviolet light, certain drugs or chemicals, or the existence of disease. Therapeutic interventions include whitening agents, chemical peels, lasers, and physical methods. Many skin-lightening agents cause skin irritation and require months of use before results appear, and some agents are only partly effective. Although multiple interventions are available, skin-whitening agents, due to their simplicity and convenience, continue to be the mainstay of approach to either lighten skin (individuals who wish to change or modify their skin color) in the cosmetic field or depigment skin (treatment for abnormal hyperpigmentation skin such as melasma, freckles, and actinic lentigines) in the clinical therapy. Chromameter measurements are useful in measuring skin tone and color in products claiming evenness of skin tone or skin whitening as well as the reduction of redness when measuring anti-irritant and anti-inflammatory benefits. There are two types of whitening creams – those that 'lighten', and those that 'bleach'. Bleaching creams contain harsh chemicals that inhibit the production of melanin, and quite rapidly make the skin whiter. Lightening creams, however, don't necessarily contain these chemicals, but will promise to whiten the skin with long-term use. Skin whitening is a lucrative business in many countries where beauty clinics proliferate and skin-whiteners account for more than half of the sales in facial creams. The ideal depigmentation compound should have a potent, rapid, and selective bleaching effect on hyperactivated melanocytes, carry no short- or long-term side effects, and lead to a permanent removal of undesired pigment. Depigmentation can be achieved by regulating (a) the transcription and activity of tyrosinase, tyrosinase related protein-1 (TRP-1), tyrosinase related protein-2 (TRP-2), and/or peroxidase, (b) the uptake and distribution of melanosomes in recipient keratinocytes, and (c) melanin and melanosome degradation and turnover of "pigmented keratinocytes.

3.4 GLOBAL DEMAND FOR SKIN LIGHTENING

Global industry analysts (GIA) have predicted that the universal market for skin lighteners will reach $23 billion by 2020, driven by new markets in Asia, particularly India, Japan and China. This industry is one of the fastest- growing segments of the global beauty industry, particularly in Asia and Africa, with marketing forecasters predicting it will be worth an estimated $US 31.2 billion by 2024. Approximately $13 billion spent on skin care products and cosmetics in Asia Pacific's. This is particularly relevant in Asian countries, including India, Japan, Korea, China, and Thailand, where skin fairness has been understood to be a cultural marker of class, wealth, and social status for centuries. Studies located in Asia, USA, U.K., India, China and the Caribbean indicate the prevalence of a thriving skin lightening cream industry. The regular and sustained use of skin bleaching products has been practiced in African and Asian contexts for decades, with prevalence estimates from 25% to 96%. China accounts for about 40% of sales in Asia, Japan 21% and Korea approximately 18%. Whitening creams account for half of the $320 million Thai market for facial creams, according to research firm Nielsen. The preference to have white skin has driven the skin lightening industry. This phenomenon was reflected in the domination of skin lightening products in the Asian skincare market with 60% of sales. A WHO survey found that nearly 40% of women polled in nations including China, Malaysia, the Philippines, and South Korea said they regularly used whitening products. In India, 60% of the skincare market consisted of whitening products, with estimates of its worth varying between $US 450–535 million. A nearly 40% of the sample reported currently using skin fairness products, with women being two times more likely to use these products. Among current users, 17% reported past experiences of adverse side effects, and "Media/TV/Adverts" were the most common prompts for using fairness products, followed by "Friends" and "Family." Men were significantly more likely than women to endorse beliefs about fairness being more attractive and were more likely to perceive family and peers as viewing fairness as beneficial for cultural capital. A recent survey showed that 80% of Indian men use fairness creams and the number of consumer's are growing 18% annually. There were no differences between women and men currently using products in their desire to look as fair as media celebrities. Among non-users, women were significantly more likely than men to report concerns about product efficacy and side effects as reasons for non-use, while men were significantly more likely to report socioeconomic reasons for non-use. In three different African countries, the statistics demonstrate that 25% of women in Bamako, Mali a further 52% in Dakar, Senegal, and 77% in Lagos, Nigeria use skin lighteners. Such practices are reinforced by a belief that fairer skin is associated with beauty, self-esteem, and financial and social advantages among Saudi women. Aside from how gender plays an important role in practicing skin lightening, the range of age is also an important factor. A study shows that the majority of samples focus on female age ranging between 20 and 30 years (more than 50% in one study and more than 70% in another one). The sales of skin lightening products increase by 100% every year (2007-2012) in Malaysia. In a study of 450 Nigerians who confessed the use of lightening creams, a nearly 70% were women and around 30% were men. Lighter skin not only enhances the perception of greater attraction but also enhances the appearances of tattoos on skin as the darker colored tattoos contrasts better with light skin than dark skin [1-10].

3.5 SKIN BRIGHTENING VS. LIGHTENING VS. WHITENING

The terms lightening, whitening, brightening and bleaching are often used interchangeably. Skin bleaching is a term that was more popular in the 80's than it is today, and is essentially the same as skin whitening. The difference between skin lightening and whitening is largely based on the degree/severity with which melanin production is reduced. *Skin lightening* is used when the method is more gradual and the effect less obvious while whitening is used to describe a more aggressive technique. Both techniques use tyrosinase inhibitors to block the skin's production of melanin. Lightening creams work to reduce the melanin pigmentation in a particular area on the skin. It has to do with discoloration and evening of skin tone. Skin lighteners can be both over-the-counter products or skin care products that target brown spots, dark spots, age spots, freckles, etc. Instead of affecting the whole face, skin lightening agents seek to reduce the darkness in one area or spot on the face. These spots usually occur from sun damage, so it can take time to see results. Lightening reduces pigmentation, lightens discoloration and evens skin tone. Skin lightening products target particular areas of discolorations like age spots and hyperpigmentation from acne breakouts and bruising. Lightening products are best used for a limited time. *Skin whitening* uses stronger inhibitors such as hydroquinone or mercury to strip the skin of its melanin. Skin Brightening is an entirely different concept. Our skin is continuously creating new skin cells to replace older skin cells, and often, these dead skin cells remain on the skin's surface and can cause it to appear dull. Exfoliation removes these dead skin cells from the skin's surface, thereby revitalizing it and making it look more radiant and "brighter". Brightening here is achieved with ingredients such as alpha and beta hydroxy acids, vitamins A, E and C that help the skin to naturally shed dead skin cells. Some brightening products may also contain natural extracts and antioxidants that have lightening properties e.g. licorice root extract to help gradually fade dark spots. *Skin brighteners* are skin care products that make skin brighter and more even throughout the entire face. Brightening is more about restoring vibrancy to the skin. Hydroquinone, Kojic Acid, Arbutine, Vitamin C, retinol, Niacinamide, Licorice Extract act as skin brighteners. Brightening can also be used to describe products that help to increase cell turnover and therefore speed up the flaking away of damaged upper layers of the skin to reveal the beautiful baby-soft skin below. There is overlap between ingredients for both. Using all those ingredients can address both issues. In addition to stimulating collagen production, which will soften lines and wrinkles, peels firm skin and even our skin tone. Repetitive peels can also help to reduce pore size, fade discolorations, improve rosacea, as well as treat and prevent acne [11-17].

3.6 SKIN PIGMENTATION

Visible pigmentation of the skin, hair, and eyes depends primarily on the functions of melanocytes, a very minor population of cells that specialize in the synthesis and distribution of the pigmented biopolymer melanin. Melanocytes are melanin-producing precursor cells (called melanoblasts) cells embryological development found in skin, hair follicles, eyes, inner ear, bones, heart and brain of humans. They arise from pluripotent neural crest cells and differentiate in response to a complex network of interacting regulatory pathways. Melanins are pigment molecules that are endogenously synthesized by melanocytes. The light absorption of melanin in skin and hair leads to photoreceptor shielding, thermoregulation, photoprotection, camouflage and display coloring. Melanins are also powerful cation chelators and may act as free radical sinks [18,19]. The number of melanocytes is relatively comparable among different ethnicities and variations in skin color are mainly dependent on the type (the relative quantity of pheo and eumelanins) and the amount of melanin produced within melanosomes. Size, quantity, distribution and degradation of these structures in the surrounding keratinocytes are also determinants in ethnic color differences. In light skin, melanosomes are smaller and mainly at an early stage of maturation (stages I and II). They are transferred to keratinocytes (**Figure 3.1**) as clusters and are degraded at the level of the spinous layer. In dark skin, these structures are larger, at stage IV and are singly transferred to the surrounding cells. Their degradation appears also slower than that in the light skin, being some melanins yet observed in the stratum corneum. Moreover, the ratio between pheo and eumelanins appears higher in dark versus light skins [20].

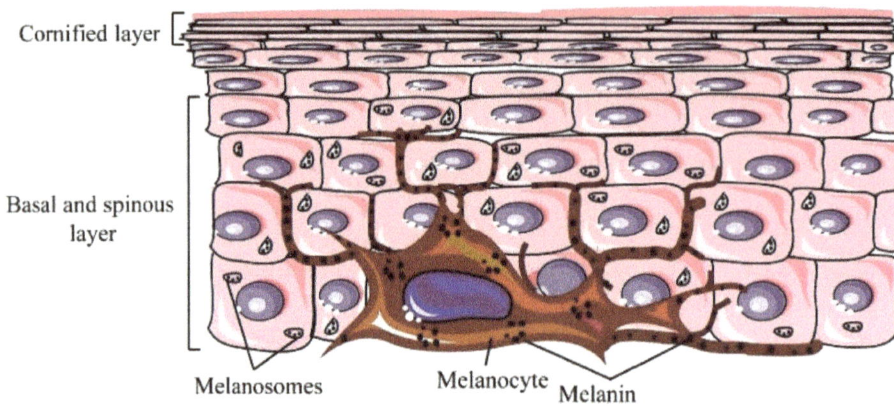

Figure 3.1 Association of keratinocytes and melanocytes [18]. The dendritic melanocyte is located in the basal layer of skin and produces melanin. Melanin pigments in melanosomes are transferred to keratinocytes.

Cutaneous melanin pigment plays a critical role in camouflage, mimicry, social communication, and protection against the harmful effects of solar radiation. Pigmentation in skin is determined by various physiological processes occurring at different stages:

(a) Development of melanocytes
(b) Density of melanocytes
(c) Expression of the enzymatic and structural constituents of melanosomes
(d) Synthesis of melanin
(e) Transport of melanosomes to dendrites
(f) Transfer of melanosomes to keratinocytes
(g) Distribution of melanin in the supra basal layers of the skin [21]

Maranduca et.al, 2019 stated that the melanin molecule plays a role in the skin pigmentation and offers photoprotection to the organism by absorbing the sun ultraviolet radiation, due to its specific chemical structure. The color of the skin, hair and eyes is determined by the melanic pigments, and more precisely the ratio between the two types of melanic pigment. The quantity of melanic pigment offers the skin the color from white (lack of melanic pigment) to black (increased melanin density), and the ratio eumelanin-pheomelanin determines the differences in pigmentation of the human skin (**Figure 3.2**). If the quantity of pheomelanin produced by the epidermal melanocytes is higher compared to the quantity of eumelanin, then the skin is of lighter color and has a higher susceptibility to the sun burns. In the skin containing a higher quantity of pheomelanin, following the exposure of the sun ultraviolet radiation, a higher quantity of reactive species of oxygen is produced, leading to a cellular lesion and initiating the carcinogen process [22]. The general geographic patterns of skin pigmentation show a strong correlation with latitude and UVR intensity. Skin pigmentation tends to be darker in equatorial and tropical regions (Sub-Saharan Africa, South Asia, Australia and Melanesia) where UVR levels are higher than in regions distant to the equator [23].

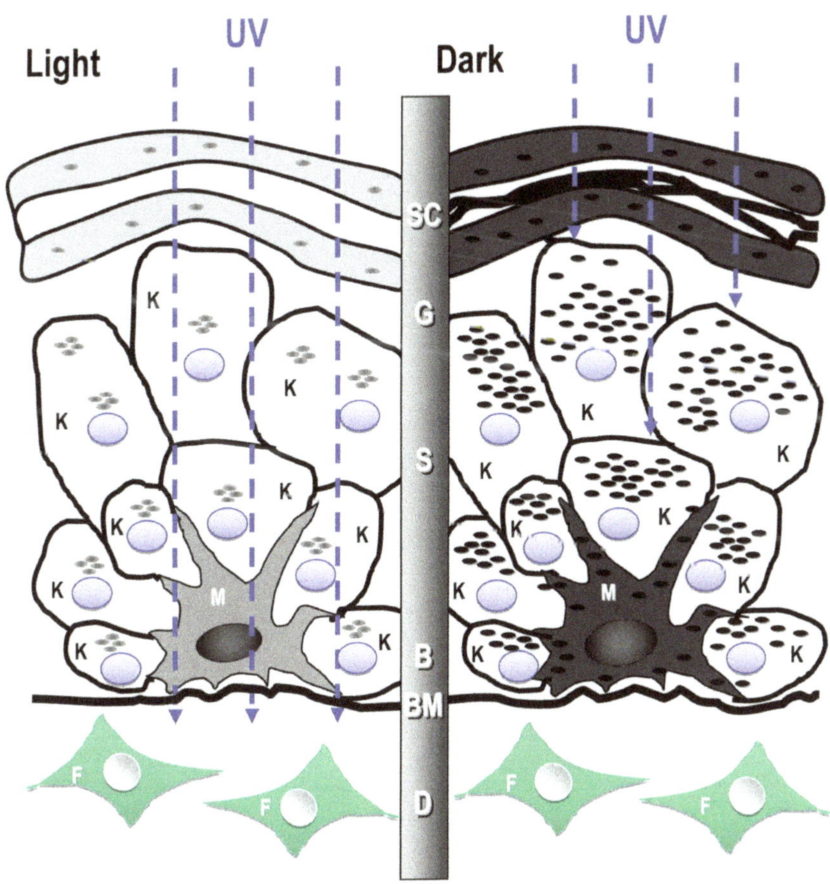

Figure 3.2 Schematic of human skin architecture from light- and dark-pigmented skin types [18]. From top to bottom: SC, stratum corneum; G, stratum granulosum; S, stratum spinosum; B, stratum basale; BM, basement membrane; D, dermis. Cell types: K, keratinocyte; M, melanocyte; F, fibroblast; shaded oval, melanin granule.

The first step of the biosynthesis of both eumelanin and pheomelanin begins the same way. Tyrosine is converted into dihydroxyphenylalanine (DOPA), which requires tyrosine hydroxylase and tetrahydrobiopterin as a cofactor. The enzyme tyrosinase then converts dihydroxyphenylalanine into dopaquinone, which can follow a variety of pathways to form the eumelanin or pheomelanin. The primary stimulus for melanogenesis and subsequent melanosome production is UV radiation, which upregulates melanocyte production of pro-opiomelanocortin (POMC) and its downstream products, alpha-melanocyte-stimulating hormone (alpha-MSH) and adrenocorticotropic hormone (ACTH). The overall effect is to increase eumelanin production (**Figure 3.3**). (Interestingly, people with pro-opiomelanocortin mutations have red hair and Fitzpatrick skin type 1 due to the relative increase in pheomelanin to eumelanin expression) [24,25].

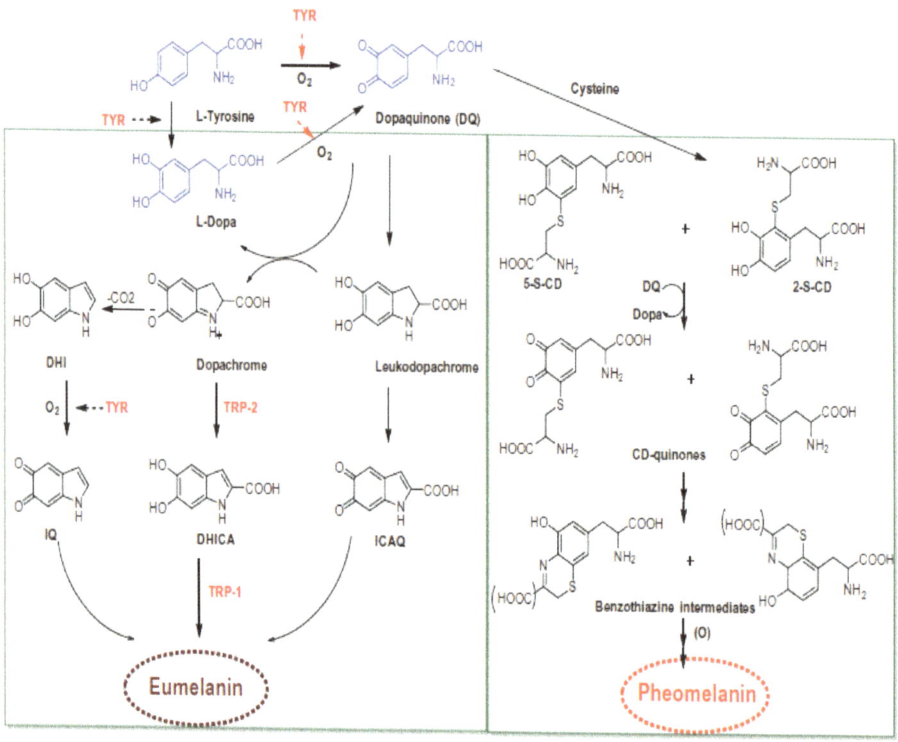

Figure 3.3 Melanogenesis pathway (production of eumelanin and pheomelanin) [1]. (Tyr: tyrosinase; DQ: dopaquinone; L-Dopa: L-3:4-dihydroxyphenylalanine; DHICA: 5,6-dihydroxyindole-2 carboxylic acid; DHI: 5,6-dihydroxyindole; ICAQ: indole-2-carboxylic acid-5,6-quinone; IQ: indole-5,6-quinone; HBTA: 5-hydroxy-1,4-benzothiazinylalanine).

3.7 REGULATION OF SKIN PIGMENTATION

Given that melanocytes are present in a variety of tissues in the body, the initiation and extent of pigmentation or melanogenesis can be influenced several intrinsic and extrinsic factors. In addition, melanogenesis can also be influenced by predetermined genetic factors such as age and ethnicity, and this process has evolved to provide protection and maintenance of homeostasis. Extrinsic factors include UVR and certain chemical compounds, while intrinsic factors include molecules secreted by surrounding keratinocytes, fibroblasts, inflammatory, neural or endocrine cells which are affected by conditions such as pregnancy and diabetes [18].

A. Intrinsic regulation of skin pigmentation

In human skin, melanogenesis is a tightly regulated process. Indeed, several extracellular signals are transduced via dedicated signaling pathways and mostly converge to MITF, a transcription factor integrating upstream signaling and regulating downstream genes involved in the various inherent mechanisms modulating melanogenesis. The synthesis of melanin pigments occurs in melanocytes inside melanosomes where melanogenic enzymes (tyrosinase and related proteins) are addressed with the help of specific protein complexes. The melanosomes loaded with melanin are then transferred to keratinocytes. Melanocytes produce Proopiomelanocortin (POMC) peptides, cytokines, NO, prostaglandins, and leukotrienes, which act via an autocrine or paracrine way on keratinocytes, and are involved in immune and inflammatory responses. Keratinocytes also produce several factors in response to UVR exposure, with paracrine action on melanocytes, which may stimulate or inhibit melanogenesis. The increase in estrogen levels during pregnancy can cause hyperpigmentation (melasma, areolar hyperpigmentation and line nigricans). Catecholamines may be produced by keratinocytes from L-DOPA, the melanin precursor, and can bind to α1 and β2 adrenergic receptors in melanocytes, stimulating melanogenesis via the cAMP pathway and Protein kinase C-β (PKC-β). Besides this canonical regulation, melanogenesis can also be modulated by other non-specific intrinsic pathways (hormonal environment, inflammation) and by extrinsic factors (solar irradiation such as ultraviolet irradiation, environmental pollution) [26,27]. MITF has been investigated intensively among the many transcription factors known to regulate melanocyte function. MITF itself is regulated by many other transcription factors, including PAX3 (a neural-crest-associated transcription factor), SOX9, SOX10, LEF-1/TCF (a downstream regulator of Wnt signaling pathway), and CREB (cAMP responsive-element-binding protein, which is phosphorylated by signals via MC1R, melanocortin-1 receptor) [28].

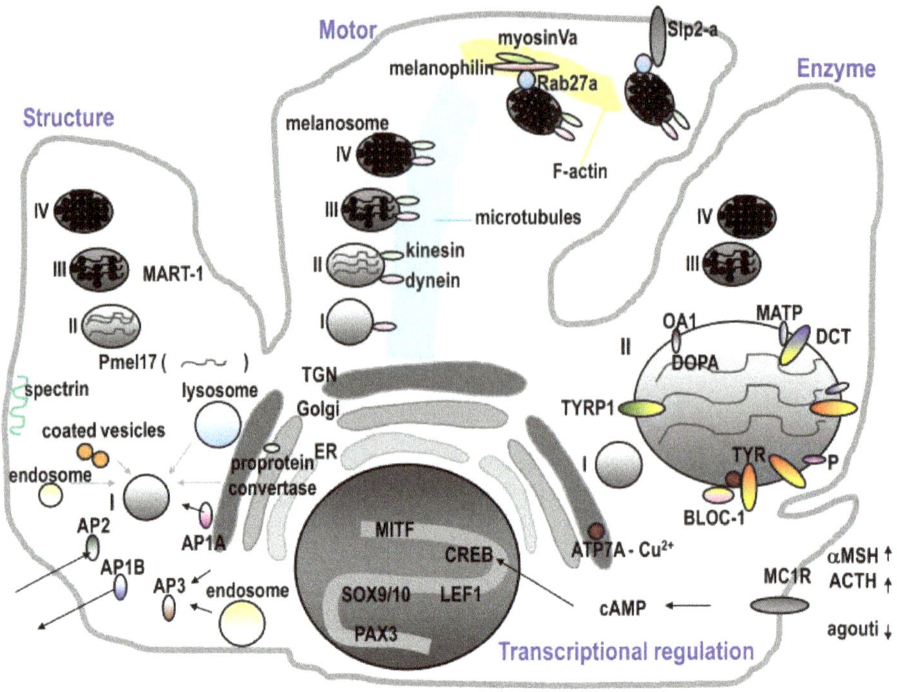

Figure 3.4 Factors that affect skin pigmentation within melanocytes [29]. Schemes show components involved in melanosome structure (left), transport (middle), enzyme (right) and transcriptional (bottom) related factors. Abbreviations: Microphthalmia-associated transcription factor (MITF); Adrenocorticotropic hormone (ACTH); α-Melanocyte-stimulating hormone (α-MSH); melanocortin type 1 receptor (MC1R).

B. Extrinsic regulation of skin pigmentation by ultraviolet radiation (UVR)

UVR increases proliferation and/or recruitment of melanocytes, the number of dendrites, and the transfer of melanosomes to a supranuclear location on the keratinocytes for DNA photoprotection. On the other hand, the expression of POMC peptides, MC1-R, and melanogenic enzymes increases in keratinocytes and melanocytes respectively. UVR has numerous effects on the skin, including DNA damage, tanning, vitamin D synthesis, carcinogenesis, and immunomodulation. In keratinocytes, UV-mediated DNA damage activates p53, which then binds and activates the POMC gene. The POMC polypeptide is post-translationally cleaved, producing adrenocorticotropic hormone, α-MSH, and β-endorphin. Secreted keratinocyte-derived α-MSH then signals to melanocytes via the MC1R, a G protein-coupled receptor. The pigmentation (tanning) response is an adaptation that provides some delayed protection against further DNA damage and carcinogenesis, while the opioid response may be an evolutionary adaptation for promoting sun-seeking behavior to prevent vitamin D deficiency [27], [30,31].

Exhibit 1. Management of Hyperpigmented Disorders Linked to Sun Light [23]
The first line of treatment is to avoid the causative or aggravating factor, i.e., sun light exposure, by using sun- blocking agents. Such protection has shown to reduce the incidence or relapse of melasma. In association with UV blocking agents, the second line of treatment may be physical therapies (cryotherapy, laser, IPD, dermoabrasion) or chemical peels which are quite efficient for the treatment of hyperpigmentation. However, they are usually not sustainable and associated with relapses. The risks of side effects such as hypo- or hyperpigmentation (PIH) specially in dark skins phototypes is also high with these procedures. Alternatively, less invasive and costly than physical modalities, topical or oral treatments, combining depigmenting agents with different modes of action may be useful. They may contain different molecules acting at different level of melanogenesis: (1) inhibitors of tyrosinase (e.g., hydroquinone, mequinol, rucinol, arbutin, kojic acid, azelaic acid or natural extracts such as pomegranate extract rich in ellagic acid); (2) inhibitors of tyrosinase maturation (e.g., N-acetyl glucosamine); (3) inhibitors of melanosome transfer (e.g., niacinamide, soybeans, lectins). Other agents can be used to complete the action of melanogenesis such as agents accelerating epidermal desquamation and melanin turn over (e.g., retinoids, salicylic acid, hydroxy acids) or agents acting by other modes such as anti-inflammatory and/or anti-vasculature agents (e.g., dexamethasone, fluocinolone acetate, and tranexamic acid) or antioxidants (e.g., vitamin C, resveratrol, vitamin E, ferulic acid, natural agents such as grapeseed extract, and gGngko biloba).

3.8 SKIN WHITENERS

Pigmentation of the skin occurs as a result of increased melanin production or deposition due to various reasons including age, hormonal imbalances, endocrine disease, inflammation, and/or exposure to damaging radiation, resulting in dermatologic conditions such as lentigines, melasma, or post-inflammatory hyperpigmentation. The enzymatic breakdown of tyrosine into DOPA and then dopaquinone leads to the synthesis of two types of skin pigment (melanin), eumelanin and pheomelanin. These skin pigments (of which eumelanin is the more abundant and which regularly correlates with the visual phenotype) are produced by melanocytes, which use melanosomes to transport the pigments to keratinocytes. One melanocyte is typically attached to approximately 30 keratinocytes. Melanosomes are surrounded by keratinocytes, which absorb the melanin after activation of the protease-activated receptor (PAR)-2. Expressed in keratinocytes but not melanocytes, PAR-2 is a seven transmembrane G-protein coupled trypsin/tryptase receptor activated by a serine protease cleavage. PAR-2 is believed to regulate pigmentation via exchanges between keratinocytes and melanocytes. Notably, melanogenesis can also be initiated by UV irradiation. Under these conditions, melanogenesis is a defensive manifestation to protect the skin and is characterized by accelerated melanin. synthesis and transfer to keratinocytes, leading to darkening of the skin in the exposed areas. Melanocytes synthesize more melanin in darker-skinned people, and their larger melanosomes accommodate this comparatively greater abundance of melanin and consequently break down more slowly than in lighter-skinned people. Inhibiting tyrosinase, thus preventing melanin formation, and blocking the transfer of melanin into keratinocytes represent the two main pathways through which the development of skin pigmentation can be hindered. Hydroquinone, vitamin C, kojic acid, arbutin, mulberry extract, and licorice extract are the most effective tyrosinase inhibitors. Skin pigmentation is also thought to be inhibited by two small proteins contained in soy—soybean trypsin inhibitor (STI) and Bowman–Birk inhibitor (BBI). Both STI and BBI have been shown in vitro and in vivo to exhibit depigmenting activity and to prevent UV-induced pigmentation by inhibiting the cleavage of PAR-2. Consequently, STI and BBI are thought to influence melanosome transfer into keratinocytes, thereby exerting an effect on pigmentation. Niacinamide, a vitamin B3 derivative, has also been demonstrated to hinder the melanosome transfer from melanocytes to keratinocytes. Soy and niacinamide, the most effective PAR-2 blockers, are the main agents for preventing this transfer. There are three classes of topical agents used within the two pathways of inhibiting melanin formation. In addition to the inhibitors of tyrosinase and PAR-2, exfoliating products (e.g., a-hydroxy acids, b-hydroxy acid, retinoids) have the capacity to increase cell turnover to outpace the rate of melanin production. Such exfoliation can also be achieved through microdermabrasion and the use of facial scrubs. Broad-spectrum sunscreens should also be employed in any skin care program intended to reduce or eliminate undesired pigmentation. The most effective way of preventing pigmentary alterations remains the avoidance of chronic sun exposure. Although numerous topical therapies exist for skin lightening, they are limited by efficacy and pigmentation recurrence after treatment cessation. The use of OTC lightening agents is widespread among those patients with hyperpigmentation disorders who reside in the United States. Those with melasma and PIH were more likely to use an OTC lightening cream. The majority of patients believed that OTC creams were safe to use without physician supervision. In those who had also tried prescription products, triple combination was deemed most effective compared to other lightening agents. Multiple systemic therapies for skin lightening exist including oral carotenoids, glutathione, melatonin, *Polypodium leucotomos* (tropical fern that has long been used for the treatment of inflammatory disorders by Native Americans) hydrophilic extract, procyanidin, and tranexamic acid. Preliminary data for the treatment of hyperpigmentation are promising, and currently, these oral treatments appear safe. Among the natural extracts, mulberry and licorice are popular components added to the skin whiteners. Also, lemon extract is used in preparations like Skin Bright, Lucederm and Meladerm as a potent skin bleaching ingredient. However, it can only be used at low concentrations because it easily causes skin irritation [15], [32], [42], [56].

Exhibit 2. Classification of depigmenting agents and their mechanism of action [193]

Stage of melanin synthesis	Deposition	Active molecules
Before melanin synthesis	Tyrosinase transcription	Tretinoin, c-2 ceramide
	Tyrosinase glycosylation	$PaSSO_3Ca$
	Inhibition of plasmin	Tranexamic acid
During melanin synthesis	Tyrosinase inhibition	Hydroquinone, mequinol, azelaic acid, kojic acid, arbutin, deoxyarbutin, licorice extract, rucinol, 2,5-dimethyl-4-hydroxy-3(2H)-furanone, *N*-acetyl glucosamine, resveratrol, oxyresveratrol, ellagic acid, methyl gentisate, 4-hydroxyanisole
	Peroxidase inhibition	Phenolic compounds
	Reactive oxygen species scavengers	Ascorbic acid, ascorbic acid palmitate, thiotic acid, hydrocumarins
After melanin synthesis	Tyrosinase degradation	Linoleic acid, α-linoleic acid
	Inhibition of melanosome transfer	Niacinamide, serine protease inhibitors, retinoids, lecithins, neoglycoproteins, soybean trypsin inhibitor
	Skin turnover acceleration	Lactic acid, glycolic acid, linoleic acid, retinoic acid
	Regulation of melanocyte environment	Corticosteroids, glabiridin
	Interaction with copper	Kojic acid, ascorbic acid
	Inhibition of melanosome maturation	Arbutin and deoxyarbutin
	Inhibition of protease activated receptor 2	Soybean trypsin inhibitor

3.8.1 TYROSINASE INHIBITION

Tyrosinase, a rate-limiting enzyme in melanogenesis, is a melanocyte-specific copper-containing glycoprotein located within specialized organelles called melanosomes [216]. Since tyrosinase is a crucial enzyme in synthesizing melanin through melanogenesis, it becomes the most prominent and successful target for melanogenesis inhibitors that directly inhibit the tyrosinase catalytic activity. Most of cosmetics or skin lightening agents commercially available are tyrosinase inhibitors [1]. Depigmentation can be achieved by regulating (i) the transcription and activity of tyrosinase, tyrosinase related protein-1 (TRP-1), tyrosinase related protein-2 (TRP-2), and/or peroxidase, (ii) the uptake and distribution of melanosomes in recipient keratinocytes, and (iii) melanin and melanosome degradation and turnover of "pigmented keratinocytes". Tyrosinase is a copper enzyme, which catalyses both the hydroxylation of monophenols to o-diphenols and the oxidation of o-diquinones to o-quinones. Most whitening agents act specifically to reduce the function of this enzyme through the following mechanisms: (i) interference with its transcription and/or glycosylation, (ii) inhibition by different modalities, (iii) reduction of by-products, and (iv) post-transcriptional control [33].

A. Hydroquinone

Hydroquinone (HQ) is a dihydric phenol with two important derivatives viz. monobenzyl and monomethyl ether of hydroquinone. Hydroquinone competitively inhibits melanin synthesis by inhibiting sulfhydryl groups and acting as a substrate for tyrosinase. Melanosomes and melanocytes are damaged by the semiquinone free radicals released during the above reaction. The effectiveness of HQ is related directly to the concentration of the preparation [34]. Sun screens, sun avoidance and bleaching agents, such as 4% hydroquinone alone or in combination with retinoid and topical steroids are conventional treatments [52]. Clinically, it is used to treat areas of dyschromia, such as melasma, chloasma, solar lentigines, freckles, post-inflammatory hyperpigmentation [35]. Concentrations of HQ vary from 2% (over the counter) to as high as 10% that are prescribed extemporaneously for resistant cases. It was known that the higher concentrations of HQ were more effective, but the irritating and toxin for melanocytes sign were obvious. There was a reduction in the effectiveness of HQ preparation due to oxidation so that stabilizing agents like sodium bisulphate and ascorbic acid were used as antioxidants. The most suitable vehicle for the formulation is a hydroalcoholic solution (equal parts of propylene glycol and absolute ethanol) or a hydrophilic ointment, or a gel containing 10% alpha-hydroxy acids (AHAs), taking into consideration the desired 3% to 5% HQ concentration in ethanol and propylene glycol 1:1 (or in a cream base or an AHA 10% gel) [33]. The FDA has even proposed banning over-the counter skin bleaching agents containing hydroquinone in 2006 [36]. It is also banned in EU since 2001 [37]. Due to the side-effect and safety profile, hydroquinone is not used as a component of cosmeceuticals available in the market for the treatment of hyperpigmentation.

Possible long-term effects such as carcinogenesis may be expected as well. Metabolites of hydroquinone formed in the liver, e.g., p-benzoquinone and glutathione conjugates of hydroquinone, are mainly responsible for this. In the bone marrow, hydroquinone is oxidized into p-benzoquinone because of the high myeloperoxidase activity. Topically applied hydroquinone-containing creams may give rise to the accumulation of these compounds, which can cause DNA damage and mutations [38]. Although, HQs exhibits *In Vitro* and *In Vivo* Anti-Cancer Activity in Cancer Cells and Mice [39] is reported However, other chronic adverse effects include exogenous ochronosis, cataract, pigmented colloid milia, sclera, and nail pigmentation, loss of elasticity of the skin, impaired wound healing and exuding an offensive fish odor. Topical Silymarin cream might serve as an effective and safe treatment modality [40]. Shankar et.al, 2014 concluded that fluorinated steroid containing 2-4% HQ-based triple combination for first line, with additional selective peels if required in second line treatment for melasma. Lasers are a last resort [193].

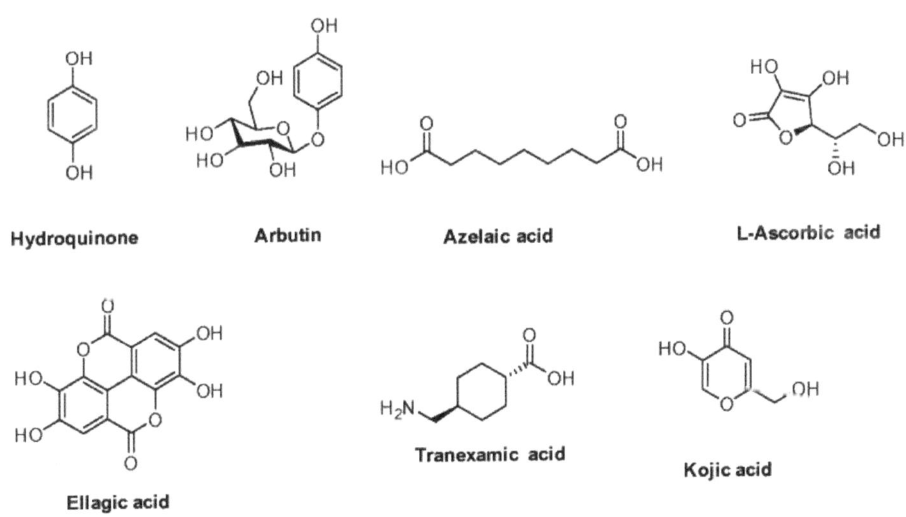

Figure 3.5 Chemical structure of well-known tyrosinase inhibitors as skin lightening agents [1].

Exhibit 3. Common lightening agents with brief M/A & S/E [41]		
Name	**Mechanism of action**	**Side effects**
Hydroquinone	Tyrosinase inhibition	Erythema, irritation, exogenous ochronosis
Azelaic acid	Tyrosinase inhibition	Stinging, burning, itching, dryness

Contd...

Name	Mechanism of action	Side effects
Kojic acid	Tyrosinase inhibition	Irritation, contact dermatitis
Ascorbic acid	Inhibition of reactive oxygen species	No significant adverse event
Retinoids	Downregulation of Tyrosinase	Irritant reaction, dryness, hyperpigmentation
Corticosteroid treatments	Anti-inflammatory and nonselective inhibition of melanogenesis	Telangiectasias, epidermal atrophy, steroid-induced acne, striae, hypopigmentation
Niacinamide	Inhibition of melanasome transfer	Irritation
Licorice	Melanin dispersion, tyrosinase inhibition	No significant adverse event
Undecylenoyl phenylalanine	Antagonist of α-melanocyte-stimulating hormone, β-adrenergic, stem cell receptors	No significant adverse event
4-N-butylresorcinol	Tyrosinase inhibition, antioxidant, anti-inflammatory	Mild erythema and itching
Soybean	Inhibits melanosome transfer to keratinocytes	No significant adverse event
Arbutin	Inhibition of tyrosinase	Skin irritation
Glucosamine	Inhibition of tyrosinase activation	Skin rash
Mequinol	Inhibition of tyrosinase	Skin irritation, redness, peeling

B. Kojic Acid

Kojic acid (5-hydroxy-2 hydroxymethyl-4-pyrone), crystalline white powder, is increasingly being used as a skin-lightening agent in skin care products marketed in Japan since 1988. It is a naturally occurring hydrophilic fungal product derived from certain species of *Acetobacter*, *Aspergillus*, and *Penicillium*. It was first isolated from Aspergillus in 1907. Kojic acid (KA) suppresses free tyrosinase, mainly attributable to chelation of its copper, and it is shown to be responsible for therapy and prevention of pigmentation, both in vitro and in vivo. In Japan, it is used in nonprescription skin care products up to a concentration of 1%. To increase percutaneous absorption and thus therapeutic activity, it is usually used at the highest concentration allowed.

Since it is used intensively in foods (such as bean paste, soy, and sake) in some countries, particularly Japan, it was thought to be safe [42]. This has been used for a long time in Japan in the form of an alternative to hydroquinone. American Academy of Dermatologists have clinically proven that KA can be effective for the treatment of hyper-pigmentation. KA functions similar to Arbutin and inhibits the activity of the enzyme tyrosinase. Like mentioned earlier, tyrosinase is responsible for the production of melanin [43]. It reduces hyperpigmentation by inhibiting the production of free tyrosinase and is also a potent antioxidant. KA is used at concentrations ranging from 1% to 4% [34]. Montazeri et. al, 2019 detailed potent anti-Toxoplasma activity with direct and indirect effects on the parasite [44]. Kojic acid is most commonly used in cosmetic products, such as creams, lotions, and serums. It is also used in some soaps. Many products with kojic acid are intended for use on the hands or face [45]. The major applications of KA and its derivatives in medicine are based on their biocompatibility, antimicrobial and antiviral, antitumor, antidiabetic, anticancer, anti-speck, anti-parasitic, and pesticidal and insecticidal properties. In addition, KA and its derivatives are used as anti-oxidant, anti-proliferative, anti-inflammatory, radio protective and skin-lightening agent in skin creams, lotions, soaps, and dental care products [46]. Burnett et.al, 2010 stated that KA was not a toxicant in acute, chronic, reproductive, and genotoxicity studies [47]. Contact dermatitis is the most common side effect of topical KA use. Even if KA does not initially irritate the skin, there's a risk of developing allergic contact dermatitis with continued use. However, KA does not find a place in the cosmeceuticals available. This could be due to the side effect profile of this drug [34], [48].

C. Azelaic Acid

Azelaic Acid (AA) is derived from the fungus *Pityrosporum ovale* and can be found in rye, wheat, and barley. The effect of AA can be attributed to its ability to inhibit the energy production and/or DNA synthesis of hyperactive melanocytes, and partially to its anti-tyrosinase activity. This may also account for the beneficial effect on post-inflammatory hyperpigmentation [49], [55]. It brightens the skin tone while visibly improving the evenness of skin texture and reducing the look of blemishes. It is a multi-functional support ingredient for all skin types and also acts as an effective antioxidant, antibacterial, keratolytic and comedolytic [50,51]. Faghihi et.al, 2017 demonstrates that triple-combination of 20% azelaic acid + 10% resorcinol + 6% phytic acid was found to be an effective and safe peeling agent in the treatment of melasma and it was as effective as 50% glycolic acid peel [52]. In a similar study, Dayal et.al, 2017 stated that Glycolic acid (GA) peel alone or in combination with topical hypopigmenting agents (GA peel every 3 weeks with twice daily 20% AA cream) has shown encouraging results for treatment of melasma, improvement in melasma quality of life (MELASQOL) scores without serious side effects [53]. AA-loaded nano-emulsion with hyaluronic acid as a double targeting strategy to increase drug retention and tyrosinase inhibition activity reached the deeper layers of the skin while improving in vitro tyrosinase inhibition; hence, it could be a promising treatment to dermic melasma [54]. This agent preferentially targets abnormal and highly active melanocytes with minimal effect on uninvolved skin [55]. Topical potent steroids and 20% AA cream combines the beneficial effects of both besides perhaps increasing the compliance of the patients. AA with tretinoin caused more skin lightening after three months than AA alone, and a higher proportion of excellent responders at the end of treatment. The combination of AA 20% cream and glycolic acid 15% or 20% lotion was as effective as HQ 4% cream in the treatment of hyperpigmentation in darker skinned patients, with only a slightly higher rate of mild local irritation. Particular advantages of AA therapy include its favorable safety and side effect profile. It is non-teratogenic, is not associated with systemic adverse events or photodynamic reactions and exhibits excellent local tolerability. Adverse effects from the AA included irritant contact dermatitis that was usually mild and transient, but occasionally was pronounced [33]. However, Tehranchinia et.al, 2018 demonstrates that common therapeutic approaches for melasma include topical HQ, AA, steroids, chemical peels, and lasers, most of which could not induce remarkable and constant satisfying outcomes [57].

D. Glutathione

Glutathione (GSH), being a strong antioxidant with additional anti-melanogenic properties, has recently become the most popular "systemic skin lightening molecule." In addition to be one of the richest antioxidants, it is being promoted as a skin-lightening agent, following the discovery of its anti-melanogenic properties. GSH is one of agents that is commonly used to lighten skin color in Asia as a dietary supplement. The most "popular" and controversial route of administration of glutathione for skin lightening has been intravenous (IV). GSH, an LMW thiol-tripeptide (component of cysteine, glutamate and glycine) is central to the maintenance of intracellular redox balance [58]. The proposed mechanisms of action include (a) direct inactivation of the enzyme tyrosinase by binding with the copper-containing active site of the enzyme, (b) mediating the switch mechanism from eumelanin to phaeomelanin production, (c) quenching of free radicals and peroxides that contribute to tyrosinase activation and melanin formation, and (d) modulation of depigmenting abilities of melanocytotoxic agents [33], [59]. Orally administered GSH, 500 mg per day for 4 weeks, resulted in a lightening of skin color in a small number of subjects [60] and 250 mg/d, in both reduced and oxidized forms effectively influences skin properties. Overall, glutathione in both forms are well tolerated [61]. In its reduced form, GSH is an antioxidant and also is involved in pheomelanin formation. Although glutathione is present in its both reduced (GSH) and oxidized (GSSG) states, the majority of it found in the body is in the reduced form. GSH conducts antioxidant activity by scavenging free-radicals during reductive detoxification of hydrogen peroxide and lipid peroxide. Chung et.al, 2016 reported that GSH monoethyl ester (GSH-MEE) was effective for anti-melanogenesis, whereas GSH itself was not. Particularly GSH-MEE (but not GSH itself), was effective without affecting cellular viability for reducing melanin and tyrosinase activity and raising the suggested pheomelanin/ eumelanin ratio. Taken together, this novel esterified GSH derivative could be developed as a safe and efficient agent for the treatment of hyperpigmentary skin disorders (Figure 3.6) [62].

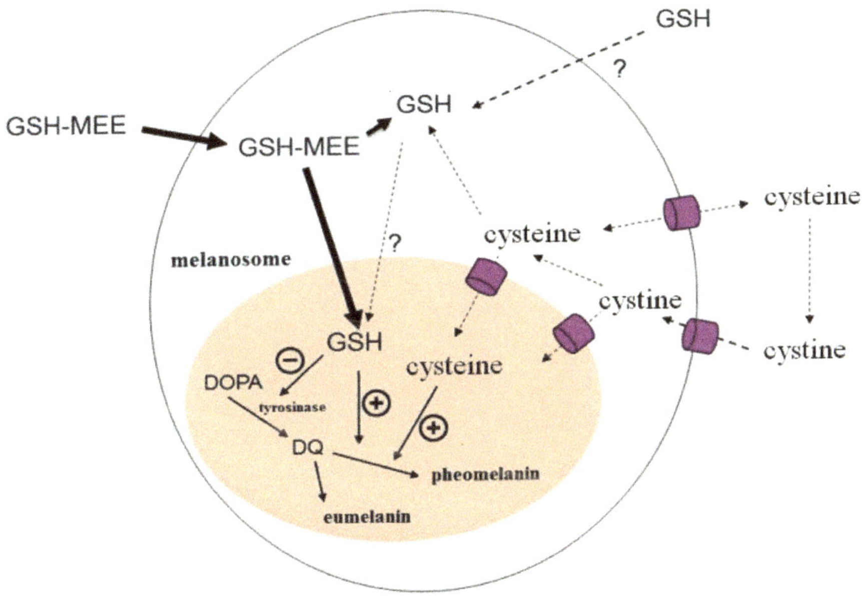

Figure 3.6 Possible effects of GSH-MEE, GSH, and cysteine on melanogenesis [62]. GSH synthesize intracellularly and exported to extracellular space. Cellular uptake of GSH itself is not probable. GSH-MEE cross the biological membranes by simple diffusion and metabolize intracellularly to generate GSH. Cysteine is readily transported across cell membranes but potentially toxic at high concentrations due to generation of reactive oxygen species and depletion of pyridoxal phosphate. GSH-MEE (but not GSH itself) could suppress the melanin production and tyrosinase activity and raise the suggested pheomelanin/eumelanin ratio. black arrows, melanin synthesis process flow; dotted black arrows, transport process flows of GSH, cysteine, and cysteine, bold black arrows, transport process flow of GSH-MEE; question marks, not yet confirmed; +, positive effects (activation); −, negative effects (suppression); purple shape, membrane channel. GSH, reduced glutathione; GSH-MEE, GSH monoethyl ester; DOPA, dihydroxyphenylalanine; DQ, dopaquinone.

Multiple articles have been published in the lay press on the use of GSH for a variety of diseases including melasma. IV use of GSH has been associated with severe life-threatening reactions including Stevens–Johnson syndrome and anaphylaxis [41]. According to Dilokthornsakul et.al, 2019 skin whitening effect of glutathione is still inconclusive due to the quality of included studies and inconsistent findings [63]. Cosmetic doctors have called on the UK government to warn consumers about the dangers of skin whitening antioxidant glutathione. However, concern is growing over the use of the antioxidant by unqualified or unlicensed practitioners, including in some salons, to lighten the color of the skin [64]. Finally, there is little convincing evidence in favor of GSH as a therapy for hyperpigmentation at the present time, and there are many unresolved controversies that surround its use, as reported by Sonthalia et.al, 2018 [58]. FDA clarified that only glutathione tablets are approved by the agency, and not glutathione injectables. Antioxidant's main use is to counter the A/Es of cancer treatments, but is now being used by consumers seeking whiter skin. Its side effect is the whitening of skin as it deactivates tyrosinase, the enzyme that helps produce melanin, the pigment that determines skin color. Glutathione may cause kidney failure and blood poisoning [65,66].

E. Arbutin

Arbutin, the b-D-glucopyranoside derivative of hydroquinone, is a naturally occurring plant- derived compound found in the dried leaves of several different plant species including, bearberry (Arctostaphylos uva-ursi), blueberry, cranberry, and pear trees [34], [67]. Hydroquinone occurs in nature as the b-glucopyranoside conjugate (arbutin). Uva-ursi folium (bearberry leaf) has been traditionally used in Japan (contained in the leaves of pear trees and certain herbs) to treat symptoms of lower urinary tract infections. The most representative constituent of this herbal drug is arbutin that is rapidly absorbed in the small intestine and undergoes hepatic conjugation to form HQ conjugates [68]. Arbutin is a mild agent for treating cutaneous hyperpigmentation, including melasma and UV-induced ephelides. Arbutin was first discovered in Arctostapylos uva-ursi (L.) Spreng and then in the leaves of Vaccinicum vitis-idaca L., Pyrus pyrifolia (Burm.f.) Kakai. and Saxifraga stolonifera (L.) Meerb. In both normal human melanocytes and melanoma, arbutin induces a decrease of tyrosinase activity without affecting mRNA expression, inhibits the 5,6-dihydroxyindole-2-carboxylic acid (DHICA) polymerase activity, and exerts an inhibitory effect on melanosome maturation. This phenotypic change was associated with the inhibition of tyrosinase and DHICA polymerase activities, and the degree of inhibition was dose dependent [67]. Higher concentrations are more efficacious than lower concentrations, but they may also result in a paradoxical hyperpigmentation [33]. The depigmentation effect of arbutin works through an inhibition of the melanosomal tyrosinase activity, rather than by suppression of the expression and synthesis of tyrosinase in human melanocytes [69]. It was found to inhibit the oxidation of l-tyrosine catalyzed by mushroom tyrosinase. The kinetics and mechanism for inhibition of tyrosinase confirms the reversibility of arbutin as a competitive inhibitor of this enzyme [33], [42]. The Scientific Committee on Consumer Safety (SCCS) assessed the use safety of alpha arbutin (for concentrations greater than 2% in facial creams and greater than 0.5% for body lotions) and of beta arbutin (for concentrations greater than 7% in facial creams) [70,71]. Treatment of the human skin model with 250 mcg of α-arbutin did not inhibit cell viability, while melanin synthesis was reduced to 40% of that in the control. These results indicate that alpha-arbutin is an effective and safe ingredient for skin-lightening [72]. Arbutin was less cytotoxic than hydroquinone to cultured human melanocytes [73,74]. Miao et.al, 2016 reported that deoxy-arbutin possesses a potent ability in skin lightening and antioxidation with less melanosome cytotoxicity [74]. Hamed et al, 2006 reported the efficacy and safety of deoxyarbutin, a new tyrosinase inhibiting agent both in vitro and in vivo on human skin. They demonstrated that deoxyarbutin has the potential to be as safe and effective as a depigmenting agent and suggested that it may act an as an alternative agent to hydroquinone [75].

F. Ellagic Acid

Ellagic acid (EA) is a phenolic compound related to flavonoids that is structurally a condensed dimer of gallic acid. It has been described as a tyrosinase inhibitor and is used in the cosmetic industry as a whitening agent. It is present either in free form or as part of more complex molecules (ellagitannins), which can be metabolized to liberate ellagic acid and several of its metabolites, including urolithins. Only a small portion of EA is found in the free form. EA is usually conjugated with a glycoside moiety such as glucose, rhamnose, arabinose, or bound in the form of ellagitannins. Phenolic compounds possess benzene ring and hydroxyl group substituents and are able to quench free radicals and prevent cellular damage, thereby functioning as effective antioxidants. While EA 's antioxidant properties are doubtless responsible for many of its pharmacological activities, other mechanisms have also been implicated in its various effects, including its ability to reduce the lipidemic profile and lipid metabolism, alter pro-inflammatory mediators (tumor necrosis factor-α, IL-1β, IL-6), and decrease the activity of nuclear factor κB while increasing nuclear factor erythroid 2-related factor 2 expression. Frozen apple, raspberry and blackberry are good sources of EA [76-78]. It is capable of preventing pigmentation caused by sunburn, found in trees, nuts, and fruit. It inhibits tyrosinase non-competitively in a dose-dependent manner, through its capacity to chelate copper, even if other mechanisms, such as a scavenger effect have been suggested [33], [55]. EA has been demonstrated to have melanogenic inhibitory activity both in vitro and in vivo. A topical product containing 0.5% ellagic acid and 0.1% salicylic acid appears to have better esthetics (texture, pleasantness to use, skin feel) than the 4% HQ product [79]. EA is oxidized by tyrosinase, producing reactive o-quinones. As an antioxidant it can inhibit the melanogenesis process. This first aspect should be taken into consideration in its application as a cosmetic ingredient due to the toxicity of o-quinones and its ability to modify the redox status of the cell [80]. Dietary and pharmacological interventions with berries rich in ellagic acid may be promising treatment strategies interrupting skin wrinkle and inflammation associated with chronic UV exposure leading to photoaging [81]. The antioxidant efficiency of EA is directly correlated with its degree of hydroxylation and decreases with the presence of a sugar moiety. Many health benefits of EA are attributed to its antioxidant properties because oxidative stress is involved in the pathogenesis of different diseases [78] EA is a plausible candidate used as a natural resource for manufacturing anti-photoaging cosmetics, which may have similar or enhanced activities with fewer side effects [82].

G. Aloesin

Aloesin, a natural hydroxymethylchromone derivative isolated from Aloe Vera, acts by two different mechanisms of action on tyrosinase activity, e.g., aloesin inhibits the formation of DOPA quinone by competitive inhibition at the DOPA oxidation site, reduction of copper ions at the hydroxylase site, and consequently tyrosine hydroxylation by noncompetitive inhibition. In comparison with other depigmenting agents, aloesin shows no cytotoxicity in cell-based assays, no skin irritation in preliminary human studies and any genotoxicity or mutagenicity in the Ames assay. Cultured cells used in tyrosinase activity assays show no morphologic abnormalities when treated with aloesin, and human melanocytes appear normal with multiple dendrites. Thus, aloesin is a potent inhibitor of human tyrosinase. However, because of the hydrophilic nature of the compound and moderately high molecular weight, penetration of human skin was poor. At non-cytotoxic concentration aloesin probably acting as a competitive inhibitor on DOPA oxidation and as a non-competitive on tyrosine hydroxylase activity [33]. Aloesin performed more inhibitory activity toward crude murine tyrosinase than mushroom tyrosinase and has been recently used in topically applied cosmetics due to its natural source and multifunctional activity in skin care. Aloesin treatment showed pigmentation suppression in a dose- dependent manner; thus, aloesin might be used as an agent that inhibits melanin formation induced by UV radiation. In vivo, aloesin and arbutin co-treatment inhibits UV induced melanogenesis in a synergistic manner [83-86]. The hydrophilic nature of the compound reduces the skin penetration of aloesin. Hence, combination treatment of aloesin with arbutin has been studied to assess the synergistic effects on tyrosinase activity. The two adhere to different mechanisms of action where aloesin exhibits noncompetitive inhibition while arbutin inhibits competitively. Studies of aloesin revealed no cytotoxicity, which makes it a good alternative to HQ [87]. The mixture of aloesin and arbutin can significantly inhibit the tyrosinase activity and melanogenesis of cultured human melanocytes. It showed the effects of aloesin and arbutin in a synergistic manner [88]. Even though aloesin appears to be an important component in the armamentarium against hyperpigmentation disorders, its hydrophilic nature renders it less able than hydroquinone to penetrate the skin [89]. However, some believe that its slower penetration of the skin endows aloesin with greater potential as a skin-lightening agent for cosmetic purposes [90].

H. Tranexamic Acid

Tranexamic acid (TXA) is commonly being used to reduce melanin synthesis in patients with melasma and also used as a raw material for functional whitening cosmetics. The mechanism of TXA, which is a lysine analog, in the treatment of UV-induced pigmentation includes interfering with the structure of plasminogen and preventing the binding of plasminogen to the lysine-binding sites of keratinocytes (**Figure 3.7**). The consequences of such an event are less free arachidonic acid so a reduced ability to produce prostaglandins and thus decreased melanocyte tyrosinase activity and melanogenesis [91]. However, Cho et.al., 2017 reported that TXA can reduce melanin synthesis in melanoma B16-F1 cells by activating the extracellular signal-regulated kinase (ERK) signaling pathway and the autophagy system [92]. Histological and immunohistochemical evaluation following oral TXA has shown decrease in epidermal pigmentation as well as melasma-associated dermal changes such as number of vessels and mast cells, according to evidence-based review by Sharma et.al, 2017 [101]. Kim et.al, 2016 reported the downregulation of Endothelin (ET)-1 by TXA for the same. The number of CD31-positive vessels and the expression of the vascular endothelial growth factor both tended to decrease. This immunohistochemical study found that suppression of ET-1 could be one of the mechanisms of action of TXA on melasma [100]. TXA 5%, topically twice a day for 12 weeks in the location of the melasma significantly reduced both melanin level and MASI score. Given its high efficiency and low drug side effects, this regimen results in high patient satisfaction compared with topical hydroquinone [93]. In a similar study with the Asian population, Kanechorn et.al, 2012 reported topical TXA 5% produced erythema as side effects [98]. TXA has been found to lighten melasma by interfering with the interaction of melanocytes and keratinocytes by inhibiting the plasminogen/plasmin system. Tan et.al, 2017 reported (study results from a tertiary dermatological center in Singapore between 1 August 2009 and 31 March 2011) that low-dose oral TXA can serve as a safe and useful adjunct in the treatment of refractory melasma [94].

TXA is easily available (5 mL ampoule containing 500 mg of the drug) and affordable. Better therapeutic response to treatment in the micro-needling group could be attributed to the deeper and uniform delivery of the medication through microchannels created by micro-needling. EMLA Cream (lidocaine 2.5% and prilocaine 2.5%) was used as an anesthetic in this study. Budamakuntla et.al, 2013 reported more than 50% improvement without major adverse events observed in both the treatment groups. The MASI scores, physician global assessment (PGA) and patient global assessment (PtGA) score showed a significant decreasing trend from the baseline to the fourth, eighth, and twelfth

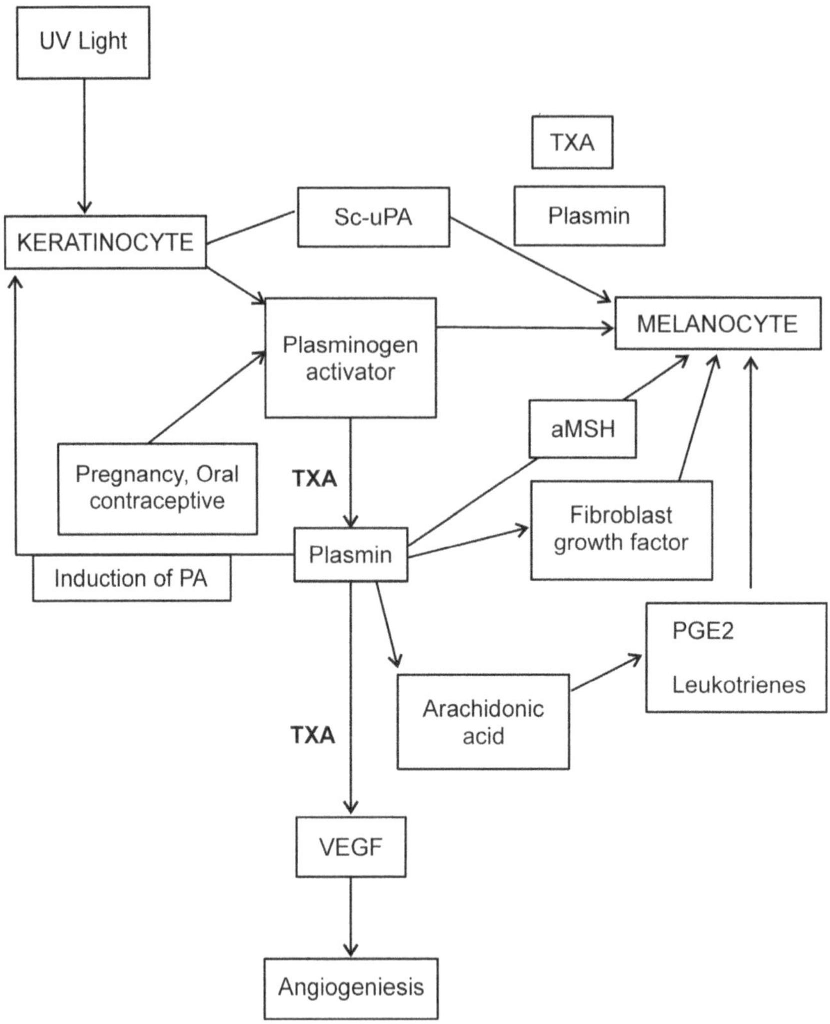

Figure 3.7 Pathogenesis of Melasma and Role of Tranexemic Acid [93]. TXA, a synthetic derivative of lysine, is a fibrinolytic agent that blocks the conversion of plasminogen to plasmin and thereby impedes the binding of plasminogen to keratinocytes. Human keratinocytes secrete the urokinase-type plasminogen activator, which increases the activity of melanocytes in vitro. The blockade of this effect may be due to the mechanism by which TXA reduces hyperpigmentation in melasma patients. The consequences of such event are less free arachidonic acid leading to a reduced ability to produce prostaglandins and thus decreased melanocyte tyrosinase activity and melanogenesis. Tranexamic acid does effect on non-sun exposed healthy skin. Also, action of TXA on angiogenesis via plasmin could play a contributory role in its action on melasma. Blocking of the Sc-uPA pathway may be another mechanism through which TXA reduces hyperpigmentation. TXA: Tranexemic acid, PA: Plasminogen activator, Sc-uPA: Single Chain urokinase Plasminogen Activator, VEGF: Vascular Endothelial Growth Factor.

week of treatment with TXA [95]. Melasma relapse was found to be 72% as reported by Tan et.al, 2017. TXA treatment should not be short-term, but needs to be maintained for an extended period.. However, TXA is used as a haemostatic treatment, it is prescribed at a dosage of 1,000 mg 3 times daily. For melasma, it is commonly used at a dosage of 250 mg twice daily, which is only one-sixth of the normal dosage of TA as a haemostatic agent. Kim et.al, 2017 reported that ADEs were minor, with a few cases reporting hypo-menorrhoea, mild abdominal discomfort, and transient skin irritation. These results support the efficacy and safety of TXA, either alone or as an adjuvant to routine treatment modalities for melasma [96]. Hair follicles are important reservoirs for co-drug delivery. Hsieh et.al, 2013 reported TXA to be a superior candidate as a co-drug. Daily administration of co-drugs (both TXA and HQ) to the skin did not generate irritation for up to 7 days [97]. An eight-week, prospective, randomized, double-blind, vehicle-controlled clinical study evaluated a combination of niacinamide and TXA as a topical moisturizer in the treatment of 42 Korean women with irregular facial hyperpigmentation. This formulation was significantly more effective in reducing hyperpigmentation than vehicle control, providing an effect beyond that achieved with sunscreen [99]. Role of oral TXA as adjuvant to other therapies such as fluocinolone based TC (fluocinolone acetonide 0.01%, HQ 4%, tretinoin 0.05%), HQ, and laser were assessed in RCTs. All these studies reported significantly enhanced efficacy with addition of TXA to TC (LOE 2), IPL and LASER treatment (LOE 2, 4) in melasma [101]. Zhang et.al, 2018 review shows that both single and adjuvant TA treatments showed a significant reduction of MASI and MI scores while incurring minimal side effects [102]. It can also be used when other topical treatments fail [103].

I. Ascorbic Acid

Ascorbic acid may inhibit melanin production by reducing o-quinones, so that melanin cannot be formed by the action of tyrosinase until all vitamin C is oxidized. It interferes with the different steps of melanization, by interacting with copper ions at the tyrosinase active site and reducing dopaquinone and DHICA oxidation. Melanin can be changed from jet black to light tan by the reduction of oxidized melanin. Because vitamin C is quickly oxidized and decomposes in aqueous solution, it is not generally useful as a depigmenting agent (Figure 3.8). Ascorbic acid is an effective reducing agent, which, at high concentrations, can momentarily retard the melanin-biosynthesis pathway, but never eliminate it. On the contrary, the resultant accumulation of diphenol produces an indirect activation on this pathway when the reductant is completely depleted. However, ascorbic acid is highly unstable, being quickly oxidized and decomposed in aqueous solution and, because of its prevalent hydrophilic nature, has a low degree of penetration into the skin. Stable derivatives of vitamin C have been synthesized to minimize this problem. Magnesium-L-ascorbyl-2-phosphate (VC-PMG) is a vitamin C derivative that is stable in water, especially in neutral or alkaline solution containing boric acid or its salt. The more stable ascorbate ester VC-PMG (QD approval was obtained by the Takeda Pharmaceutical Company Limited in 1988) is more lipophilic and has a greater permeation through the stratum corneum. VC-PMG is hydrolyzed by phosphatases of the liver or skin to vitamin C and thus exhibits vitamin C– reducing activity. VC-PMG is hydrolyzed by phosphatases of liver or skin to ascorbic acid and thus exhibits vitamin C-reducing activity. It significantly suppressed melanin formation on purified tyrosinase or cultured cells and inhibited melanin formation without cell growth suppression on cultured human melanoma cells. The inhibition of melanogenesis was stronger when the activity of melanogenic enzymes was relatively high. VC-PMG is absorbed percutaneously, stays in the skin, and inhibits tyrosinase activity of melanocytes. The addition of 1% to 3% 1,1-methyleneglycol-bis increases the absorption of VC-PMG. In situ experiments demonstrated that 10% VC-PMG cream was absorbed into the epidermis and that 1.6% remained 48 hours after application [33], [42]. Al-Niaimi et.al, 2017 reported that a concentration above 20% does not increase its biological significance and, conversely, might cause some irritation. Reputable products of vitamin C available today are, therefore, in the range of 10 to 20% [105]. A study compared 5% ascorbic acid and 4% HQ shows that situation improved more than 90% but ADEs were around 70% in melasma patients. Author concluded that vitamin C may play a role as it is devoid of any side-effects, can be used alone or in combination therapy [106].

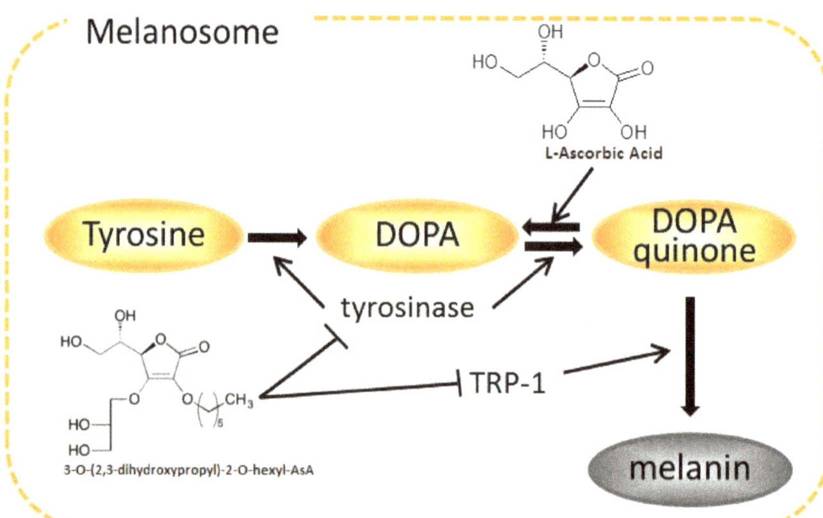

Figure 3.8 Plausible mechanisms of action of alkylglyceryl-Ascorbic acid derivatives on melanogenesis inhibitory activity [104].

High-frequency ultrasound radiation, when combined with skin lightening gel (ascorbyl glucoside with niacinamide) caused reduction in hyperpigmentation by causing enhanced transepidermal transport of the gel [107]. Tai et.al, 2009 stated that VC-PMG and ascorbic acid-2-glucoside (AA2G) (**Figure 3.9**) are very safe compounds for human use and also the most famous skin-whitening ingredients used in commercial cosmetics, compared to KA [108]. Vitamin C iontophoresis may be an effective treatment modality for melasma [109]. In this double-blind, placebo-controlled RCT, vitamin C solution was applied to one half of the face and distilled water (control) was applied to the other half. After 12 weeks of iontophoresis treatment, the colorimeter recorded a clinically significant reduction in luminance value on the treated side compared to the control side [55]. Both microphthalmia-associated transcription factor–siRNA (MITF-siR) cream and VC-PMG demonstrated significant improvement in the skin lesions compared to adjacent normal skin in melasma in a study. The total efficiency rate was 20% in the VC-PMG group, which was significantly lower than the MITF-siR group [110]. Taira et.al, 2018 reported that 3-O-Glyceryl-2-O-hexyl ascorbate (VC-HG), having an added glyceryl group and a hexyl group had an impact on skin lightening/whitening by inhibiting tyrosinase protein synthesis and interfering with intracellular melanosome transport [111]. Ascorbic acid and its QDs are the most popular skin lightening quasi- drugs that have ever been used in Japan. A 2% L-ascorbic acid 2-glucoside-containing cream was shown to accelerate the disappearance of ultraviolet light B (UVB) (280–320 nm)—induced hyperpigmentation of the skin [112]. However, Puvabanditsin et.al, 2006 reported that administration of topical 10% vitamin C derivative (VC-PMG) and topical 5% vitamin E had no bleaching effects observed after 2, 4, 6, 8, 10 and 12 weeks compared to the placebo [113].

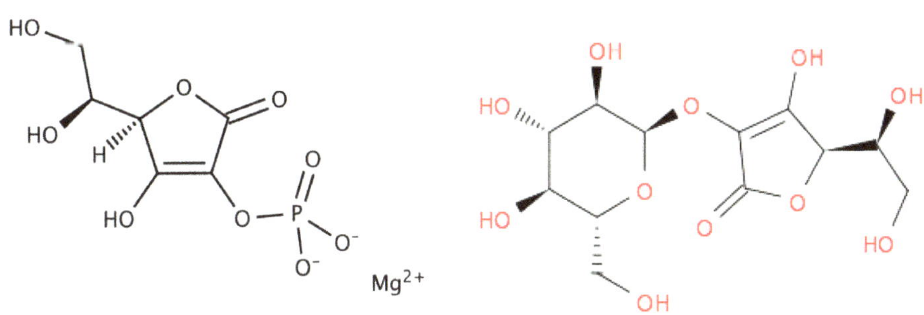

(a) Magnesium-L-ascorbyl-2-phosphate (VC-PMG) (b) ascorbic acid-2-glucoside (AA2G)

Figure 3.9 Ascorbic acid derivatives in hyperpigmentation management

J. Mulberry Extract

The leaves of the white mulberry (*Morus alba*, Moraceae) have been used for many years in traditional medicine in China, Korea, Japan, and Thailand. Fever-reducing, liver-protecting, and blood pressure-lowering properties are attributed to them [114]. Studies have shown that mulberry fruits possess several potential pharmacological health benefits including anti-cholesterol, anti-obesity and hepatoprotective effects which might be associated with the presence of some of these bioactive compounds. Volatile compounds found in mulberry fruits grown in Spain included acetic acid, 3-hydroxyl-2-butanone, ethyl butyrate, ethyl acetate, 3-methylbutanal, 2-methybutanal, heptanal, methional, hexanal, trans-2-hexanal, 2-octenone,hexanoic acid, benzaldehyde, methyl hexanoate, 2-ethylhexanal, octanal, limonene, 6-methyl-5-hepten-2on, ethyl hexanoate, 2,4-nonanadienal, phenylacetaldehyde, trans-2-octenal, cis-α-ocimene, terpinonene, 2-nonanone, nonanal, octanoic acid, cis-2-nonenal, dodecanoic acid, terpinen-4-ol, ethyl octanoate, ethyl dodecanoate, decanal, decanoic acid and ethyl decanoate [115]. Yuan et.al, 2017 also reported its antioxidant, neuroprotective, immunomodulative and antitumor activities [116]. An in vitro anti-tyrosinase activity study of the extracts from a hybrid Mulberry plant obtained from *Morus alba* L. and *Morus rotundiloba* Koidz, is shown to prove as new source of Thai whitening agent. The presence of betulinic acid, as an anti-inflammatory and anti-tyrosinase activity agent, is also reported [117]. Mulberry (*Morus alba* L.) leaves containing many nutritional components are the best food for silkworms. *Morus alba* L. also contains rutin, isoquercitrin, and astragalin. The root bark of *Morus alba* has been shown to have a skin whitening effect. But its activity was low and weaker than that of KA [33]. Yang et.al, 2014 reported the polyphenols contained in the leaves have depigmentation properties that have been demonstrated in vitro [114]. Lim et.al, 2019 reviewed anti-melanogenic property of all its stem, root, leaf, twig and fruit [118]. However, the anti-tyrosinase activity could be due to inhibition of DOPA oxidase activity of tyrosinase and superoxide scavenging activity. IC50 (concentration causing 50% inhibition of activity of tyrosinase) was very low (0.396%) as compared to 5.5% for hydroquinone and 10.0% for kojic acid. A patch test using 1% paper mulberry extract revealed no significant skin irritation at 24 h and 28 h [34]. 2,4,2',4'-tetrahydroxy-3-(3-methyl-2-butenyl)-chalcone (TMBC) (**Figure 3.10**) obtained from M. nigra significantly reduced the melanin content and cellular tyrosinase activity in B16 melanoma cells, although it increased mRNA levels of cellular tyrosinase [119]. Zheng et al, 2010 screened tyrosinase inhibitory properties of a total of 29 constituents isolated from roots of M. nigra (Black Mulberry). Among them, nine compounds (5'-geranyl-5,7,2',4'-tetrahydroxyflavone, steppogenin-7-O-β-d-glucoside, 2,4,2',4'-tetrahydroxy-chalcone, moracin N, kuwanon H, mulberrofuran G, morachalcone A, oxyresveratrol-3'-O-β-d-glucopyranoside and oxyresveratrol-2-O-β-d-glucopyranoside) showed better tyrosinase inhibitory activities than kojic acid (IC50 value 46.95 ± 1.72

μM, with 2,4,2',4'-tetrahydroxychalcone having the highest activity (IC50 value 0.062 ± 0.002 μM, 757-fold lower IC50 than kojic acid) [120]. Fresh fruits of M. nigra microwave assisted extractions were investigated by Koyu et.al, 2017. The highest tyrosinase inhibitory activity (IC50 value 1.44 mg/mL) was observed in the optimum microwave extraction system yielding the highest amount of anthocyanin content (13.28 mg/g cyanidin-3-glucoside equivalent) (**Figure 3.10**), suggesting the important potential of anthocyanins on tyrosinase inhibition [121].

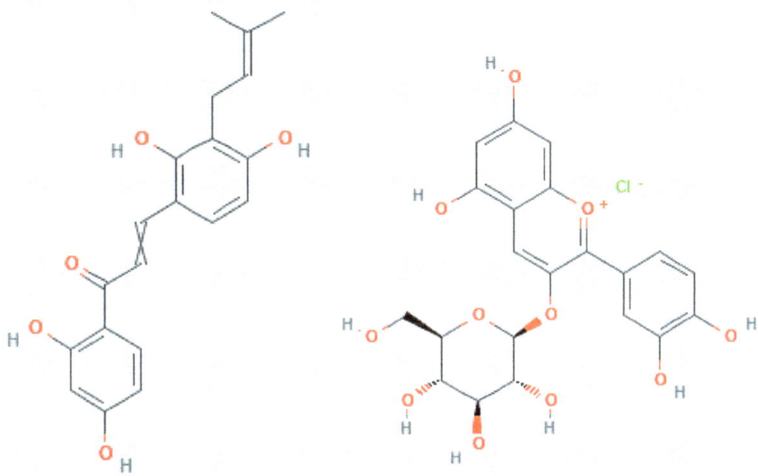

(a) TMBC (b) Cyanidin-3-glucoside

Figure 3.10 Important tyrosinase inhibitors from Mulberry extract

K. Licorice

Licorice extract is obtained from the root of Glycyrrhia Glabra L, legume native to Europe and Asia. It is cultivated extensively in India. Liquorice root offers skin depigmenting, lightening, emollient, anti-acne, photo protection, antiaging, antimicrobial and antioxidant properties, all helpful for healthy skin. Role of G. glabra on skin is mainly attributed to its antioxidant activity of phytochemicals namely triterpene, saponins (Glycyrrhizin-salts of glycyrrhizic acid) and flavonoids. Glycyrrhizetic acid controls the secretion of melanin in skin and it has the effect of reducing dark pigmentation and making the complexion fairer. Methanolic extract of its rhizome has been reported to be a potent tyrosinase inhibitor in human skin with more than 75% inhibition. The IC50 value was found to be within range when compared to well-known skin whitening agent i.e. Kojic acid. Therefore, it is likely to be useful for cosmetic applications [125]. The licorice extract includes liquiritin, isoliquertin (a chalcone) that occurs as a glycoside and during drying is partly converted into liquiritin (**Figure 3.11**), liquiritigenin, isoliquiritigenin, and other compounds [33], [87]. Liquiritin causes depigmentation by two mechanism: (i) via melanin dispersibility by means of the pyran ring of the color dispersing flavonoidal nucleus of liquiritin, and (ii) via amelanodermic and epidermal stain removing property. Acute and chronic toxicity studies have been carried out with no adverse effects. Glabrene and isoliquiritigenin (20, 40, 4-trihydroxychalcone) in the licorice extract can inhibit both mono- and diphenolase tyrosinase activities. The IC50 values for glabrene and isoliquiritigenin were 3.5 and 8.1 mM, respectively, when tyrosine was used as substrate. The effects of glabrene (**Figure 3.11**) and isoliquiritigenin on tyrosinase activity were dose-dependent and correlated to their ability to inhibit melanin formation in melanocytes [33]. Glabrene and isoliquiritigenin exert varying degrees of inhibition on tyrosinase-dependent melanin biosynthesis, suggesting that isoflavenes and chalcones may serve as candidates for skin-lightening agents [122]. Glabridin (**Figure 3.11**), a polyphenolic flavonoid is the main component of licorice extract [87], [123]. This ingredient has been shown to scavenge ROS, inhibit UVB-induced pigmentation and tyrosinase without affecting DNA synthesis, and possess anti-inflammatory properties [127]. Glabridin has been shown in vitro to have a skin lightening effect 16 times greater than that of hydroquinone and might reduce UVB pigmentation [34]. Licorice extracts also influence pigmentation by removing epidermal melanin, inhibiting the biosynthesis of melanin and inhibiting the activity of tyrosinase in a dose-dependent manner. Licorice extract has been tested in the treatment of melasma with good results and very mild irritation [87]. Costa et.al, 2010 stated that the association of Emblica, Licorice, and Belides is a safe and efficient alternative for the treatment of melasma [124]. Licochalcone A, an active ingredient in licorice extract, was shown in vitro to decrease prostaglandin E2, leukotriene B4, interleukin-6, and tumor necrosis factor- alpha in human keratinocytes. Licochalcone A (**Figure 3.11**) may also effectively reduce sunburn erythema. Patients treated with 0.05% of the Licochalcone A -rich licorice extract and vehicle immediately and 5 hours after exposure to UVB irradiation had significantly less erythema where the Licochalcone A was applied [126].

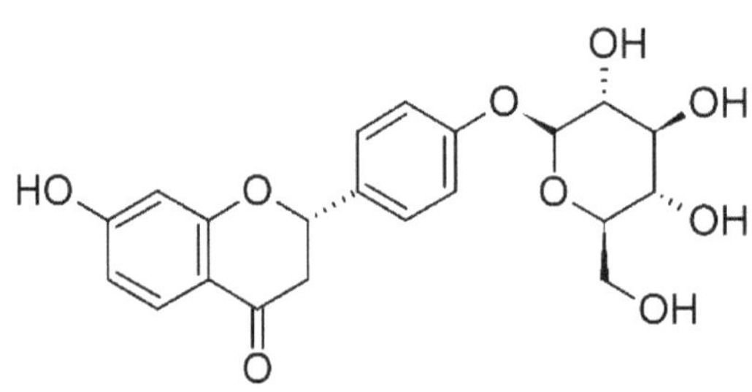

(a) Liquiritin

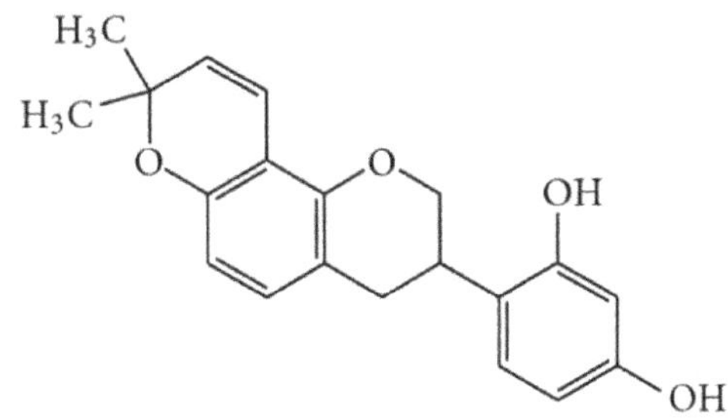

(b) Glabridin

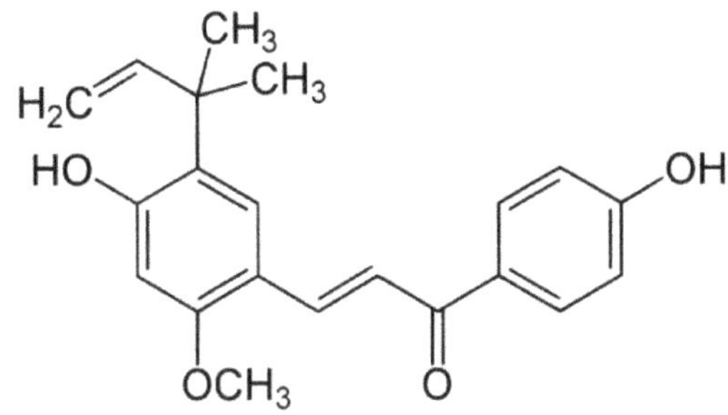

(c) Licochalcone A

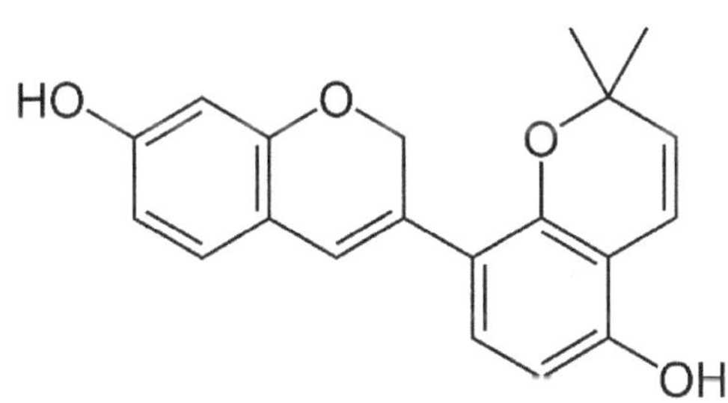

(d) Glabrene

Figure 3.11 Important Licorice ingredients for skin depigmenting, lightening

L. Alpha-Tocopherol

Vitamin E is the major lipophilic antioxidant in plasma, membranes, and tissues. The term "vitamin E" includes eight naturally occurring molecules (four tocopherols and four tocotrienols) that have vitamin E activity. In humans, alpha tocopherol (α-Toc) is the most abundant vitamin E derivative, followed by gamma tocopherol [128]. There is a large body of experimental evidence proving its photo-protective effects. It has been shown to cause depigmentation by interference with lipid peroxidation of melanocyte membranes, increase in intracellular glutathione content, and inhibition of tyrosinase [129].

Antioxidants such as vitamin B, vitamin C or vitamin E can also reduce the photooxidation of pre-existing melanin particles. Hence, these vitamins with antioxidant activity are commonly applied in skin-whitening cosmetic formulations [87]. The antioxidant properties of α-Toc, which interferes with lipid peroxidation of melanocyte membranes and increases the intracellular glutathione content, could explain its depigmenting effect. α-Toc has a more effective and long-lasting antioxidant response. Topical application of α-Toc and ascorbic acid, in vivo, decreases the tanning response inhibiting the UV-induced melanogenesis and proliferation of melanocytes. An alternative compound is alpha-Tocopherol ferulate (α -Toc-F), a derivative of α-Toc linked by an ester bond to ferulic acid, an antioxidant, which provides stabilization to α-Toc, similar to ascorbic acid. α-Toc inhibited melanogenesis in cultured normal human melanocytes, although it did not influence melanin synthesis in enzyme solution prepared as cell homogenates. Also, α-Toc stimulated intracellular GSH synthesis [33]. Although, topical alpha-tocopherol is mostly used at concentration of 5% or less, products with varying concentrations have been marketed. Side-effects such as allergic or irritant reactions are rare with topical vitamin E and hence, it is a component of cosmeceuticals preparations. Kamei et.al, 2009 reported that both d-β-tocopherol and d-γ-tocopherol might be useful as effective ingredients in whitening cosmetics with lower skin toxicity to prevent or improve skin pigmentation such as skin spots and freckles caused by UV exposure. Analysis by reverse transcription-polymerase chain reaction showed that the mechanism of melanogenesis inhibition by d-beta- and d-gamma-tocopherols in cells might be attributed to reduced expression of tyrosinase and tyrosinase related protein-2 mRNA in addition to direct inhibition of the tyrosinase [130]. Kuwabara et.al, 2006 reported that gamma-tocopheryl-N,N-dimethylglycinate hydrochloride (gamma-TDMG) or KA (250 microM) were added to homogenates of B16 melanoma cells, their tyrosinase activity was significantly inhibited by approximately 40% and 75%, respectively [131]. However, Keen et.al, 2016 commented that Vitamin E alone has shown minimal efficacy in the treatment of melasma [132]. Oral procyanidin + vitamins A, C, E proved to be safe and effective among Filipino women with epidermal melasma, after an 8-week trial period. There was a significant reduction in MASI scores and pigmentation by mexametry in malar regions [133]. Daily use of a facial lotion containing niacinamide, panthenol, and tocopheryl acetate improved skin tone and texture and was well tolerated in Indian women with facial signs of aging [134]. Experimental evidence suggests that topical and oral vitamin E has anticarcinogenic, photoprotective, and skin barrier-stabilizing properties [135]. Mice treated with each form of vitamin E showed no signs of toxicity and had significantly less acute and chronic skin damage induced by UV irradiation, as indicated by reduced inflammation and pigmentation and by later onset and lesser incidence of skin cancer [136]. Topical L-selenomethionine alone and combined with vitamin E gave the best protection against UV-induced blistering and pigmentation. In protecting against skin cancer, topical RRR-alpha-tocopherol (Oral) and topical L-selenomethionine (Lotion) plus oral RRR-alpha-tocopheryl acetate were (Lotion) best. A significant synergy of L-selenomethionine with vitamin E was not observed [137]. Appreciable photoprotection can be obtained from the combination of topical stable aqueous solution of 15% L-ascorbic acid (vitamin C) and 1% alpha-tocopherol (vitamin E) to pig skin daily for 4 days [138].

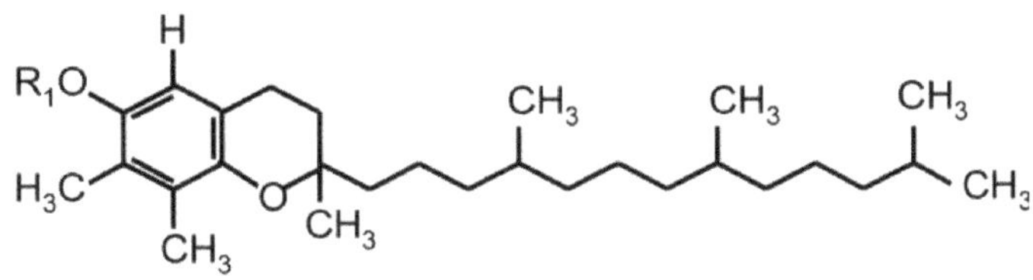

(a) γ- TDMG

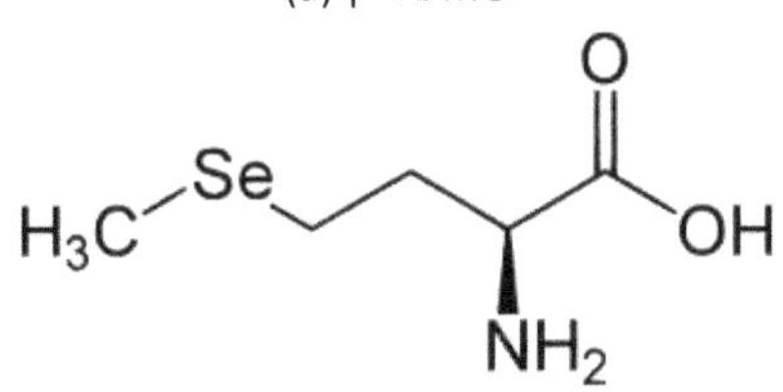

(b) L-selenomethionine

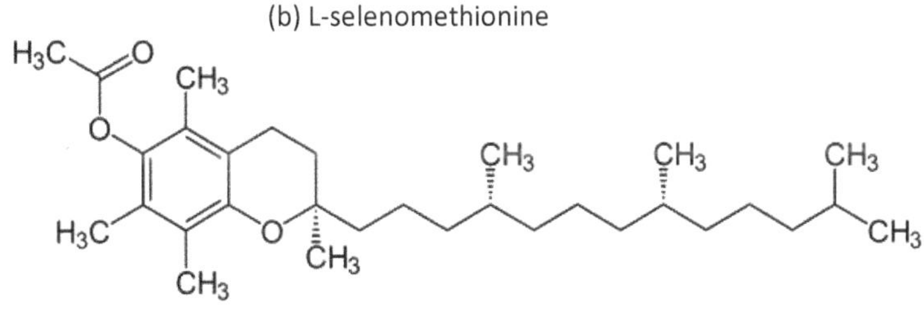

(c) Tocopheryl acetate

Figure 3.12 Vitamin E associated compounds for hyperpigmentation management.

M. Polypodium leucotomos

Polypodium leucotomos (PL) is used as an adjunct photoprotective agent in melasma. Polypodium is a fern of the Polypodiaceae family that is unique to Central and South America. PL's mechanisms of action include the promotion of the p53 suppressor gene expression, modulation of inflammatory cytokines, upregulation of endogenous antioxidant systems, and blockade of UV radiation-induced cyclooxygenase–2 expression [41]. Various extracts of PL applied topically or taken orally have been shown to have several beneficial antioxidants, photo-protectant, antimutagenic, and immunoregulatory effects [140]. The most significant differences between this extract and conventional anti-oxidants refer to its capacity as a superoxide anion scavenger. The majority of traditional anti-oxidants such as vitamin C, E, carotenoids are good quenchers of singlet oxygen; however, PL also exhibits excellent anti-oxidant properties against superoxide anion. In addition to its anti-oxidant activity, PL shows promise in the prevention of photodamage and photo-carcinogenesis because it enhances DNA repair and modulates the inflammatory and immune responses [149]. Fernblock® (IFC, Madrid, Spain), an aqueous extract of PL, is a potent antioxidant ingredient with demonstrated photo- and immune-protective activities against UVA and UVB radiations. It is available in over-the-counter formulations in topical and oral sunscreens and has been used since the 1970s for the treatment or adjunctive treatment of various skin conditions [142]. For many years, extracts of this fern have been used for treating a variety of skin conditions, including psoriasis, atopic dermatitis, vitiligo, polymorphic light eruption, and melasma. Growing evidence indicates the oral administration of oral PL extract can provide effective protection against solar UV radiation. PL extract 240mg taken twice daily for 60 days was a safe and effective means for reducing the damaging effects of UV radiation [139]. Phenolic components of PL extract include chlorogenic acid, coumaric acid, vanillic acid, caffeic acid and ferulic acid (Figure 3.13), the latter two being the most potent inhibitors of oxidation in vitro [145]. Coumaric, ferulic and vanillic acids were metabolized by CYP450-dependent mono-oxygenases and partially conjugated to glucuronic acid and sulfate. These phenolic compounds may contribute to the health benefits afforded by this oral photo-protectant [146]. Winkelmann et.al, 2015 concluded that PL is well tolerated at all doses administered and associated with a negligible risk of side effects [140]. Extracts of PL, topically applied or orally taken, have been shown to have a variety of potentially beneficial properties. Administration of PL leads to a significant reduction of sensitivity to UVR ($p<0.05$) in all patients. Dark-eye patients and patients with higher UVR sensibility (lower basal MED) would be the most benefited from oral PL treatment [141]. PL appears to be a useful adjunctive treatment for melasma [142] and may have the potential to help with post-inflammatory hyperpigmentation [143], even with just once-daily application during summer months, results in mild improvement of melasma [144]. PL is an effective chemo-photoprotector against PUVA-induced skin phototoxicity and leads to substantial benefits of skin protection against the damaging effects of PUVA as evidenced by histology [147]. PL suppressive effects on UVB-induced erythema within 2 hours of administration which demonstrates the potential correlation between non-invasive colorimetry outcomes and UVB induced molecular damage [148]. Wistar rats using doses of 0, 2000, 3500, and 5000 mg/kg bw/day Fernblock® by gavage for 28 consecutive days. No mortality or toxic effects were observed and no target organs were identified. The no observed adverse effect level was determined to be 5000 mg/kg bw/day, the highest dose tested [150].

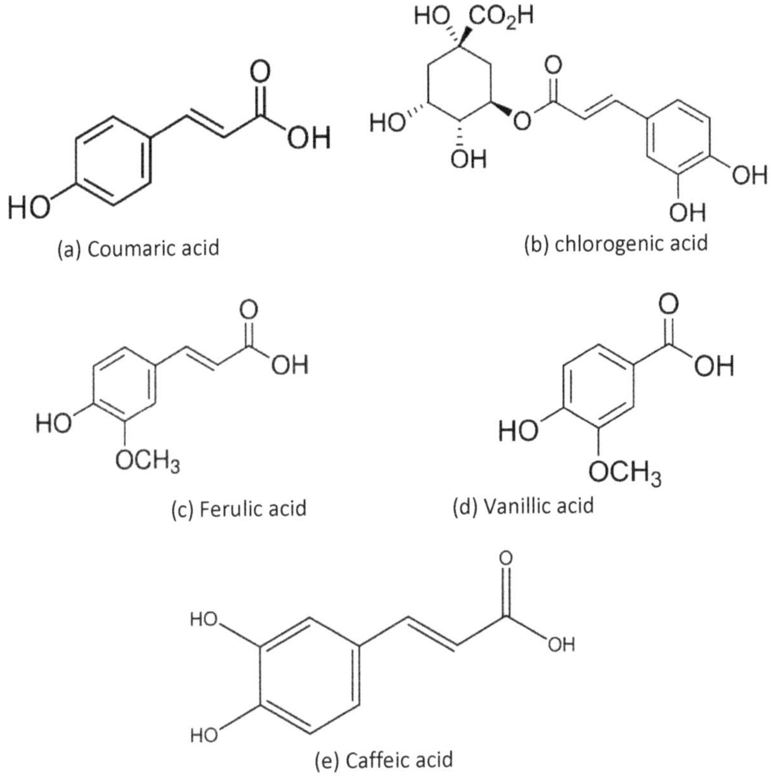

Figure 3.13 Phenolic components of *Polypodium leucotomos*

3.8.2 BLOCKING OF MELANOSOME TRANSFER

The activation of protease-activated receptor-2 (PAR-2), a seven trans-membrane G-protein coupled receptor, which is expressed in keratinocytes and not in melanocytes, was found to activate keratinocyte phagocytosis, enhancing the melanosome transfer. Inhibition of PAR-2 cleavage by serine protease inhibitor, such as RWJ-50353, completely avoids the UVB-induced pigmentation of epidermal analogs [33].

A. Niacinamide

Given a sufficient bioavailability, niacinamide has antipruritic, antimicrobial, vasoactive, photo-protective, sebostatic and lightening effects depending on its concentration [155]. Niacinamide is an effective skin lightening compound that works by inhibiting melanosome transfer from melanocytes to keratinocytes [152]. Niacinamide or nicotinamide is a biologically active form of niacin (vitamin B3) involved in over 200 enzyme reactions in the form of nicotinamide adenine dinucleotide and nicotinamide adenine dinucleotide phosphate [33].

Topical application of niacinamide at concentrations that do not affect cell viability are reversible inhibitors of melanosome transfer, resulted in a dose-dependent and reversible reduction in hyperpigmented lesions [151]. Niacinamide had no effect on the catalytic activity of mushroom tyrosinase or on melanogenesis in cultured melanocytes. Hakozaki et al.,2002 found that niacinamide decreased melanocyte transfer by 35-68% in a keratinocyte/melanocyte coculture method [152]. Clinical trials using 2% niacinamide have shown that it significantly reduces the total area of hyperpigmentation and increases skin lightness after 4 weeks of treatment. The study also showed that the daily use of niacinamide with sunscreen was effective in reducing hyperpigmentation and in increasing lightness of basal skin color compared with sunscreen alone [34]. Niacinamide interferes in melanosome transfer to keratinocytes is used in the formulations of Meladerm and Lucederm [15]. The lightening effect of Niacinamide 4% versus HQ 4% was apparent at 4 weeks of treatment, whereas it was more evident at 8 weeks in melasma patients. HQ had the disadvantage of moderate adverse effects in 18% of patients, compared to milder in 7% with niacinamide. Treatment with niacinamide showed no significant side effects and was well tolerated; therefore, it could be used for longer periods, as part of the initial hyperpigmentation treatment and as maintenance drug [153]. There is a strong need for the improvement of hyperpigmentation especially among Asian women. Ultrasound radiation enhanced the absorption of skin-lightening agents in the stratum corneum in a radiation-time-dependent manner. In the facial clinical trial, use of ultrasound radiation together with the skin-lightening gel (coupling gel of ascorbyl glucoside and niacinamide) significantly reduced facial hyperpigmented spots compared with both no treatment and skin-lightening gel alone after 4 weeks [154]. A formulation containing the combination of niacinamide + TXA reduced the appearance of irregular pigmentation, providing an effect beyond that achieved with sunscreen [99].

Bissett et.al, 2009 reported that combination of 5% niacinamide and 1% N-undecylenoyl phenylalanine is an effective anti-aging technology for use on facial skin. The combination formulation was significantly more effective than the vehicle and the 5% niacinamide formulation alone in reducing the appearance of hyperpigmentation after 8 weeks [156]. Bissett et.al, 2007 reported that topical combination of 2% N-acetyl glucosamine with 4% niacinamide ensured greater effect on facial hyperpigmentation that N-acetyl glucosamine alone [157]. A similar study by Kimball et.al, 2010 detailed that a formulation containing the combination of niacinamide + NAG reduced the appearance of irregular pigmentation including hypermelaninization, providing an effect beyond that achieved with SPF 15 sunscreen [158]. Bissett et.al, 2004 reported that 5% niacinamide was well tolerated by the skin and provided significant improvements in fine lines/wrinkles, hyperpigmentation spots, texture, skin yellowing (sallowness) and red blotchiness. In addition, skin yellowing (sallowness) versus control was significantly improved [159]. In addition to previously observed benefits for topical niacinamide, additional effects were identified by Bissett et.al, 2005, which was improved the appearance of skin wrinkles, yellowing and improved elasticity [160].

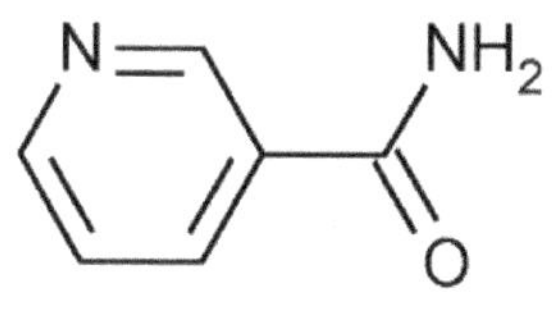

Figure 3.14 Niacinamide

B. Soy

Glycine max/Soybean, a legume commonly grown in East Asia, consists of many biologically active substances, including isoflavones and serine protease inhibitors. Glycine max, known as the soybean or soya bean, is a species of legume native to East Asia. Soybean (*Glycine max* L. Merrill) is one of the major crops containing antioxidant components such as phenolic acids, tocopherols, phytic acids, trypsin inhibitor, amino acid and isoflavones containing quercetin, genistein, daidzein and glycitein; small proteins (Bowman-Birk inhibitor, soybean trypsin inhibitor) tannins, and proanthocyanidins [161,162]. Daidzein and genistein are two major components of soy isoflavones [168]. The aglycone group (daidzein, genistein and glycitein) and acetylglucoside group (acetyldaidzin, acetylgenistin and acetylglycitin) of soy isoflavones, could inhibit UVB-induced death of human keratinocytes and reduce the level of desquamation, transepidermal water loss (TEWL), erythema and epidermal thickness in mouse skin [169]. Supplementation with 160 mgs/day of soybean isoflavone can reduce total AV lesion as a result of decreased DHT level [170]. The Supplement to Compendium of Materia Medica states that black beans can be beneficial to sperm and bone marrow production, muscle strength, hair growth, and the immune system. Modern scientific research shows that black beans have hypolipidemic and antioxidant properties and can be used to beautify the skin [163]. In-vitro studies have unleashed the anti-aging, antioxidant, pigment-reducing, photoprotective, and melanosome transfer inhibiting properties of soybean extract [55]. It has been reported that these nutritional components in soybean were associated with human health benefits such as decreased risks of various cancers, heart disease, cardiovascular disease, and increased antioxidative effects [161]. The fatty acids in soy inhibit trypsin which is a known activator of PAR-2, may be used as a natural alternative to skin lightening [165]. Furthermore, the isoflavones inhibit the DOPA oxidase activity thus inhibiting melanogenesis [34]. Soybean trypsin inhibitor (STI) inhibited PAR-2 cleavage, and completely inhibited the UVB-induced pigmentation of the epidermal equivalents containing melanocytes [33]. Although, Lai et.al, 2012 reported that black bean extracts have good antioxidant and tyrosinase-inhibitor properties, particularly in the bud rather than the dry seeds, where the budding process can improve the antioxidant and whitening properties of black soybean [163]. The major components of soy are phospholipids (45-60%), and essential fatty oils (30-35%). It also contains active ingredients like isoflavones, vitamin E and serine protease inhibitors-soybean trypsin inhibitor (STI) and Bowman-Birk protease inhibitor (BBI). The protease inhibitors inhibit PAR-2 activation, thereby inhibiting melanosome transfer. Soy has proven to be both efficacious and safe. Several skin care products containing soy are available to improve hyperpigmentation. Skin lightening benefit can be seen after 12 weeks of twice daily application. The de-pigmenting effect of soymilk is reversible and daily topical treatments for 7 months result in no adverse effects [34]. Zhao et.al, 2009 reported that non-denatured *Glycine max* extracts induced elastin promoter activity, inhibited elastase activity and protected elastic fibers from degradation by exogenous elastases in vitro, may be used as skin care agents to reduce the signs of skin ageing [164]. Evaluation through clinical observation, self-assessment, colorimetry, and photography over a 12-weeks demonstrated the soy-containing moisturizer to have a more favorable outcome in terms of improving mottled pigmentation, blotchiness, dullness, fine lines, overall texture, overall skin tone, and overall appearance than the vehicle alone. Another study involving Caucasian and Hispanic women found that the application of soy extract to melasma lesions once daily for three months led to an average reduction of hyperpigmentation of 12% [55]. Soy isoflavone is an attractive source of functional cosmetic materials with anti-wrinkle, whitening and skin hydration effects. After consumption, the majority of soy isoflavones are converted to their metabolites in the human gastrointestinal tract. Lim et.al, 2014 reported that isoflavone daidzein metabolite 6,7,4'-Trihydroxyisoflavone pretreatment significantly reduced UV induced matrix metalloproteinases (MMPs) in normal human dermal fibroblasts that are responsible for akin aging [166]. Liu-Smith et.al, 2016 reported that genistein and quercetin targeted tyrosinase directly or indirectly (**Figure 3.15**).

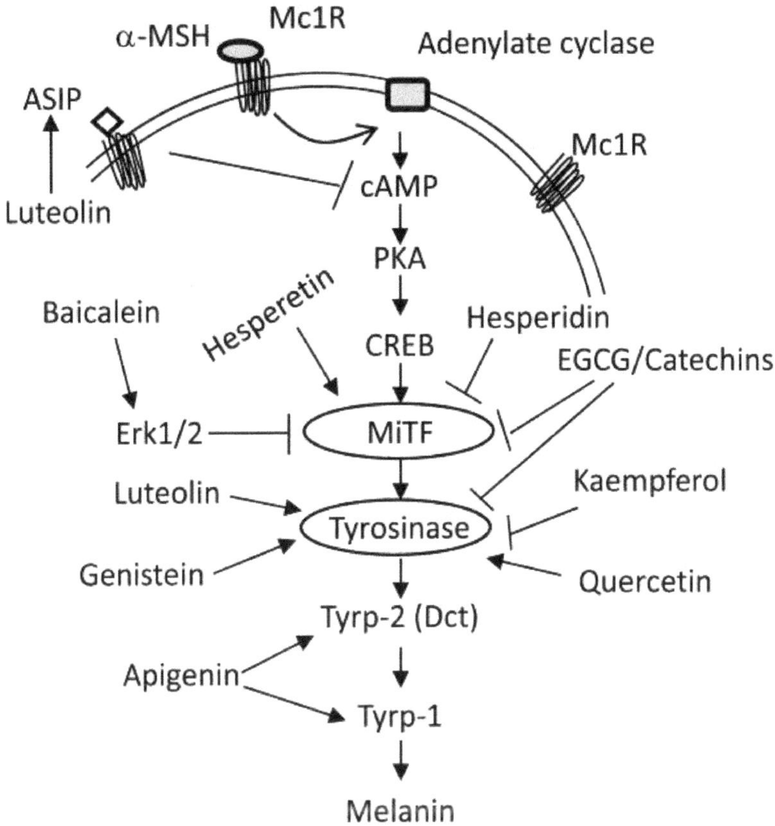

Figure 3.15 Molecular mechanisms of flavonoids on melanin synthesis [167]. Mushroom tyrosinase has been widely used as a substitute for mammalian tyrosinase to screen for tyrosinase inhibitors as it is inexpensive and commercially available in a purified form. Soy isoflavones are attractive source of functional cosmetic materials with anti-wrinkle, whitening and skin hydration effects. For quercetin, two studies showed a stimulatory effect and one showed an inhibitory effect for melanogenesis. Genistein also exhibited melanogenic effect. So, the skin whitening of soya bean may be explained by some other mechanism(s).

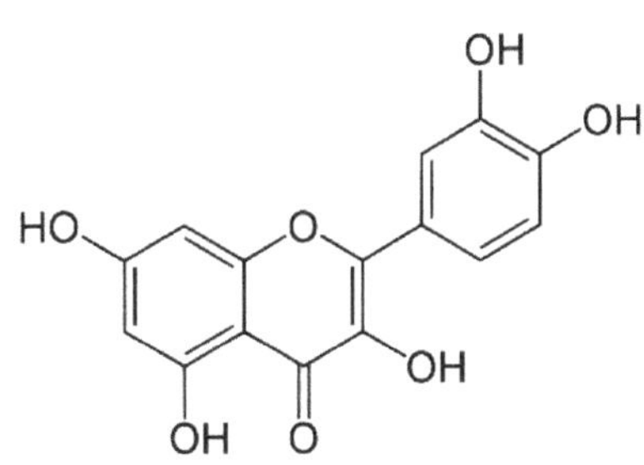

(a) Quercetin

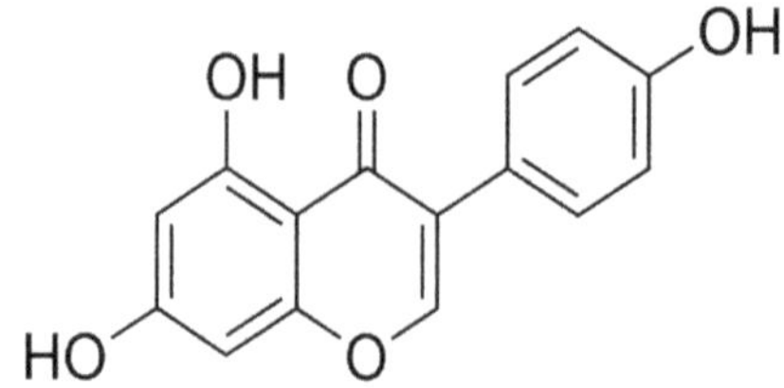

(b) Genistein

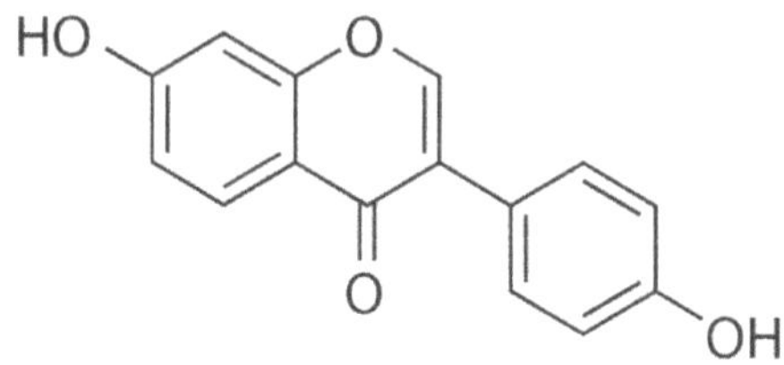

(c) Daidzein

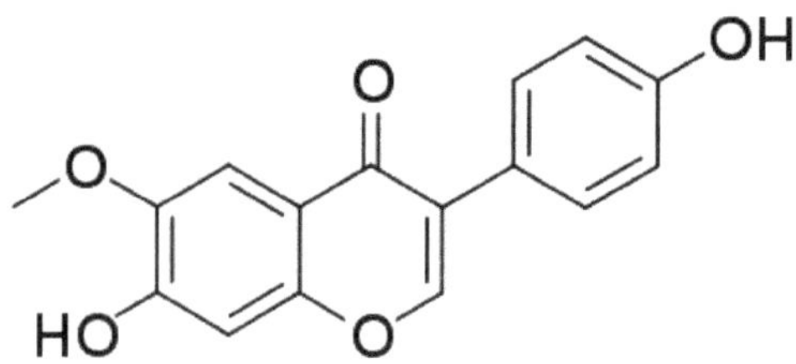

(d) Glycitein

Figure 3.16 Soy isoflavones (aglycones) of skin care prospect

C. Lectins and Neoglycoproteins

Lectins are proteins found in certain foods such as whole grains, beans and some vegetables. Potatoes, eggplant, soybeans, lentils, capsicum, wheat germ, red kidney beans, peas, tomatoes, peanuts are rich in lectins. Oral consumptions may cause problems like inflammation, leaky gut, blocking the absorption of some minerals, immune response and toxicity and digestive complaints [171]. Lectins and neoglycoproteins have been explored as candidates that are involved in this phenomenon, because of their influence in cellular processes including intracellular trafficking, endocytosis and cell-cell recognition. Lectins and neoglycoproteins interrupt melanocyte and keratinocyte contact and interaction, by binding their specific plasma membrane receptors, inhibiting melanosome transfer. This inhibition is reversible and is shown to be enhanced by the presence of niacinamide [87]. Minwalla et.al, 2001 reported fusion of keratinocyte and melanocyte plasma membranes with the formation of tunneling nanotubes. Molecules involved in transfer are being identified. Transfer is influenced by the interactions of lectins and glycoproteins and, probably, by the action of E-cadherin, SNAREs, Rab and Rho GTPases [172].

3.8.3 ACCELERATING EPIDERMAL DESQUAMATION AND MELANIN TURN OVER

The capacity of several compounds to disperse melanin pigment and/or accelerate epidermal turnover can result in skin lightening. Chemical substances used as exfoliates, such as Alpha Hydroxy Acids (AHAs), free fatty acids, and retinoic acid, stimulate cell renewal facilitating the removal of melanized keratinocyte, leading to melanin granules loss. Topical application has been shown to reduce the visibility of age spots without reducing their size or number, and can be useful in the treatment of melasma. Unsaturated fatty acid, such as oleic acid, linoleic acid, or alpha-linolenic acid, suppress pigmentation, in vitro, whereas saturated fatty acids, such as palmitic acid, increase the rate of melanogenesis. Alpha hydroxy acid (AHA) and beta hydroxy acid (BHA) are two main classes of hydroxy acids.

A. Alpha Hydroxy Acids

Hydroxy acids, also called fruit acids, are among non-organic acids which have been used in the treatment of skin disorders since about 40 years ago. The driving force behind the increase in HAs use in cosmetic dermatology and skin care systems has been their antiaging effects [195]. They are some of the most widely used and studied anti-aging skincare compounds. Clinical trials have shown the effectiveness of these ingredients in reversing the effects of photoaging and improving wrinkles, skin elasticity, tone and hydration. The benefits of AHAs have long been recognized. AHAs including glycolic acid, lactic acid, malic acid, tartaric acid, and citric acid (**Figure 3.17**) are often used extensively in cosmetic formulations. AHAs have been used as superficial peeling agents as well as to ameliorate the appearance of keratoses and acne in dermatology. However, caution should be exercised with certain adverse reactions among patients using products with AHAs, including swelling, burning, and pruritus [174]. AHA is used in the treatment of several skin conditions such as acne, scar, pigmentation, skin dryness and wrinkles. They involve in metabolic pathways and essential cell cycles, including Krebs cycle, glycolysis and biosynthesis of serin. AHAs act on both the epidermal and the dermal levels. When applied to the skin, AHAs stimulate the exfoliation of epidermal cells in the stratum corneum by interfering with the ionic bonding between these cells. This results in the sloughing off dull and rough skin and promotes cellular renewal. Initially used for treatment of hyperkeratosis and other skin conditions affecting subcutaneous turnover, AHAs were found to promote softer, smoother skin, faded wrinkles, lightened age spots, and decreased blemishes. AHAs also improve the subcutaneous barrier function, increase epidermal proliferation and thickness, and restore hydration and pursiness through an increase in hyaluronic acid. The well-known benefits of AHA's include exfoliation, moisturization, reduction of fine lines and wrinkles, collagen synthesis, firming and skin lightening. Glycolic acid is the smallest at AHA compounds, extracted from sugar. Formulations containing 10-15% GA are currently used topically, vaginally and rectally or as ophthalmic preparations for treatment at skin aging and hyper pigmentation due to sunlight. A negative side effect of AHAs may be a sensation of stinging or burning immediately after application, particularly on people with sensitive skin. New more lipophilic AHAs will be utilized more in the future, especially when targeting oily skins [173]. Sour milk (LA) and sugarcane juice (GA) were applied to the face. In low concentrations, AHAs decreased corneocyte cohesion, leading to sloughing of dead cells and stimulation of new cell growth in the basal layer. In higher concentrations, they cause epidermilysis. AHAs have been reported to be effective in treating pigmentary lesions such as melasma, solar lentigines, and post-inflammatory hyperpigmentation. The mechanism of this effect might be due to epidermal remodeling and accelerated desquamation, which would result in quick pigment dispersion. GA and LA might work on pigmentary lesions not only by accelerating the turnover of the epidermis but also by directly inhibiting melanin formation by inhibiting tyrosinase in melanocytes. GA or LA (at doses of 300 or 500 mg/ml) inhibited melanin formation in similar dose-dependent manner, without affecting cell growth. The bioavailability of AHAs increases as the pH decreases (desirable pH 2.8–4.8), and they are the only peels that are time-dependent and can be neutralized easily [33]. The most common indications for chemical peeling are chronic photoaging and hyperpigmentation. Chemical peels are the third most commonly performed noninvasive cosmetic procedure in the US, with over 1,300,000 procedures performed in 2016 alone. There has been a paradigm shift in recent years, with lasers largely supplanting deep peels. Despite this shift, superficial peels have proliferated in both popularity and product diversity [190].

Glycolic acid peels are commercially available as free acids, partially neutralized (higher pH), buffered, or esterified solutions. They are available in various concentrations ranging from 20%–70%. The higher the concentration and lower the pH, the more intense the peeling will be. In general, gel formulations have a slower penetration time and are easier to control. Fabbrocini et.al, 2009, classified glycolic peels as: very superficial (30%–50% GA, applied for 1–2 minutes); superficial (50%–70% GA, applied for 2–5 minutes); and medium depth (70% GA, applied for 3–15 minutes) [175]. GA peels have antiinflammatory, keratolytic, and antioxidant effects. GA targets the corneosome by enhancing breakdown and decreasing cohesiveness, causing desquamation. The intensity of GA peel is determined by the concentration of the acid. GA peels need to be properly neutralized to stop acidification of the skin. Priming the skin with hydroquinone, or topical retinoids, before performing a peel has been found to increase peel efficacy and reduce the risk of post-inflammatory hyperpigmentation. After the skin has been cleansed and degreased, GA solution is applied using cotton buds or a brush in a sequential manner starting from the forehead to the left cheek, chin, right cheek to cover the entire face [176]. When properly used, superficial exfoliation with glycolic acid at concentrations of 30 to 50% has demonstrated excellent clinical efficacy in the treatment of superficial hyperpigmentation, mild-to-moderate chrono- and photoaging, and fine rhytides [190]

Exhibit 4. Glycolic Acid in Melasma Management

Study	Result	Reference
Concentrations of 20%–70% GA were administered every 3 weeks, either alone or in combination with a topical regimen of 2% hydroquinone plus 10% GA	There was significant improvement in melasma and fine facial wrinkling in patients who received the combination of creams and peeling.	Lim et.al, 1997[177]
55%–75% GA versus 10%–15% trichloroacetic acid (TCA) peels in 100 patients with recalcitrant melasma. The peels were conducted at 15-day intervals in both groups.	Response to TCA was rapid, and produced better results than GA. However, relapse was more common in the TCA group (25%) than in the GA group	Kella et.al, 2001 [178]
Using 50% GA, once-monthly for 3 months, peeling was performed upon 15 Indian females with melasma	An improvement in MASI score was observed in 91% of patients. A better response was seen in patients with epidermal melasma, compared to those with mixed melasma	Javaheri et.al, 2001 [178]
20 Indian patients received serial GA peels (30% GA for the first three sittings; 40% GA for the next three sittings), combined with the modified Kligman's formula (2% hydroquinone, 0.025% tretinoin, and 1% mometasone). A further 20 Indian patients received only the modified Kligman's formula, with no peeling.	In both groups, a significant decrease in the MASI score was observed from baseline to 21 weeks. However, the GA peel group showed more rapid and greater improvement.	Sarkar et.al, 2002 [180]*

Contd...

Study	Result	Reference
21 Hispanic women with bilateral, epidermal, and mixed melasma to assess the efficacy of 4% hydroquinone cream versus 4% hydroquinone cream combined with GA peels. Patients received GA peels (20%–30% GA) every 2 weeks to one side of the face only, in addition to twice-daily application of 4% hydroquinone cream to the other side of the face	Pigmentation was measured objectively using a Mexameter® (Courage + Khazaka electronic GmbH, Cologne, Germany) and the MASI, and measured subjectively using a linear analog scale and physician and patient global evaluation. Both sides of the face showed a reduction of pigmentation, and there was no significant difference.	Hurley et.al, 2002 [181]*
Patients with melasma were treated with a 70% GA peel on one half of the face, while the other half was treated with a 1% tretinoin peel.	A significant decrease in the modified MASI score was observed on both facial sides from baseline to 6 weeks, and then from 6 to 12 weeks.	Khunger et.al, 2004 [182]
Same as above, melasma patients were treated with a 70% GA peel on one half of the face, and with a 1% tretinoin peel on the other one.	Two peels to be equally effective and well tolerated.	Kligman et.al, 2004 [183]
In 15 cases of melasma (epidermal: 80%; dermal: 13.3%; and mixed: 6.6%), 52.5% GA concentration was applied for 3 minutes.	There was good to fair response in patients with epidermal and mixed melasma, while no significant improvement was seen in dermal melasma.	Grover et.al, 2003 [184]
Serial GA peels (from 35%–50%, and 70% every second peel) plus combination topical therapy (azelaic acid and adapalene) in 28 women with melasma	Better results in the group receiving chemical peel plus topical therapy, but only when the GA concentration was 50% or higher.	Ebril et.al, 2007 [185]
A triple combination cream consisting of fluocinolone acetonide 0.01%, hydroquinone 4%, and tretinoin 0.05% was used in an alternating sequential treatment pattern, cycling with a series of GA peels, for the treatment of moderate to severe melasma.	Hyperpigmentation was significantly reduced at 6 and 12 weeks, compared with baseline, with evaluations showing improvement of 90% or more by week 12.	Rendon et.al, 2008 [186]

Contd...

Study	Result	Reference
In a comparative study of 10%–20% TCA versus 20%–35% GA peels for the treatment of melasma, similar improvement was seen with both peels.	GA peel was seen to be associated with fewer side effects than the TCA peel, and gave the added benefit of facial rejuvenation.	Kumari et.al, 2010 [187]
A similar study as above, 15% TCA peel versus 35% GA peel for the treatment of melasma, there was no statistically significant difference in efficacy.	Both peels significantly reduced MASI scores, and both were found to be equally effective in the treatment of melasma. It was also seen that adverse effects were more common with TCA than with GA peels.	Puri et.al, 2012 [188]

* The concentration of GA used by Hurley et.al, 2002 was low (20%–30%), compared to the 30%–40% GA used by Sarkar et.al, 2002. This could be a reason for the difference in the results they observed.

AHAs		structure	Molecular weight
Glycolic acid	C_2H4O3	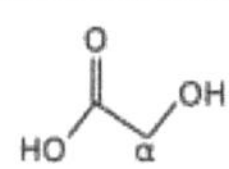	72
Lactic acid	$C_3H_6O_3$	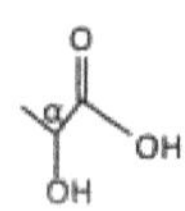	90
Malic acid	$C_4H_6O_5$	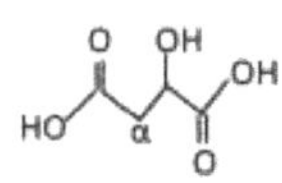	134
Tartaric acid	$C_4H_6O_6$	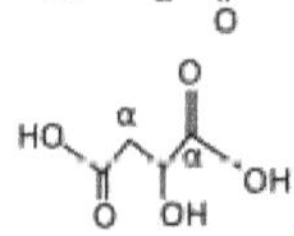	150
Citric acid	$C_6H_8O_7$	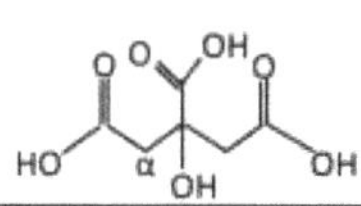	192

Figure 3.17 The structures of AHAs commonly used in dermatology [174].

Lactic acid, especially the L isomer, increases ceramide biosynthesis in vitro and in vivo. Presumably lactic acid achieves this by acting as a general lipid precursor by providing acetate and providing more reducing power in the form of NADH or NADPH [33]. Glycolic acid and lactic acid suppress melanin synthesis by inhibiting tyrosinase activity, the critical enzyme involved in melanin synthesis, inhuman and in mouse melanoma cells. Both the transcription and translation of tyrosinase were decreased significantly, which resulted in the reduced enzyme function but with no significant effect on cell growth. Based on that in vitro analysis, increased epidermal turnover and inhibition of melanin formation were surmised to be the effects of glycolic acid and lactic acid treatment [195]. Lactic acid peels being relatively inexpensive and having shown equally good results in a few studies. Pure lactic acid, full strength (92%; pH 3.5), was used 3 weeks until the desired response was achieved, but not more than six sessions. Follow-up was carried out for 6 months after the last session. All patients had skin type IV. Patients showed marked improvement, as calculated by the MASI score before and after treatment, and the response was highly statistically significant. No side effect was recorded in all treated patients [189]. Clinically, lactic acid has demonstrated comparable efficacy in the treatment of photodamage, superficial hyperpigmentation, and fine rhytides compared to standard glycolic acid peels. Because lactic acid has a lower pH than glycolic acid, a lower concentration is often used to achieve an equivalent depth of keratocoagulation compared to glycolic acid, which allows a favorable side effect profile and recovery time [190]. Further, lactic acid was compared with a well-established peeling agent, Jessner's solution in a split-face design, and similar improvement was seen on both the sides with no relapse at a follow-up after six months [191]. Puri et.al, 2015 reported that Jessner's solution (comprising 14g resorcinol, 14g salicylic acid, 14mL lactic acid in ethanol constituted to 100mL) can be an adjuvant treatment with TCA in the treatment of acne scars, improving the results and minimizing post inflammatory hyperpigmentation [192]. Histological differences in skin treated with glycolic, lactic, citric and acetic acids once daily for 6 weeks were investigated by Yamamoto et.al, 2006. The melanin pigments in the basal layer were less prominent in the glycolic and lactic acid-treated skin than in the citric and acetic acid-treated skin. The melanin deposits in the horny layers were equal for all AHA. However, the melanin deposits in the squamous layers were less prominent in the glycolic and lactic acid-treated skins than in the citric and acetic acid-treated skins [194].

B. Beta Hydroxy Acid

Salicylic acid (SA) peels have been shown useful in PIH, including for patients with darker skin types [196]. It is also a phytohormone, a plant product that acts similar to a hormone and regulates cell growth and differentiation. SA functions as a desquamating agent that penetrates and dissolves the intercellular matrix of the stratum corneum [87]. Being a lipophilic agent and having an ability to concentrate in the pilosebaceous apparatus, SA peels are a good therapeutic option for comedonal acne and hyperpigmentation. Pre-peel regimens differ between acne vulgaris, photodamage, and hyperpigmentation, including melasma and post-inflammatory hyperpigmentation. The combination of pre-peel application of 4% hydroquinone twice daily with peeling produces substantial decreases in the intensity of hyperpigmentation in both post-inflammatory hyperpigmentation and melasma [197]. Superficial SA peels are both safe and efficacious for the treatment of acne vulgaris, oily skin, textural changes, melasma, and post-inflammatory hyperpigmentation in patients with skin types V and VI. In an open- label trial, 25 patients were treated with five salicylic acid peels (20-30% concentration) provided at two-week intervals. Patients underwent two weeks of pretreatment with hydroquinone 4%. Four out of five patients with Fitzpatrick type V or VI had greater than 75% improvement in pigmentation [198]. Fifty patients attending the outpatient clinic of Dermatology Department, with clinically evident periorbital hyperpigmentation were included. All patients were divided randomly into two groups of 25 each and one group was treated with 4% HQ and another group with 30% SA for 12 weeks. Separately, both the treatments significantly improved the dermatological life quality index of the patients although there was no significant difference found between the two groups [199]. A combination of SA peel 20-30% and topical tretinoin 0.1% treatment showed significant clinical improvement of PIH than each treatment alone with no complications [200]. SA peels are beneficial in whitening the face of Asian patients with acne. The whitening effect would be an important factor in choosing the superficial peeling agent for them [201]. Clinical efficacy of SA 33% peeling once in a month, for a total of 4 times in patients with melasma reveals statistically significant values comparing MASI score obtained by digital photo and MASI score obtained clinically [202].

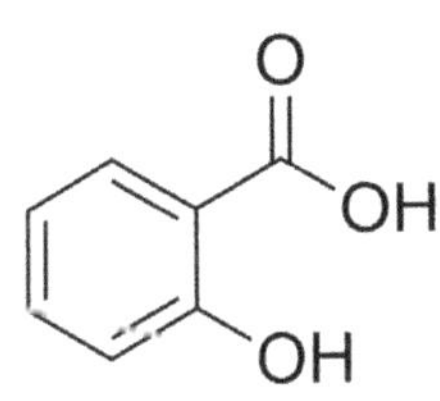

Figure 3.18 Salicylic Acid

C. Linolenic Acid

Unsaturated fatty acids including oleic acid (C18:1), linoleic acid (C18:2) or α-linolenic acid (C18:3) suppresses melanogenesis and tyrosinase activity, while saturated fatty acids such as palmitic acid (C16:0) or stearic acid (C18:0) increases it. Omega-3 polyunsaturated fatty acids (PUFAs) like *Linoleic acid* (LnA) reduces the activity of tyrosinase in melanocytes, while mRNA levels remain unchanged. α-LnA and LnA were reported to reveal skin-whitening capability through the mechanism of tyrosinase inhibition by Anso et.al, 1999 [205]. This may influence the enzyme's degradation via a physiologic proteasome-dependent mechanism, altering the tyrosinase protein content in hyperactive melanocytes [87]. LnA is known to have a whitening effect on hyperpigmented skin, and is encapsulated in liposomes for topical application because of its low solubility in aqueous solution. Topical application of alpha-linolenic acid to UV-stimulated hyperpigmented dorsal skin of brownish guinea pigs. The number of melanocytes in the treated skin was similar to the number in the skin of the pigmented control, indicating that the pigment-lightening effect was not due to the depletion of melanocytes. Linoleic acid also influences skin pigmentation by stimulating epidermal turnover and increased desquamation of melanin pigment from the epidermis [203]. Liposomal LnA (0.1%) showed a whitening effect comparable to 10.0% non-liposomal LA and was far more effective than 3.0% non-liposomal LnA [204]. Ko et.al, 2018 reported LnA ester, ethyl linoleate decreased melanin production and tyrosinase activity through the reduction of tyrosinase and TRP1 expression. Ethyl linoleate may be used as a non-cytotoxic and skin-whitening agent as a cosmetic and medicine [206]. In a 6-week, double-blind, RCT among 60 patients, LnA in combination with lincomycin and betamethasone valerate was found to result in higher improvement than a combination of the latter two or vehicle [101].

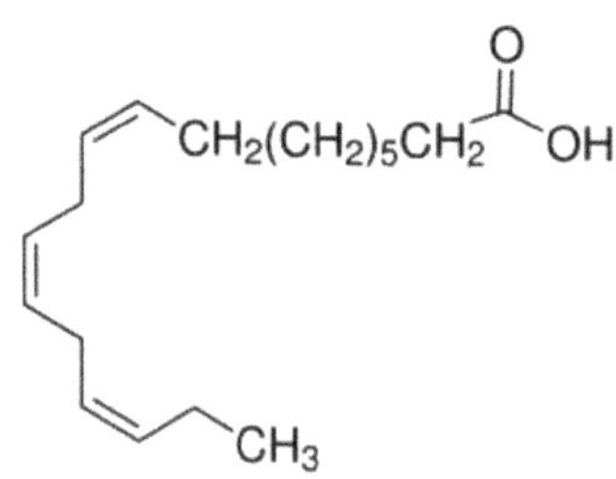

Figure 3.19 Linolenic Acid

D. Retinoids

Topical retinoids such as all-trans-retinoic acid (RA), 13-cis-retinoic acid (isotretinoin), retinol, retinaldehyde, tazarotene, and adapalene have been shown to improve dyspigmentation of photodamaged skin including mottling and actinic lentigines. RA monotherapy has also been demonstrated to improve melasma and post-inflammatory hypermelanosis [208]. Irritant reactions can result from long-term daily use of 4% or higher HQ, particularly when used in combination with irritants such as retinoids. An early formulation, Kligman's formula containing 5% HQ, 0.1% tretinoin, and 0.1% dexamethasone, is one such combination that was effective yet problematic due to its use of high concentrations of tretinoin and a potent fluorinated steroid. 4% HQ, 0.05% tretinoin, and 0.01% fluocinolone acetonide triple- combination agent has been shown to be both safe and effective in the treatment of melasma and photoaging in skin of color and is used successfully in clinical practice to treat PIH. Topical tretinoin, all-trans-retinoic acid, is a naturally occurring metabolite of retinol and first-generation retinoid. Concentrations range from 0.01 to 0.1% and tretinoin can be formulated in creams, gels, and microsphere gels, which allows for the controlled release of tretinoin leading to less irritation. Tretinoin was significantly more effective than vehicle in lightening PIH lesions when assessed by clinical and colorimetric analysis after a 40-week trial with 54 black patients to determine the safety and efficacy of 0.1% tretinoin in the treatment of PIH. However, 50% of patients developed retinoid dermatitis, which is the concern with using retinoids in skin of color. Third-generation retinoids, adapalene and tazarotene, are synthetic topical agents that are also effective in the treatment of PIH. Adapalene is formulated in creams or gels in 0.1 to 0.3% concentrations; whereas, formulations of tazarotene include 0.05 and 0.1% creams or gels. Both agents have been shown in clinical studies to safely and effectively treat PIH, particularly acne-induced PIH, in darker skinned individuals. Isotretinoin (13-cis-retinoic acid) is a naturally occurring, first-generation retinoid that is available in both oral and topical formulations [209]. These cosmetic products are suspected to contain illegal active substances (in particular hydroquinone, tretinoin and corticosteroids) that may provoke as well local as systemic toxic effects, being the reason for their banning from the EU market [210].

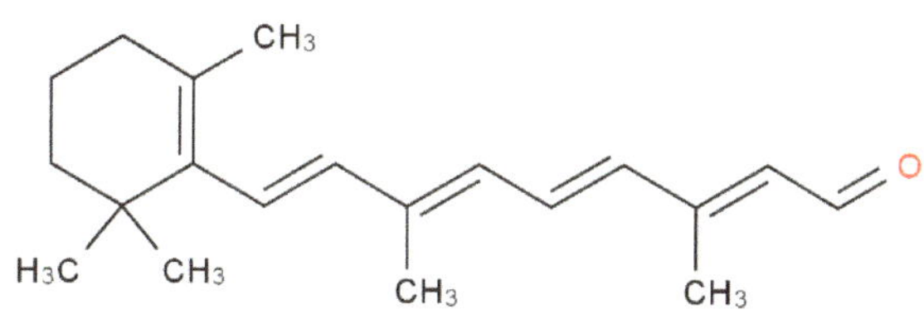

(a) Retinaldehyde

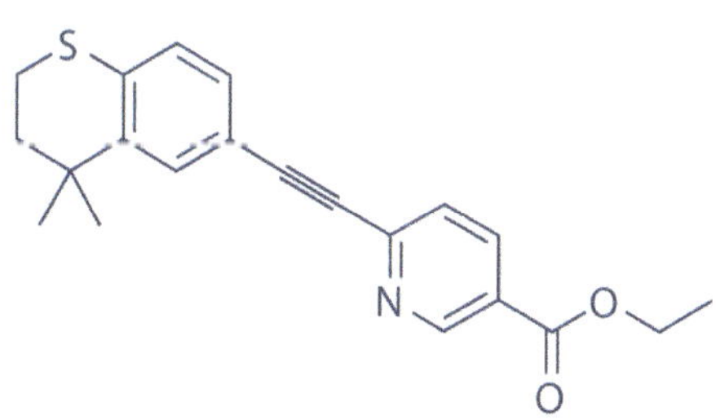

(b) Tazarotene

Figure 3.20 Topical retinoids

E. Antioxidants

Oxidative stress is an integral element that influences a variety of biochemical reactions throughout the body and is known to play a notable role in melanogenesis. Exogenous triggers of oxidative stress, such as UVR and VL, lead to pigment formation through somewhat different pathways, but both share a common endpoint-the potential to generate cosmetically undesirable hyperpigmentation [211]. There is evidence that situations of mild stress, such as caloric restriction or physical activity, can modulate the aging process since they increase mitochondrial activity, also increasing the generation of ROS - which would provoke an adaptive response, with improvement of defense mechanisms and consequent better response and resistance to stress. Antioxidant molecules employed that have proven utility also have whitening action by inhibition of tyrosinase (for example, ascorbic acid and ellagic acid) or anti-inflammatory (for example, pycnogenol) (Figure 3.21) [212]. Schalka et.al, 2017 concluded that UV, VL and IR light induce pigmentation. To prevent hyperpigmentation, protection using adequate sunscreens on exposed areas is needed. To date, no efficient protection from IR light exists, but topical antioxidants may be able to provide some protection [213]. Antioxidants neutralize free radicals produced by various environmental insults such as ultraviolet radiation, cigarette smoke and air pollutants, thereby preventing cellular damage [214]. For example, grape seed extract rich in monomers of flavanols, vitamin C, and zinc has a beneficial effect on skin radiance (improvement of luminosity, reduction of imperfections, and improvement of skin firmness) in women [222]. Snail slime (SS) is currently revolutionizing the world of cosmetics and human skin care. The efficacy of SS in wound healing has been proven both in vitro and by clinical studies. SS reduced melanin content and tyrosinase activity on B16F10 cells with IC50 values of 288 μg/mL and 286 μg/mL, respectively, without altering cell viability [223].

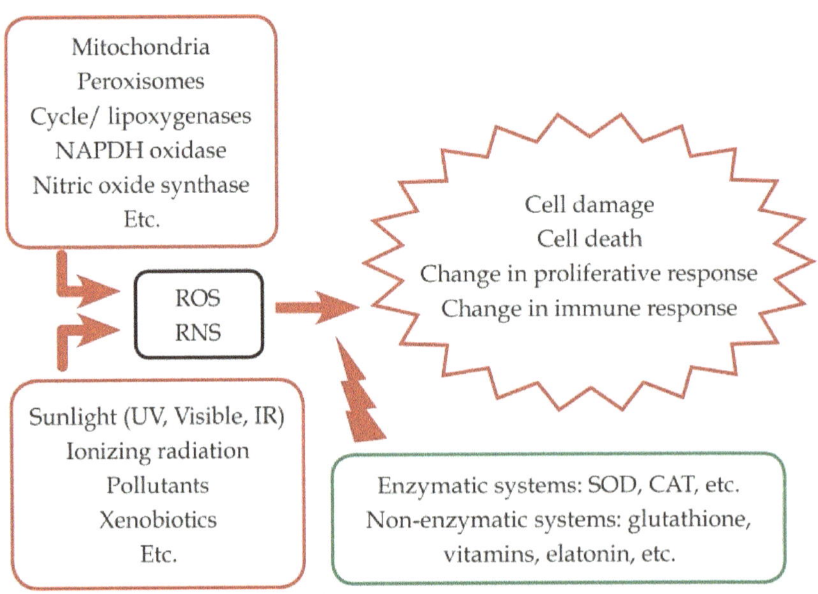

Figure 3.21 Diagram of the redox balance in the skin [212].

F. Tea

Green tea has long been studied for its antioxidant and anti-inflammatory properties. Fresh tea leaves contain polyphenols, primarily the catechins epigallocatechin (EGC), epicatechin (EC), epigallo-catechin-3-gallate (ECGC), and epicatechin gallate (ECG) [217,218]. These four catechins, of which EGCG is the most abundant, accounting up to 30% of tea leaf dry weight [215]. The irradiation of green tea polyphenol did not change and even increased its anti-wrinkle, skin-whitening and anticancer effects on the human skin [221]. According to the abstract of a single RCT, green tea has shown clinical efficacy in treating melasma [55]. Tea and its components have been shown to inhibit intracellular and cell-extracted tyrosinase activities. EGCG causes such inhibition in mushrooms, and oolong tea reduces tyrosinase activity in B16 mouse melanoma cells. Tea flavonoids have metal chelation abilities. For example, proanthocyanidins, which are flavonoids from grape seeds, inhibit tyrosinase by chelating tyrosinase-bound copper. Black tea theaflavins and Green Tea flavonols are also known to exert antioxidant effects by radical scavenging and metal chelation. White tea was also reported to have higher levels of antioxidant activity than green tea [34], [215]. EGCG significantly inhibits cell growth as well as the migration and invasion of melanoma cells [220]. EGCG reduced melanin secretion and production in melanoma cells [217].

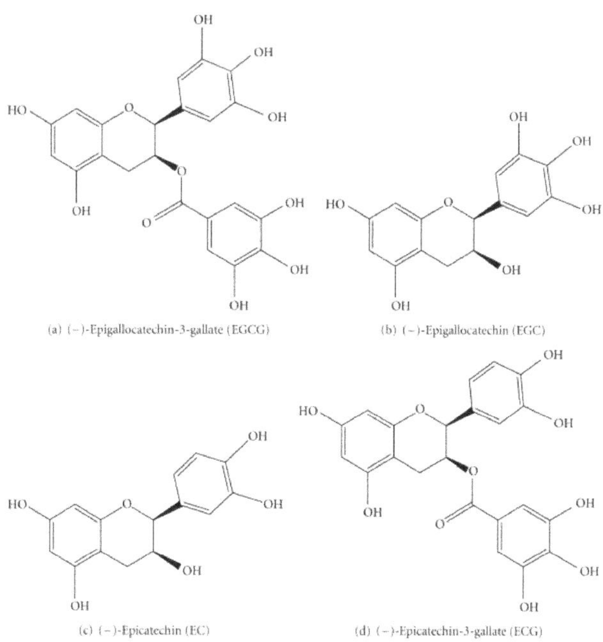

Figure 3.22 Structure of green tea polyphenols [219].

G. Ginseng

Panax ginseng has been used traditionally in eastern Asia to treat various diseases, due to its immunomodulatory, neuroprotective, antioxidative, and antitumor activities. Recently, several reports have shown that extract, powder, or some constituents of ginseng could inhibit melanogenesis in vivo or in vitro. The underlying mechanisms of antimelanogenic properties in ginseng or its components include the direct inhibition of key enzymes of melanogenesis, inhibition of transcription factors or signaling pathways involved in melanogenesis, decreasing production of inducers of melanogenesis, and enhancing production of antimelanogenic factor. Cinnamic acid, one of the major components of *Cinnamomum cassia* Blume, is found in the root and seed of P. ginseng. Cinnamic acid is reported to have inhibitory activity on mushroom tyrosinase. Cinnamic acid significantly reduced melanin production, tyrosinase activity, and tyrosinase expression in the melan-a cells. In addition, cinnamic acid showed depigmenting activity on the UVB-tanned skin of brown guinea pigs [224].

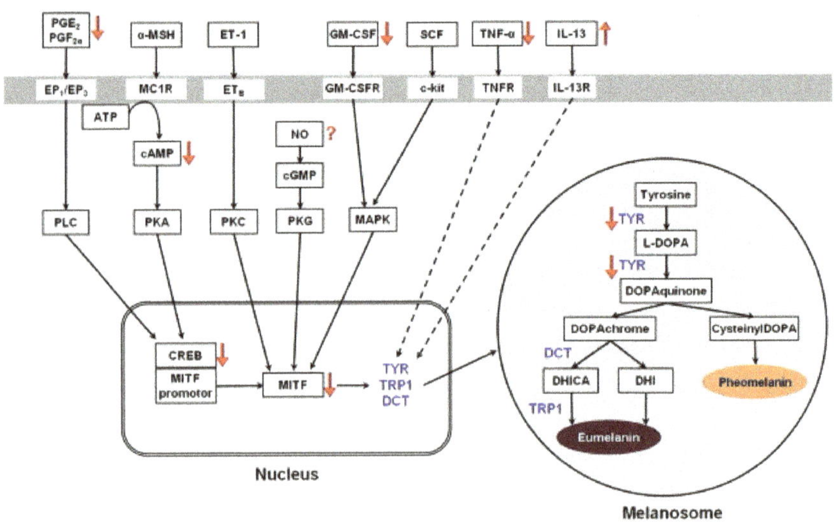

Figure 3.23 Schematic view of the effects of ginseng on melanogenesis [224]. Black solid arrow indicates activation, black dashed arrow indicates inhibition, red upward arrow indicates increase by ginseng components, and red downward arrow indicates decrease by ginseng components. α-MSH, α-melanocyte stimulating factor; CREB, cAMP response element-binding protein; DCT, dopachrome tautomerase; DHI, 5,6-dihydroxyindole; DHICA, 5,6-dihydroxyindole-2-carboxylic acid; DOPA, 3,4-dihydroxyphenylalanine; EP1, prostaglandin E receptor 1; ET-1, endothelin-1; ETB , endothelin receptor type B; GM-CSF, granulocyte-macrophage colony-stimulating factor; IL-13, interleukin 13; MAPK, mitogen-activated protein kinases; MC1R, melanocortin 1 receptor; MITF, micropthalmia-associated transcription factor; NO, nitric oxide; PGE2, prostaglandin E2; PGF2α, prostaglandin F2α; PKA, protein kinase A; PKG, protein kinase G; PLC, phospholipase C; SCF, stem cell factor; TNF-α, tumor necrosis factor-α; TRP1, tyrosinase-related protein-1; TYR, tyrosinase.

Exhibit 5. Direct effects of ginseng and its components on melanogenesis in vivo and in vitro [224]

Reagent	Experimental model	Dose	Effects on melanogenesis
Powder of KRG	Melasma lesion of female patients	3 g/d oral 24 wk	MASI: decreased MELASQoL: improved Patient- and investigator-rated global improvement scale: improved
Ethanol extract of ginseng seed	Melan-a cells cultured with phorbol-12 myristate 13-acetate	100 ppm 3 d	Melanin content: decreased tyrosinase activity: decreased
Extract of KRG and FKRG	Mushroom tyrosinase		Tyrosinase activity: decreased
Aglycone of ginsenoside Rh4	B16 cells stimulated by a-MSH	20e50mM 5 d	Melanin content: decreased Tyrosinase activity: decreased MITF expression: decreased
p-Coumaric acid	Mushroom tyrosinase		Tyrosinase activity: decreased
Ginsenoside Rb1	B16 cells stimulated by a-MSH	125e500mM 2 d	Melanin content: decreased Tyrosinase activity: decreased
Ginsenoside F1	Human skin artificially tanned by UV irradiation	0.1% cream topical 8 wk	Luminosity values: increased

*α-MSH, α-melanocyte stimulating factor; FKRG, fermented Korean Red Ginseng; KRG, Korean Red Ginseng; MASI, melasma area and severity index; MELASQoL, melasma quality of life scale; MITF, micropthalmia-associated transcription factor

Lee et.al, 2019 reported that Ginsenoside Rg1 increases melanogenesis and tyrosinase activity in human melanocytes. In contrast, ginsenoside F1 (GF1), a metabolite produced by the hydrolysis of Rg1, is reported to inhibit visible pigmentation. GF1 has the potential for development as an effective whitening reagent for the treatment of pigmentary disorders and lightening of darkened

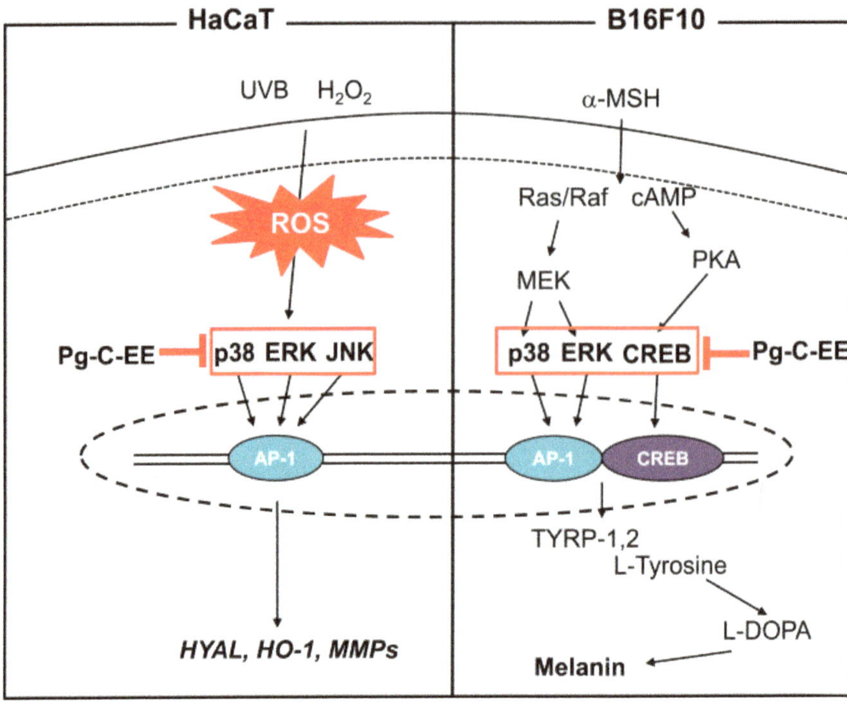

Figure 3.24 Pathway by which Pg-C-EE inhibits melanogenesis and ROS generation [228]. α-MSH, α-melanocyte–stimulating hormone; AP-1, activator protein 1; cAMP, cyclic adenosine monophosphate; CREB, cAMP response element- binding; ERK, extracellular signal-regulated kinase; HO-1, heme oxygenase-1; HYAL, hyaluronidase; JNK, c-Jun N-terminal kinase; L-DOPA, L-dopamine; MMP, matrix metalloproteinase; Pg-C-EE, Panax ginseng calyx ethanol extract; PKA, Protein kinase A; ROS, reactive oxygen species; TYRP, tyrosinase-related protein; UVB, ultraviolet B.

skin color as a cosmetic ingredient [225]. Ginsenoside Rb2 (Gin-Rb2) decreased potent melanogenesis in melan-a cells, with 23.4% at 80 μM without cytotoxicity. Gin-Rb2 also decreased tyrosinase and MITF protein expression in melan-a cells. Furthermore, Gin-Rb2 presented inhibition of the body pigmentation in the zebrafish in vivo system and reduced melanin contents and tyrosinase activity [230]. The ethanol extract of ginseng seed showed an excellent inhibitory effect on melanin production (due to presence of arbutin) and demonstrated low cytotoxicity when applied to melanocytes, compared to the ethanol extracts of ginseng root and ginseng leaf [226]. Jiménez et.al, 2018 reported that P. ginseng berry mediated gold nanoparticles, significantly reduced melanin content and suppress tyrosinase activity in α-MSH-stimulated B16BL6 cells. In addition, P. ginseng berry mediated gold nanoparticles exhibited moisture retention capacity [227]. Lee et.al, 2018 reported that P. ginseng berry calyx (Pg-C-EE) exerted skin-protective effects through antimelanogenesis activity in α-MSH–induced B16F10 cells (a murine melanoma cell line from the C57BL/6J mouse), antiphotoaging activity in UVB-irradiated HaCaT cells (immortalized human keratinocytes and have been extensively used to study the epidermal homeostasis and its pathophysiology), and antioxidant activity in hydrogen peroxide–induced HaCaT cells. In addition, Pg-C-EE inhibited Activator Protein-1 (AP-1) and cAMP response element binding (CREB) transcription factors and their upstream activation pathway (mitogen-activated protein kinases, MAPK and CREB) **(Figure 3.25)** [228]. Yang et.al, 2017 reported that fermented red ginseng is believed to be more effective in reducing wrinkles and enhance whitening compared to unfermented red ginseng [229]. Song et.al, 2011 reported 3 g of Korean red ginseng powder was orally administered for a 24-weeks in 25 women resulted improvement in 74% of the patients and it was tolerated by most of the patients [231].

Exhibit 6. Summary of clinical studies evaluating the efficacy of natural ingredients as hypo pigmenting agents [55]

Natural Ingred-ients	Hypo pigmenting Mechanism	Comparison	Pigmentation Disorder	Conclusion
Azelaic Acid (AA)	Mitochondrial oxidoreductase inhibition, DNA synthesis inhibition, Tyrosinase inhibition	20% AA vs. 4% HQ cream	Melasma	Melasma responded better to AA during second treatment month
		None	PIH	15% AA gel applied twice daily reduced PIH over 16 week period
		GA peel with twice daily 20% AA cream vs. 20% AA cream	Melasma	At 12 weeks, AA/GA combination has a statistically significant decrease in MASI score compared with AA alone
		None	PIH	Dermocosmetics containing AA showed improvement in pigmentation
Aloesin	Tyrosinase inhibition, tyrosine hydroxylase, DOPA oxidase	Aloesin vs. Arbutin vs. Aloesin/Arbutin	UVR-induced hyperpigmentation	Dose-dependent suppression in pigmentation with application of aloesin; synergism between arbutin and aloesin

Contd...

Natural Ingred-ients	Hypo pigmenting Mechanism	Comparison	Pigmentation Disorder	Conclusion
Mulberry	Tyrosinase inhibition, melanogenesis inhibition, ROS Scavenger	75% mulberry extract	Melasma	Compared to placebo, 75% mulberry extract showed significant improvement in MASI score, average Mexamater measurements, and MelasQoL scores
Licorice Extracts	Tyrosinase inhibition (glabridin)	None	Melasma	Sixteen out of 20 patients had an "excellent response" to 20% liquitin cream applied BID for four weeks Glabridin was more efficacious compared to HQ
	ROS cavenger (glabridin)	None	UVR-induced hyperpigmentation	Skin brightener contain-ing glabridin was shown to be clinically efficacious
	Disperses melanin (liquiritin)	Cream with belides, emblica, and licorice vs. 2% HQ	Melasma	Although depigmentation was seen in both groups, no statistical difference in efficacy
	Disperses melanin (liquiritin)	4% liquiritin vs. 2% liquiritin and HQ	Melasma	4% liquiritin significantly more effective than combination group
Lignin Pero-xidase	Oxidizes and breaks down melanin	Lignin peroxidase cream vs. placebo or 2% HQ	Mottled hyperpigmentation	According to Mexameter evaluation, lignin per-oxidase had more rapid and observable skin-lightening effect com-pared to placebo or HQ
		Lignin peroxidase cream vs. none, lignin peroxidase cream vs. 4% HQ	Facial dyspigmentation	Lignin peroxidase was more effective than applying nothing at all based on dermato-spectrophotometer. Lignin peroxidase was superior to 4% HQ in aesthetics when including skin texture, lack of clarity and radiance, roughness, and overall appearance. Parity was demonstrated between both agents when evaluating skin lightening efficacy.

Contd...

Natural Ingred-ients	Hypo pigmenting Mechanism	Comparison	Pigmentation Disorder	Conclusion
Kojic Acid (Ka)	ROS scavenger, tyrosinase inhibition	0.75% KA with 2.5% Vitamin C vs. 4% HQ	Melasma	Patients responded faster and better to HQ
		Compound (KA, emblica extract, glycolic acid) vs. 4% HQ	Facial dyschromia	Both treatments equally efficacious
		1% KA vs. KA with 2% HQ vs, KA with 0.1% betamethasone vs. combination of products	Melasma	KA with HQ was most effective combination
Niacina-mide	Inhibits melanosome transfer to keratinocytes	Cream containing 2% niacinamide with 2% tranexamic acid vs. vehicle control	Irregular facial hyperpigmentation	Niacinamide with TXA combination product showed efficacy
		Niacinamide 4% vs. desonide 0.05% vs. control	Axillary hyperpigmentation	4% Niacinamide with 0.05% desonide emulsion showed significant colorimetric improvement, though desonide alone was more effective
		None	PIH	Skin brightening compound containing retinol 0.5%, niacinamide 4.4%, resveratrol 1%, and hexylresorcinol 1.1% improved hyperpigmentation

Contd...

Natural Ingred-ients	Hypo pigmenting Mechanism	Comparison	Pigmentation Disorder	Conclusion
Ellagic Acid	Tyrosinase inhibition	1% arbutin vs. synthetic 1% ellagic acid vs. synthetic 1% ellagic acid with plant extracts containing natural ellagic acid	Melasma	All three treatments show efficacy
		0.5% ellagic acid combined with 0.1% salicylic acid vs. 4% HQ	Hyperpigmentation and dark spots	Based on clinical grading, physical measurement of spot size by Chroma Meter, and patient questionnaire analysis, the compound had comparable efficacy to HQ but better aesthetics
Arbutin	Tyrosinase inhibition	1% arbutin vs. synthetic 1% ellagic acid vs. synthetic 1% ellagic acid with plant extracts	Melasma	All three treatments show efficacy
		None	Melasma	7% alpha arbutin in conjunction with the MedLite C6 Q-switched Nd:YAG laser showed favorable results
Green Tea	Antioxidant	2% analogue of green tea extract vs. placebo control	Melasma	2% analogue of green tea extract in hydrophilic cream shows clinical efficacy
Turmeric	Antioxidant	Turmeric extract cream formulation vs. unknown control	Facial hyperpigmentation	Formulation improved areas of hyperpigmentation by 14.16% (P<.0001) at four weeks

Contd...

Natural Ingred-ients	Hypo pigmenting Mechanism	Comparison	Pigmentation Disorder	Conclusion
Soy	Anticarcinogenic (Isofla-vones), inhibits melanosome transfer to keratinocytes (serine protease inhibitors)	Azelaic acid vs. glycolic acid vs. soy extract	Facial hypermelanosis	Soybean extract showed clinical efficacy based on video camera analysis
		None; authors compared affected vs. unaffected areas	Melasma	Application of soy extract to melasma lesions once daily for 3 months led to an average reduction of hyperpigmentation of 12%
		Soy moisturizer vs. vehicle control	Facial photo-damage	Application of soy-containing moisturizer improved mottled pigmentation, blotchiness, dullness, fine lines, overall texture, overall skin tone, and overall appearance
Ascorbic Acid	UVA-mediated catalase inactivation	Topical AA with trichloro-acetic acid peel vs. trichloro-acetic acid peel	Severe melasma	Melasma peel (alpha-hydroxy acid, AA, and oxygen) showed improvement in 95 percent of patients at eight weeks
	Glutathione depletion, oxidant formation	Combined trichloro-acetic acid peel and topical ascorbic acid vs. trichloro-acetic acid peel	Bilateral epidermal melasma	According to digital photography and MASI score, combination product showed greater improvement
	Nitrous oxide production	Vitamin C vs. distilled water	Melasma	After 12 weeks of vitamin C iontophoresis treatment, the colorimeter recorded a clinically significant reduction in luminance value on the treated side

Contd...

Natural Ingred-ients	Hypo pigmenting Mechanism	Comparison	Pigmentation Disorder	Conclusion
	ROS scavenger, tyrosinase inhibition	None	Melasma and post-inflammatory hyperpigmen tation	Novel full-face iontophoresis mask and ascorbyl glucoside preparation over a 1 to 2 months period showed clinical efficacy. *In conjunction to the treatment, patients adhered to a regimen of mandelic/malic acid skin care regimen, broad-spectrum UVA/UVB sunblock, and basic sun protection.

3.9 DARK SIDE OF WHITENERS

Hydroquinone, mercury, and bleaching agents such as hydrogen peroxide are considered high risk ingredients used in cosmetics. These agents act in different ways to lighten skin, but generally work by suppressing the production of melanin, the pigment which gives human skin its color. Lartey et.al, 2017 reported the practice of skin lightening has been reported from North America, Europe, Asia, and Africa. In literature, some prevalence rates exceed 50%, and both sexes are involved. Common agents used include hydroquinone, mercury, corticosteroids, and caustic agents. The agents are easily accessible and affordable with very little regulation. Cutaneous and systemic side effects occur but do not appear to be a deterrent, as the notion of light skin as a surrogate for beauty is strong [238]. While effective in lightening skin color, the products are also associated with health risks, such as dermatitis, impaired wound healing and adrenal suppression. Mercury is associated with adverse neurological, psychological and renal effects and organic mercury compounds can cross the placenta with toxic effects for the fetus. Cosmetic use of hydroquinone and corticosteroids were extensively prevalent among pregnant women and with a negative impact on birth and placenta weights [5]. Among the toxic components, heavy metals are one of the major ingredients, which are used in them intentionally. Among the heavy metal impurities, mercury, arsenic, lead, cobalt, antimony, cadmium, nickel and chromium are highly toxic and are banned in cosmetics to be added intentionally as ingredients in European Union and United States [243]. However, Shroff et.al, 2018 reported side effects of skin fairness products containing hydroquinone, steroids, or mercury can include irritation, inflammation, thinning of skin, scarring, abnormalities among newborn babies if used during pregnancy and breast-feeding, and kidney, liver, or nerve damage. Skin-bleaching agents also increase susceptibility to infections including bacteria, fungus, parasites, and viruses. Some countries (e.g., Ghana, Ivory Coast, Nigeria, South Africa, and Zimbabwe) have banned the import of fairness products that contain hydroquinone and mercury. Nevertheless, many countries, including the two biggest markets, India and China, do not have regulations on ingredients contained within these products. The widespread use of skin fairness products presents a growing public health concern, particularly in Asia [2]. Many skin lightening creams also contain steroids in doses up to 1,000 times higher than in creams used to treat eczema and other skin conditions. Steroid use can cause all sorts of complications such as thinning of the skin, acne, red stretch marks and discoloration. Worse still, the steroids in these creams can act like cortisol, a hormone made by the body to deal with stress. Too much cortisol can cause a myriad of problems, including swelling of the face and abdomen, weight gain, thin skin that bruises easily, stretch marks, weak muscles, high blood pressure, diabetes, osteoporosis and depression [232]. Sharma et.al, 2017 detailed about new entity known as "Topical Steroid Damaged/Dependent face (TSDF)", that has been coined to encompass the various symptoms aggravated such as erythema or burning sensation on attempted cessation of topical steroid application [233]. In the Indian market, topical corticosteroids are easily available; pharmacists are using it as OTC medicine, bypassing the need for a prescription [235]. Hence, misuse and prolonged use of the medicine without medical supervision particularly on the face produce different adverse effects such as steroid rosacea, acneiform eruption, hypertrichosis, demodicidosis, steroid addiction, dermatitis rosaceaformis steroidica, and red face syndrome. Red face syndrome is a condition where any attempted cessation of the application of topical corticosteroids on the face after prolonged use, leads to rebound erythema, burning, and scaling on the face [234]. Coondoo et.al, 2014 commented on the use of topical steroids as “double edged sword”. The end-users of topical corticosteroids are hapless patients. They tend to overuse topical corticosteroids beyond the time limit set by clinicians by repeating prescriptions. Of more concern is the mass use of topical corticosteroids as fairness creams. Vast sections of the Indian society have willingly or unknowingly become victims to the craze of beautification [236]. A Senegalese cohort study of 147 women showed a statistically significant increase in the risk of hypertension and diabetes linked to the use of skin-lightening agents. Other systemic adverse effects attributed to skin-lightening cosmetics include Cushing's syndrome, adrenal insufficiency, nephrotic syndrome, neurological disorders, and ocular disorders. Hypersensitivity reactions, including anaphylaxis, have also been attributed to these products. Many skin-lightening cosmetics contain substances that can harm the unborn child. For example, tretinoin is teratogenic while salicylic acid is feto-toxic. In practice, users are often unaware of the risk of severe adverse effects associated with skin-lightening cosmetics. Users should be informed of these adverse effects and encouraged to stop using these products, especially when skin disorders appear [237]. Mistry et.al, 2011 reported that cultural practice of skin bleaching is highly prevalent in Africa.

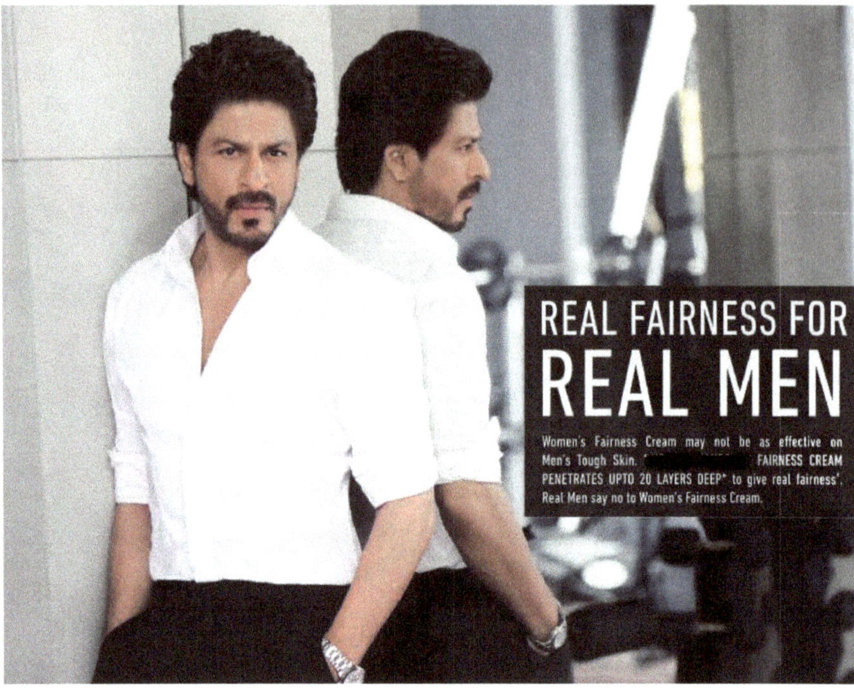

Figure 3.25 An Indian film star posing for a "Men Fairness Cream" [2], [244]. The trend seems to be changing with many new-age celebrities saying no to endorse problematic products like alcohol, tobacco, fairness creams, aerated drinks etc. A recent survey showed that 80% of Indian men use fairness creams and the number of consumers are growing 18% annually. There were no differences between women and men currently using products in their desire to look as fair as media celebrities (Courtacy: Business Standard).

Most reported cases of toxic effects of skin-lightening products occur in this region [239]. Legally, bleaching products might be drugs that are misused; however, more often, their presentations are those of true cosmetic brands, which are numerous. The active ingredients might be indicated on the packages, which could give the true information or not, but are often withheld. These products appear to be available in every country where they are used, including Northern countries, through well-organized networks of distribution. Despite these reports, surprisingly sparse epidemiological studies are available regarding the health impacts of skin-bleaching practices on Afro-Caribbean immigrant groups in the US [241]. All products are used as milks, creams or gel creams, or soaps. Caustic compounds (lemon juice, high concentration acid salicylic preparations, etc.) are sometimes used on certain areas that are more difficult to lighten (such as hands and feet).The compounds are commonly applied on the entire surface of the body, once or twice daily, often for decades because of the rapid reversibility of the lightening after stopping the use of the product [240]. Skin-lightening products are used by a third of African and Indian women in South Africa Cultural and historical perceptions equating a fairer skin with social advantage are pervasive and strongly reinforced by the media. There is a poor understanding of the risks associated with the use of these products. Public education campaigns are required to teach consumers about these risks and the importance of concomitant use of sunscreens with these products [242].

EPILOGUE

Disorders of hyperpigmentation (including melasma, post-inflammatory hyperpigmentation, lentigo, etc.) are commonly seen in office-based dermatology practices worldwide. Their management is challenging and requires a long-term treatment plan. Facial and neck pigmentations are the most cosmetically important. They are common in middle-aged women, and are related to endogenous (hormones) and exogenous factors (such as use of cosmetics and perfumes, and exposure to sun radiation). The results are often unsatisfactory and topical agents may sometimes cause significant adverse reactions. An improved understanding of melanogenesis has also led to new pathways as targets for topical therapy. Multiple topical agents available act upon different steps of the pigmentation pathway. Cosmeceuticals for hyperpigmentation are in great demand and most of them target the key regulatory steps in melanin synthesis. Successful treatment typically involves a combination of topical agents with or without in-office procedures, exploiting the different mechanisms of action of each agent or treatment modality. Sunscreen use and minimizing sun exposure are crucial in all cases. Treatment of melasma and other facial pigmentations has always been challenging and discouraging. It is important to avoid exposure to the Sun or ultraviolet lamps, and to use broad-spectrum sunscreens. Topical applications are the mainstay of treatment and include phenols, retinoids, corticosteroids, and their combinations. Additionally, many studies have addressed the safety and efficacy of chemical peels and laser/light sources for pigment reduction in melasma. Such procedures are most often considered second- and third-line therapeutic approaches. In order to identify any underlying causes of hyperpigmentation or identify any factors that may hinder treatment, it is essential to obtain a detailed medication history for all patients. It is also important to assess any family history and/or personal history of melasma. If the patient has been treated for melasma in the past, ascertain what therapies were used and how the patient responded. Allergic reactions to cosmetics and/or fragrance-based products may contribute to PIH. Serial photography is essential in the clinical management of hyperpigmentation. With the advent of laser technology, the treatment options have increased especially for dermal or mixed melasma. Lasers have been tried in the treatment of various pigmentary disorders with variable success. In contrast, laser therapies have not produced completely satisfactory results, because they can induce hyperpigmentation and recurrences can occur. Combining topical therapy with procedures such as chemical peels, intense pulsed light (IPL), fractional non-ablative lasers or radiofrequency, pigment lasers (microsecond, picosecond, Q-switched), and micro-needling, enhances results. Patients are savvy consumers who often present to physicians asking about the latest treatments and breakthroughs. With proper treatment, melasma can be controlled, improved, and maintained. With the patient population seeking effective systemic treatments for skin pigmentation, it is important for dermatologists to understand the properties, the efficacy, and the adverse events profile of each compound, thus ensuring proper use by patients, and that patients are appropriately counseled regarding treatment expectation and safety.

SUMMARY

Hyperpigmentation is one of the most common skin disorders that affect both men and women of all ethnic groups, caused by several factors, such as UV exposure and skin inflammation. Topical whitening agents were found to be the best and the least aggressive therapy for treating hyperpigmentation compared to instrumental approaches. However, topical treatment faces several obstacles due to the low stability of the whitening agents. The number of patients that visit dermatologists with pigmentary disorders is significant. Patients are often overwhelmed with numerous OTC skin lightening agents, many without clinical evidence of efficacy. However, evidence-based studies on many of these agents are still lacking. The treatment of melasma should include a multimodality approach that incorporates photoprotective agents, antioxidant treatments, skin lighteners, exfoliants, and resurfacing procedures, as needed. Evidence-based studies suggest that first line therapies for melasma encompass intense photoprotection and topical lightening agents. Second-line treatments, such as chemical peels and lasers, are efficacious in some patients, but these approaches can be associated with acute and long-term complications, particularly in individuals with darker skin types. Given the global negative impact of melasma on the quality of life, a quest to find more efficacious treatments that offer sustained long-term remission for patients with this frustrating and therapeutically challenging disorder is ongoing.

ABBREVIATIONS

Tyrosinase related protein-1 (TRP-1); Global industry analysts (GIA); Proopiomelanocortin (POMC); Microphthalmia-associated transcription factor (MITF); Adrenocorticotropic hormone (ACTH); α-Melanocyte-stimulating hormone (α-MSH); melanocortin type 1 receptor (MC1R); alpha-hydroxy acids (AHAs); melasma quality of life (MELASQOL); 5,6-dihydroxyindole-2-carboxylic acid (DHICA); Scientific Committee on Consumer Safety (SCCS); Melasma Area and Severity Index (MASI); physician global assessment (PGA); patient global assessment (PtGA); Level of evidence (LOE); protease-activated receptor (PAR); soybean trypsin inhibitor (STI); Bowman–Birk inhibitor (BBI); quasi-drugs (QDs); Soybean trypsin inhibitor (STI); post-inflammatory hyperpigmentation (PIH); omega-3 polyunsaturated fatty acids (PUFAs)

BIBLIOGRAPHY AND WEBLIOGRAPHY

1. Pillaiyar T, Manickam M, Namasivayam V. Skin whitening agents: medicinal chemistry perspective of tyrosinase inhibitors. J Enzyme Inhib Med Chem. 2017 Dec;32(1):403-425. doi: 10.1080/14756366.2016.1256882. Review. PubMed PMID: 28097901; PubMed Central PMCID: PMC6010116.
2. Shroff H, Diedrichs PC, Craddock N. Skin Color, Cultural Capital, and Beauty Products: An Investigation of the Use of Skin Fairness Products in Mumbai, India. Front Public Health. 2018 Jan 23;5:365. doi: 10.3389/fpubh.2017.00365. eCollection 2017. PubMed PMID: 29410952; PubMed Central PMCID: PMC5787082.
3. Jacobs M, Levine S, Abney K, Davids L. Fifty Shades of African Lightness: A Bio-psychosocial Review of the Global Phenomenon of Skin Lightening Practices. J Public Health Afr. 2016 Dec 31;7(2):552. doi: 10.4081/jphia.2016.552. eCollection 2016 Dec 31. Review. PubMed PMID: 28299156; PubMed Central PMCID: PMC5345401.
4. Rusmadi SZ, Syed Ismail SN, Praveena SM. Preliminary study on the skin lightening practice and health symptoms among female students in Malaysia. J Environ Public Health. 2015;2015:591790. doi: 10.1155/2015/591790. Epub 2015 Nov 26. PubMed PMID: 26693230; PubMed Central PMCID: PMC4674599.
5. Darj E, Infanti JJ, Ahlberg BM, Okumu J. "The fairer the better?" Use of potentially toxic skin bleaching products. Afr Health Sci. 2015 Dec;15(4):1074-80. doi: 10.4314/ahs.v15i4.4. PubMed PMID: 26958006; PubMed Central PMCID: PMC4765398.
6. Mohammed T, Mohammed E, Bascombe S. The evaluation of total mercury and arsenic in skin bleaching creams commonly used in Trinidad and Tobago and their potential risk to the people of the Caribbean. J Public Health Res. 2017 Oct 9;6(3):1097. doi: 10.4081/jphr.2017.1097. eCollection 2017 Dec 13. PubMed PMID: 29291194; PubMed Central PMCID: PMC5736993.PubMed Central PMCID: PMC4765398.
7. Tai C and Sukumaran T. Asia is obsessed with skin whitening – but the backlash is beginning. Web InkStone News.
8. Liu M. Skin whiteners are still in demand, despite health concerns. CNN, September 3, 2018.
9. Karmali N. Thailand's Richest 2018: Skin-Whitening Craze Continues To Surge Across Asia. Forbes, May 2, 2018.
10. Alrayyes SF, Alrayyes SF, Farooq Dar U. Skin-lightening practices behind the veil: An epidemiological study among Saudi women. J Cosmet Dermatol. 2019 May 6. doi: 10.1111/jocd.12972. [Epub ahead of print] PubMed PMID: 31058398.

11. Gruber JV, Holtz R. Examining the impact of skin lighteners in vitro. Oxid Med Cell Longev. 2013;2013:702120. doi: 10.1155/2013/702120. Epub 2013 Apr 28. PubMed PMID: 23738040; PubMed Central PMCID: PMC3655678.
12. de Suisse M. Do you know the difference between Skin Lightening vs. Skin Brightening? Natural Skin Care Blog, October 19, 2017.
13. The 411: Brightening vs. Whitening vs. Lightening. Bolden Blog, USA May 19, 2018.
14. Spradley N. This Is The Real Difference Between Skin Brightening and Skin Lightening. Essence, September 30, 2016.
15. Smit N, Vicanova J, Pavel S. The hunt for natural skin whitening agents. Int J Mol Sci. 2009 Dec 10;10(12):5326-49. doi: 10.3390/ijms10125326. Review. PubMed PMID: 20054473; PubMed Central PMCID: PMC2801997.
16. Malathi M, Thappa DM. Systemic skin whitening/lightening agents: What is the evidence?. Indian J Dermatol VenereolLeprol2013;79:842-6
17. The Different Meanings Between: Skin Lightening, Brightening, & Whitening. http://skinlighteningbeautyguide.com
18. D'Mello SA, Finlay GJ, Baguley BC, Askarian-Amiri ME. Signaling Pathways in Melanogenesis. Int J Mol Sci. 2016 Jul 15;17(7). pii: E1144. doi: 10.3390/ijms17071144. Review. PubMed PMID: 27428965; PubMed Central PMCID: PMC4964517.
19. Yamaguchi Y, Brenner M, Hearing VJ. The regulation of skin pigmentation. J Biol Chem. 2007 Sep 21;282(38):27557-61. Epub 2007 Jul 16. Review. PubMed PMID: 17635904.
20. Bastonini E, Kovacs D, Picardo M. Skin Pigmentation and Pigmentary Disorders: Focus on Epidermal/Dermal Cross-Talk. Ann Dermatol. 2016 Jun;28(3):279-89. doi: 10.5021/ad.2016.28.3.279. Epub 2016 May 25. Review. PubMed PMID: 27274625; PubMed Central PMCID: PMC4884703.
21. Kamakshi R. Fairness via formulations: a review of cosmetic skin-lightening ingredients. J Cosmet Sci. 2012 Jan-Feb;63(1):43-54. Review. PubMed PMID: 22487451.
22. MaranducaMA, Branisteanu D, Serban DN, Branisteanu DC, Stoleriu G, Manolache N, Serban IL. Synthesis and physiological implications of melanic pigments. Oncol Lett. 2019 May;17(5):4183-4187. doi: 10.3892/ol.2019.10071. Epub 2019 Feb 25. Review. PubMed PMID: 30944614; PubMed Central PMCID: PMC6444329.
23. Del Bino S, Duval C, Bernerd F. Clinical and Biological Characterization of Skin Pigmentation Diversity and Its Consequences on UV Impact. Int J Mol Sci. 2018 Sep 8;19(9). pii: E2668. doi: 10.3390/ijms19092668. Review. PubMed PMID: 30205563; PubMed Central PMCID: PMC6163216.
24. Schlessinger DI, Schlessinger J. Biochemistry, Melanin. [Updated 2019 Apr 21]. In: StatPearls [Internet]. Treasure Island (FL): StatPearls Publishing; 2019 Jan-. Available from: https://www.ncbi.nlm.nih.gov/books/NBK459156/
25. Sunar, K., Kumar, U., Deshmukh, S., 2016. Recent Applications of Enzymes in Personal Care Products. In: Dhillon, G.Singh, Kaur, S. (Eds.), Agro-Industrial Wastes as Feedstock for Enzyme Production: Apply and Exploit the Emerging

and Valuable Use Options of Waste Biomass. Academic Press, 279–298. ISBN: 9780128023921

26. Serre C, Busuttil V, Botto JM. Intrinsic and extrinsic regulation of human skin melanogenesis and pigmentation. Int J Cosmet Sci. 2018 Aug;40(4):328-347. doi: 10.1111/ics.12466. Epub 2018 Jul 19. Review. PubMed PMID: 29752874.
27. Videira IF, Moura DF, Magina S. Mechanisms regulating melanogenesis. An Bras Dermatol. 2013 Jan-Feb;88(1):76-83. Review. PubMed PMID: 23539007; PubMed Central PMCID: PMC3699939.
28. Yamaguchi Y, Hearing VJ. Melanocytes and their diseases. Cold Spring HarbPerspect Med. 2014 May 1;4(5). pii: a017046. doi: 10.1101/cshperspect.a017046. Review. PubMed PMID: 24789876; PubMed Central PMCID: PMC3996377.
29. Yamaguchi Y, Hearing VJ. Physiological factors that regulate skin pigmentation. Biofactors. 2009 Mar-Apr;35(2):193-9. doi: 10.1002/biof.29. Review. PubMed PMID: 19449448; PubMed Central PMCID: PMC2793097.
30. Nguyen NT, Fisher DE. MITF and UV responses in skin: From pigmentation to addiction. Pigment Cell Melanoma Res. 2019 Mar;32(2):224-236. doi: 10.1111/pcmr.12726. Epub 2018 Aug 3. Review. PubMed PMID: 30019545; PubMed Central PMCID: PMC6336527.
31. Tran TT, Schulman J, Fisher DE. UV and pigmentation: molecular mechanisms and social controversies. Pigment Cell Melanoma Res. 2008 Oct;21(5):509-16. doi: 10.1111/j.1755-148X.2008.00498.x. Review. PubMed PMID: 18821855; PubMed Central PMCID: PMC2733367.
32. Juhasz MLW, Levin MK. The role of systemic treatments for skin lightening. J Cosmet Dermatol. 2018 Dec;17(6):1144-1157. doi: 10.1111/jocd.12747. Epub 2018 Aug 21. Review. PubMed PMID: 30133125.
33. Zhu-WY, Zhang RZ. Chapter 13. Skin Lightening Agents. In: Zoe Diana Draelos, Lauren A. Thaman. Cosmetic Formulation of Skin Care Products. Published by CRC Press, June 19, 2005. ISBN 9780849339684
34. Sarkar R, Arora P, Garg KV. Cosmeceuticals for Hyperpigmentation: What is Available? J CutanAesthet Surg. 2013 Jan;6(1):4-11. doi: 10.4103/0974-2077.110089. PubMed PMID: 23723597; PubMed Central PMCID: PMC3663177.
35. Schwartz C, Jan A. Hydroquinone. [Updated 2019 Mar 8]. In: StatPearls [Internet]. Treasure Island (FL): StatPearls Publishing; 2019 Jan-. Available from: https://www.ncbi.nlm.nih.gov/books/NBK539693/
36. Tse TW. Hydroquinone for skin lightening: safety profile, duration of use and when should we stop? J Dermatolog Treat. 2010 Sep;21(5):272-5. doi: 10.3109/09546630903341945. Review. PubMed PMID: 20095963.
37. Godse KV. Triple combination of hydroquinone, tretinoin and mometasone furoate with glycolic acid peels in melasma. Indian J Dermatol. 2009;54(1):92-3. doi: 10.4103/0019-5154.49005. PubMed PMID: 20049286; PubMed Central PMCID: PMC2800888.
38. Westerhof W, Kooyers TJ. Hydroquinone and its analogues in dermatology - a potential health risk. J Cosmet Dermatol. 2005 Jun;4(2):55-9. PubMed PMID: 17166200.

39. Byeon SE, Yi YS, Lee J, Yang WS, Kim JH, Kim J, Hong S, Kim JH, Cho JY. Hydroquinone Exhibits In Vitro and In Vivo Anti-Cancer Activity in Cancer Cells and Mice. Int J Mol Sci. 2018 Mar 19;19(3). pii: E903. doi: 10.3390/ijms19030903. PubMed PMID: 29562668; PubMed Central PMCID: PMC5877764.
40. Nofal A, Ibrahim AM, Nofal E, Gamal N, Osman S. Topical silymarin versus hydroquinone in the treatment of melasma: A comparative study. J Cosmet Dermatol. 2019 Feb;18(1):263-270. doi: 10.1111/jocd.12769. Epub 2018 Aug 26. PubMed PMID: 30146802.
41. Grimes PE, Ijaz S, Nashawati R, Kwak D. New oral and topical approaches for the treatment of melasma. Int J Womens Dermatol. 2018 Nov 20;5(1):30-36. doi: 10.1016/j.ijwd.2018.09.004. eCollection 2019 Feb. PubMed PMID: 30809577; PubMed Central PMCID: PMC6374710.
42. Zhai H, Maibach HI. Skin-Whitening Agents. In: André O. Barel, Marc Paye, Howard I. Maibach. Handbook of Cosmetic Science and Technology, 3rd Edition, published by CRC Press, 2014. ISBN 9781842145647
43. Natural Skin Whitening Ingredients That Work. Available From: https://www.beskinformed.com/skin-lightening-products/natural-skin-whitening-ingredients-work/
44. MontazeriM, Emami S, Asgarian-Omran H, Azizi S, Sharif M, Sarvi S, Rezaei F, Sadeghi M, Gohardehi S, Daryani A. In vitro and in vivo evaluation of kojic acid against Toxoplasma gondii in experimental models of acute toxoplasmosis. Exp Parasitol. 2019 May;200:7-12. doi: 10.1016/j.exppara.2019.03.009. Epub 2019 Mar 20. PubMed PMID: 30904693.
45. de Pietro MA.Kojic acid: What you need to know? MedicalNewsToday, 3 October 2017.
46. Saeedi M, Eslamifar M, Khezri K. Kojic acid applications in cosmetic and pharmaceutical preparations. Biomed Pharmacother. 2019 Feb;110:582-593. doi: 10.1016/j.biopha.2018.12.006. Epub 2018 Dec 8. Review. PubMed PMID: 30537675.
47. Burnett CL, Bergfeld WF, Belsito DV, Hill RA, Klaassen CD, Liebler DC, Marks JG Jr, Shank RC, Slaga TJ, Snyder PW, Andersen FA. Final report of the safety assessment of Kojic acid as used in cosmetics. Int J Toxicol. 2010 Nov-Dec;29(6 Suppl):244S-73. doi: 10.1177/1091581810385956. Review. PubMed PMID: 21164073.
48. Stirner M. Kojic Acid Side Effects. Available From: https://www.livestrong.com/article/102302-kojic-acid-side-effects/
49. Breathnach AS. Melanin hyperpigmentation of skin: melasma, topical treatment with azelaic acid, and other therapies. Cutis. 1996 Jan;57(1 Suppl):36-45. Review. PubMed PMID: 8654129.
50. Azelaic Acid Suspension 10% 30ml. Web theordinary.com
51. National Center for Biotechnology Information. PubChem Database. Azelaic acid, CID=2266, https://pubchem.ncbi.nlm.nih.gov/compound/2266 (accessed on May 12, 2019)
52. FaghihiG, Taheri A, Shahmoradi Z, Nilforoushzadeh MA. Solution of Azelaic Acid (20%), Resorcinol (10%) and Phytic Acid (6%) Versus Glycolic Acid (50%)

Peeling Agent in the Treatment of Female Patients with Facial Melasma. Adv Biomed Res. 2017 Feb 22;6:9. doi: 10.4103/2277-9175.200784. eCollection 2017. PubMed PMID: 28299301; PubMed Central PMCID: PMC5343614.

53. DayalS, Sahu P, Dua R. Combination of glycolic acid peel and topical 20% azelaic acid cream in melasma patients: efficacy and improvement in quality of life. J Cosmet Dermatol. 2017 Mar;16(1):35-42. doi: 10.1111/jocd.12260. Epub 2016 Aug 8. PubMed PMID: 27500896.
54. Jacobus Berlitz S, De Villa D, Maschmann Inácio LA, Davies S, Zatta KC, Guterres SS, Külkamp-Guerreiro IC. Azelaic acid-loaded nanoemulsion with hyaluronic acid - a new strategy to treat hyperpigmentary skin disorders. Drug Dev Ind Pharm. 2019 Apr;45(4):642-650. doi: 10.1080/03639045.2019.1569032. Epub 2019 Jan 28. PubMed PMID: 30642209.
55. Hollinger JC, Angra K, Halder RM. Are Natural Ingredients Effective in the Management of Hyperpigmentation? A Systematic Review. J Clin Aesthet Dermatol. 2018 Feb;11(2):28-37. Epub 2018 Feb 1. Review. PubMed PMID: 29552273; PubMed Central PMCID: PMC5843359.
56. Saade DS, Maymone MBC, Secemsky EA, Kennedy KF, Vashi NA. Patterns of Over-the-counter Lightening Agent Use among Patients with Hyperpigmentation Disorders: A United States-based Cohort Study. J Clin Aesthet Dermatol. 2018 Jul;11(7):26-30. Epub 2018 Jul 1. PubMed PMID: 30057662; PubMed Central PMCID: PMC6057735.
57. TehranchiniaZ, Saghi B, Rahimi H. Evaluation of Therapeutic Efficacy and Safety of Tranexamic Acid Local Infiltration in Combination with Topical 4% Hydroquinone Cream Compared to Topical 4% Hydroquinone Cream Alone in Patients with Melasma: A Split-Face Study. Dermatol Res Pract. 2018 Jul 2;2018:8350317. doi: 10.1155/2018/8350317. eCollection 2018. PubMed PMID: 30079087; PubMed Central PMCID: PMC6051262.
58. SonthaliaS, Jha AK, Lallas A, Jain G, Jakhar D. Glutathione for skin lightening: a regnant myth or evidence-based verity? Dermatol Pract Concept. 2018 Jan 31;8(1):15-21. doi: 10.5826/dpc.0801a04. eCollection 2018 Jan. PubMed PMID: 29445569; PubMed Central PMCID: PMC5808366.
59. Villarama CD, Maibach HI. Glutathione as a depigmenting agent: an overview. Int J Cosmet Sci. 2005 Jun;27(3):147-53. doi: 10.1111/j.1467-2494.2005.00235.x. PubMed PMID: 18492181.
60. Arjinpathana N, Asawanonda P. Glutathione as an oral whitening agent: a randomized, double-blind, placebo-controlled study. J Dermatolog Treat. 2012 Apr;23(2):97-102. doi: 10.3109/09546631003801619. Epub 2010 Jun 5. PubMed PMID: 20524875.
61. Weschawalit S, Thongthip S, Phutrakool P, Asawanonda P. Glutathione and its antiaging and antimelanogenic effects. Clin CosmetInvestig Dermatol. 2017 Apr 27;10:147-153. doi: 10.2147/CCID.S128339. eCollection 2017. PubMed PMID: 28490897; PubMed Central PMCID: PMC5413479.
62. Chung BY, Choi SR, Moon IJ, Park CW, Kim YH, Chang SE. The Glutathione Derivative, GSH Monoethyl Ester, May Effectively Whiten Skin but GSH Does

Not. Int J Mol Sci. 2016 Apr 27;17(5). pii: E629. doi: 10.3390/ijms17050629. PubMed PMID: 27128906; PubMed Central PMCID: PMC4881455.

63. DilokthornsakulW, Dhippayom T, Dilokthornsakul P. The clinical effect of glutathione on skin color and other related skin conditions: A systematic review. J Cosmet Dermatol. 2019 Mar 20. doi: 10.1111/jocd.12910. [Epub ahead of print] Review. PubMed PMID: 30895708.
64. Dadzie OE. Unethical skin bleaching with glutathione. BMJ. 2016 Aug 31;354:i4386. doi: 10.1136/bmj.i4386. PubMed PMID: 27581922.
65. Galarpe C. 'Glutathione injectables not legal' – FDA. ABS-CBN News, Jun 01 2011.
66. Cosmetic doctors raise concerns over skin bleacher glutathione. COSMEICS BUSINESS (Regulatory), 5-Sep-2016.
67. Chakraborty AK, Funasaka Y, Komoto M, Ichihashi M. Effect of arbutin on melanogenic proteins in human melanocytes. Pigment Cell Res. 1998 Aug;11(4):206-12. PubMed PMID: 9711535.
68. de Arriba SG, Naser B, Nolte KU. Risk assessment of free hydroquinone derived from Arctostaphylos Uva-ursi folium herbal preparations. Int J Toxicol. 2013 Nov-Dec;32(6):442-53. doi: 10.1177/1091581813507721. Review. PubMed PMID: 24296864.
69. Inoue Y, Hasegawa S, Yamada T, Date Y, Mizutani H, Nakata S, Matsunaga K, Akamatsu H. Analysis of the effects of hydroquinone and arbutin on the differentiation of melanocytes. Biol Pharm Bull. 2013;36(11):1722-30. PubMed PMID: 24189417.
70. Degen, G.H. Opinion of the Scientific Committee on Consumer Safety (SCCS)—Opinion on the safety of the use of α-arbutin in cosmetic products. Regul. Toxicol. Pharmacol. 2016, 74, 75–76.
71. SCCS, Degen GH. Opinion of the Scientific Committee on Consumer Safety (SCCS)--Opinion on the safety of the use of β-arbutin in cosmetic products. RegulToxicolPharmacol. 2015 Dec;73(3):866-7. doi: 10.1016/j.yrtph.2015.10.008. Epub 2015 Oct 19. PubMed PMID: 26482403.
72. Sugimoto K, Nishimura T, Nomura K, Sugimoto K, Kuriki T. Inhibitory effects of alpha-arbutin on melanin synthesis in cultured human melanoma cells and a three-dimensional human skin model. Biol Pharm Bull. 2004 Apr;27(4):510-4. PubMed PMID: 15056856.
73. Bandyopadhyay D. Topical treatment of melasma. Indian J Dermatol. 2009;54(4):303-9. doi: 10.4103/0019-5154.57602. PubMed PMID: 20101327; PubMed Central PMCID: PMC2807702.
74. Miao F, Shi Y, Fan ZF, Jiang S, Xu SZ, Lei TC. Deoxyarbutin Possesses a Potent Skin-Lightening Capacity with No Discernible Cytotoxicity against Melanosomes. PLoS One. 2016 Oct 24;11(10):e0165338. doi: 10.1371/journal.pone.0165338. eCollection 2016. PubMed PMID: 27776184; PubMed Central PMCID: PMC5077105.
75. Hamed SH, Sriwiriyanont P, deLong MA, Visscher MO, Wickett RR, Boissy RE. Comparative efficacy and safety of deoxyarbutin, a new tyrosinase-inhibiting agent. J Cosmet Sci. 2006 Jul-Aug;57(4):291-308. PubMed PMID: 16957809.

76. Chapter 9. Accessory Nutrients and Phytochemicals. In: Michael T. Murray, Joseph Pizzorno. The Encyclopedia of Healing Foods, published by Simon and Schuster, May 11, 2010. ISBN 1439103445, 9781439103449, Page 142
77. Ríos JL, Giner RM, Marín M, Recio MC. A Pharmacological Update of Ellagic Acid. Planta Med. 2018 Oct;84(15):1068-1093. doi: 10.1055/a-0633-9492. Epub2018 May 30. Review. PubMed PMID: 29847844.
78. Shakeri A, Zirak MR, Sahebkar A. Ellagic Acid: A Logical Lead for Drug Development? Curr Pharm Des. 2018;24(2):106-122. doi: 10.2174/1381612823666171115094557. PubMed PMID: 29141541.
79. Dahl A, Yatskayer M, Raab S, Oresajo C. Tolerance and efficacy of a product containing ellagic and salicylic acids in reducing hyperpigmentation and dark spots in comparison with 4% hydroquinone. J Drugs Dermatol. 2013 Jan;12(1):52-8. PubMed PMID: 23377328.
80. Ortiz-Ruiz CV, Berna J, Tudela J, Varon R, Garcia-Canovas F. Action of ellagic acid on the melanin biosynthesis pathway. J Dermatol Sci. 2016 May;82(2):115-22. doi: 10.1016/j.jdermsci.2016.02.004. Epub 2016 Feb 12. PubMed PMID: 26899308.
81. Bae JY, Choi JS, Kang SW, Lee YJ, Park J, Kang YH. Dietary compound ellagic acid alleviates skin wrinkle and inflammation induced by UV-B irradiation. Exp Dermatol. 2010 Aug;19(8):e182-90. doi: 10.1111/j.1600-0625.2009.01044.x. PubMed PMID: 20113347.
82. Baek B, Lee SH, Kim K, Lim HW, Lim CJ. Ellagic acid plays a protective role against UV-B-induced oxidative stress by up-regulating antioxidant components in human dermal fibroblasts. Korean J PhysiolPharmacol. 2016 May;20(3):269-77. doi: 10.4196/kjpp.2016.20.3.269. Epub 2016 Apr 26. PubMed PMID: 27162481; PubMed Central PMCID: PMC4860369.
83. Yagi A, Takeo S. [Anti-inflammatory constituents, aloesin and aloemannan in Aloe species and effects of tanshinon VI in Salvia miltiorrhiza on heart]. YakugakuZasshi. 2003 Jul;123(7):517-32. Review. Japanese. PubMed PMID: 12875235.
84. Chang TS. An updated review of tyrosinase inhibitors. Int J Mol Sci. 2009 May 26;10(6):2440-75. doi: 10.3390/ijms10062440. Review. PubMed PMID: 19582213; PubMed Central PMCID: PMC2705500.
85. Jones K, Hughes J, Hong M, Jia Q, Orndorff S. Modulation of melanogenesis by aloesin: a competitive inhibitor of tyrosinase. Pigment Cell Res. 2002 Oct;15(5):335-40. PubMed PMID: 12213089.
86. Jin YH, Lee SJ, Chung MH, Park JH, Park YI, Cho TH, Lee SK. Aloesin and arbutin inhibit tyrosinase activity in a synergistic manner via a different action mechanism. Arch Pharm Res. 1999 Jun;22(3):232-6. PubMed PMID: 10403123.
87. Ebanks JP, Wickett RR, Boissy RE. Mechanisms regulating skin pigmentation: the rise and fall of complexion coloration. Int J Mol Sci. 2009 Sep 15;10(9):4066-87. doi: 10.3390/ijms10094066. Review. PubMed PMID: 19865532; PubMed Central PMCID: PMC2769151.

88. Yang ZQ, Wang ZH, Tu JB, Li P, Hu XY. [The effects of aloesin and arbutin on cultured melanocytes in a synergetic method]. Zhonghua Zheng Xing Wai Ke Za Zhi. 2004 Sep;20(5):369-71. Chinese. PubMed PMID: 15623110.
89. Draelos ZD. Skin lightening preparations and the hydroquinone controversy. Dermatol Ther. 2007 Sep-Oct;20(5):308-13. Review. PubMed PMID: 18045355.
90. Solano F, Briganti S, Picardo M, Ghanem G. Hypopigmenting agents: an updated review on biological, chemical and clinical aspects. Pigment Cell Res. 2006 Dec;19(6):550-71. Review. PubMed PMID: 17083484.
91. Ebrahimi B, Naeini FF. Topical tranexamic acid as a promising treatment for melasma. J Res Med Sci. 2014 Aug;19(8):753-7. PubMed PMID: 25422661; PubMed Central PMCID: PMC4235096.
92. Cho YH, Park JE, Lim DS, Lee JS. Tranexamic acid inhibits melanogenesis by activating the autophagy system in cultured melanoma cells. J Dermatol Sci. 2017 Oct;88(1):96-102. doi: 10.1016/j.jdermsci.2017.05.019. Epub 2017 Jun 7. PubMed PMID: 28669590.
93. Atefi N, Dalvand B, Ghassemi M, Mehran G, Heydarian A. Therapeutic Effects of Topical Tranexamic Acid in Comparison with Hydroquinone in Treatment of Women with Melasma. Dermatol Ther (Heidelb). 2017 Sep;7(3):417-424. doi: 10.1007/s13555-017-0195-0. Epub 2017 Jul 26. PubMed PMID: 28748406; PubMed Central PMCID: PMC5574746.
94. Tan AWM, Sen P, Chua SH, Goh BK. Oral tranexamic acid lightens refractory melasma. Australas J Dermatol. 2017 Aug;58(3):e105-e108. doi: 10.1111/ajd.12474. Epub 2016 May 13. PubMed PMID: 27173008.
95. BudamakuntlaL, Loganathan E, Suresh DH, Shanmugam S, Suryanarayan S, Dongare A, Venkataramiah LD, Prabhu N. A Randomised, Open-label, Comparative Study of Tranexamic Acid Microinjections and Tranexamic Acid with Microneedling in Patients with Melasma. J CutanAesthet Surg. 2013 Jul;6(3):139-43. doi: 10.4103/0974-2077.118403. PubMed PMID: 24163529; PubMed Central PMCID: PMC3800287.
96. Kim HJ, Moon SH, Cho SH, Lee JD, Kim HS. Efficacy and Safety of Tranexamic Acid in Melasma: A Meta-analysis and Systematic Review. Acta DermVenereol. 2017 Jul 6;97(7):776-781. doi: 10.2340/00015555-2668. Review. PubMed PMID: 28374042.
97. Hsieh PW, Chen WY, Aljuffali IA, Chen CC, Fang JY. Co-drug strategy for promoting skin targeting and minimizing the transdermal diffusion of hydroquinone and tranexamic acid. Curr Med Chem. 2013;20(32):4080-92. PubMed PMID: 23931279.
98. KanechornNa Ayuthaya P, Niumphradit N, Manosroi A, Nakakes A. Topical 5% tranexamic acid for the treatment of melasma in Asians: a double-blind randomized controlled clinical trial. J Cosmet Laser Ther. 2012 Jun;14(3):150-4. doi: 10.3109/14764172.2012.685478. PubMed PMID: 22506692.
99. Lee DH, Oh IY, Koo KT, Suk JM, Jung SW, Park JO, Kim BJ, Choi YM. Reduction in facial hyperpigmentation after treatment with a combination of topical niacinamide and tranexamic acid: a randomized, double-blind, vehicle-

controlled trial. Skin Res Technol. 2014 May;20(2):208-12. doi: 10.1111/srt.12107. Epub 2013 Sep 5. PubMed PMID: 24033822.

100. Kim SJ, Park JY, Shibata T, Fujiwara R, Kang HY. Efficacy and possible mechanisms of topical tranexamic acid in melasma. Clin Exp Dermatol. 2016 Jul;41(5):480-5. doi: 10.1111/ced.12835. Epub 2016 May 2. PubMed PMID: 27135282.

101. Sarma N, Chakraborty S, Poojary SA, Rathi S, Kumaran S, Nirmal B, Felicita J, Sarkar R, Jaiswal P, D'Souza P, Donthula N, Sethi S, Ailawadi P, Joseph B. Evidence-based Review, Grade of Recommendation, and Suggested Treatment Recommendations for Melasma. Indian Dermatol Online J. 2017 Nov-Dec;8(6):406-442. doi: 10.4103/idoj.IDOJ_187_17. PubMed PMID: 29204385; PubMed Central PMCID: PMC5707834.

102. Zhang L, Tan WQ, Fang QQ, Zhao WY, Zhao QM, Gao J, Wang XW. Tranexamic Acid for Adults with Melasma: A Systematic Review and Meta-Analysis. Biomed Res Int. 2018 Nov 6;2018:1683414. doi: 10.1155/2018/1683414. eCollection 2018. PubMed PMID: 30533427; PubMed Central PMCID: PMC6247725.

103. Sarkar R, Gokhale N, Godse K, Ailawadi P, Arya L, Sarma N, Torsekar RG, Somani VK, Arora P, Majid I, Ravichandran G, Singh M, Aurangabadkar S, Arsiwala S, Sonthalia S, Salim T, Shah S. Medical Management of Melasma: A Review with Consensus Recommendations by Indian Pigmentary Expert Group. Indian J Dermatol. 2017 Nov-Dec;62(6):558-577. doi: 10.4103/ijd.IJD_489_17. PubMed PMID: 29263529; PubMed Central PMCID: PMC5724303.

104. Taira N, Katsuyama Y, Yoshioka M, Muraoka O, Morikawa T. Structural Requirements of Alkylglyceryl-l-Ascorbic Acid Derivatives for Melanogenesis Inhibitory Activity. Int J Mol Sci. 2018 Apr 10;19(4). pii: E1144. doi: 10.3390/ijms19041144. PubMed PMID: 29642633; PubMed Central PMCID: PMC5979531.

105. Al-Niaimi F, Chiang NYZ. Topical Vitamin C and the Skin: Mechanisms of Action and Clinical Applications. J Clin Aesthet Dermatol. 2017 Jul;10(7):14-17. Epub 2017 Jul 1. Review. PubMed PMID: 29104718; PubMed Central PMCID: PMC5605218.

106. Espinal-Perez LE, Moncada B, Castanedo-Cazares JP. A double-blind randomized trial of 5% ascorbic acid vs. 4% hydroquinone in melasma. Int J Dermatol. 2004 Aug;43(8):604-7. PubMed PMID: 15304189.

107. Hakozaki T, Takiwaki H, Miyamoto K, Sato Y, Arase S. Ultrasound enhanced skin-lightening effect of vitamin C and niacinamide. Skin Res Technol. 2006 May;12(2):105-13. PubMed PMID: 16626384.

108. Tai SS, Lin CG, Wu MH, Chang TS. Evaluation of depigmenting activity by 8-hydroxydaidzein in mouse B16 melanoma cells and human volunteers. Int J Mol Sci. 2009 Nov 20;10(10):4257-66. doi: 10.3390/ijms10104257. PubMed PMID: 20057943; PubMed Central PMCID: PMC2790106.

109. Huh CH, Seo KI, Park JY, Lim JG, Eun HC, Park KC. A randomized, double-blind, placebo-controlled trial of vitamin C iontophoresis in melasma. Dermatology. 2003;206(4):316-20. PubMed PMID: 12771472.

110. Yi X, Zhao G, Zhang H, Guan D, Meng R, Zhang Y, Yang Q, Jia H, Dou K, Liu C, Que F, Yin JQ. MITF-siRNA formulation is a safe and effective therapy for human melasma. Mol Ther. 2011 Feb;19(2):362-71. doi: 10.1038/mt.2010.263. Epub 2010 Nov 30. PubMed PMID: 21119619; PubMed Central PMCID: PMC3034856.

111. Taira N, Katsuyama Y, Yoshioka M, Okano Y, Masaki H. 3-O-Glyceryl-2-O-hexyl ascorbate suppresses melanogenesis by interfering with intracellular melanosome transport and suppressing tyrosinase protein synthesis. J Cosmet Dermatol. 2018 Dec;17(6):1209-1215. doi: 10.1111/jocd.12451. Epub 2017 Nov 7. PubMed PMID: 29115012.

112. Ando H, Matsui MS, Ichihashi M. Quasi-drugs developed in Japan for the prevention or treatment of hyperpigmentary disorders. Int J Mol Sci. 2010 Jun 18;11(6):2566-75. doi: 10.3390/ijms11062566. Review. PubMed PMID: 20640168; PubMed Central PMCID: PMC2904932.

113. PuvabanditsinP, Vongtongsri R. Efficacy of topical vitamin C derivative (VC-PMG) and topical vitamin E in prevention and treatment of UVA suntan skin. J Med Assoc Thai. 2006 Sep;89 Suppl 3:S65-8. PubMed PMID: 17722304.

114. Yang, Z.; Wang, Y.; Wang, Y.; Zhang, Y. Bioassay-guided screening and isolation of
-glucosidase and tyrosinase inhibitors from leaves of Morus alba. Food Chem. 2012, 131, 617–622.

115. Yuan Q, Zhao L. The Mulberry (Morus alba L.) Fruit-A Review of Characteristic Components and Health Benefits. J Agric Food Chem. 2017 Dec 6;65(48):10383-10394. doi: 10.1021/acs.jafc.7b03614. Epub 2017 Nov 20. Review. PubMed PMID: 29129054.

116. Zhang H, Ma ZF, Luo X, Li X. Effects of Mulberry Fruit (Morus alba L.) Consumption on Health Outcomes: A Mini-Review. Antioxidants (Basel). 2018 May 21;7(5). pii: E69. doi: 10.3390/antiox7050069. Review. PubMed PMID: 29883416; PubMed Central PMCID: PMC5981255.

117. Nattapong S, Omboon L. A new source of whitening agent from a Thai Mulberry plant and its betulinic acid quantitation. Nat Prod Res. 2008 Jun 15;22(9):727-34. doi: 10.1080/14786410601130794. PubMed PMID: 18569714.

118. Lim SH, Choi CI. Pharmacological Properties of Morusnigra L. (Black Mulberry) as A Promising Nutraceutical Resource. Nutrients. 2019 Feb 20;11(2). pii: E437. doi: 10.3390/nu11020437. Review. PubMed PMID: 30791521; PubMed Central PMCID: PMC6412198.

119. Zhang X, Hu X, Hou A, Wang H. Inhibitory effect of 2,4,2',4'-tetrahydroxy-3-(3-methyl-2-butenyl)-chalcone on tyrosinase activity and melanin biosynthesis. Biol Pharm Bull. 2009 Jan;32(1):86-90. PubMed PMID: 19122286.

120. Zheng ZP, Cheng KW, Zhu Q, Wang XC, Lin ZX, Wang M. Tyrosinase inhibitory constituents from the roots of Morusnigra: a structure-activity relationship study. J Agric Food Chem. 2010 May 12;58(9):5368-73. doi: 10.1021/jf1003607. PubMed PMID: 20297841.

121. Koyu H, Kazan A, Demir S, Haznedaroglu MZ, Yesil-Celiktas O. Optimization of microwave assisted extraction of Morusnigra L. fruits maximizing tyrosinase inhibitory activity with isolation of bioactive constituents. Food Chem. 2018 May

15;248:183-191. doi: 10.1016/j.foodchem.2017.12.049. Epub 2017 Dec 14. PubMed PMID: 29329842.

122. Nerya O, Vaya J, Musa R, Izrael S, Ben-Arie R, Tamir S. Glabrene and isoliquiritigenin as tyrosinase inhibitors from licorice roots. J Agric Food Chem. 2003 Feb 26;51(5):1201-7. PubMed PMID: 12590456.

123. Leyden JJ, Shergill B, Micali G, Downie J, Wallo W. Natural options for the management of hyperpigmentation. J Eur Acad Dermatol Venereol. 2011 Oct;25(10):1140-5. doi: 10.1111/j.1468-3083.2011.04130.x.Epub 2011 May 31. Review. PubMed PMID: 21623927.

124. Costa A, Moisés TA, Cordero T, Alves CR, Marmirori J. Association of emblica, licorice and belides as an alternative to hydroquinone in the clinical treatment of melasma. An Bras Dermatol. 2010 Sep-Oct;85(5):613-20. PubMed PMID: 21152784.

125. Sharma K, Joshi N, Goyal C. Critical review of Ayurvedic Varṇya herbs and their tyrosinase inhibition effect. Anc Sci Life. 2015 Jul-Sep;35(1):18-25. doi: 10.4103/0257-7941.165627. Review. PubMed PMID: 26600663; PubMed Central PMCID: PMC4623628.

126. Quay ER, Chang YC, Graber E. Evidence for Anti-Aging South Korean Cosmeceuticals. J Drugs Dermatol. 2017 Apr 1;16(4):358-363. PubMed PMID: 28403270.

127. Binic I, Lazarevic V, Ljubenovic M, Mojsa J, Sokolovic D. Skin ageing: natural weapons and strategies. Evid Based Complement Alternat Med. 2013;2013:827248. doi: 10.1155/2013/827248. Epub 2013 Jan 29. PubMed PMID: 23431351; PubMed Central PMCID: PMC3569896.

128. Thiele JJ, Hsieh SN, Ekanayake-Mudiyanselage S. Vitamin E: critical review of its current use in cosmetic and clinical dermatology. Dermatol Surg. 2005 Jul;31(7 Pt 2):805-13; discussion 813. Review. PubMed PMID: 16029671.

129. Badreshia-Bansal S, Draelos ZD. Insight into skin lightening cosmeceuticals for women of color. J Drugs Dermatol. 2007 Jan;6(1):32-9. Review. PubMed PMID: 17373159.

130. Kamei Y, Otsuka Y, Abe K. Comparison of the inhibitory effects of vitamin E analogues on melanogenesis in mouse B16 melanoma cells. Cytotechnology. 2009 Apr;59(3):183-90. doi: 10.1007/s10616-009-9207-y. Epub 2009 Jul 1. PubMed PMID: 19568943; PubMed Central PMCID: PMC2774566.

131. Kuwabara Y, Watanabe T, Yasuoka S, Fukui K, Takata J, Karube Y, Okamoto Y, Asano S, Katoh E, Tsuzuki T, Kobayashi S. Topical application of gamma-tocopherol derivative prevents UV-induced skin pigmentation. Biol Pharm Bull. 2006 Jun;29(6):1175-9. PubMed PMID: 16755012.

132. Keen MA, Hassan I. Vitamin E in dermatology. Indian Dermatol Online J. 2016 Jul-Aug;7(4):311-5. doi: 10.4103/2229-5178.185494. PubMed PMID: 27559512; PubMed Central PMCID: PMC4976416.

133. Handog EB, Galang DA, de Leon-Godinez MA, Chan GP. A randomized, double-blind, placebo-controlled trial of oral procyanidin with vitamins A, C, E for melasma among Filipino women. Int J Dermatol. 2009 Aug;48(8):896-901. doi: 10.1111/j.1365-4632.2009.04130.x. PubMed PMID: 19659873.

134. Jerajani HR, Mizoguchi H, Li J, Whittenbarger DJ, Marmor MJ. The effects of a daily facial lotion containing vitamins B3 and E and provitamin B5 on the facial skin of Indian women: a randomized, double-blind trial. Indian J Dermatol VenereolLeprol. 2010 Jan-Feb;76(1):20-6. doi: 10.4103/0378-6323.58674. PubMed PMID: 20061726.

135. Thiele JJ, Hsieh SN, Ekanayake-Mudiyanselage S. Vitamin E: critical review of its current use in cosmetic and clinical dermatology. Dermatol Surg. 2005 Jul;31(7 Pt 2):805-13; discussion 813. Review. PubMed PMID: 16029671.

136. Burke KE, Clive J, Combs GF Jr, Commisso J, Keen CL, Nakamura RM. Effects of topical and oral vitamin E on pigmentation and skin cancer induced by ultraviolet irradiation in Skh:2 hairless mice. Nutr Cancer. 2000;38(1):87-97. PubMed PMID: 11341050.

137. Burke KE, Clive J, Combs GF Jr, Nakamura RM. Effects of topical L-selenomethionine with topical and oral vitamin E on pigmentation and skin cancer induced by ultraviolet irradiation in Skh:2 hairless mice. J Am Acad Dermatol. 2003 Sep;49(3):458-72. PubMed PMID: 12963910.

138. Lin JY, Selim MA, Shea CR, Grichnik JM, Omar MM, Monteiro-Riviere NA, Pinnell SR. UV photoprotection by combination topical antioxidants vitamin C and vitamin E. J Am Acad Dermatol. 2003 Jun;48(6):866-74. PubMed PMID: 12789176.

139. Nestor MS, Berman B, Swenson N. Safety and Efficacy of Oral Polypodium leucotomos Extract in Healthy Adult Subjects. J Clin Aesthet Dermatol. 2015 Feb;8(2):19-23. PubMed PMID: 25741399; PubMed Central PMCID: PMC4345929.

140. Winkelmann RR, Del Rosso J, Rigel DS. Polypodium leucotomos extract: a status report on clinical efficacy and safety. J Drugs Dermatol. 2015 Mar;14(3):254-61. Review. PubMed PMID: 25738847.

141. Aguilera P, Carrera C, Puig-Butille JA, Badenas C, Lecha M, González S, Malvehy J, Puig S. Benefits of oral Polypodium Leucotomos extract in MM high-risk patients. J Eur Acad Dermatol Venereol. 2013 Sep;27(9):1095-100. doi: 10.1111/j.1468-3083.2012.04659.x.Epub 2012 Jul 31. PubMed PMID: 22849563; PubMed Central PMCID: PMC4556114.

142. Goh CL, Chuah SY, Tien S, Thng G, Vitale MA, Delgado-Rubin A. Double-blind, Placebo-controlled Trial to Evaluate the Effectiveness of Polypodium Leucotomos Extract in the Treatment of Melasma in Asian Skin: A Pilot Study. J Clin Aesthet Dermatol. 2018 Mar;11(3):14-19. Epub 2018 Mar 1. PubMed PMID: 29606995; PubMed Central PMCID: PMC5868779.

143. Nestor M, Bucay V, Callender V, Cohen JL, Sadick N, Waldorf H. Polypodium leucotomos as an Adjunct Treatment of Pigmentary Disorders. J Clin Aesthet Dermatol. 2014 Mar;7(3):13-7. Review. PubMed PMID: 24688621; PubMed Central PMCID: PMC3970827.

144. Ahmed AM, Lopez I, Perese F, Vasquez R, Hynan LS, Chong B, Pandya AG. A randomized, double-blinded, placebo-controlled trial of oral Polypodium leucotomos extract as an adjunct to sunscreen in the treatment of melasma. JAMA Dermatol. 2013 Aug;149(8):981-3. doi: 10.1001/jamadermatol.2013.4294. PubMed PMID: 23740292.

145. Berman B, Ellis C, Elmets C. Polypodium Leucotomos--An Overview of Basic Investigative Findings. J Drugs Dermatol. 2016 Feb;15(2):224-8. Review. PubMed PMID: 26885792; PubMed Central PMCID: PMC5189711.

146. Gombau L, García F, Lahoz A, Fabre M, Roda-Navarro P, Majano P, Alonso-Lebrero JL, Pivel JP, Castell JV, Gómez-Lechon MJ, González S. Polypodium leucotomos extract: antioxidant activity and disposition. Toxicol In Vitro. 2006 Jun;20(4):464-71. Epub 2005 Nov 2. PubMed PMID: 16263237.

147. Middelkamp-Hup MA, Pathak MA, Parrado C, Garcia-Caballero T, Rius-Díaz F, Fitzpatrick TB, González S. Orally administered Polypodium leucotomos extract decreases psoralen-UVA-induced phototoxicity, pigmentation, and damage of human skin. J Am Acad Dermatol. 2004 Jan;50(1):41-9. PubMed PMID: 14699363.

148. Kohli I, Shafi R, Isedeh P, Griffith JL, Al-Jamal MS, Silpa-Archa N, Jackson B, Athar M, Kollias N, Elmets CA, Lim HW, Hamzavi IH. The impact of oral Polypodium leucotomos extract on ultraviolet B response: A human clinical study. J Am Acad Dermatol. 2017 Jul;77(1):33-41.e1. doi: 10.1016/j.jaad.2017.01.044. Epub 2017 Mar 22. PubMed PMID: 28341348; PubMed Central PMCID: PMC5730054.

149. Parrado C, Philips N, Gilaberte Y, Juarranz A, González S. Oral Photoprotection: Effective Agents and Potential Candidates. Front Med (Lausanne). 2018 Jun 26;5:188. doi: 10.3389/fmed.2018.00188. eCollection 2018. Review. PubMed PMID: 29998107; PubMed Central PMCID: PMC6028556.

150. Murbach TS, Glávits R, Hirka G, Endres JR, Clewell AE, Szakonyiné IP. A 28-day oral toxicology study of an aqueous extract of Polypodium leucotomos (Fernblock(®)). Toxicol Rep. 2017 Sep 12;4:494-501. doi: 10.1016/j.toxrep.2017.09.002. eCollection 2017. PubMed PMID: 28959679; PubMed Central PMCID: PMC5615158.

151. Greatens A, Hakozaki T, Koshoffer A, Epstein H, Schwemberger S, Babcock G, Bissett D, Takiwaki H, Arase S, Wickett RR, Boissy RE. Effective inhibition of melanosome transfer to keratinocytes by lectins and niacinamide is reversible. Exp Dermatol. 2005 Jul;14(7):498-508. PubMed PMID: 15946237.

152. Hakozaki T, Minwalla L, Zhuang J, Chhoa M, Matsubara A, Miyamoto K, Greatens A, Hillebrand GG, Bissett DL, Boissy RE. The effect of niacinamide on reducing cutaneous pigmentation and suppression of melanosome transfer. Br J Dermatol. 2002 Jul;147(1):20-31. PubMed PMID: 12100180.

153. Navarrete-Solís J, Castanedo-Cázares JP, Torres-Álvarez B, Oros-Ovalle C, Fuentes-Ahumada C, González FJ, Martínez-Ramírez JD, Moncada B. A Double-Blind, Randomized Clinical Trial of Niacinamide 4% versus Hydroquinone 4% in the Treatment of Melasma. Dermatol Res Pract. 2011;2011:379173. doi: 10.1155/2011/379173. Epub 2011 Jul 21. PubMed PMID: 21822427; PubMed Central PMCID: PMC3142702.

154. Hakozaki T, Takiwaki H, Miyamoto K, Sato Y, Arase S. Ultrasound enhanced skin-lightening effect of vitamin C and niacinamide. Skin Res Technol. 2006 May;12(2):105-13. PubMed PMID: 16626384.

155. Wohlrab J, Kreft D. Niacinamide - mechanisms of action and its topical use in dermatology. Skin Pharmacol Physiol. 2014;27(6):311-5. doi: 10.1159/000359974. Epub 2014 Jun 27. Review. PubMed PMID: 24993939.
156. Bissett DL, Robinson LR, Raleigh PS, Miyamoto K, Hakozaki T, Li J, Kelm GR. Reduction in the appearance of facial hyperpigmentation by topical N-undecyl-10-enoyl-L-phenylalanine and its combination with niacinamide. J Cosmet Dermatol. 2009 Dec;8(4):260-6. doi: 10.1111/j.1473-2165.2009.00470.x. PubMed PMID: 19958429.
157. Bissett DL, Robinson LR, Raleigh PS, Miyamoto K, Hakozaki T, Li J, Kelm GR. Reduction in the appearance of facial hyperpigmentation by topical N-acetyl glucosamine. J Cosmet Dermatol. 2007 Mar;6(1):20-6. Review. PubMed PMID: 17348991.
158. Kimball AB, Kaczvinsky JR, Li J, Robinson LR, Matts PJ, Berge CA, Miyamoto K, Bissett DL. Reduction in the appearance of facial hyperpigmentation after use of moisturizers with a combination of topical niacinamide and N-acetyl glucosamine: results of a randomized, double-blind, vehicle-controlled trial. Br J Dermatol. 2010 Feb 1;162(2):435-41. doi: 10.1111/j.1365-2133.2009.09477.x.Epub 2009 Aug 28. PubMed PMID: 19845667.
159. Bissett DL, Miyamoto K, Sun P, Li J, Berge CA. Topical niacinamide reduces yellowing, wrinkling, red blotchiness, and hyperpigmented spots in aging facial skin. Int J Cosmet Sci. 2004 Oct;26(5):231-8. doi: 10.1111/j.1467-2494.2004.00228.x. PubMed PMID: 18492135.
160. Bissett DL, Oblong JE, Berge CA. Niacinamide: A B vitamin that improves aging facial skin appearance. Dermatol Surg. 2005 Jul;31(7 Pt 2):860-5; discussion 865. PubMed PMID: 16029679.
161. Chae GY, Ha BJ. The Comparative Evaluation of Fermented and Non-fermented Soybean Extract on Antioxidation and Whitening. Toxicol Res. 2011 Dec;27(4):205-9. doi: 10.5487/TR.2011.27.4.205. PubMed PMID: 24278573; PubMed Central PMCID: PMC3834387.
162. Waqas MK, Akhtar N, Mustafa R, Jamshaid M, Khan HM, Murtaza G. Dermatological and cosmeceutical benefits of Glycine max (soybean) and its active components. Acta Pol Pharm. 2015 Jan-Feb;72(1):3-11. Review. PubMed PMID: 25850195.
163. Lai J, Xin C, Zhao Y, Feng B, He C, Dong Y, Fang Y, Wei S. Study of active ingredients in black soybean sprouts and their safety in cosmetic use. Molecules. 2012 Oct 1;17(10):11669-79. doi: 10.3390/molecules171011669. PubMed PMID: 23027368; PubMed Central PMCID: PMC6268251.
164. Zhao R, Bruning E, Rossetti D, Starcher B, Seiberg M, Iotsova-Stone V. Extracts from Glycine max (soybean) induce elastin synthesis and inhibit elastase activity. Exp Dermatol. 2009 Oct;18(10):883-6. doi: 10.1111/j.1600-0625.2009.00862.x.Epub 2009 Mar 10. PubMed PMID: 19469891.
165. Paine C, Sharlow E, Liebel F, Eisinger M, Shapiro S, Seiberg M. An alternative approach to depigmentation by soybean extracts via inhibition of the PAR-2 pathway. J Invest Dermatol. 2001 Apr;116(4):587-95. PubMed PMID: 11286627.

166. Lim TG, Kim JE, Lee SY, Park JS, Yeom MH, Chen H, Bode AM, Dong Z, Lee KW. The daidzein metabolite, 6,7,4'-Trihydroxyisoflavone, is a novel inhibitor of PKCα in suppressing solar UV-induced matrix metalloproteinase 1. Int J Mol Sci. 2014 Nov 19;15(11):21419-32. doi: 10.3390/ijms151121419. PubMed PMID: 25415304; PubMed Central PMCID: PMC4264233.
167. Liu-Smith F, Meyskens FL. Molecular mechanisms of flavonoids in melanin synthesis and the potential for the prevention and treatment of melanoma. Mol Nutr Food Res. 2016 Jun;60(6):1264-74. doi: 10.1002/mnfr.201500822. Epub 2016 Mar 21. Review. PubMed PMID: 26865001; PubMed Central PMCID: PMC4900912.
168. Chang TS. Isolation, bioactivity, and production of ortho-hydroxydaidzeinand ortho-hydroxygenistein. Int J Mol Sci. 2014 Apr 3;15(4):5699-716. doi: 10.3390/ijms15045699. Review. PubMed PMID: 24705463; PubMed Central PMCID: PMC4013590.
169. Huang CC, Hsu BY, Wu NL, Tsui WH, Lin TJ, Su CC, Hung CF. Anti-photoaging effects of soy isoflavone extract (aglycone and acetylglucoside form) from soybean cake. Int J Mol Sci. 2010;11(12):4782-95. doi: 10.3390/ijms11124782. Epub 2010 Nov 24. PubMed PMID: 21614173; PubMed Central PMCID: PMC3100816.
170. Riyanto P, Subchan P, Lelyana R. Advantage of soybean isoflavone as antiandrogen on acne vulgaris. Dermatoendocrinol. 2015 Jul 20;7(1):e1063751. doi: 10.1080/19381980.2015.1063751. eCollection 2015 Jan-Dec. PubMed PMID: 26413190; PubMed Central PMCID: PMC4579974.
171. Naturopath. Lectins in Food. Superpharmacy, August 5, 2018.
172. MinwallaL, Zhao Y, Cornelius J, Babcock GF, Wickett RR, Le Poole IC, Boissy RE. Inhibition of melanosome transfer from melanocytes to keratinocytes by lectins and neoglycoproteins in an in vitro model system. Pigment Cell Res. 2001 Jun;14(3):185-94. PubMed PMID: 11434566.
173. Moghimipour E. Hydroxy Acids, the Most Widely Used Anti-aging Agents. Jundishapur J Nat Pharm Prod. 2012 Winter;7(1):9-10. Epub 2012 Jan 4. PubMed PMID: 24624144; PubMed Central PMCID: PMC3941867.
174. Tang SC, Yang JH. Dual Effects of Alpha-Hydroxy Acids on the Skin. Molecules. 2018 Apr 10;23(4). pii: E863. doi: 10.3390/molecules23040863. Review. PubMed PMID: 29642579; PubMed Central PMCID: PMC6017965.
175. Fabbrocini G, De Padova MP, Tosti A. Chemical peels: what's new and what isn't new but still works well. Facial Plast Surg. 2009 Dec;25(5):329-36. doi: 10.1055/s-0029-1243082. Epub 2009 Dec 18. Review. PubMed PMID: 20024875.
176. Sharad J. Glycolic acid peel therapy - a current review. Clin CosmetInvestig Dermatol. 2013 Nov 11;6:281-8. doi: 10.2147/CCID.S34029. Review. PubMed PMID: 24399880; PubMed Central PMCID: PMC3875240.
177. Lim JT, Tham SN. Glycolic acid peels in the treatment of melasma among Asian women. Dermatol Surg. 1997 Mar;23(3):177-9. PubMed PMID: 9145959.
178. Kalla G, Garg A, Kachhawa D. Chemical peeling--glycolic acid versus trichloroacetic acid in melasma. Indian J Dermatol VenereolLeprol. 2001 Mar-Apr;67(2):82-4. PubMed PMID: 17664715.

179. Javaheri SM, Handa S, Kaur I, Kumar B. Safety and efficacy of glycolic acid facial peel in Indian women with melasma. Int J Dermatol. 2001 May;40(5):354-7. PubMed PMID: 11555002.
180. Sarkar R, Kaur C, Bhalla M, Kanwar AJ. The combination of glycolic acid peels with a topical regimen in the treatment of melasma in dark-skinned patients: a comparative study. Dermatol Surg. 2002 Sep;28(9):828-32; discussion 832. PubMed PMID: 12269877.
181. Hurley ME, Guevara IL, Gonzales RM, Pandya AG. Efficacy of glycolic acid peels in the treatment of melasma. Arch Dermatol. 2002 Dec;138(12):1578-82. PubMed PMID: 12472345.
182. Khunger N, Sarkar R, Jain RK. Tretinoin peels versus glycolic acid peels in the treatment of Melasma in dark-skinned patients. Dermatol Surg. 2004 May;30(5):756-60; discussion 760. PubMed PMID: 15099320.
183. Kligman DE. Tretinoin peels versus glycolic acid peels. Dermatol Surg. 2004 Dec;30(12 Pt 2):1609. PubMed PMID: 15606862.
184. Grover C, Reddu BS. The therapeutic value of glycolic acid peels in dermatology. Indian J Dermatol VenereolLeprol. 2003 Mar-Apr;69(2):148-50. PubMed PMID: 17642863.
185. Erbil H, Sezer E, Taştan B, Arca E, Kurumlu Z. Efficacy and safety of serial glycolic acid peels and a topical regimen in the treatment of recalcitrant melasma. J Dermatol. 2007 Jan;34(1):25-30. PubMed PMID: 17204097.
186. Rendon M, Cardona LM, Bussear EW, Benitez AL, Colón LE, Johnson LA. Successful treatment of moderate to severe melasma with triple-combination cream and glycolic acid peels: a pilot study. Cutis. 2008 Nov;82(5):372-8. PubMed PMID: 19090343.
187. Kumari R, Thappa DM. Comparative study of trichloroacetic acid versus glycolic acid chemical peels in the treatment of melasma. Indian J Dermatol VenereolLeprol. 2010 Jul-Aug;76(4):447. doi: 10.4103/0378-6323.66602. PubMed PMID: 20657143.
188. Puri N. Comparative study of 15% TCA peel versus 35% glycolic acid peel for the treatment of melasma. Indian Dermatol Online J. 2012 May;3(2):109-13. doi: 10.4103/2229-5178.96702. PubMed PMID: 23130283; PubMed Central PMCID: PMC3481880.
189. Sharquie KE, Al-Tikreety MM, Al-Mashhadani SA. Lactic acid as a new therapeutic peeling agent in melasma. Dermatol Surg. 2005 Feb;31(2):149-54; discussion 154. PubMed PMID: 15762205.
190. Soleymani T, Lanoue J, Rahman Z. A Practical Approach to Chemical Peels: A Review of Fundamentals and Step-by-step Algorithmic Protocol for Treatment. J Clin Aesthet Dermatol. 2018 Aug;11(8):21-28. Epub 2018 Aug 1. PubMed PMID: 30214663; PubMed Central PMCID: PMC6122508.
191. Sharquie KE, Al-Tikreety MM, Al-Mashhadani SA. Lactic acid chemical peels as a new therapeutic modality in melasma in comparison to Jessner's solution chemical peels. Dermatol Surg. 2006 Dec;32(12):1429-36. PubMed PMID: 17199649.

192. Puri N. Efficacy of Modified Jessner's Peel and 20% TCA Versus 20% TCA Peel Alone for the Treatment of Acne Scars. J CutanAesthet Surg. 2015 Jan-Mar;8(1):42-5. doi: 10.4103/0974-2077.155082. PubMed PMID: 25949022; PubMed Central PMCID: PMC4411592.

193. Shankar K, Godse K, Aurangabadkar S, Lahiri K, Mysore V, Ganjoo A, Vedamurty M, Kohli M, Sharad J, Kadhe G, Ahirrao P, Narayanan V, Motlekar SA. Evidence-based treatment for melasma: expert opinion and a review. Dermatol Ther (Heidelb). 2014 Dec;4(2):165-86. doi: 10.1007/s13555-014-0064-z. Epub 2014 Oct 1. PubMed PMID: 25269451; PubMed Central PMCID: PMC4257945.

194. Yamamoto Y, Uede K, Yonei N, Kishioka A, Ohtani T, Furukawa F. Effects of alpha-hydroxy acids on the human skin of Japanese subjects: the rationale for chemical peeling. J Dermatol. 2006 Jan;33(1):16-22. PubMed PMID: 16469079.

195. Kornhauser A, Coelho SG, Hearing VJ. Effects of cosmetic formulations containing hydroxyacids on sun-exposed skin: current applications and future developments. Dermatol Res Pract. 2012;2012:710893. doi: 10.1155/2012/710893. Epub 2012 May 20. PubMed PMID: 22675344; PubMed Central PMCID: PMC3362829.

196. Desai SR. Hyperpigmentation therapy: a review. J Clin Aesthet Dermatol. 2014 Aug;7(8):13-7. PubMed PMID: 25161755; PubMed Central PMCID: PMC4142815.

197. Arif T. Salicylic acid as a peeling agent: a comprehensive review. Clin CosmetInvestig Dermatol. 2015 Aug 26;8:455-61. doi: 10.2147/CCID.S84765. eCollection 2015. Review. PubMed PMID: 26347269; PubMed Central PMCID: PMC4554394.

198. Grimes PE. The safety and efficacy of salicylic acid chemical peels in darker racial-ethnic groups. Dermatol Surg. 1999 Jan;25(1):18-22. PubMed PMID: 9935087.

199. Ranjan R, Sarkar R, Garg VK, Gupta T. A Comparative Study of Two Modalities, 4% Hydroquinone Versus 30% Salicylic Acid in Periorbital Hyperpigmentation and Assessment of Quality of Life Before and After Treatment. Indian J Dermatol. 2016 Jul-Aug;61(4):413-7. doi: 10.4103/0019-5154.185707. PubMed PMID: 27512187; PubMed Central PMCID: PMC4966400.

200. Mohamed Ali BM, Gheida SF, El Mahdy NA, Sadek SN. Evaluation of salicylic acid peeling in comparison with topical tretinoin in the treatment of postinflammatory hyperpigmentation. J Cosmet Dermatol. 2017 Mar;16(1):52-60. doi: 10.1111/jocd.12301. Epub 2016 Dec 15. PubMed PMID: 27976510.

201. Ahn HH, Kim IH. Whitening effect of salicylic acid peels in Asian patients. Dermatol Surg. 2006 Mar;32(3):372-5; discussion 375. PubMed PMID: 16640681.

202. Fabbrocini G, De Vita V, Marasca C, Palmisano F, Monfrecola G. Salicylic acid for the treatment of melasma: new acquisitions for monitoring the clinical improvement. Skin Res Technol. 2013 Nov;19(4):466-73. doi: 10.1111/srt.12070. Epub 2013 Mar 25. PubMed PMID: 23527534.

203. Ando H, Ryu A, Hashimoto A, Oka M, Ichihashi M. Linoleic acid and alpha-linolenic acid lightens ultraviolet-induced hyperpigmentation of the skin. Arch Dermatol Res. 1998 Jul;290(7):375-81. PubMed PMID: 9749992.

204. Shigeta Y, Imanaka H, Ando H, Ryu A, Oku N, Baba N, Makino T. Skin whitening effect of linoleic acid is enhanced by liposomal formulations. Biol Pharm Bull. 2004 Apr;27(4):591-4. PubMed PMID: 15056874.

205. Ando H, Funasaka Y, Oka M, Ohashi A, Furumura M, Matsunaga J, Matsunaga N, Hearing VJ, Ichihashi M. Possible involvement of proteolytic degradation of tyrosinase in the regulatory effect of fatty acids on melanogenesis. J Lipid Res. 1999 Jul;40(7):1312-6. PubMed PMID: 10393216.

206. Ko GA, Kim Cho S. Ethyl linoleate inhibits α-MSH-induced melanogenesis through Akt/GSK3β/β-catenin signal pathway. Korean J PhysiolPharmacol. 2018 Jan;22(1):53-61. doi: 10.4196/kjpp.2018.22.1.53. Epub 2017 Dec 22. PubMed PMID: 29302212; PubMed Central PMCID: PMC5746512.

207. Lee MH, Kim HJ, Ha DJ, Paik JH, Kim HY. Therapeutic effect of topical application of linoleic acid and lincomycin in combination with betamethasone valerate in melasma patients. J Korean Med Sci. 2002 Aug;17(4):518-23. PubMed PMID: 12172049; PubMed Central PMCID: PMC3054896.

208. Ortonne JP. Retinoid therapy of pigmentary disorders. Dermatol Ther. 2006 Sep-Oct;19(5):280-8. Review. PubMed PMID: 17014483.

209. Davis EC, Callender VD. Postinflammatory hyperpigmentation: a review of the epidemiology, clinical features, and treatment options in skin of color. J Clin Aesthet Dermatol. 2010 Jul;3(7):20-31. PubMed PMID: 20725554; PubMed Central PMCID: PMC2921758.

210. Desmedt B, Van Hoeck E, Rogiers V, Courselle P, De Beer JO, De Paepe K, Deconinck E. Characterization of suspected illegal skin whitening cosmetics. J Pharm Biomed Anal. 2014 Mar;90:85-91. doi: 10.1016/j.jpba.2013.11.024. Epub2013 Nov 28. PubMed PMID: 24334193.

211. Nahhas AF, Abdel-Malek ZA, Kohli I, Braunberger TL, Lim HW, Hamzavi IH. The potential role of antioxidants in mitigating skin hyperpigmentation resulting from ultraviolet and visible light-induced oxidative stress. PhotodermatolPhotoimmunolPhotomed. 2018 Sep 10. doi: 10.1111/phpp.12423. [Epub ahead of print] Review. PubMed PMID: 30198587.

212. Addor FAS. Antioxidants in dermatology. An Bras Dermatol. 2017 May-Jun;92(3):356-362. doi: 10.1590/abd1806-4841.20175697. Review. PubMed PMID: 29186248; PubMed Central PMCID: PMC5514576.

213. SchalkaS. New data on hyperpigmentation disorders. J Eur Acad Dermatol Venereol. 2017 Sep;31 Suppl 5:18-21. doi: 10.1111/jdv.14411. Review. PubMed PMID: 28805937.

214. Pai VV, Shukla P, Kikkeri NN. Antioxidants in dermatology. Indian Dermatol Online J. 2014 Apr;5(2):210-4. doi: 10.4103/2229-5178.131127. PubMed PMID: 24860765; PubMed Central PMCID: PMC4030358.

215. Kim YC, Choi SY, Park EY. Anti-melanogenic effects of black, green, and white tea extracts on immortalized melanocytes. J Vet Sci. 2015;16(2):135-43. Epub 2015 Jan 30. PubMed PMID: 25643794; PubMed Central PMCID: PMC4483495.

216. Mallick S, Singh SK, Sarkar C, Saha B, Bhadra R. Human placental lipid induces melanogenesis by increasing the expression of tyrosinase and its related proteins in vitro. Pigment Cell Res. 2005 Feb;18(1):25-33. PubMed PMID: 15649149.
217. Kim E, Hwang K, Lee J, Han SY, Kim EM, Park J, Cho JY. Skin Protective Effect of Epigallocatechin Gallate. Int J Mol Sci. 2018 Jan 6;19(1). pii: E173. doi: 10.3390/ijms19010173. PubMed PMID: 29316635; PubMed Central PMCID: PMC5796122.
218. Choi SY, Kim YC. Whitening effect of black tea water extract on brown Guinea pig skin. Toxicol Res. 2011 Sep;27(3):153-60. doi: 10.5487/TR.2011.27.3.153. PubMed PMID: 24278566; PubMed Central PMCID: PMC3834380.
219. OyetakinWhite P, Tribout H, Baron E. Protective mechanisms of green tea polyphenols in skin. Oxid Med Cell Longev. 2012;2012:560682. doi: 10.1155/2012/560682. Epub 2012 Jun 26. Review. PubMed PMID: 22792414; PubMed Central PMCID: PMC3390139.
220. Zhang J, Lei Z, Huang Z, Zhang X, Zhou Y, Luo Z, Zeng W, Su J, Peng C, Chen X. Epigallocatechin-3-gallate(EGCG) suppresses melanoma cell growth and metastasis by targeting TRAF6 activity. Oncotarget. 2016 Nov 29;7(48):79557-79571. doi: 10.18632/oncotarget.12836. PubMed PMID: 27791197; PubMed Central PMCID: PMC5346735.
221. An BJ, Kwak JH, Son JH, Park JM, Lee JY, Park TS, Kim SY, Kim YS, Jo C, Byun MW. Physiological activity of irradiated green tea polyphenol on the human skin. Am J Chin Med. 2005;33(4):535-46. PubMed PMID: 16173528.
222. Dumoulin M, Gaudout D, Lemaire B. Clinical effects of an oral supplement rich in antioxidants on skin radiance in women. Clin CosmetInvestig Dermatol. 2016 Oct 18;9:315-324. eCollection 2016. PubMed PMID: 27799805; PubMed Central PMCID: PMC5076548.
223. Ellijimi C, Ben Hammouda M, Othman H, Moslah W, Jebali J, Mabrouk HB, Morjen M, Haoues M, Luis J, Marrakchi N, Essafi-Benkhadir K, Srairi-Abid N. Helix aspersa maxima mucus exhibits antimelanogenic and antitumoral effects against melanoma cells. Biomed Pharmacother. 2018 May;101:871-880. doi: 10.1016/j.biopha.2018.03.020. Epub 2018 Mar 22. PubMed PMID: 29635896.
224. Kim K. Effect of ginseng and ginsenosides on melanogenesis and their mechanism of action. J Ginseng Res. 2015 Jan;39(1):1-6. doi: 10.1016/j.jgr.2014.10.006. Epub 2014 Nov 24. Review. PubMed PMID: 25535470; PubMed Central PMCID: PMC4268563.
225. Lee CS, Nam G, Bae IH, Park J. Whitening efficacy of ginsenoside F1 through inhibition of melanin transfer in cocultured human melanocytes-keratinocytes and three-dimensional human skin equivalent. J Ginseng Res. 2019 Apr;43(2):300-304. doi: 10.1016/j.jgr.2017.12.005. Epub 2018 Jan 31. PubMed PMID: 30962737; PubMed Central PMCID: PMC6437421.
226. Lee Y, Kim KT, Kim SS, Hur J, Ha SK, Cho CW, Choi SY. Inhibitory effects of ginseng seed on melanin biosynthesis. Pharmacogn Mag. 2014 Apr;10(Suppl 2):S272-5. doi: 10.4103/0973-1296.133271. PubMed PMID: 24991102; PubMed Central PMCID: PMC4078335.

227. Jiménez Z, Kim YJ, Mathiyalagan R, Seo KH, Mohanan P, Ahn JC, Kim YJ, Yang DC. Assessment of radical scavenging, whitening and moisture retention activities of Panax ginseng berry mediated gold nanoparticles as safe and efficient novel cosmetic material. Artif Cells NanomedBiotechnol. 2018 Mar;46(2):333-340. doi: 10.1080/21691401.2017.1307216. Epub 2017 Apr 9. PubMed PMID: 28393568.
228. Lee JO, Kim E, Kim JH, Hong YH, Kim HG, Jeong D, Kim J, Kim SH, Park C, Seo DB, Son YJ, Han SY, Cho JY. Antimelanogenesis and skin-protective activities of Panax ginseng calyx ethanol extract. J Ginseng Res. 2018 Jul;42(3):389-399. doi: 10.1016/j.jgr.2018.02.007. Epub 2018 Feb 21. PubMed PMID: 29983620; PubMed Central PMCID: PMC6026384.
229. Yang Y, Ren C, Zhang Y, Wu X. Ginseng: An Nonnegligible Natural Remedy for Healthy Aging. Aging Dis. 2017 Dec 1;8(6):708-720. doi: 10.14336/AD.2017.0707. eCollection 2017 Dec. Review. PubMed PMID: 29344412; PubMed Central PMCID: PMC5758347.
230. Lee DY, Jeong YT, Jeong SC, Lee MK, Min JW, Lee JW, Kim GS, Lee SE, Ahn YS, Kang HC, Kim JH. Melanin Biosynthesis Inhibition Effects of Ginsenoside Rb2 Isolated from Panax ginseng Berry. J Microbiol Biotechnol. 2015 Dec 28;25(12):2011-5. doi: 10.4014/jmb.1505.05069. PubMed PMID: 26437949.
231. Song M, Mun JH, Ko HC, Kim BS, Kim MB. Korean red ginseng powder in the treatment of melasma: an uncontrolled observational study. J Ginseng Res. 2011 Jun;35(2):170-5. doi: 10.5142/jgr.2011.35.2.170. PubMed PMID: 23717059; PubMed Central PMCID: PMC3659531.
232. Time for a reality check on skin lightening creams. The Conversation, September 11, 2012.
233. Sharma R, Abrol S, Wani M. Misuse of topical corticosteroids on facial skin. A study of 200 patients. J Dermatol Case Rep. 2017 Mar 31;11(1):5-8. doi: 10.3315/jdcr.2017.1240. eCollection 2017 Mar 31. PubMed PMID: 28539982; PubMed Central PMCID: PMC5439689.
234. Pal D, Biswas P, Das S, De A, Sharma N, Ansari A. Topical Steroid Damaged/Dependent Face (TSDF): A Study from a Tertiary Care Hospital in Eastern India. Indian J Dermatol. 2018 Sep-Oct;63(5):375-379. doi: 10.4103/ijd.IJD_218_17. PubMed PMID: 30210157; PubMed Central PMCID: PMC6124224.
235. Ashique KT, Chandrasekhar D. Role of Clinical Pharmacist in Cosmeto-vigilance of Misuse and Abuse of Topical Corticosteroids. Indian J Dermatol. 2017 Mar-Apr;62(2):213. doi: 10.4103/ijd.IJD_686_16. PubMed PMID: 28400646; PubMed Central PMCID: PMC5363150.
236. CoondooA, Phiske M, Verma S, Lahiri K. Side-effects of topical steroids: A long overdue revisit. Indian Dermatol Online J. 2014 Oct;5(4):416-25. doi: 10.4103/2229-5178.142483. Review. PubMed PMID: 25396122; PubMed Central PMCID: PMC4228634.
237. Skin-lightening cosmetics: frequent, potentially severe adverse effects. Prescrire Int. 2011 Sep;20(119):209-13, 215. Review. PubMed PMID: 21954516.

238. Lartey M, Krampa FD, Abdul-Rahman M, Quarcoo NL, Yamson P, Hagan PG, Tettey Y, Gyasi R, Adjei AA. Use of skin-lightening products among selected urban communities in Accra, Ghana. Int J Dermatol. 2017 Jan;56(1):32-39. doi: 10.1111/ijd.13449. PubMed PMID: 27943305.
239. Mistry N, Shapero J, Kundu RV, Shapero H. Toxic effects of skin-lightening products in Canadian immigrants. J Cutan Med Surg. 2011 Sep-Oct;15(5):254-8. PubMed PMID: 21962184.
240. Mahé A. The practice of skin-bleaching for a cosmetic purpose in immigrant communities. J Travel Med. 2014 Jul-Aug;21(4):282-7. doi: 10.1111/jtm.12106. Epub 2014 Mar 11. Review. PubMed PMID: 24612323.
241. Benn EK, Alexis A, Mohamed N, Wang YH, Khan IA, Liu B. Skin Bleaching and Dermatologic Health of African and Afro-Caribbean Populations in the US: New Directions for Methodologically Rigorous, Multidisciplinary, and Culturally Sensitive Research. Dermatol Ther (Heidelb). 2016 Dec;6(4):453-459. Epub 2016 Nov 11. PubMed PMID: 27837412; PubMed Central PMCID: PMC5120641.
242. Dlova N, Hamed SH, Tsoka-Gwegweni J, Grobler A, Hift R. Women's perceptions of the benefits and risks of skin-lightening creams in two South African communities. J Cosmet Dermatol. 2014 Sep;13(3):236-41. doi: 10.1111/jocd.12104. PubMed PMID: 25196692.
243. Jose, A., & Ray, J. G. (2018). Toxic content of certain commercially available fairness creams in Indian market. Cogent Medicine, 5(1), 1433104. https://doi.org/10.1080/2331205X.2018.1433104
244. Not Just Virat Kohli, Here Are Other Celebs Who Said No To Endorsements On Ethical Grounds. SCOOPWHOOP, Sep 14, 2017.

CHAPTER 4

SKIN AGING AND MODERN AGE ANTI-AGING STRATEGIES

4.1 BACKGROUND

Skin is the barrier that segregates the body from the outer environment. Besides protecting the body from water loss and microorganism infection, it has an important cosmetic role. Young and beautiful appearance may have a positive influence on people's social behavior and reproductive status. Cleopatra, the Egyptian queen is said to have indulged in daily donkey-milk baths, a practice that apparently required over 700 donkeys to accomplish. The alpha hydroxy acids in the milk is believed to be anti-aging and skin-softening agents. Tang-dynasty ruler and sole female emperor of China, Wu Zetian, maintained a lifelong interest in skincare formulas. She mixed her "fairy powder" (made of carefully harvested and prepared Chinese motherwort) with cold water to wash her face each morning. The empress was a famed beauty well into her old age. The most hair-raising entrant in this list, 16th century Hungarian countess Elizabeth Báthory is infamous for being one of the world's first documented female serial killers. Most of her life is shrouded in mystery and legend—the most famous story being that she would regularly bathe in the blood of her female victims. Mary, Queen of Scots, the ill-fated and attractive adversary of Elizabeth I, spent her sixteenth-century happier days on her estate in Edinburgh, Scotland, where her beauty regimen was said to include white-wine baths. In addition to wine's antiseptic alcohol content, it was also was thought to improve complexion in general. Crème Céleste, a favorite product of empress Elisabeth (Sisi) of Austria, was a concoction of spermaceti (a wax found in the head of sperm whales), sweet almond oil, and rosewater. She would apply this daily and at night, she was known to coat her face in raw veal and crushed strawberries, kept in place with a custom-made leather mask. The skin folds are indicative of an aged personality, but not youthfulness. So, everyone wants to look younger for the whole of life, which lead to the discovery of many surgical and non-surgical treatment modalities to improve the youthfulness. Since the introduction of Botox in 2002 after FDA approval more aesthetic procedures using Botox were performed by aestheticisms involving plastic surgeons and dermatologists. However, many scientists are now starting to view physical aging as a disease process. The cellular and molecular mechanisms involved in aging reveal an intricate series of signals, markers, and pathways, all of which are programmed to monitor and control the lifespan of a cell as it ages. By studying these molecular events and pathways, the field of anti-aging will be furthered by the use of more and more cosmetics.

4.2 ABSTRACT

As the most voluminous organ of the body that is exposed to the outer environment, the skin suffers from both intrinsic and extrinsic aging factors. Skin aging is characterized by features such as wrinkling, loss of elasticity, laxity, and rough-textured appearance. This aging process is accompanied by phenotypic changes in cutaneous cells as well as structural and functional changes in extracellular matrix components such as collagens and elastin. With intrinsic aging, structural changes occur in the skin as a natural consequence of the biological changes over time and produce a certain number of histological, physiological, and biochemical modifications. Intrinsic aging is determined genetically (influence of gender and ethnic group), variable in function of skin site, and also influenced by hormonal changes. Visually it is characterized by fine wrinkles. By comparison, "photoaging" is the term used to describe the changes occurring in the skin, resulting from repetitive exposure to sunlight. The histological, physiological, and biochemical changes in the different layers of the skin are much more drastic. From a mechanical point of view, human skin appears as a layered composite containing the stiff thin cover layer presented by the stratum corneum, below which are the more compliant layers of viable epidermis and dermis and further below the much more compliant adjacent layer of subcutaneous white adipose tissue. Upon exposure to a strain, such a multi-layer system demonstrates structural instabilities in its stiffer layers, which in its simplest form is the wrinkling. These instabilities appear hierarchically when the mechanical strain in the skin exceeds some critical values. Their appearance is mainly dependent on the mismatch in mechanical properties between adjacent skin layers or between the skin and subcutaneous white adipose tissue, on the adhesive strength and thickness ratios between the layers, on their bending and tensile stiffness as well as on the value of the stress existing in single layers. Gradual reduction of elastic fibers in aging significantly reduces the skin's ability to bend, prompting an up to 4-fold reduction of its stability against wrinkling, thereby explaining the role of these fibers in skin aging. Anti-aging medicine is practiced by physicians, scientists, and researchers dedicated to the belief that the process of physical aging in humans can be slowed, stopped, or even reversed through existing medical and scientific interventions. This specialty of medicine is based on the very early detection and prevention of age-related diseases. Physicians practicing anti-aging medicine seek to enhance the quality of life as well as its length, limiting the period of illness and disability toward the end of one's life. Anti-aging medicine encompasses lifestyle changes (diet and exercise); hormone replacement therapies, as needed, determined by a physician through blood testing (DHEA, melatonin, thyroid, human growth hormone, estrogen, testosterone); antioxidants and vitamin supplements; and testing protocols that can measure not only hormone levels and blood chemistry but every metabolic factor right down to the cellular level.

Keywords: skin care; anti-aging; photoaging; wrinkles; antioxidants; keratinocytes; retinoids

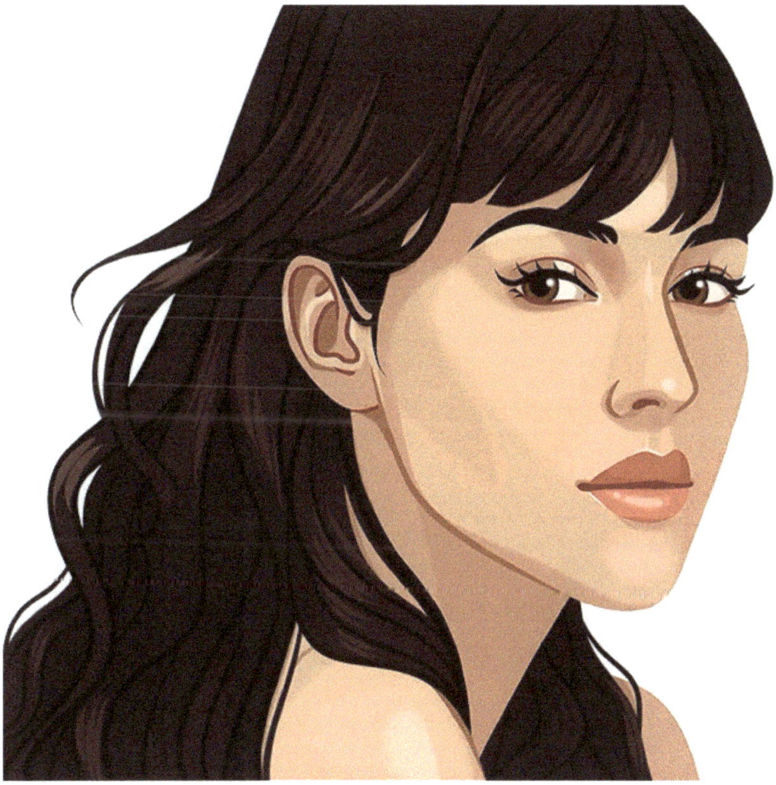

Figure 4.1 Evergreen Monica Bellucci [227,228]. One of the hottest Italian beauties, although she is 54 years old, starts taking a cold shower to the day. Cold shower, the skin maintains the elasticity and argues that tightens. She uses thermal water and revitalizing spray for her face. The actress is totally against all sorts of plastic surgery, but don't forget to constantly clean and moisturize the skin. She says, noting that eating and drinking can be anything, the main thing in small amounts and never blame themselves for the food. She never denied that sport is important for health and toned figure. Drinking plenty of water is another good thing that Bellucci follows as her regular activities (Courtacy: Dribbble).

4.3 INTRODUCTION

Skin aging is a complex biological process influenced by a combination of endogenous or intrinsic and exogenous or extrinsic factors. Because skin health and beauty is considered one of the principal factors representing overall "well-being" and the perception of "health" in humans, several anti-aging strategies have been developed during the last years. In contrast to thin and atrophic, finely wrinkled and dry intrinsically aged skin, premature photoaged skin typically shows a thickened epidermis, mottled discoloration, deep wrinkles, laxity, dullness and roughness. Gradual loss of skin elasticity leads to the phenomenon of sagging. Slowing of the epidermal turnover rate and cell cycle lengthening coincides with a slower wound healing and less effective desquamation in older adults. This fact is important when esthetic procedures are scheduled. On the other side, many of these features are targets to product application or procedures to accelerate the cell cycle, in the belief that a faster turnover rate will yield improvement in skin appearance and will speed wound healing. A marked loss of fibrillin-positive structures as well as a reduced content of collagen type VII (Col-7), may contribute to wrinkles by weakening the bond between dermis and epidermis of extrinsically age skin. Sun-exposed aged skin is characterized by the solar elastosis. The sparse distribution and decrease in collagen content in photoaged skin can be due to increased collagen degradation by various matrix metalloproteinases, serine, and other proteases irrespective of the same collagen production. The overall collagen content per unit area of the skin surface is known to decline approximately 1%/year. Glycosaminoglycans (GAGs) are among the primary dermal skin matrix constituents assisting in binding water. In photo-aged skin, GAGs may be

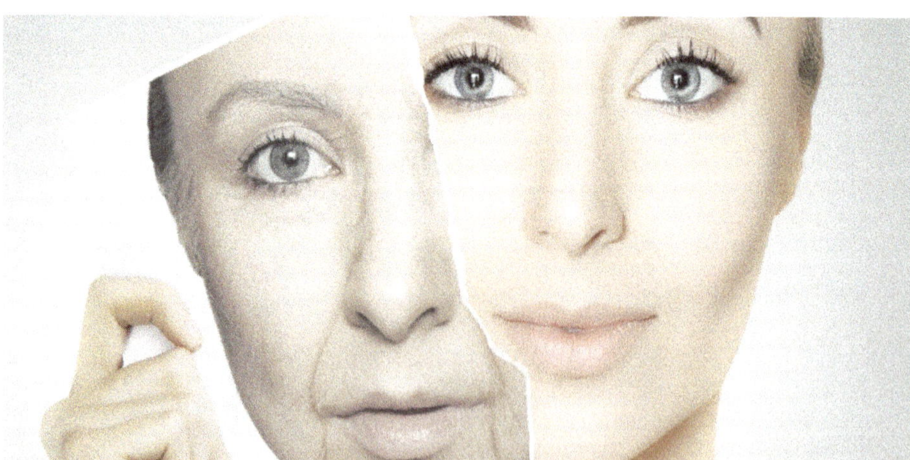

Figure 4.2 Desired effect of anti-aging treatment (Courtacy: peernest.org)

associated with abnormal elastotic material and thus be unable to function effectively. The total hyaluronic acid (HA) level in the dermis of the skin that age intrinsically remains stable; however, epidermal HA diminishes markedly. Decreased estrogen levels may play a role in skin aging in women and compounds stimulating estrogen receptors could potentially counteract some of the visible signs of aging. As people live longer, women spend a larger portion of their lives in a post-menopausal state, with a deficiency of estrogen as compared to their younger selves. Changes in diet and increasing exercise, together with a regimen of antioxidants, nutritional supplements, and growth factors, can alter how the genes express themselves. Both factors can greatly enhance the healing capability of the skin and can improve the results of cosmetic surgeries.

4.4 THE AGING PROCESSES

Aging can be viewed as the accumulation of changes in cells and tissues resulting from a greater disorderliness of regulatory mechanisms that result in reduced robustness of the organism to encountered stress and disease. The notion of greater disorderliness in aging is illustrated by the erosion of the orderly neuroendocrine feedback regulation of the secretion of luteinizing hormone (LH), follicle stimulating hormone (FSH), adrenocorticotropic hormone (ACTH) and growth hormone (GH). These changes are manifested as menopause, andropause, adrenopause, and somatopause. Skin aging is part of the slow decline in appearance and function that appears to be attributed in large part to the drastic decline of hormones in the body after adulthood. At the cellular level, several processes are involved in the physiology of aging and the development of some age-related diseases. The process of apoptosis signifies the process of nontraumatic and noninflammatory cell death. Dysregulation of apoptosis has been implicated in the increased incidence of cutaneous malignancies that are more prevalent in older individuals, such as basal cell carcinoma, squamous cell carcinoma, and malignant melanoma. Cell senescence limits cell divisions in normal somatic cells and may play a central role in age-related diseases. Telomeres are thought to play a role in cellular aging and might contribute to the genetic background of human aging and longevity. It has been speculated that the limited proliferation potential of human cells is a result of the telomere shortening that occurs during DNA synthesis at each cell division. Photoaging may accelerate the shortening of telomeres and push cells into senescence sooner. That could be the reason why various growth factors may affect the speed and quality of wound healing. Biochemical insults also arise within aging cells, in part from the action of reactive oxygen species generated and scavenged incompletely throughout the cell cycle. Aging-associated changes also occur between and among cells via alterations in the intercellular matrix, the intercellular exchange of trophic factors, the release of inflammatory cytokine mediators, and the degree of infiltration by other associated cell types. In addition, the quantity and distribution of various growth factors may affect wound healing. The decline of DNA repair in combination with loss of melanin increases the risk of photo-carcinogenesis and can also cause the decline of enzymatically active melanocytes (10–20% each decade) that contributes to increased sensitivity to UV radiation. However, it is not known why free radical damage does not adversely affect all of the body's cells (e.g., gonadal germ cells) [1].

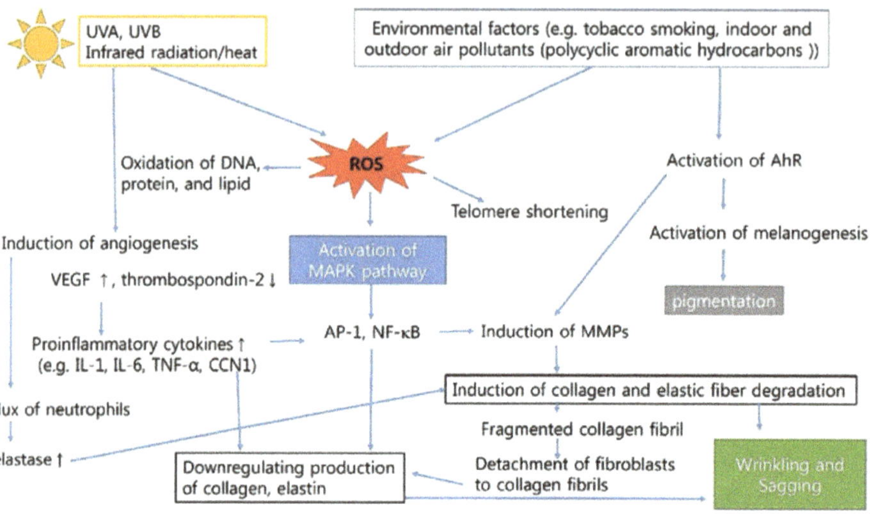

Figure 4.3 Schematic representation of pathogenesis of premature/extrinsic skin aging [226]. ROS: reactive oxygen species, AhR: arylhydrocarbon receptor, NF-kB: nuclear factor kappa-B, IL-1: interleukin-1, TNF-α: tumor necrosis factor, CCN1: cysteine-rich protein 61, MAPK: mitogen-activated protein kinase, AP-1: activator protein 1, and MMPs: matrix metalloproteinases.

4.5 FACTORS INVOLVED IN SKIN AGING

Skin aging is a complex biological process influenced by a combination of endogenous or intrinsic (genetics, cellular metabolism, hormone and metabolic processes) and exogenous or extrinsic (chronic light exposure, pollution, ionizing radiation, chemicals, toxins) factors. These factors lead together to cumulative structural and physiological alterations and progressive changes in each skin layer as well as changes in skin appearance, especially, on the sun-exposed skin areas [2]. Facial skin wrinkles can be considered as a marker for intrinsic aging (**See wrinkle classification in Exhibit 1**). The major perceived risk factors are unhealthy eating habits, stress, less exercise, dehydration, diseased state and sleeping habits. Although the main factor responsible for extrinsic aging is UVR [3]. Beyond sun damage factors such as smoking and atmospheric pollution have also been studied and considered in extrinsic aging. Studies have shown a clear correlation between these factors and the appearance of melanosis and wrinkles. Both of these factors contribute to aging through a common mechanism called oxidative stress and harms cellular processes, such as DNA replication. In addition to the UV region of solar radiation that contributes to cellular injury, visible radiation has an oxidative effect similar to that of infrared radiation via heat generation. The effects of comorbidities, such as metabolic illnesses common in the elderly, nutritional deficiencies, and the use of drugs such as corticosteroids, and even cancer treatments, should be assessed by dermatologists attending to skin conditions associated with aging [4]. Good skin condition can be maintained to some extent by changes in modifiable lifestyle factors such as smoking and sunscreen use [5]. Human skin cells respond to instructions from highly specialized proteins or hormones referred to as growth factors. The growth differentiation factor GDF11, a TGF-β family member, has been associated with the maintenance of youth phenotypes in different human tissues and organs, and in the skin has been related to an inhibition of the inflammatory response. The production of elastin and collagen dermal connective fibers slows, and, with age, the regenerative rates of GAGs become delayed [6.7].

Exhibit 1. Pierard Classification of Wrinkles [26]

- Atrophic wrinkles develop in exposed and non-exposed skin, disappear with skin traction, change in orientation with body posture, and are due to atrophy of the extracellular matrix.
- Elastotic wrinkles develop in sun exposed skin, exhibit solar elastosis, become progressively permanent, and do not disappear with perpendicular traction.
- Expressional wrinkles due to subdermal muscle contraction, become permanent with repeated wrinkling.
- Gravitational wrinkles due to skin sagging in response to gravitational forces and inelasticity.

4.5.1 PHOTODAMAGE

Chronic repetitive exposure of human skin to solar UV rays causes marked morphological, histological, biochemical, and biophysical changes that are described as photoaging. the clinical signs of photoaging are fine and coarse wrinkles, actinic keratoses, solar elastosis, yellowing, pigmentation disorders and premalignant lesions, skin atrophy, senile purpura, freckles, solar comedones, telangiectasia, laxity, roughness, and extreme dryness [8]. UV damage can also cause significant changes in some of the mechanical properties of the stratum corneum, reducing its cell cohesion and mechanical integrity; the UV radiation also affects the molecular structure of cell proteins and lipids [4].

According to Leccia et.al, 2019, at the cellular level DNA damage is the main event following UV exposure. The kind of lesions produced depends on the wavelength and the energy profile of the radiation, with different photoproducts being formed as a result. Although endogenous DNA repair mechanisms are somewhat effective in repairing DNA, some DNA damage persists and can accumulate with chronic exposure [9]. Through ROS formation, UVB induces activator protein-1 (AP-1) overexpression along with the upregulation of collagen-degrading enzymes like matrix metalloproteinases (MMPs) **(Figure 4)**. Overall, UVB stimulates collagen degradation and inhibits procollagen biosynthesis resulting in loss of collagen content and wrinkle formation, thus inducing skin photoaging, as reported by Karapetsas et.al, 2019 [10]. Sun damage also creates a state of chronic inflammation, with the release of proteolytic enzymes by the inflammatory system, disrupting the dermal matrix [8]. UV protection strategies, such as sunscreen use, are important in limiting further DNA damage [9]. Exposure to UV radiation is the primary factor of extrinsic skin aging; it accounts for about 80% of facial aging [11].

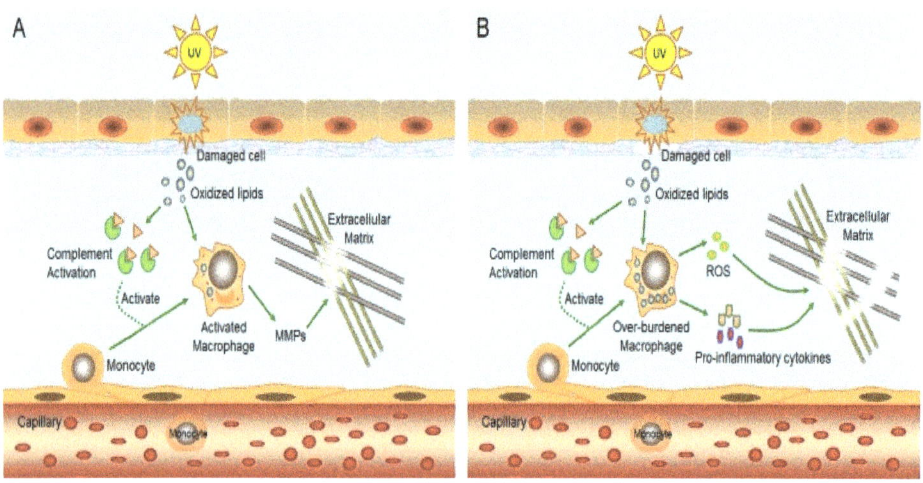

Figure 4.4 A model proposed to explain the mechanism of inflammaging in skin [11]. (A) UV radiation induces oxidative stress in epidermal cells, resulting in damaged cells with oxidized lipids. Oxidation-specific epitopes on damaged cells and oxidized lipids activate complement systems and cause inflammation, leading to infiltration and activation of macrophages. Activated macrophages release MMPs to degrade extracellular matrix. (B) Repeated UV radiation over-activates the complement system, causing damage to the dermis–epidermis junction, on which they deposit, and macrophages are overburdened with oxidized lipids. Overburdened macrophages release proinflammatory cytokines and ROS, the former of which cause chronic inflammation and long-term damage to the dermis, while the latter triggers the oxidative stress-induced damages to the dermal extracellular matrix.

Exhibit 2. Comparison of Intrinsic Aging and Photoaging [8], [91]		
Feature	**Intrinsic aging**	**Photoaging**
Clinical appearance	Fine wrinkles, some deepening of skin surface markings, some loss of elasticity, redundant skin; Skin is smooth, unblemished, but shows saggy appearance	Nodular, leathery surface sallow complexion, yellowish mottled pigmentation, coarse wrinkles, severe loss of elasticity, reddened appearance with initially light wrinkles, which later deepen, thus showing loss of collagen fibers
Epidermis	Thin and viable; Thinner than normal with lower cell growth, minor abnormalities in keratinocyte regularity; Normal stratum corneum There is loss of rete pegs here as well	Marked acanthosis, cellular atypia; Thick skin, with acanthosis followed by atrophy of the cells; High basal keratinocyte irregularity; Stratum corneum appears compact; There is loss of rete pegs here as well
Elastic tissue	Increased, but almost normal	Tremendous increase, degenerates into amorphous mass
Reticular dermis	Thinner, fibroblasts decreased, inactive mast cells decreased, no inflammation; Elastin fibers appear irregular in their arrangement, whereas collagen fibers begin to lower in number and thickness	Thickened, elastosis, fibroblasts increased, hyperactive mast cells; Excessive production of elastin fibers in an improper orientation, collagen fibres appear to thicken and then wear out soon; Appearance of grenzzone
Collagen	Bundles thick, disoriented	Marked decrease of bundles and fibers
Glycosaminoglycans	Slightly decreased	Markedly increased
Papillary dermis	No grenz zone	Solar elastosis with grenz zone,
Microvasculature	Moderate loss	Great loss, abnormal and telangiectatic

Effects of UVR on the Dermal white adipose tissue (dWAT) in vitro: UVR can significantly modulate sWAT metabolism. This effect is observable not only in chronically sun-damaged human skin, but even after a single UV exposure of a non-damaged skin. Free fatty acid and triglyceride content in sWAT of sun-exposed skin (forearm) is significantly lower than in the buttocks (sun-protected area) of the same subjects. At the same time, young subjects did not demonstrate such differences, which points to the UV-induced effect and not just to the regional variations in fat metabolism. Additionally, both chronic and single UVR exposure significantly reduces master adipogenic factors such as peroxisome proliferator-activated receptor γ (PPARγ); this reduction was rapid and remained stable for at least 72 h after acute UVR exposure.According to this point of view, dWAT content correlates with a much more pronounced extrinsic aging process in the dorsal hand comparing to the palm area. Chronological skin aging demonstrates similar but not as pronounced differences in aging processes in palmar and dorsal regions of the hand. This can be an indication that UVR accelerates the processes of skin aging, whereas their basic components are determined by some other factors, one of which could be the local dWAT content. This can make skin aging not only body area dependent, but also spatially heterogeneous in the same body area, since dWAT can have a spatially heterogeneous structure [78].

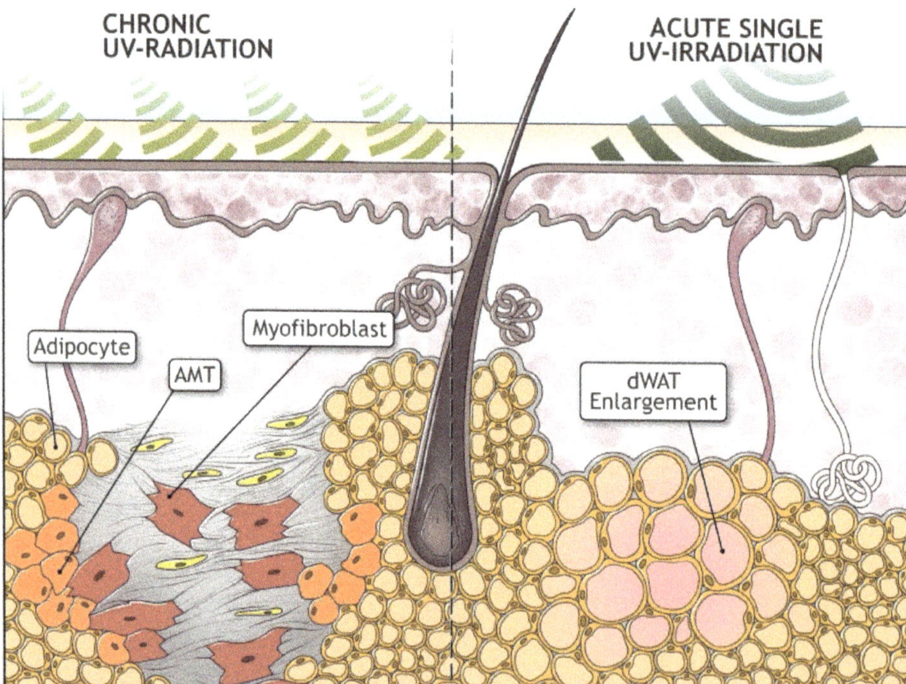

Figure 4.5 Possible role of adipocyte-myofibroblast transition in extrinsic aging [78]. Absorption of UV radiation in the skin causes acute enlargement of the dWAT layer. However, upon chronic overexposure to UV radiation, it causes the depletion of dWAT and a concurrent development of cutaneous fibrosis, presumably through adipocyte-myofibroblast transition (AMT). Replacement of dWAT volume with fibrosis leads to production of mechanically heterogeneous skin structures and to the loss of the effective skin volume (Courtacy: aging-us.com).

4.5.2 ENVIRONMENTAL FACTORS BEYOND UV RADIATION

Infrared radiation and heat: Visible light (400–740 nm) and IR radiation have long been considered to minimally impact the skin, apart from the heat sensation provided by IR radiation [12]. IR radiation accounts for approximately 40% of the solar radiation energy reaching the earth's surface, subsequently generating heat and increased skin temperature. IR thermogenic radiation can reach the dermis (65%) and hypodermis (10%), and its capacity to induce metalloproteinase expression in the dermis is well known along with its oxidative role. In human skin, IR radiation and heat can lead to macrophage recruitment like UVR. Heat can induce various cytokines in human skin and was found to increase tropoelastin mRNA and protein expression in the epidermis and in the dermis. Both IR and heat-induced acute stress increase in the number of mast cells and expression of tryptase. Chronic IR and heat exposure each induce cutaneous angiogenesis and inflammatory cellular infiltration, disrupts the dermal extracellular matrix by inducing matrix metalloproteinases, and alters dermal structural proteins, thereby adding to premature skin aging [4], [13]. Erythema ab igne, a cutaneous rash characterized by a reticulated pattern of erythema and hyperpigmentation, is caused by repeated exposure of direct heat or infrared radiation to a person's skin, often from occupational exposures or use of heating pads [14].

Pollution: The damaging effects of skin exposure to pollutants may result in skin disorders and pathologies, including xerotic skin, sensitive skin, premature skin aging and accelerated aging symptoms, such as wrinkle formation, abnormal pigmentation and skin dryness. Pollutants may also be involved in acne, eczema, skin rashes and skin cancers. Prolonged and repetitive daily exposure to high levels of pollutants impairs the skin's natural defense capacity to some extent. Moreover, some pollutants (e.g., ozone) can induce damage via signal transduction mechanism even when there is no percutaneous penetration to deeper skin layers [230]. There is solid evidence that skin pathologies such as premature aging, atopic dermatitis (AD), and psoriasis are associated with pollutant exposure; all of these skin conditions are also associated with an altered redox status. Some of the most noxious pollutants that humans are exposed to include ozone (O3), particulate matter and cigarette smoke. Pecorelli et.al, 2019 reported that increased levels of 4-hydroxy-2-nonenal (HNE) in the skin, in response to pollutants, likely accelerates skin aging and exacerbates existing skin inflammatory conditions [15]. When ozone exposure precedes UV exposure, there is an enhancement of UV-induced depletion of protective vitamin E from the skin's stratum corneum [16]. Even in indoor conditions, particulate matter (PM2.5) exposure levels were positively associated with skin aging manifestation. Particles can serve as carriers for organic chemicals and metals that are capable of localizing in mitochondria and generating ROS directly in mitochondria leading to collagen degradation in human skin [17]. In line with this, cosmetic anti-pollution products containing anti-oxidants, but also aryl hydrocarbon receptor (AHR) antagonists are effective in reducing or preventing an increase in skin pigmentation [18].

4.5.3 LIFESTYLE-RELATED FACTORS

Smoking: It is now well established that smoking has an aggravating effect on skin aging. Even external exposure to cigarette smoke (secondhand cigarette smoke) prematurely ages the skin [4]. Particularly owing to nicotine, smoking negatively affects the dermal microvasculature and hinders the healing process. It also has a toxic effect on keratinocytes and fibroblasts by increasing the expression of metalloproteins and tropoelastin. Furthermore, smoking increases the expression of small proteoglycans and reduces the synthesis of procollagen. The clinical manifestations of these phenomena are pale and wrinkled skin; DNA mutations also result from oxidative effects or direct toxic damage [8]. Smoking provokes elastosis, telangiectasia, skin roughness, and premature wrinkles on facial skin due to the vascular constriction of nicotine. A clear dose-response relationship has been observed between smoking and wrinkling [4]. Park et.al, 2018 reported that cigarette smoke induces both ROS production (oxidative stress) and autophagy [19]. It has been observed that the skin of smoking addicts at the age of 40 years resembles skin of non-smoking 70-year-old adults. Skin damage due to tobacco smoke is irreversible, where further damage can be avoided by stopping smoking [20]. Wang et.al, 2018 reported that application of tobacco extracts to skin and oral fibroblasts in vitro triggered several hallmarks of senescence including premature cell cycle arrest, oxidative DNA damage, secretion of inflammatory cytokines and MMPs, and downregulation of cell junction proteins E-cadherin and Zonula occludens-1 (ZO-1, tight junction protein) [21].

Sleep: Restricted sleep affects facial appearance negatively and decreases others' willingness to socialize with the sleep-restricted person [22]. An estimated 50–70 million American adults suffer from one or more sleep disorders [23]. Sleep is important for the growth and renewal of multiple physiological systems. Oyetakin-White et.al, 2015 reported that good sleepers had significantly lower intrinsic skin ageing scores (by SCINEXA^{TM}). Sleep deprivation is associated with increased signs of intrinsic skin aging (fine lines, uneven pigmentation, reduced elasticity), with much slower recovery rates after skin barrier disruption and lower satisfaction with appearance [24,25]. The sleep deprived individuals were noted to have hanging eyelids, swollen eyes, darker circles and more droopy corners of the mouth [23]. Wrinkles occur where fault lines develop in aging skin. Those fault lines may be due to skin distortion resulting from facial expression or may be due to skin distortion from mechanical compression during sleep. Expression wrinkles and sleep wrinkles differ in etiology, location, and anatomical pattern. Compression, shear, and stress forces act on the face in lateral or prone sleep positions (**Figure 4.6**) [26].

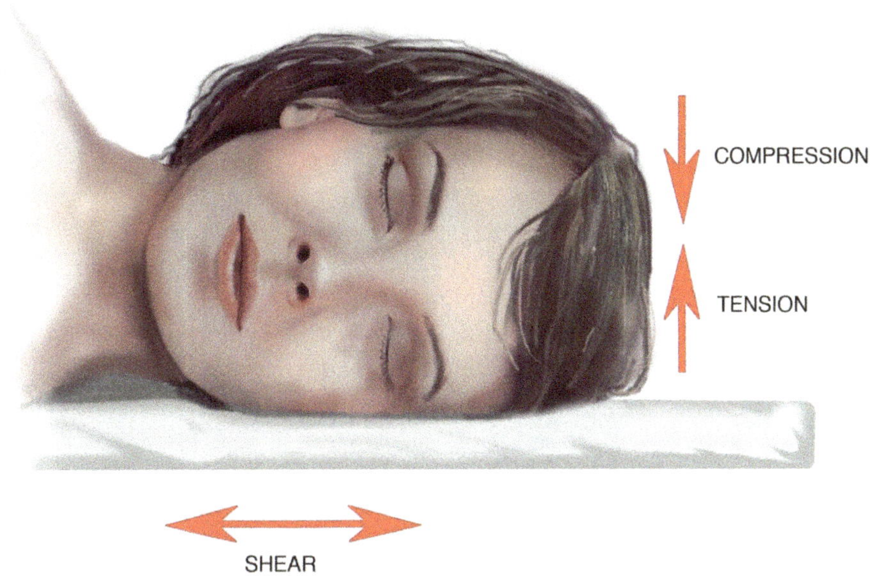

Figure 4.6 External forces (including compression, tension, and shear) act on facial tissue in lateral or prone sleep positions [26]. During side or stomach sleeping, facial tissue is subject to shear, compression, and tensile mechanical forces. The skin is stretched and pulled in all directions with changes in sleep position. These forces become significant when we consider the amount of time spent in sleep and sleep position (Courtacy: Reddit).

Diet and Nutrition: Rhytides, sagging of skin, and loss of elasticity are all related to changes in the collagen and elastic fibers of the skin, which are themselves impacted by diet. Ingestion of sugar, in particular, can accelerate these signs of aging, as it promotes cross-linking of collagen fibers. This process is accelerated by hyperglycemia. Research indicates that once established, the body is unable to repair these cross-links. With the accumulation of advanced glycation end products (AGEs), structural changes in the skin can occur, resulting in increased stiffness and reduced elasticity. Cooking processes that lead to higher levels of AGEs include grilling, frying, and roasting. Herbs and spices, such as oregano, cinnamon, cloves, ginger, and garlic, as well as substances found naturally in certain fruits and vegetables, such as lipoic acid inhibit the production of AGEs [27]. Frequently researched antioxidants such as carotenoids, tocophenols and flavonoids, as well as vitamins (A, C, D and E), essential omega-3-fatty acids, some proteins and *lactobacilli* have been referred as agents capable of promoting skin health and beauty [28]. The WHO and Food and Agriculture of the UN reports recommend adults to consume at least five servings of fruits and vegetables per day excluding starchy vegetables [29]. National Health and Nutrition Examination Surveys (NHANES) 2007-2010 indicate that among US population 75% consumed less fruit and 87% consumed fewer vegetables than recommended

[30]. The accumulation of glycoxidation products such as carboxymethyl lysine (CML) and pentosidine in cutaneous collagen promotes skin aging. Bragazzi et.al, 2019 reported that chronic caloric restriction decreased the glycation rate of skin proteins, resulting in the reduction of age-related accumulation of these metabolites in cutaneous collagen [31]. Mekić et.al, 2019 reported that better adherence to the Dutch Healthy Diet Index (DHDI) was significantly associated with less wrinkles among women but not in men. In women, a red meat and snack-dominant PCA pattern was associated with more facial wrinkles, whereas a fruit-dominant principal component analysis (PCA) pattern was associated with fewer wrinkles [32]. Higher intakes of vitamin C and linoleic acid and lower intakes of fats and carbohydrates are associated with better skin-aging appearance [33].

Inappropriate/Harsh soaps: Dry skin often occurs in the elderly and tends to worsen in association with hot baths and the use of standard alkaline bar soaps [4]. Skin dryness, scaling and roughness-lipid solvents such as acetone, alcohols and even nonionic surfactants can cause dryness of the skin [34]. Each cleansing agent, even normal tap water, influences the skin surface. The increase of the skin pH irritates the physiological protective 'acid mantle', changes the composition of the cutaneous bacterial flora and the activity of enzymes in the upper epidermis, which have an acid pH optimum. The dissolution of fat from the skin surface may influence the hydration status leading to a dry and squamous skin [35]. Accordingly, to lower the skin damage, cleansings with neutral pH and pH close to 5.5 are recommended [36].

4.5.4 SYSTEMIC MORBIDITIES

From a biochemical standpoint, chronological aging induces increased markers of oxidation, glycoxidation, lipoxidation, and glycation in skin collagen. In particular, skin collagen's cross-linking lysine residues undergo significant oxidative changes with age. Lysine oxidase, a copper-dependent enzyme, converts lysine to allysine at all ages. Recently it has been shown that allysine is further oxidized to a stable end product, 2-aminoadipic acid. This oxidative change results in significant accumulation of 2-aminoadipic acid in the collagen of aged skin; increased oxidative end product is also seen in diabetes, renal failure, and sepsis. Obesity and overweight are risk factors for various disorders, including diabetes [38].

Diabetes mellitus (DM): Yoon et.al, 2002 reported that elasticity of facial skin was decreased in patients with diabetes. Decrease of the fine flakes of the diabetes patients reflect that irritation and xerotic changes are aggravated in skins of diabetic patients [44]. DM is among the most common aging-related comorbidities, and the generation of advanced glycation end products is intimately related to dermal damage since it changes the properties of collagen types I and IV. Clinically, reductions in flexibility and rigidity and an increase in susceptibility to mechanical stimulation are observed [4]. 30-70% of patients with DM, both type 1 and type 2, will present with a cutaneous complication of DM at some point during their lifetime. The prevalence of ichthyosiform changes of the shins ("fish scale" skin) in those with type 1 diabetes has been reported to be between 25-50%. Xerosis is one of the most common skin presentations (abnormally dry skin) in patients with diabetes and has been reported to be present in as many as 40% of patients with diabetes [37]. Uruska et.al, 2019 reported a two-way relationship between insulin resistance and AGE accumulation in the skin in people with Type 1 diabetes [39] which is related with increased stiffness and reduced elasticity. Moreover, not only collagen, but also elastin, is affected by AGEs, resulting in a reduction of skin elasticity. Pageon et.al., 2014 reported that the imbalance between synthesis and degradation that results from glycation, may contribute to skin aging [40]. Noordam et.al, 2013 reported higher glucose levels are associated with a higher perceived age among non-diabetic subjects also. Several studies have shown that culturing human fibroblasts under hyperglycemic conditions results in both an increased amount of ROS at a cellular level as well as an increased induction of premature cellular senescence which in turn may cause premature skin aging and a higher perceived age (**Figure 4.7**) [41-43].

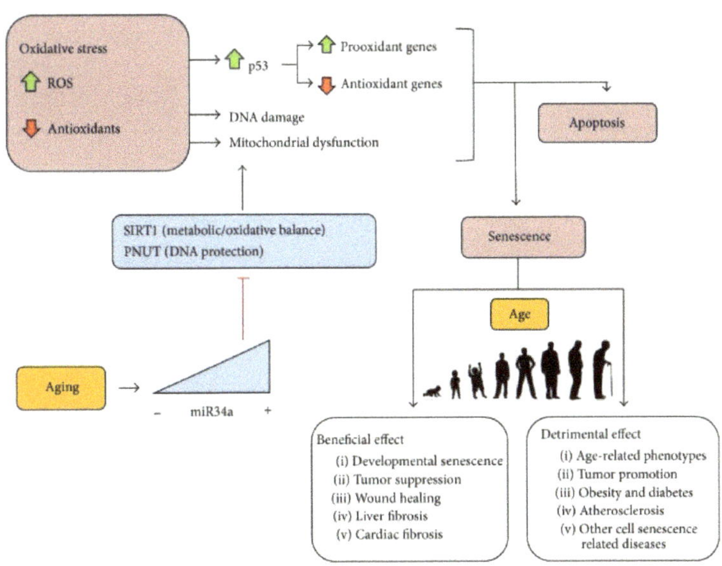

Figure 4.7 ROS-mediated senescence [42]. Besides causing DNA damage and mitochondria dysfunction, OS activates p53 that, in turn, induces prooxidant genes and imbalances antioxidant genes induction. The set of alterations caused by ROS lead to induction of cell senescence, which, in turn, can develop both positive and negative effects; miR34a expression increases with aging in many tissues downregulating SIRT1 protein activity (a longevity promoting factor) and PNUT protein (a DNA protecting factor which prevents telomere attrition and is involved in tissues repairs).

Obesity: A hyperglycemic state is common in obesity and is associated with peripheral resistance to insulin and a higher risk of glycation [45]. Also, Sami et.al, 2015 reported that skin of the patients with massive weight loss is weak due to lower density and thickness of collagen fibers and damage to its elastic fibers. It usually occurs because of damage of collagen and elastin, which allows for no skin retraction after weight loss [46]. Striae distensae (striae or stretch marks) is a common dermatosis in patients with obesity, representing linear atrophic plaques which are created due to tension and skin stretching from expanding fat deposits. Due to excessive sweating and increased friction between skin surfaces, a number of skin infections are more frequent in obesity including oppositional intertrigo (inflammation-rash in body folds), candidiasis, candida folliculitis, folliculitis and less often cellulitis, erysipelas or fasciitis [47]. Ibuki et.al, 2017 reported that obese-diabetes patients have decreased stratum corneum hydration, increased transepidermal water loss, higher skin advanced glycation end-products and decreased dermal collagen fiber density compared with normal-weight subjects. These results indicate that the ordinary age-related physiological skin changes seen in the elderly can also occur in obese-diabetes patients aged in their 40s [48].

Menopause: The effects of estrogen deficiency on the skin are an important endogenous cause of aging skin in women. Estrogen's key role in maintaining the skin's structural and functional integrity is well established with evidence that shows that estrogens are essential for skin hydration, sebum production, improved barrier function of the stratum corneum, and increased collagen and elastin content [49]. Following menopause many women detect a swift commencement of skin aging; skin becomes thinner with decreased collagen content, decreased elasticity, increased wrinkling and increased dryness [50]. Reduced estrogen levels during menopause affect skin components with estrogen receptors, particularly in epidermal cells and sebaceous glands. By contrast, androgenic hormone levels do not decline significantly during this period [4]. Accordingly, dermal cellular metabolism is influenced by the hypoestrogenoemic state of menopause leading to changes in the collagen content, alterations in the concentration of glycoaminoglycans and most importantly the water content. Consequently, changes in these basic components leads to an alteration in function compatible with skin aging. Changes in the skin collagen leads to diminished elasticity and skin strength. Collagen content may be measured by various methods such as direct skin biopsy, skin blister assessment for collagen markers and skin thickness measurement. All these variables indicate a reduction in collagen content following menopause. This may be reversed with the administration of estrogen given both topically and systemically. A reduction in hydrophilic glycoaminglycans leads to a direct reduction in water content, which influences the skin turgor [51]. A study of elderly males and females has confirmed that the administration of topical estrogen increases keratinocyte proliferation and epidermal thickness after only two weeks. In the estrogen deficient women skin thickness is reduced by 1.13% and collagen content by 2% per postmenopausal year. Type I and III skin collagen is thought to decrease by as much as 30% in the first five years after menopause. This decrease in skin thickness and collagen content in elderly females correlates with the period of estrogen deficiency rather than chronological age [50]. The highest loss (of up to 30%) is observed in the first 5 years, followed by a 1%–2% loss of collagen annually [171].

Acne scarring: Skin with acne scarring has reduced elasticity due to scar fibrosis and shows a worsened appearance of furrows and wrinkles. Atrophic facial acne scarring is a widely prevalent condition that can have a negative impact on a patient's quality of life. The appearance of these scars is often worsened by the normal effects of aging. Facial aging often exacerbates the effects of acne scarring. Inflammation associated with moderate to severe acne can result in dermal collagen and fat loss, leading to atrophic scarring. Both acne scarring and the normal aging process can result in the loss of dermal collagen and facial lipoatrophy, such that patients already suffering from the negative impact of facial acne scarring may find the appearance of these scars worsening over time as they approach their 40s and 50s [52].

Emotional stress and depression: Evidence suggests that chronic psychological stress stimulates the autonomic nervous system, renin-angiotensin system, and the hypothalamic-pituitary-adrenal axis when the body attempts to resolve perceived threats to homeostasis. Prolonged activation of these pathways can result in chronic immune dysfunction, increased production of ROS, and DNA damage, which are known to contribute to the again of skin and other tissues [53]. Maarouf et.al, 2019 reported similar observation of aberrant barrier dysfunction, characterized by decreased epidermal lipid and structural protein production, decreased stratum corneum hydration and increased transepidermal water loss [54]. Liu et.al, 2018 reported that early life adversity is associated with both persistent disruptions in the hypothalamic-pituitary-adrenal (HPA) axis and psychiatric symptoms. Glucocorticoid receptors (GRs), which are encoded by the NR3C1 gene, bind to cortisol and other glucocorticoids to create a negative feedback loop within the HPA axis to regulate the body's neuroendocrine response to stress. Excess methylation of a promoter sequence within NR3C1 that attenuates GR expression, however, has been associated with both early life adversity and psychopathology. As critical regulators within the HPA axis, GRs and their epigenetic regulation may mediate the link between early life adversity and the onset of psychopathology [55].

4.5.5 HORMONE AND METABOLIC PROCESSES

All endocrine glands are affected by the global aging process. A few direct consequences interfere with skin aging. They are mostly related to the declined activity of the pituitary gland, adrenal glands, ovaries, and testes [56]. The most important endocrine compound produced by the skin is vitamin D, which is a regulator of the calcium metabolism and exhibits other systemic effects as well. Vitamin D3 and its analogues regulates several physiological processes in the skin-like proliferation, differentiation, and apoptosis of keratinocytes and maintenance of normal skin barriers and immune system [57]. Extension of health-span in experimental animals and analysis of survival curves suggest that in the absence of Growth hormone (GH), aging is slowed down or delayed. The peripheral effects of GH are mainly exerted by insulin-like growth factor (IGF), produced by the liver upon GH stimulation. The circulating IGF-1 is bioavailable and functionally active depending upon its binding with the IGF-binding proteins (IGF-BPs) [58]. Eto et.al, 2018 reported severe GH deficiency results in early aging, such as wrinkling and dryness of skin [59]. Hypopituitary adults are usually described as having dry and thin skin, an increase in skin thickness was demonstrated after GH treatment in normal elderly males selected based on low IGF-I levels [60]. The progressive decline in dehydroepi-androsterone (DHEA) serum concentration with age, and conversely its supplementation has not demonstrated prominent effects on the skin except on sebum production [56]. DHEA is the major steroid produced by the adrenal zona reticularis and, in contrast to cortisol and aldosterone, its secretion declines with ageing [61]. DHEA and its sulfate (DHEA-S) are the most abundant steroids in humans whose low levels are related to aging, greater incidence of various cancers, immune dysfunction, atherosclerosis, and osteoporosis [62]. Calvo et.al, 2008 strongly suggested the possibility that DHEA could exert an anti-aging effect in the skin through stimulation of collagen biosynthesis, improved structural organization of the dermis while modulating keratinocyte metabolism [63]. Estrogen, alone or together with progesterone, prevents or reverses skin atrophy, dryness, and wrinkles associated with chronological aging or photoaging. Estrogen and progesterone stimulate proliferation of keratinocytes while estrogen suppresses apoptosis and thus prevents epidermal atrophy. Estrogen also enhances collagen synthesis, and estrogen and progesterone suppress collagenolysis by reducing MMP activity in fibroblasts, thereby maintaining skin thickness. Estrogen maintains skin moisture by increasing hyaluronic acid levels in the dermis; progesterone increases sebum excretion [64]. Several reports suggest positive correlations between the levels of circulating estrogens and: (1) perceived age, (2) attractiveness, (3) enhanced skin health, and (4) facial coloration in women [65]. Topical corticosteroids have been shown to reduce cutaneous CD44 expression, correlated with skin atrophy if there's a CD44 deficiency. Corticosteroids can also induce dermatoporotic changes through modulating gene expression of collagen I, collagen III, collagen IV, and matrix metalloproteinases (MMPs) [66]. The corticosteroid-induced atrophy can be one of the most severe forms of skin aging corresponding to dermatoporosis.

Exhibit 3. Neuroendocrine Receptors Active in the Skin [56]
• Adrenergic receptors • Androgen and estrogen receptors • Calcitonin gene-related peptide receptor • Cholinergic receptors • Corticotropin-releasing hormone and urocortin receptors • Glucocorticoid and mineralocorticoid receptors • Glutamate receptors • Growth hormone receptor • Histamine receptors • Melanocortin receptors • Miscellaneous neuropeptide receptors • Miscellaneous receptors • Neurokinin receptors • Neutrophin receptors • Opioid receptors • Parathormone and PTH-related protein receptors • PRL and LH-CG receptors • Serotonin receptors • Thyroid hormone receptors • Vasoactive intestinal peptide receptor • 21. Vitamin D receptor

* CGRP-R, calcitonin gene-related peptide receptor; CRH-R, corticotropin-releasing hormone and urocortin receptors; GH-R, growth hormone receptor; MC-R, melanocortin receptors; NK R, neurokinin receptors; NT-R, neutrophin receptors; PTH, parathormone; PTHrP, PTH-related protein receptors; LH/CG-R, PRL and LH-CG receptors; VIP-R, vasoactive intestinal peptide receptor; VDR, vitamin D receptor.

Exhibit 4. Hormones and Neurotransmitters Produced by the Skin [56]
• Hypothalamic and pituitary hormones • Neuropeptides and neurotrophins • Neurotransmitters/neurohormones • Other steroid hormones • Parathormone-related protein • Sex steroid hormones • Thyroid hormones

4.5.6 OTHER INTRINSIC ISSUES OF AGING

Anatomical Skin Sites: Large variations in some skin properties (hydration, transepidermal water loss, epidermal lipids, sebum secretion, and mechanical properties) have been observed with respect to the studied body site. There are also large differences in skin thickness in the function of the body site, ranging from very thin on the eyelids to more than 5 mm on the sole of the feet. A regional variation is observed when considering the quantity and composition of lipids in the stratum corneum. Because of thickness and sebum secretion, the viscoelastic properties of the skin is very different at the forehead, nose, and cheeks compared with the forearm [8]. Human skin retains water mostly through the outermost stratum corneum layer. Loss of hydration in aged skin, due to a decline in function of the stratum corneum, results in a sagging and wrinkling appearance [77].

Ethnicity: Campiche et.al, 2019 reported that Africans from the African continent show delayed signs of aging compared to Caucasians [67]. Facial wrinkles and acne lines appear later in African Americans than in Caucasians and may not appear until late in the fifth or sixth decade. White women self-reported more signs of moderate and severe facial aging than Asian and Hispanic women beginning in the fourth decade. When comparing the severity of facial features against photo-numeric rating scales, the mean severity of crow's feet lines was most severe in Fitzpatrick skin type I and least severe in Fitzpatrick skin types IV and V [68]. Asians are a population with various skin phototypes, ranging from type III to IV Fitzpatrick's classification in Chinese and Japanese to type IV and V in Indian and Pakistani people. Chan et.al, 2019 reported that Asian skin tends to present post-inflammatory hyperpigmentation, melasma, lentigines and freckles, nevus of Ota, and Hori nevus. The main skin diseases reported in Asians are acne, atopic dermatitis, and viral infections. Wrinkles and skin thickness, early signs of aging in Caucasians, are less evident in Asian skin. However, pigmentary changes occur earlier [69]. Asian and black skin has thicker and more compact dermis than white skin, with the thickness being proportional to the degree of pigmentation. This likely contributes to the lower incidence of facial rhytides in Asians and blacks [70]. Signs of facial aging in individuals with skin of color tend to be most pronounced in the periorbital and midface region with less prominent features of skin aging in the upper third of the face and a decreased tendency toward perioral rhytides and radial lip lines [71]. Darker skin types are better protected regarding sun exposure due to the higher melanin content in their skin. In fair-skinned persons, the skin appears severely atrophic with multiple teleangiectasis and a variety of premalignant lesions such as actinic keratosis, whereas in dark-skinned persons deep furrows and severe solar elastosis occur [72].

Gender: Sugawara et.al, 2019 reported cauliflower-shaped sebaceous glands in males while young females had somewhat more cylindrical and smaller sebaceous glands than the young males [73]. There are significant morphological differences according to sex: total skin thickness is greater for men on most skin sites [56]. Also, increased sebum and decreased skin elasticity were mostly correlated with facial pore development in male [74]. Rahrovan et.al, 2018 reported SC rehydration capacity in sun-exposed aged female subjects was significantly lower than that of age-matched male subjects. The skin parameters of hydration, transepidermal water loss, sebum, microcirculation, pigmentation, and thickness are generally higher in men but skin pH is higher in women [75]. Trojahn et.al, 2015 reported that changes in skin elasticity, wrinkling, sagging, and yellowness seem to be caused by additional extrinsic ageing in women. Intrinsic ageing has a very strong influence on facial skin characteristics in Caucasian women in general [76].

4.6 SKIN AGING PREVENTION AND THERAPY

Anti-aging in dermatology primarily focuses on the prevention of skin aging with UV protection (clothing and sunscreens), free radical scavengers (synthetic or botanic), and cell-protecting agents such as vitamin B3. For the correction of signs of early skin aging, retinoic acid derivatives in dermatological prescriptions are the best studied substances. Topical hormonal prescriptions are also an option if UV damage has not been the leading culprit for aging. Chemical peeling leads to a marked increase in collagen formation, the deeper the better. Ingredients in cream preparations can reduce superficial skin folds (polyphenols, amino acid peptides). Modulators of regular pigmentation are important for anti-aging preparations [79]. There are no proven effective topical antiaging ingredients/or treatment that completely eliminates the symptoms of skin photoaging, but there are products and treatments that can visibly reduce or slow down these symptoms. it is more correct to consider reduction of the appearance of aged skin. Many cosmetic products claim to reduce the clinical signs of photoaged skin; however, there are very few scientific, randomized, double-blind, placebo-controlled, clinical studies to support these claims. Generally speaking, the quality control testing on ingredients and safety testing are of good quality, and the used ingredients are mostly safe. However, these ingredients may not be as efficient as claimed, and the concentrations used in these formulations will not necessarily correspond to an "effective" concentration. This can be the case with many plant extracts with antioxidant properties [8]. Indeed, product testing may also be warranted by the companies to document claimed efficacy and to support marketing. Finally, many antiaging claims are based on in vivo testing on cells or simple skin models but not in vivo on a sufficient number of human subjects.

Exhibit 5. Skin antiaging approaches [2]	
Cosmetological care	Daily skin care, Correct sun protection, Aesthetic non-invasive procedures, Chemical peelings, visible light devices, intense pulsed light (IPL), ablative and non-ablative laser photo–rejuvenation, radiofrequency (RF)
Topical medical agents or topical agents	Antioxidants, Cell regulators
Invasive procedures	Injectable skin bio-stimulation and rejuvenation, prevention of dynamic wrinkles, correction of static, anatomical wrinkles, restoration (redistribution) of fat and volume loss, skin augmentation and contouring, restoration (redistribution) of fat and volume loss, skin augmentation and contouring
Systemic agents	Hormone replacement therapy (HRT)
Avoiding of exogenous factors of aging, correction of life style and habits	Smoking, Pollution, Solar UV irradiation. Stress, Nutrition, diet restriction and alimentary supplementation, Physical activity, Control of general health
Preventive medicine	

4.6.1 COSMETOLOGICAL CARE

A. Daily skin care

Healthy and functioning skin barrier is an important protector against dehydration, penetration of various microorganisms, allergens, irritants, reactive oxygen species and radiation. The skin barrier may be specifically adjusted to allow penetration. For this reason, daily skin care may increase skin regeneration, elasticity, smoothness, and thus temporarily change the skin condition [2]. Protection, prevention, cleansing, and moisturizing are the key components of an effective skincare routine. Because most sun damage results from every day, incidental UV exposure, rather than occasional bursts while on vacation, dermatologists recommend daily use of sunscreens. In general, gel-based and bar cleansers are best for oily complexions, whereas cream or lotion-based ones are better for normal to dry skin. Moisturizers supply humectant agents, which draw water into the stratum corneum from the environment and dermis below. Moisturizers also include occlusive agents that act as a barrier to trans-epidermal water loss. In almost all cases, products contain both humectants, like hyaluronic acid, urea, and allantoin, and occlusives, including petrolatum, mineral oil, and lanolin. The classical moisturizers are used for treating dryness in the photoaged skin: polyols (glycerin, propylene glycol, butylene glycol and sorbitol), urea, lactic acid and salts, hyaluronic and salts, pyrrolodone-5-carboxylic acid and salts, panthenol, amino acids and proteins (collagen and proteins from wheat, rice, silk, soybean, and oat). More sophisticated peptides and proteins are presently used as moisturizers. It concerns generally more lipophylic quaternary N-alkyl derivatives of proteins or small polypeptides with long side chains (ester binding) to increase the lipophilic character: binding to the horny layer and a better percutaneous absorption. Recently, the use of small peptides, which mimic the amino acid sequence of collagen or enzymes (biomimetic peptides), has been proposed as moisturizers [56]. Surface-smoothing silicone derivatives or filmogen proteins such as quaternized proteins or silk, rice and oat, and skin feel agents are used in antiaging products. The high adsorption to the skin surface provokes a smoothing of the skin surface and is at the same time humectant. For a better percutaneous penetration, small fragments of hyaluronic acid were also suggested. Humectants are present in the water phase of a formula; occlusives are in the oil phase. Oil in water formulations tend to be lightweight gels, lotions, and serums and are best suited for normal to dry skin. Water in oil formulations may be ointments or creams and offer superior hydration for dry skin [80]

B. Correct Sun-Protection

Singer et.al, 2019 reported that avoidance of sun exposure at peak times and textile sun protection are important pillars of a modern prophylactic approach. Besides, antioxidants and DNA repair enzymes may be added to topical sunscreens in order to enhance the protection before and even after sun exposure [81]. The FDA regulates sunscreen as an over-the-counter medication. Currently, 16 UV filters are listed, 14 organic filters and two nonorganic filters, including zinc oxide and titanium dioxide. The FDA has changed its guidelines to address broad-spectrum sunscreen use, which involves UVA and UVB coverage; water resistance, to indicate the time duration the sunscreen is effective; and sun protection factor (SPF). SPF-30 or higher is recommended and can be labeled as reducing the risk of skin cancer and early skin aging [82,83]. Nutritional antioxidants act through different mechanisms and in different compartments, but are mainly FR scavengers: (a) they directly neutralize free radicals (b) they reduce the peroxide concentrations and repair oxidized membranes (c) they quench iron to decrease ROS production (d) via lipid metabolism, short-chain free fatty acids and cholesteryl esters neutralize ROS. The most important source of antioxidants is provided by nutrition. To the most known systemic antioxidants belong vitamin C, vitamin E, carotenoids, and from the trace elements copper and selenium. There are also studies demonstrating that vitamins C and E combined with ferulic acid impart both a sunscreen and an anti-oxidant effect [2].

C. Aesthetic non-invasive procedures

Noninvasive skin tightening has become one of the most common cosmetic aesthetic procedures being performed today. According to the American Society for Aesthetic Plastic Surgery (ASAPS) surveys released in 2014 and 2015, there has been a 12% increase in the demand for cosmetic procedures, with Americans spending more than $12 billion and having 10 billion procedures in 2014 [84]. A noninvasive device combines multipolar RF and PEMFs and is referred as $(MP)^2$, which stands for "Multipolar Magnetic Pulse." The device was introduced for the non-ablative treatment of skin laxity and cellulite [85]. Lee et.al, 2014 reported that combined multi-polar radiofrequency and pulsed electromagnetic field device is safe and effective for rejuvenating aged skin in Korean subjects [88].

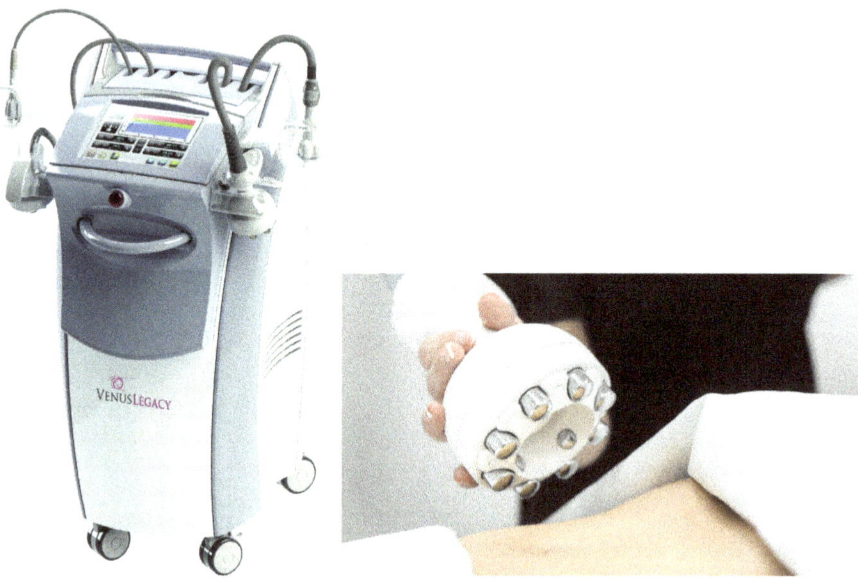

Figure 4.8 The Venus Legacy noninvasive skin tightening device [86,87]. The medical device is used in non-invasive body shaping, cellulite reduction, skin tightening, and wrinkle reduction for the face and body. The device is powered by $(MP)^2$ technology, which combines Multi-Polar Radio Frequency and Pulsed Electro Magnetic Fields, and features the advanced technology that induces lipolysis, allows for increased blood circulation, and stimulates lymphatic drainage in the treatment area (Courtacy: Elemental Esthetics).

Pulsed electromagnetic fields (PEMFs) are induced by short pulses of electrical current that penetrates into the skin and results in the stimulation of molecular and cellular activities. It has been used in medicine for bone growth, wound healing, cardiovascular disease, and other conditions. Pulsed electromagnetic fields increase collagen fiber production by dermal fibroblasts and stimulate angiogenesis, leading to wound-healing effects. *Radiofrequency* (RF) devices remain a dominant technology in the noninvasive management of skin aging, as it is a safe and effective treatment for a broad range of skin conditions. It can induce wrinkle reduction, cellulite improvement, laxity and body, and skin contouring improvement. When radiofrequency is applied by an alternating current, an electric field is generated, which achieves skin tissues, generating thermal energy. The heat is not diminished by tissue diffraction or absorption by epidermal melanin and is then appropriate for treatment of all skin types [85,86]. RF with micro-needling is effective and safe in improving skin laxity and texture. Pairing skincare cosmeceutical products pre- and post-procedure is beneficial as it enhances patient results, patient experience, and reduces patient downtime. Zahr et.al, 2019 reported that combining the multi-ingredient anti-aging facial moisturizer pre- and post-RF microneedling was safe and tolerable for the patients [229].

Exhibit 6. Classification of Noninvasive Body-Contouring Devices According to Energy Used [89]

Energy	Device (Company)
Mechanical suction	Endermologie (LPG Systems)
Mechanical suction and thermal	TriActive (Cynosure); SmoothShapes (Cynosure)
Radiofrequency	VelaShape (Syneron Candela); VelaSmooth (Syneron Candela); Thermage (Solta Medical); Accent (Alma Lasers); TiteFX (Invasix); Vanquish (BTL Industries, Inc); Exilis (BTL Industries, Inc)
Ultrasound	Ultrashape (Ultrashape); Liposonix (Solta Medical); VASERShape (Solta Medical)
Cryolipolysis	Coolsculpting (Zeltiq)
Low-level light laser	Zerona (Erchonia Medical, Inc)
Mechanical suction	Endermologie (LPG Systems)
Mechanical suction and thermal	TriActive (Cynosure); SmoothShapes (Cynosure)
Radiofrequency	VelaShape (Syneron Candela); VelaSmooth (Syneron Candela); Thermage (Solta Medical); Accent (Alma Lasers); TiteFX (Invasix); Vanquish (BTL Industries, Inc); Exilis (BTL Industries, Inc)
Ultrasound	Ultrashape (Ultrashape); Liposonix (Solta Medical); VASERShape (Solta Medical)
Cryolipolysis	Coolsculpting (Zeltiq)
Low-level light laser	Zerona (Erchonia Medical, Inc)

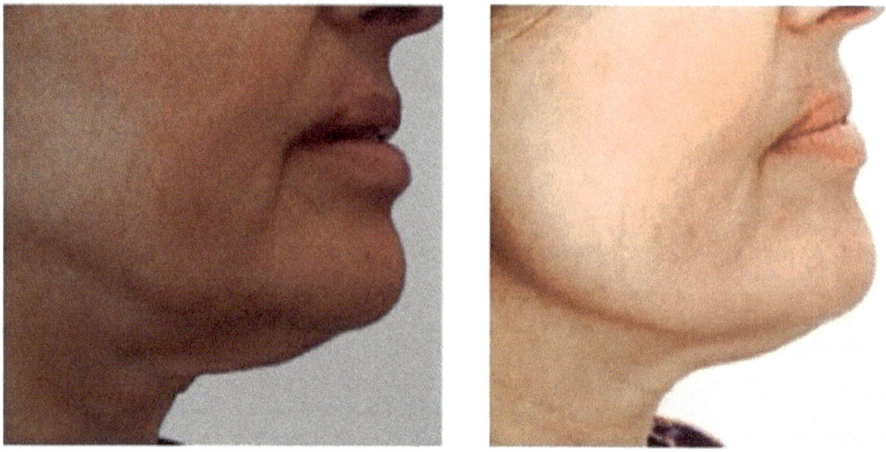

Figure 4.9 Improvements in skin condition [85]. Photographs of selected patients before (a) and after eight sessions (b) of treatment with RF and PEMFs (Courtacy: Hayes Valley Medical).

4.6.2 TOPICAL ANTI-AGING PREPARATIONS

A. Retinoids

Topical vitamin A has the ability to diminish the signs of aging by decreasing fine lines and wrinkling. In addition, there is a normalization and enhancement of elasticity. Improvement of skin tone and texture is a benefit of vitamin A, which enhances skin lightening when used in conjunction with skin lighteners [95]. The most widely utilized ones include retinol, retinyl esters (e.g., retinyl acetate, retinyl propionate, and retinyl palmitate), and retinaldehyde. Through endogenous enzymatic reactions, all of these are converted ultimately to trans-retinoic acid (trans-RA), which is an active form of vitamin A in the skin. Specifically, retinyl esters are converted to retinol via esterases. Retinol (ROL) is then converted to retinaldehyde by retinol dehydrogenase. And finally, retinaldehyde is oxidized to RA by retinaldehyde oxidase. Retinol and retinal must be metabolized in the skin to the active trans-retinoic acid. The incorporation of retinol and probably also retinal in cosmetic preparations poses the problem of stability (slow oxidation of retinol in function of time) [8], [90]. Topical natural retinoic acid precursors such as retinaldehyde or ROL are less irritant than acidic retinoids. Retinoids may be combined with other compounds with complementary actions against ageing, nutritional deficiency and cancer, such as antioxidants, to potentiate their beneficial effects in the skin [100].

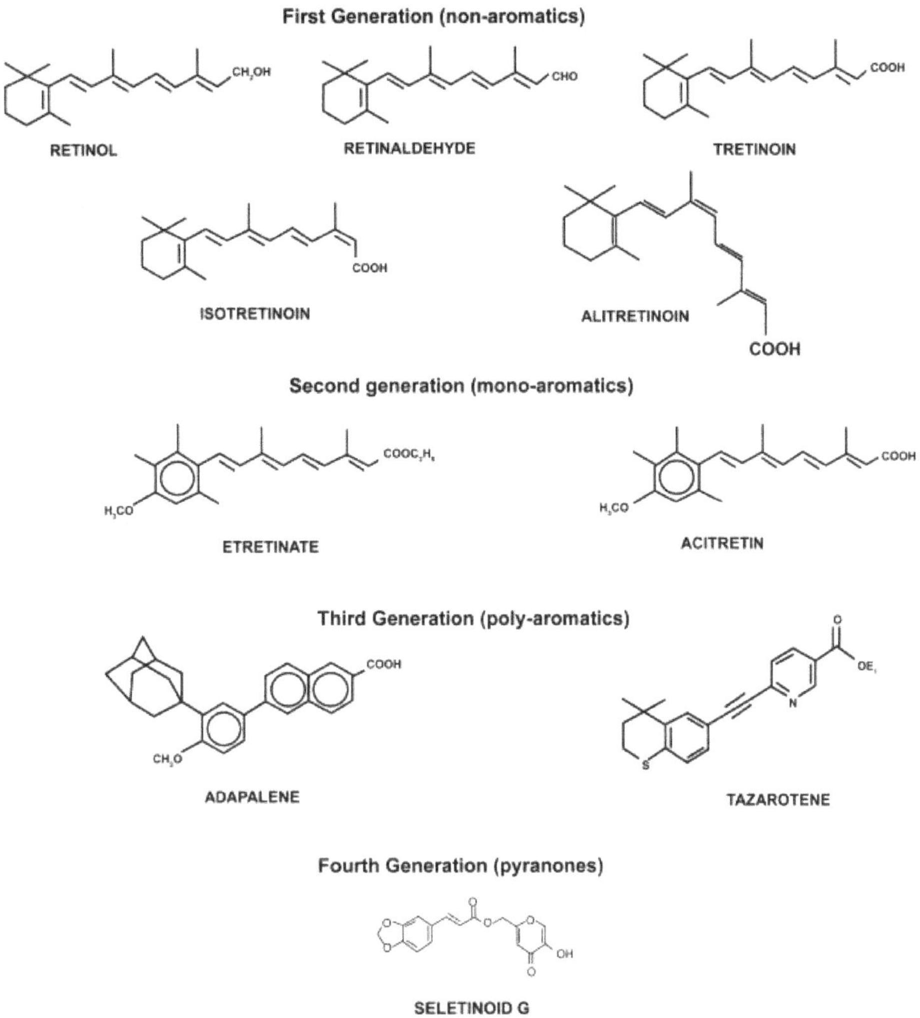

Figure 4.10 Chemical structures of retinoids [91-93]. First generation retinoids include tretinoin (all-trans RA), isotretinoin (13-cis-retinoic acid), and alitretinoin (9-cis RA). Second generation retinoids include etretinate and acitretin. Third generation retinoids include adapalene, tazarotene, and bexarotene. Kim et.al, 2005 designed synthetic retinoid, seletinoid G, by using computer-aided molecular modeling, and investigated its effects on the expression of extracellular matrix proteins in human skin *in vivo*.

The molecular mechanisms by which retinoids improve aged human skin have been difficult to investigate largely due to lack of appropriate in vitro models. Shao et.al, 2017 reported that topical application of 0.4% ROL to aged human skin leads to remarkable skin changes in both epidermis and dermis through affecting three major types of skin cells, epidermal keratinocytes, dermal endothelial cells and fibroblasts. Topical ROL significantly increases epidermal thickness by stimulating epidermal keratinocytes proliferation, which involves c-Jun transcription factor, a major deriving force for keratinocyte proliferation. In addition to epidermal changes, topical ROL significantly improves dermal ECM microenvironment; increasing dermal blood vessel formation by stimulating endothelial cells proliferation and ECM production by activating fibroblasts. Topical ROL also stimulates TGF-β/CTGF pathway, the major regulator of ECM homeostasis, and thus increased the deposition of mature collagen in aged human skin in vivo. Additionally, the restoration of dermal ECM may provide a better, more permissive environment for the proliferation of dermal endothelial cells and epidermal keratinocytes, and activation of dermal fibroblasts (TGF-β/CTGF pathway). Coupling of the proliferation of keratinocytes and endothelial cells, and dermal fibroblasts activation forms a self-enforcing environment, which might explain the remarkable anti-aging effects of ROL in aged human skin [94]. Kong et.al, 2016 reported that ROL anti-aging effects include the inhibition of UV-induction of matrix metalloproteinases, and the promotion of collagen synthesis in photoaged skin.5, 10 In clinical studies, topical retinol treatment significantly improved fine wrinkles.11 and affected markers of photoaging, including matrix metalloproteinase, collagenase, and collagen.12 Retinol was effective in producing retinoid-mediated histological changes, such as keratinocyte proliferation [96]. Bagatin et.al, 2018 reported that treatments with adapalene 0.3% gel and tretinoin 0.05% cream in cutaneous photoaging did not differ significantly regarding clinical evaluation of the following criteria: global cutaneous photoaging, periorbital wrinkles, ephelides/melanosis, forehead wrinkles, and actinic keratosis. They concluded that adapalene 0.3% gel is a safe and effective option for the treatment of mild or moderate photoaging [97]. Tretinoin is a prescription strength retinoid approved by the US FDA for acne and for the mitigation of fine facial wrinkles, mottled hyperpigmentation, and tactile roughness of facial skin. Topical application of tretinoin inhibits AP-1, thus suppressing the expression of MMPs and preventing the degradation of collagen. An increase in epidermal thickness and anchoring fibrils is observed, and intrinsically aged skin may also benefit from the topical application of retinoids. Prescription strength tretinoin affords the most potent retinoid effects, but often results in limited utility and decreased adherence due to irritation reactions (ie, burning, scaling, and dermatitis) [11], [91], [98]. Bakuchiol is a meroterpene phenol abundant in seeds and leaves of the plant *Psoralea corylifolia*. Chaudhuri et.al, 2014 reported that bakuchiol, having no structural resemblance to retinoids, can function as a functional analogue of retinol. Volcano plots showed great overall similarity of retinol and bakuchiol effects on the gene expression profile [101]. Dhaliwal et.al, 2019 reported that demonstrates that bakuchiol is comparable with retinol in its ability to improve photoageing and is better tolerated than retinol. Bakuchiol is promising as a more tolerable alternative to retinol (bakuchiol 0·5% cream twice daily or retinol 0·5% cream daily) [102]. Kwon et.al, 2018 reported that retinaldehyde 0.1% and 0.05% creams used to treat photoaged skin both were well tolerated and improved skin hydration and texture. Retinaldehyde 0.1% cream improved the melanin index as well [99]. An improvement of the photoaged dermal matrix by topical application of a cosmetic "antiaging" product containing a lipoentapeptide, white lupin, and retinyl palmitate was reported by Watson et. al, 2008 [142]. Also, synthetic retinyl-N-formyl aspartame has also been demonstrated to improve skin roughness and wrinkles. However, studies of retinyl esters, such as retinyl palmitate and retinyl propionate fail to show good efficacy [105].

B. α-Hydroxy Acids (AHAs)

Hydroxy acids, also called fruit acids, are among non-organic acids which have been used in the treatment of skin disorders since about 50 years ago. They are some of the most widely used and studied anti-aging skincare compounds. AHAs act on both the epidermal and the dermal levels. When applied to the skin, AHAs stimulate the exfoliation of epidermal cells in the stratum corneum by interfering with the ionic bonding between these cells. This results in the sloughing off dull and rough skin and promotes cellular renewal. Initially used for treatment of hyperkeratosis and other skin conditions affecting subcutaneous turnover, AHAs were found to promote softer, smoother skin, faded wrinkles, lightened age spots, and decreased blemishes. AHAs also improve the subcutaneous barrier function, increase epidermal proliferation and thickness, and restore hydration and pursiness through an increase in hyaluronic acid. The well-known benefits of AHA's include exfoliation, moisturization, reduction of fine lines and wrinkles, collagen synthesis, firming and skin lightening. Although these naturally occurring organic acids are often referred to as fruit acids because they are found in many common fruits such as citrus fruits (citric acid), apples (malic acid), and grapes (tartaric acid), the two most widely used AHAs are not components of fruit. Glycolic acid (GA) is a sugar cane derivative, and lactic acid (LA) is derived from milk [95], [103].

***Glycolic acid* (GA):** Tang et.al, 2019 demonstrated that GA reduced UVB-induced type-I procollagen expression and secretory collagen levels, when applied topically onto human keratinocytes and the C57BL/6J mice dorsal skin. The UV-induced MMP-9 level and activity were reduced by GA pre-treatment. Concomitantly, GA reverted mitogen-activated protein kinase (MMP-9) activation and inhibited the extracellular signal-regulated kinase activation (p38, pERK) triggered by UVB. Finally, GA triggers the transient receptor potential vanilloid-1 (TRPV-1) channel to initiate the anti-photoaging mechanism in keratinocytes. These findings clearly indicated that the mechanisms of GA promote skin protection against UVB-induced photoaging and wrinkle formation [104]. Application of 5% GA cream for 3 months has been shown to improve skin texture and discoloration of photoaged skin. In another study, 8%

(glycolic acid or L-lactic acid) for 22 weeks, the majority of patients (76% for glycolic acid; 71% for lactic acid) reported a noticeable improvement in the appearance and smoothness of photoaged skin [105]. In a study of 50% GA peels by Newman et al, there was improvement in mild photoaging of skin. Other significant improvements were noted, including decreases in rough texture and fine wrinkling, fewer solar keratoses, and slight lightening of solar lentigines. Histologic analysis showed thinning of the stratum corneum, granular layer enhancement, and epidermal thickening. Some specimens showed an increase in collagen thickness in the dermis. GA peels do not affect deep wrinkles or deep pigmentations [106].

***Lactic Acid* (LA):** Lactic acid (as sodium lactate) is a well-known part of the skin's natural moisturizing complex, and is considered to be an excellent moisturizer. LA also contributes to the cell cycle in human keratinocytes [107]. Treatment with 12% LA resulted in increased epidermal and dermal firmness and thickness and clinical improvement in skin smoothness and in the appearance of lines and wrinkles. Both the lactic and glycolic acid peelings were effective in reducing fine wrinkles on the external-lateral region of the eyes, after three applications (85% LA versus 70% GA) [109]. Recently more attention has been drawn to alpha hydroxy and polyhydroxy acids (AHA and PHA) due to their excellent moisturizing and antioxidant properties. Algiert-Zielińska et.al, 2019 reported maintenance of the epidermal barrier integrity during application of lactic acid (LA) and lactobionic acid and the opportunity to use them on sensitive skin types including couperose skin [112]. One of the reasons lactic acid is widely used as exfoliator and chemical peeling agent is its profound effect on desquamation of the skin. Desquamation is due to the dissociation of the cellular adhesions, which occurs as a result of reduced calcium ion concentration in the epidermis by chelating action of AHAs [113]. Yamamoto et.al, 2006 also showed that LA not only increased the production of ceramide in the stratum corneum, but also appeared to improve the ratio of ceramide 1-linoleate to oleate as compared to vehicle following 1-month topical application of 4% L-lactic acid. The increased ratio of ceramide 1-linoleate to oleate has been suggested to play an important role in increasing skin barrier function [114].

C. β-Hydroxy Acids (BHAs)

Beta Hydroxy Acids (BHAs), such as salicylic acid, are very similar to AHAs except for difference in their solubility. In the other hands, they are lipid-soluble in contrast to water solubility of AHAs. This structure allows them to penetrate into the skin through sebaceous follicles, making it appropriate for patients with oily skin and open comedones. In addition to prove anti-inflammatory effect of BHAs (e.g. salicylic acid), the skin irritancy effect of them have also been proved to be less than AHAs. Beta hydroxy acid found in skin-care products works best in a concentration of 1-2% [103]. Salicylic acid (SA) is a BHA, which has action to normal keratinization, decreases inflammation, and reduces sebum production with a comedolytic effect. The concentration of salicylic to treat acne is 0.5–5% [116]. SA has been used in the treatment of photoaging with in-office peels of 20–30%. These can be quite helpful in patients who are unable to tolerate AHAs since irritancy levels tend to be less with salicylic acid. In addition, it can be quite useful to combine or alternate both AHAs and BHAs since their mechanisms of action differ, and using both may be quite beneficial [95]. Vender et.al, 2019 reported that daily use of a ceramide containing cleanser and cream that also has SA offers an effective, easy and comfortable option for dry skin conditions. After treatment subjects reported a significant improvement in the quality of their professional life, self-image, and social life. The products were shown to be safe, comfortable, and well tolerated [115]. Shamalnasab et.al, 2018 reported that salicylates activate adenosine monophosphate-activated kinase (AMPK), which is now considered as a promising target to slow down aging and prevent age-related diseases in humans [116]. A topical combination containing 10.4% L-lactic acid, 2% salicylic acid and alpha-hydroxy acid/retinoate conjugate (ethyl lactyl retinoate) was used in the topical treatment of females of ages 20 to 58. After 4 weeks, improvement was achieved, which remained continuous and cumulative in the eighth week [97]. 2% supramolecular salicylic acid has a similar efficacy with 5% benzoyl peroxide 0.1% adapalene in mild to moderate acne treatment. The skin barrier (skin hydration value and TEWL value), skin brightness (L* value) and erythema (a* values) indicators showed similar statistical improvement [118].

D. Ascorbic Acid (AA)

Vitamin C is a water-soluble antioxidant which protects skin from oxidative damage and rejuvenates photo-aged skin. It has been utilized as a skin lightener (e.g., via tyrosinase inhibition and/or its antioxidant effect). It also has been reported to have anti-inflammatory properties since it reduces the erythema associated with post-operative laser resurfacing. In addition, AA also serves as an essential co-factor for the enzymes lysyl hydroxylase and prolyl hydroxylase, both of which are required for posttranslational processing in collagen (Types I and III) biosynthesis. Thus, by stimulating these biosynthetic steps, ascorbic acid will increase the production of collagen which will lead to wrinkle reduction [90]. Vitamin C deficient individuals may experience easy bleeding, bruising, and poor wound healing [130]. In addition, topical vitamin C increases levels of tissue inhibitors of collagen-degrading matrix metalloproteinase-1 (MMP-1) [95]. Normal skin contains high concentrations of vitamin C, which supports important and well-known functions, stimulating collagen synthesis and assisting in antioxidant protection against UV-induced photodamage. Vitamin C uptake from the plasma and transport across the skin layers is mediated by specific sodium-dependent vitamin C transporters (SVCTs) that are present throughout the body and are also responsible for transport into other tissues. Interestingly, cells in the epidermis express both types of vitamin C transporter, SVCT1 and SVCT2 (Figure 8) [131].

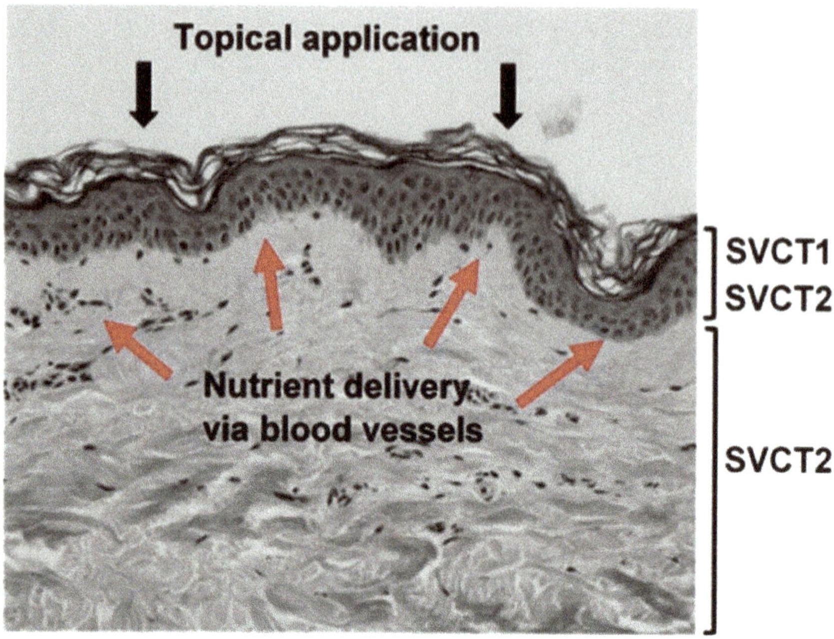

Figure 4.11 Delivery of nutrients to the skin [131]. The location of the vitamin C transport proteins SVCT1 and SVCT2 are indicated. Red arrows depict nutrient flow from the blood vessels in the dermis to the epidermal layer. Nutrients delivered by topical application would need to penetrate the barrier formed by the stratum corneum.

Exhibit 7. Skin ailments, their causes and evidence from in vitro and in vivo studies for association with vitamin C levels [131].

Type of Skin Damage	Cause	Skin Structure Affected	Evidence of Protection by Vitamin C
Sunburn	Acute and excessive UV exposure.	Cell death of all skin cells, with associated inflammation.	Improving skin vitamin C and vitamin E levels can improve resistance to UV exposure.
Photo-aging, oxidant-induced damage	Chronic UV Over exposure, cigarette smoking.	Damaged collagen and elastin matrix, thinning of the epidermal layer.	Decreased signs of aging with higher fruit and vegetable intake. Protection inferred from studies with acute UV exposure.

Contd...

Type of Skin Damage	Cause	Skin Structure Affected	Evidence of Protection by Vitamin C
Hyperpigmentation	Chronic UV exposure and environmental stresses.	Excessive pigment formation and propagation of melanocytes in the epidermis.	Nutrition studies showing improved skin color with higher fruit and vegetable intake.
Wrinkle formation	Natural aging, oxidative stress, UV exposure, smoking, medical treatments.	Dermal layer changes, deterioration of collagen and elastic fibers.	Lessening of wrinkle depth following vitamin C supplementation. Increased collagen formation by fibroblasts in cell culture.
Skin sagging	Natural aging, oxidative stress damage, extreme weight loss.	Loss of elastin and collagen fibers, thinning of skin layers, loss of muscle tone.	Improved skin tightness in individuals with higher fruit and vegetable intake.
Loss of color	Natural aging, UV exposure, illness.	Thinning of skin layers, loss of melanocytes or decreased melanin formation, loss of vasculature in dermis.	Improved skin tone with high fruit and vegetable intake.
Surface roughness	Chemical and UV exposure, physical abrasion, allergy and inflammation.	Stratum corneum, loss of skin moisture barrier function.	Vitamin C enhances production of barrier lipids in cell culture.

Garre et.al, 2018 reported that topical serum containing L-Ascorbic acid, soluble proteoglycans, low molecular weight hyaluronic acid, and a tripeptide protected against oxidative damage and dermal protein loss caused by photo- and chronological aging in human skin explants. In-vivo, the serum hydrated skin for 6 hours, and users perceived increased skin brightness, hydration, and fewer wrinkles [126]. Zasada et.al, 2019 reported that 2.5 ml of serum containing 20% L-ascorbic acid with hydrate from strawberries was used topically in every of 4 treatments. The impact of active substance on skin firmness and elasticity as well as the degree of hydration and skin tone was more efficient after micro-needle mesotherapy [127]. Wang et.al, 2019 reported 2-O-β-d-glucopyranosyl-l-ascorbic acid (AA-2βG), a unique AA derivative identified in *Lycium barbarum*, exhibited enhanced free radical scavenging activity compared with AA and its synthetic derivative AA-2αG. AA-2βG protected hydrogen peroxide-induced cell death in murine macrophage RAW264.7 cells. Treatment with AA-2βG eliminated oxidative stress and the ratio of cellular glutathione to glutathione disulfide more effectively than AA and AA-2αG [128]. Gęgotek et.al, 2019 reported three times higher antioxidant properties of than rutin, measured by the cation radical scavenging activity by the ferric-reducing activity of plasma (FRAP) test. However, the mixture of ascorbic acid and rutin (Ascorbic A. + Rutin) had approximately 20% higher antioxidant properties compared to Ascorbic A alone. The F–C test showed that AA + Rutin acted two times stronger than AA. or Rutin alone [129]. Crisan et.al, 2015 reported topically applied vitamin C (concentration of 5% and a pH of 5.5 in a novel complex with *Rosa moschata*, the musk rose oil and proteoglycans) is highly efficient as a rejuvenation therapy, inducing significant collagen synthesis in all age groups with minimal side effects [132].

E. Vitamin

The very properties that make alpha-tocopherol such a powerful antioxidant causes it to break down in the presence of oxygen or upon exposure to light. For that reason, α-tocopherol acetate, which is the more stable esterified form, is used in cosmetics. Since α-tocopherol acetate is not an antioxidant and has no antioxidant activity, it must first convert to its active alpha-tocopherol form. Years of debate questioned the ability of alpha-tocopherol acetate to be delivered to the skin and bio-converted to an active form. Finally, in 1990, the bioconversion of alpha-tocopherol acetate to free alpha-tocopherol was able to be demonstrated. The use of vitamin E in skin care has anti-aging benefits based on its moisturization properties but mostly on its protective capabilities. Vitamin E enhances the photoprotective to protective effects of sunscreen, and when combined with vitamin C, the two are even stronger as photo protectants [95]. Unfortunately, oral supplementation of vitamin C and E has proven insufficient in preventing skin aging owing to their poor solubility, inefficient skin permeability, or instability during storage [136]. Topical vitamin E (α-tocopherol) used as a component of skin products has anti-inflammatory and antiproliferative effects in concentrations between 2 and 20%. It acts by smoothing the skin and increasing the ability of the stratum corneum to maintain its humidity, to accelerate the epithelialization, and contribute to photoprotection of the skin. The effects are not as strong as with vitamins C and B3 [133]. Most of the OTC antiaging creams contain 0.5%–1% of vitamin E. Topical application of the gel containing 2% phytonadione, 0.1% retinol, 0.1% vitamin C, and 0.1% vitamin E has been seen to be fairly or moderately effective in reducing dark under-eye circles, especially in cases of hemostasis.

Topical application of vitamin E can rarely cause contact dermatitis, erythema multiforme, and xanthomatous reaction [134]. The interaction of vitamins E and C has led to the idea of "vitamin E recycling", where the antioxidant function of oxidized vitamin E is continuously restored by other antioxidants (**Figure 4.9**). This "antioxidant network" depends upon the supply of aqueous antioxidants and the metabolic activity of cells [135].

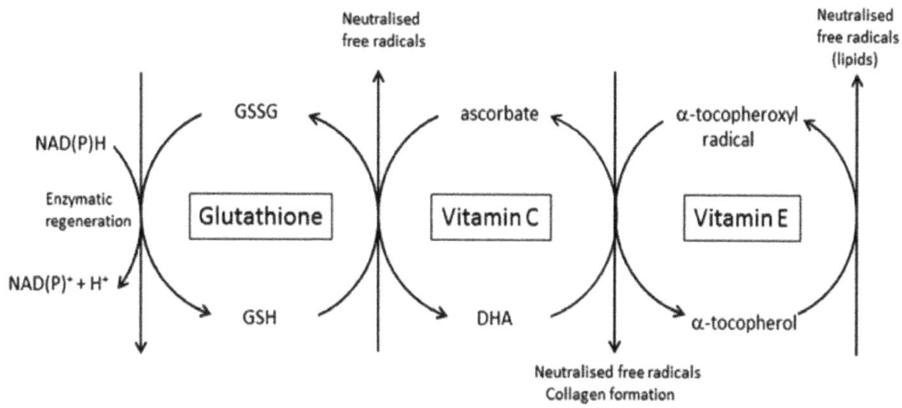

Figure 4.12 The interdependence of vitamins E and C, and glutathione, in the scavenging of free radicals and regeneration of the reduced antioxidants [131]. Vitamin E is in the lipid fraction of the cell, whereas vitamin C and glutathione are water-soluble and present in the cytosol. Vitamin C is only one player in the antioxidant arsenal that includes enzymatic defenses (catalase, glutathione peroxidase and superoxide dismutase) as well as other non-enzymatic defenses (vitamin E, glutathione, uric acid and other putative antioxidants such as carotenoids).

Vitamin E is a promising chemo-preventive and pharmacologically safe agent, which can be exploited or tested against skin cancer [137]. Experimental evidence suggests that topical and oral vitamin E has anticarcinogenic, photoprotective, and skin barrier-stabilizing properties [138]. The topical use of resveratol, a polyphenol from red grapes with great antioxidant activity in skin care formulation Farris et.al, 2014 reported that significant improvement in fine lines and wrinkles, skin firmness, skin elasticity, skin laxity, hyperpigmentation, radiance, and skin roughness over baseline in 12 weeks after using a topically applied proprietary blend containing 1% resveratrol, 0.5% baicalin, and 1% vitamin E. Ultrasound measurements in the periorbital area showed an average improvement of 18.9% in dermal thickness suggesting significant dermal remodeling [139]. Combination of vitamin E, vitamin C, and ferulic acid can reduce the incidence of oxidative stress-induced tumors, and their antioxidant effects are much better than the use of vitamin C alone [140]. Burns et.al, 2013 demonstrated that topical 5% alpha tocopherol may actually promote carcinogenesis when applied on chronically UVB-damaged skin while treating with a more stable antioxidant compound may offer therapeutic benefits [141].

F. Coenzyme Q10

Coenzyme Q10 (a ubiquinone) is a powerful free radical inhibitor that inhibits lipid peroxides from forming in plasma membranes. Q10 plays a very important role in cellular energy production and works in the mitochondrial ATP energy-producing pathway of the cell. Q10 levels diminish with age, as does cellular energy production, which may improve by adding Q10 [95]. Additionally, UVR, which leads to oxidative damage, significantly reduces skin's Q10 levels. Approximately 46% of total Q10 was found to be present in the reduced form in human epidermis. Q10 scavenges ROS and protects cells against oxidative stress. Zhao et.al, 2019 concluded that suppression of the PKA-ERK 1/2 signaling pathway may be one of the important mechanisms by which Q10 protects astrocytes from UVB-induced oxidative damage [149]. Knott et.al, 2015 reported that quinone values on the skin surface were significantly increased after treatment with Q10-containing formulas demonstrating that the powerful antioxidant Q10 can be delivered directly to the uppermost layer of the skin [143]. Q10 is an insoluble, poorly permeable antioxidant with great biological value which acts as anti-aging and anti-wrinkle agent. Q10 nano-structured lipid carrier (Q10-NLC) had greater antioxidant properties and topical skin penetration than the Q10-emulsion [144]. Also, El-Leithy et.al, 2018 reported Q10 nano-emulsion having enhanced solubility and permeability with improved anti-wrinkle efficiency [146]. The concentration of Vitamin E and Q10, which together with squalene, play a key role against external oxidative insult, has been shown to decrease significantly during ageing. Topical application was found to be more effective than oral administration in terms of sebum levels of lipophilic antioxidants and squalene [145]. Also, Žmitek et.al, 2017 reported oral supplementation with CoQ10 did not significantly affect skin hydration and dermis thickness [148]. As an effective fat-soluble antioxidant and an essential element of the mitochondrial respiratory chain, Q10 may have healing effects on wound tissues by decreasing oxidative stress and improved mitochondrial efficiency. Choi et. al, 2009 reported the anti-inflammatory and wound healing effect of Q10 in mice [146]. Despite the lack of evidence, large numbers of people in the population are taking oral Q10 and other vitamins and cofactors in the hope that these agents will slow senescence and expand longevity [150].

G. α-Lipoic Acid

Lipoic acid is a very powerful antioxidant that has the unusual advantage of being both water and fat soluble and is an important cofactor in mitochondrial dehydrogenases. α-lipoic acid (ALA) is a sulfhydryl compound found naturally in virtually all plant and animal species and in both prokaryotic and eukaryotic cells. In the human body, it is bonded to lysine residues and acts as a cofactor in various multienzyme complexes. Nevertheless, there is often little or no free ALA in tissues, so a topical antioxidant formulation containing this natural antioxidant could be used to protect the skin against the effects of ultraviolet rays, such as photoaging and skin cancer [156]. Studies have shown the ease with which lipoic acid is able to penetrate the skin, after which it converts into its active byproduct dihydrolipoic acid. Topical application of 3% lipoic acid has demonstrated its ability to decrease UVB-induced erythema, which demonstrates its photoprotective and anti-inflammatory properties. Also, a 12 - week study demonstrated that using a topical cream containing 5% ALA was quite effective in treating signs of photoaging [95]. ALA and its reduced form, dihydrolipoic acid, are powerful antioxidants that have many physiological functions, including free radical scavenging of reactive oxygen species, generation of cellular antioxidants, chelation of metal ions, and inflammatory suppression (when given orally) [155]. Though ALA is normally administered in oral or injection, it is rarely used topically because of its bad penetration. Kubota et.al, 2019 developed novel nanocapsule of ALA, named α-lipoactive (nLA), to improve skin permeability. In in vivo experiments, it was found that nLA is very effective for improving UV-induced pigmentation and epidermal thickening [151]. Sherif et.al, 2019 demonstrated application of topical 30% poloxamer gel loaded with ALA cubosomes. Reduction in facial lines, almost complete resolution of fine lines in the periorbital region and upper lip area and overall improvement in skin color and texture in most volunteers. There were no instances of irritation, peeling or other apparent adverse side effects [152]. In a similar study with 5% Cubosomal ALA significantly increased epidermal thickness with effective and safe modality for improving aging face [154]. Lin et.al, 2004 were unable to detect protection using ALA alone or together with vitamins C and E. According to them, a commercial formulation of ALA provided no protection [153]. Isaac et.al, 2015 reported that rheological features, such as viscosity, thixotropy, and compliance, and the presence of a hydrophilic polymer strongly influenced the release of ALA from topical emulsion dosage form [156].

H. β-Glucans

β-Glucan is a dietary fiber, found in many natural sources, and controls chronic metabolic diseases effectively. The in vivo cholesterol binding and reduction in the skin thickness by β-glucan were highly encouraging [160]. Although isolated from different sources, including oat, barley, and reishi mushrooms, the most biologically active are isolated from cell membranes of baker's yeast (*Saccharomyces cerevisiae*). In the epidermis, where macrophage-derived cells include both keratinocytes and Langerhans cells, β-Glucans act to stimulate the protective qualities of these cells as our first line of defense. Topical β-Glucans can accelerate wound healing and increase resistance to infection by enhancing macrophage-mediated phagocytosis. Studies have also demonstrated that β-Glucans have photoprotective properties similar to those of vitamin E by their ability to sustain levels of reduced glutathione in the skin following UVR. β-Glucans are extremely soothing and calming to the skin through their reinforcement of skin macrophages, which have implications in minimizing irritancy potential of products. The potential uses of β-Glucans in dermatology are numerous. In personal-care products for shaving, where nicks and cuts, razor burn, irritation and folliculitis are problematic, the protective, wound-healing, anti-irritating effects of β-Glucans can be quite helpful. The photoprotective effects of β-Glucans as well as their ability to soothe, moisturize, and protect the skin from potential irritation that can occur with other treatment products, makes them quite useful in anti-aging skin regimens [95]. Topical application of β-glucans is increasing, since their pluripotent activity (antioxidant, anti-inflammatory and regenerative effects, immune-modulation, radioprotection, moisturization and rejuvenation) might help as a complementary therapy in managing various skin diseases and conditions. Macrophages, keratinocytes and fibroblasts are considered the main target cells of β-glucans during wound healing. β-glucans enhance wound repair by increasing the infiltration of macrophages, which stimulates tissue granulation, collagen deposition and re-epithelialization [157].

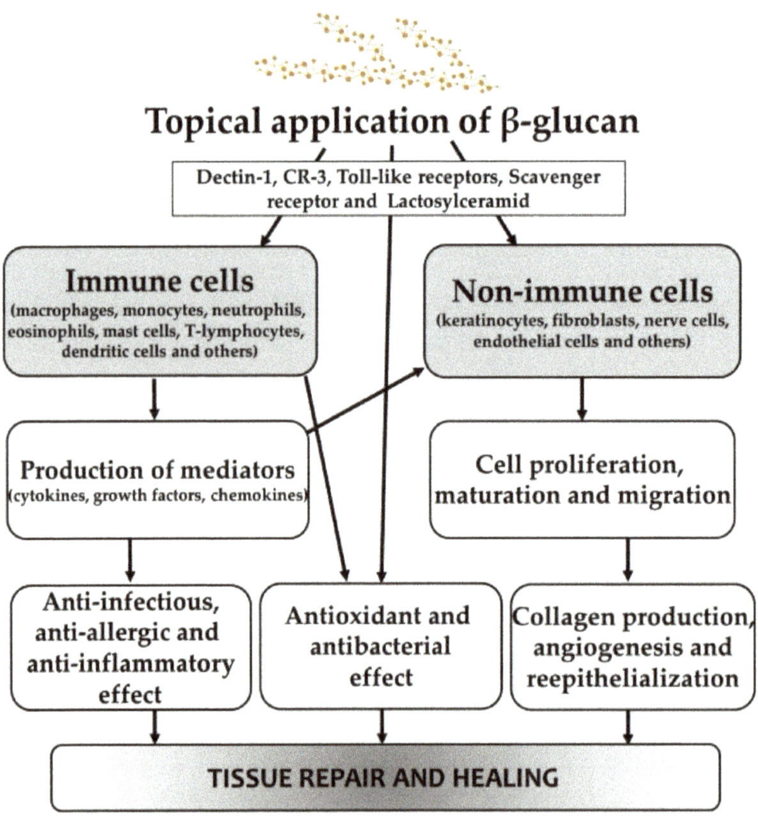

Figure 4.13 Schematic depiction of β-glucan pluripotent mechanisms in wound healing [157].

A long-term use of glucan showed reduction of wrinkle depth, height and overall roughness, which is probably caused by stimulation of fibroblast and increase production of collagen. A cell turnover and regenerative extract of βeta-glucan is believed to support healthy immunosurveillance [158]. Dammarane ginsenosides are considered to play a major role in the antiwrinkle activities of ginseng. These compounds are strongly linked with cellulose, pectin, or β-glucan [159]. Jesenak et.al, 2016 investigated the immunomodulatory and anti-inflammatory activity of an Imunoglukan P4H® cream, containing β-glucans (pleuran), in patients suffering from atopic dermatitis, where use of β-glucan-based cream as a supportive complementary therapy [161]. The topical application of Imunoglukan P4H® showed significant improvements in both subjective and objective symptoms of atopic dermatitis and a significant decline in disease severity; exacerbation was observed [162]. Sensitive skin is frequently complaint in dermatology consultation with cutaneous manifestations such as stinging, redness, dryness, and burning sensation that affect the quality of life. Its pathogenesis is mainly related to dysfunction of neurosensory, skin barrier, and also immune activity. Wang et.al, 2018 confirmed the effectiveness, tolerance and antisensitive function of a new complex cream composed by Yunnan Portulaca oleracea extract, Prinsepia utilis oil, beta-glucan, and sodium hyaluronate extracted from mushroom. The proposed daily care safe moisturizer provided a statistically significant improvement in clinical grading scores for dryness, roughness, and erythema at 28 days compared to baseline [163].

Exhibit 8. List of the Plant Extracts Mostly Used in Commercial Antiaging Cosmetics [8]
Sesamum Indicum, Prunus Amygdalis dulcis, Phyllanthus umblica, Siegesbeckia orientalis, Theobroma cacao, Bytospermum parkii, Mangifera indica, Mentha piperada, Aleurits moluccana, Glycurrhiza glabra, Arcostaphylos uva, Imperata cylindrica, Centella asiatica, Echinacea purpurea, Camelia sinensis, Thea sinensis, Hordeum vulgare, Crithium maritimum, Plantago lanceolata, Phellodendron amurense, Spirea ulmaria, Artemisia vulgaris, Santalum album, Rosmarinus officinalis, Centella asiatica, Curcuma longa, Aloe vera, Arnica calendula, Ginkgo biloba, various algae such as Fucus vesiculosus, Laminaria flexicaulis, Ascophyllum nodosum.

I. Ceramide

The stratum corneum is comprised of corneocytes surrounded by inter-celluar lipids including ceramides, free fatty acids, and cholesterol. Ceramide predominant moisturizers have become a mainstay of treatment of skin disease. Ceramides constitute (on a weight basis) approximately 47% of the SC lipids [186]. Moisturizing treatment involves a four-step process: a) repairing the skin barrier, b) increasing water content, c) reducing TEWL and d) restoring the lipid barriers' ability to attract, hold and redistribute water. Interestingly, a statistically significant higher ceramide/cholesterol ratio was found for men than for women, as reported by Vozella et.al, 2019 [183]. Jensen et.al, 2005 reported reduced activities of ceramide-generating epidermal acid sphingomyelinase (SMase) and ceramide synthase in the inner epidermis of aged skin, explaining its reduced capacity in barrier repair [182]. The effect of Ceramide cream on enhancing skin barrier function and hydration might be explained by its unique ingredients. Ceramide cream increases skin hydration and improves barrier function which may make it suitable for use on dry skin [179]. Several studies have demonstrated that ceramides play an essential role in both the barrier and water-holding functions of healthy stratum corneum, suggesting that the dysfunction of the stratum corneum associated with ageing as well that observed in patients with several skin diseases could result from a ceramide deficiency. A 2-week topical application of a sonicated Streptococcus thermophilus preparation led to significant and relevant increase of stratum corneum ceramide levels [180]. Draelos et.al, 2018 demonstrates that a proprietary combination of ceramide PC-104, palmitamide MEA, glycerrhetinic acid, and grape seed extract in a glycerin, dimethicone, and petrolatum vehicle was effective in reducing the signs and symptoms of mild-to-moderate atopic dermatitis and other types of pruritic dermatoses (e.g., senile itch, cosmetic intolerance syndrome) in children and adults [184]. Yazdanparast et.al, 2018 reported skin-identical ceramide complex cream improved contact dermatitis with a decrease in Three-Item Severity (TIS) and an increase in skin hydration, implying a repair of the skin barrier [185]. Advancements in cosmetic chemistry have resulted in the development of bio-identical synthetic ceramides that are commonly incorporated into skin care products (notably CER-1, CER-3, and CER-6), which have been shown to function similar to natural ceramides [186]. Zhang et.al, 2015 reported limited penetration of ceramide species into SC and accumulation on to the skin, suggesting that topical replenishment of CER may not be an effective approach to improve the barrier properties of healthy skin [187].

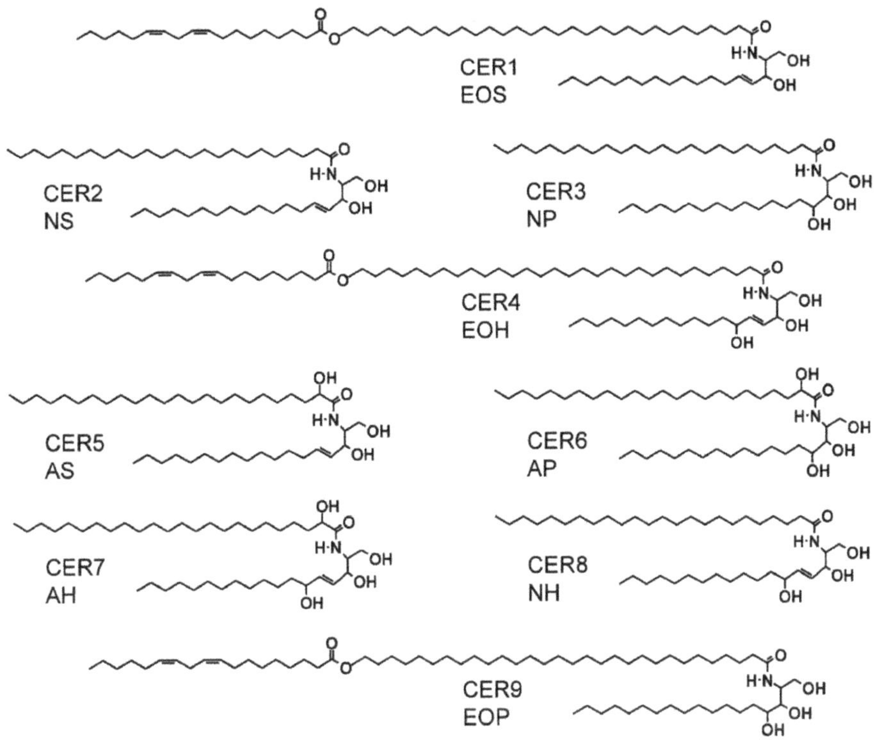

Figure 4.14 The molecular structures of the ceramides (CER) present in human stratum corneum [225], indicated according to the numbering system (based on chromatographic migration) and according to their structures. A, α-hydroxy fatty acid; H, 6-hydroxysphingosine; N, nonhydroxy fatty acid; P, phytosphingosine; S, sphingosine.

J. Nicotinamide

Niacin (vitamin B3) has two potential forms that can be used in cosmeceuticals: niacinamide (nicotinamide) and nicotinic acid [193]. Topical nicotinamide (the active form of vitamin-B3) has been shown to improve fine lines and wrinkles, hyperpigmented spots, red blotchiness and sallowness (yellowing), as well as elasticity. In addition, nicotinamide has been demonstrated to increase the skin's production of collagen and ceramides, and to stimulate keratinocyte differentiation, leading to improved barrier function and skin appearance [95], [105]. Nicotinamide cream is a more effective moisturizer than white petrolatum on atopic dry skin, and may be used as a treatment adjunct in atopic dermatitis [188]. Ashkani et.al, 2015 reported its anti-inflammatory, antioxidant, and immunomodulatory properties, as well as an epithelization inducing action. Nicotinamide also improved tissue regeneration through the increment of fibroblast proliferation, collagen synthesis, and vascularization [189]. Nicotinamide and clindamycin gels were significantly more efficacious in oily and non-oily skin types, respectively. Skin type is a significant factor in choosing between topical nicotinamide and clindamycin in patients with acne vulgaris [196]. Because topical clindamycin, like other antimicrobials, is associated with emergence of resistant microorganisms, nicotinamide 4% gel is a desirable alternative treatment for acne vulgaris [190]. Niacinamide 4% induces a decrease in pigmentation, inflammatory infiltrate, and solar elastosis. Niacinamide is a safe and effective therapeutic agent for melasma, compared to 4% hydroquinone. Niacinamide was effective in approximate 40% of patients, showing outstanding clinical results [191]. In ageing skin, topical application of niacinamide improves the surface structure, smoothens out wrinkles and inhibits photo-carcinogenesis. It is possible to demonstrate anti-inflammatory effects in acne, rosacea and nitrogen mustard-induced irritation [192]. Nicotinamide also increases the production of the epidermal proteins keratin, filaggrin, and involucrin [194]. Nicotinamide increases collagen production in fibroblast cultures and reduces the increased dermal glycoaminoglycosides in photodamaged skin. The glycation between protein and sugar resulting in the formation of cross-linked products gives a yellow color to the skin. As nicotinamide is a precursor of antioxidant NADPH, it has antiglycation effects, thus preventing shallowing of skin. In a double-blinded, split face, randomized controlled trial, 5% nicotinamide cream was compared to "vehicle only cosmetic" in 30 Japanese women on face for 8 weeks. There was a significant decrease in wrinkles and skin roughness with nicotinamide [195].

K. Zinc

The skin is the third most zinc (Zn)-abundant tissue in the body. Zn is a cofactor for over 1000 enzymatic reactions and is necessary for over 2000 transcription factors. Zn-finger proteins function for DNA interaction, RNA packaging, activation of transcription, regulation of apoptosis, folding and assembly of protein, and lipid binding. Zn also functions as an intracellular signaling molecule, like calcium, by transducing extracellular stimuli into intracellular signaling. Additionally, about 10% of human proteins binds to Zn. affects 17% of the world's population who are in the condition of general malnutrition due to starvation, severe illness, alcohol addiction [214]. The importance of zinc for humans was acknowledged in the Middle East (Iran, Egypt), in the early 1960s, in patients with growth retardation, hypogonadism, hepatomegaly, splenomegaly, dry and wrinkled skin, and severe iron deficiency anemia [215]. A Zn-deficient diet alters the expression of keratin polypeptides in rats because of impaired keratinolytic enzyme activity. Zn is required for the proliferation of keratinocytes and the suppression of inflammation in Keratinocytes. Zn facilitates the melanocyte proliferation and the autophagy. Zn promotes lipogenesis and glucose transport via its insulin-like effects on 3T3-L1 fibroblasts and adipocytes [214]. Topical preparations like zinc oxide, calamine, or zinc pyrithione have been in use as photoprotecting, soothing agents or as active ingredient of antidandruff shampoos. Its use has expanded manifold over the years for a number of dermatological conditions including infections (leishmaniasis, warts), inflammatory dermatoses (acne vulgaris, rosacea), pigmentary disorders (melasma), and neoplasias (basal cell carcinoma) [216].

L. Anti-pollution preparations

Fernández et.al, 2018 demonstrated that SIG-1273 reduced cell death by 66%, outperforming niacinamide, ascorbic acid, and α-tocopherol, commonly used actives in antipollution skin-care products [232]. Addor et.al, 2019 reported *Cryptomphalus aspersa* secretion with regenerative (hyaluronic acid, peptides) and antioxidant ingredients (ectoine, coffeeberry oil, and olive oil), according to the type and area of the face, on the improvement of signs of skin aging. Ingredients from formulations studied have been shown to reduce the signs of skin aging by the multiple extrinsic factors known today as ultraviolet, visible, and infrared solar radiation; pollutants; aridity conditions; or even endogenous factors, such as dietary factors [233]. A film-forming exopolysaccharide (EPS) called as alteromonas ferment extract was included in the formulation for its anti-adhesion effect. EPS significantly reduced particle adhesion to skin and protected keratinocyte membranes from lipid peroxidation, preserved cell integrity, and normalized the collagen network in skin exposed to heavy metals, hydrocarbons, and particulate matter. Narda et.al, 2018 reported that daily application of the facial cream containing an EPS, carnosine, and niacinamide over 5 days had a protective effect against pollution-induced changes [234]. Giacomelli et.al, 2018 reported that clinical application of a multicomponent powder, including three naturally occurring standardized extracts rich in polyphenols (grape seed extract, green tea extract, oak wood/bark extract) allows the prevention of any metal deposition within the SC following exposure in a polluted environment and plays an effective role in counteracting skin damages induced by air pollution [235].

Exhibit 9. Guidelines for formulating anti-pollution products [231]

Sr No.	Visible Skin Damage	Formulation Approach	Active Options
1.	Dull and oily skin	Deep Cleansing Exfoliation External polymer barrier Dust repellent polymer	Mild surfactant Activated charcoal Coffee beans and rice bran scrub Biosaccharide gum
2.	Dry and damaged skin	Restore natural lipid bilayer Strengthen skin's natural barrier	Long and short chain ceramides Cholesterol and behenic acid Extract of Edelweiss Extract of Red Algae

Contd...

Sr No.	Visible Skin Damage	Formulation Approach	Active Options
3.	Dehydrated rough skin	Improve skin hydration Reduce TEWL Replenish NMF in skin	Extract of Desert Rose Extract of Tremella Fuciformis
4.	Wrinkles and fine lines Loss of youthful volume	Control formation of ROS Use metal chelating agents Replenish antioxidant reserve	Chia seed oil Pink Pepper extract Extract of Malachite White Tea extract
5.	Uneven skin tone Skin darkening Formation of lentigines	Control Melanin synthesis Inhibit Tyrosinase Regulate melanosome transfer	Nature identical Reservatrol Extract of Swiss Garden Cress Marine exopolysaccharide isomerate Extract of Chinese whitening herbs
6.	Loss of skin firmness Loss of elasticity	Promote collagen/ elastin synthesis Prevent degradation of proteins	Extract f Nannochloropsis Occulata Paeonia Albiflora root extract White Tea extract Extract of Japanese Sea algae
7.	Skin redness and sensitivity Inflammation and acne	Autoinflammatory actives Use of skin soothing agent	Extract of White Peony Ginger root extract Extract of American Red Raspberry Extract of Arabian Desert Daisy

4.6.3 SYSTEMIC ANTI-AGING PREPARATIONS

A. Collagen supplementation

In 2016, the collagen market was valued at an estimated 3.71 billion USD and is projected to reach 6.63 billion USD by 2025. Collagen supplements, originating from various sources (eg, porcine, bovine, marine) and available in numerous formulations (eg, protein, gelatin, hydrolysate, peptides), are marketed as improving skin integrity and modulating skin aging. When denatured by heat, collagen forms gelatin, which has been used for centuries as a food source and traditional medicine in Europe and China. Further enzymatic hydrolysis of gelatin produces collagen hydrolysates (CH) composed of peptides of varying lengths, conveniently formulated into liquid drinks and jelly sticks for oral consumption. In the past decade, CHs have gained popularity as a nutraceutical supplement. Choi et.al, 2019 reported promising preliminary results for the short and long-term use of oral collagen supplements for wound healing and skin aging. Oral collagen supplements also increase skin elasticity, hydration, and dermal collagen density. However, even with this increase in patient interest and market share, the use of collagen supplementation in dermatology remains controversial due to the lack of regulation on the quality and quantity of ingredients in OTC collagen supplements [164], [171]. Maria et.al, 2019 reported improvement of general skin conditions, acting in different mechanisms by oral supplementation and topical application of hydrolyzed proteins [165]. Proksch et.al, 2014 reported significant improvement in after 8 weeks of supplementation in women aged 35-55 years but the study failed to reach a level of statistical significance with regard to skin moisture and skin evaporation [166]. Oral administration of Low-molecular-weight Collagen peptide (LMWCP), which is a fish-derived collagen hydrolysate, promotes recovery of collagen fibers and normal elastic fibers in the skin from degraded collagen and abnormal elastic fibers caused by UVB irradiation in hairless mice [167]. Kim et.al, 2018 reported that LMWCP is a safe health functional food ingredient with anti-skin photoaging efficacy which can effectively improve hydration, elasticity, and wrinkling in human skin at the dose of 1000 mg once daily [168].

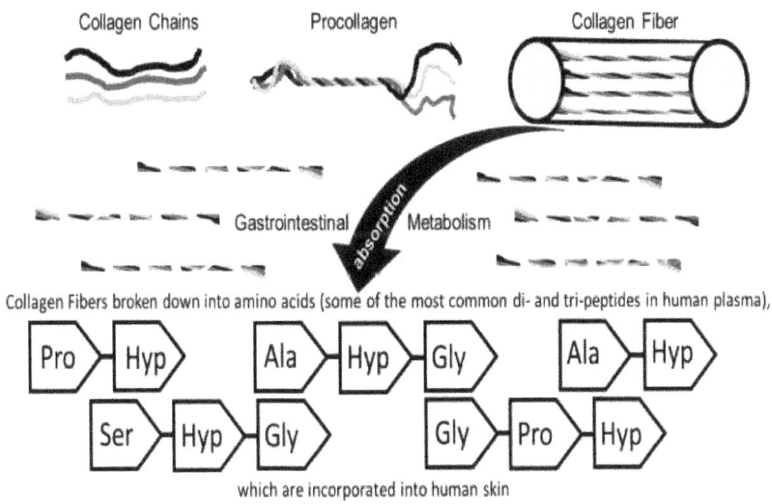

Figure 4.15 Collagen fiber structure, absorption/metabolism and deposition into skin cells and dermal layers. It is generally thought that collagen (derived products) are hydrolyzed into amino acids in the GIT prior to being absorbed into the blood circulation, which are then deposited into the skin cells and/or utilized as building block components for extracellular matrix proteins produced by fibroblasts. ALA = Alanine, HYP = Hydroxyproline, GLY = Glycine, PRO = Proline, and Ser = Serine.

Oral supplementation with collagen bioactive peptides (hydrolyzed fish collagen) combined with chondroitin sulphate, glucosamine, L-carnitine, vitamins, and minerals significantly improved the clinical parameters related to skin aging and joint health [169]. Lee et.al, 2019 reported that orally administering collagen peptide NS (CPNS) to rats, the plasma concentrations of Gly-Pro and Pro-Hyp increased dramatically. The CPNS consumption significantly attenuated UVB-induced wrinkle formation, transepidermal water loss, and epidermis thickness, and increased skin hydration [170]. An association between oral administration of collagen peptides combined with vitamin C and extracts of *Hibiscus sabdariffa* and *Aristotelia chilensis* was observed by Addor et.al, 2018. Female adult patients received an oral nutritional supplement from a sachet and were instructed to consume 1 sachet diluted in 200 mL of water once daily for 12 weeks. Clinical evaluation by high frequency ultrasound and cutometry showed significant improvement of firmness and elasticity and an increase in dermal thickness by ultrasound after 3 months of use [171]. Zague et al, 2018 reported that collagen peptides modulate the metabolism of extracellular matrix proteins by human dermal fibroblasts (in culture) that were derived from sun-protected and sun-exposed body sites [172]. Song et al, 2017 examined the effects of collagen hydrolysates from sliver carp skin on UV-induced photo-aging in mice and found that LMW peptides exerted beneficial effects when compared to high molecular weight CHs on HA levels and moisture content of the skin [173].

Exhibit 10. Summary of natural compounds and minerals used as supplement for skin health [174]

Natural Compound or Mineral	Mechanism of Action(s) Involved in Maintaining Skin Health
1. Collagen	Building block of collagen and elastin fibers-improves skin and nail health; inhibits matrix metalloproteinases (MMPs); stimulates fibroblast function
2. Ceramides	Provides the major component of the lipid "mortar" of the stratum corneum essential in the structure and maintenance of skin barrierintegrity; also involved in cell proliferation, differentiation and apoptosis
3. Beta Carotene	Provitamin A molecule, acts as an antioxidant, anti-inflammatory agent and blocks ROS formation and/or ability to quench free radicals; prevents cellular damage, premature skin aging and skin cancer

Contd...

Natural Compound or Mineral	Mechanism of Action(s) Involved in Maintaining Skin Health
4. Astaxanthin	Potent antioxidant; anti-inflammatory agent; prevents DNA damage & enhance mitochondrial function, provides UV protection; activates the Nrf2 pathway toto stimulate production of other antioxidants; inhibits MMPs; stimulates collagen production and wound healing
5. Coenzyme Q10	Antioxidant; anti-aging properties-enhances collagen; potential treatment for psoriasis; accelerates generation of ATP levels after irradiation of fibroblasts
6. Colostrum	Contains, growth factors and other immune regulatory factors that promote growth of keratinocytes and wound healing
7. Zinc	Importance for skin morphogenesis, repair and maintenance such as wound healing
8. Selenium	Acts as a cofactor for glutathione peroxidase (GPX) removing harmful peroxides; involved in DNA synthesis and repair; prevents oxidative stress and UVB-radiation; also acts as an antioxidant

B. Probiotics

Lactic acid bacteria consist of 26 genera now, and play an essential role in the food industry in the manufacture of many fermented products (cheese, yogurt, fermented vegetables, etc.). Application of these organisms is now being extended to the area of health improvement, as their probiotic activities become known. *Lactococcus lactis* H61 improved skin status in Japanese women with oral intake of heat-killed or live cells. With regard to live cells in fermented milk made by strain H61, the reported effects are attractive and it is expected that consumption of H61-fermented milk will increase [175]. It is also reported that oral intake of *Lactobacillus rhamnosus* SP1 improves the appearance of adult acne [176]. Oral intake of yoghurt made by using *Lactobacillus delbrueckii* subsp. bulgaricus 2038 plus *Streptococcus thermophilus* 1131 for 4 weeks improved skin elasticity and the degree of dryness in cheeks of women [177]. Mori et al, 2016 also reported that the intake of fermented milk containing *Bifidobacterium breve* strain Yakult plus galactooligosaccharides for 4 weeks increased hydration levels of the stratum corneum in women [178].

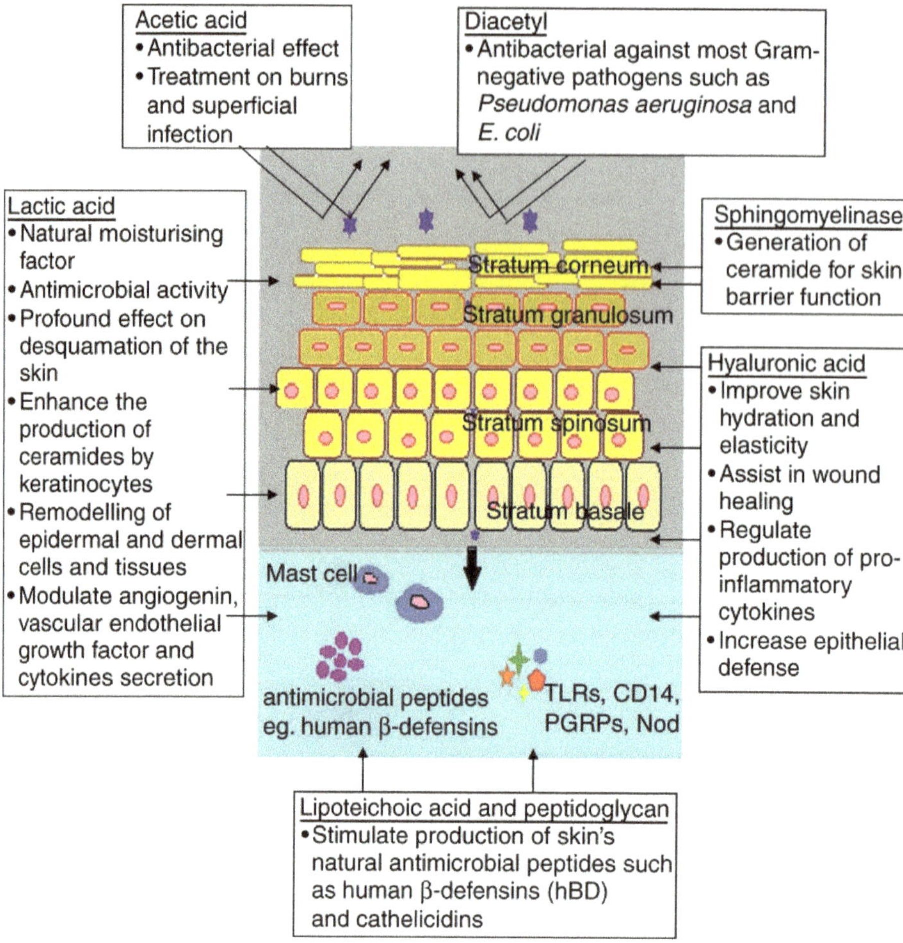

Figure 4.16 Bio-actives from probiotics for dermal applications [113].

C. Astaxanthin

Astaxanthin is ubiquitous in nature, especially found in the marine environment as a red-orange pigment common to many aquatic animals such as salmonids, shrimp, and crayfish. The ROS lead to skin aging via oxidative damage that are induced by UVR. Therefore, topical formulations which have antioxidant effect could reduce aging level [200]. Eren et.al, 2019 reported that topical formulations of astaxanthin-loaded algae extract could be suggested as topical anti-aging formulations [199]. Comparative studies examining the photoprotective effects of carotenoids have demonstrated that astaxanthin is a superior antioxidant, having greater antioxidant capacity than canthaxanthin and β-carotene in human dermal fibroblasts [200]. In particular, astaxanthin inhibits ROS formation and modulates the expression of oxidative stress-responsive enzymes such as heme oxygenase-1 (HO-1), which is a marker of oxidative stress and a regulatory mechanism involved in the cell adaptation against oxidative damage [205].

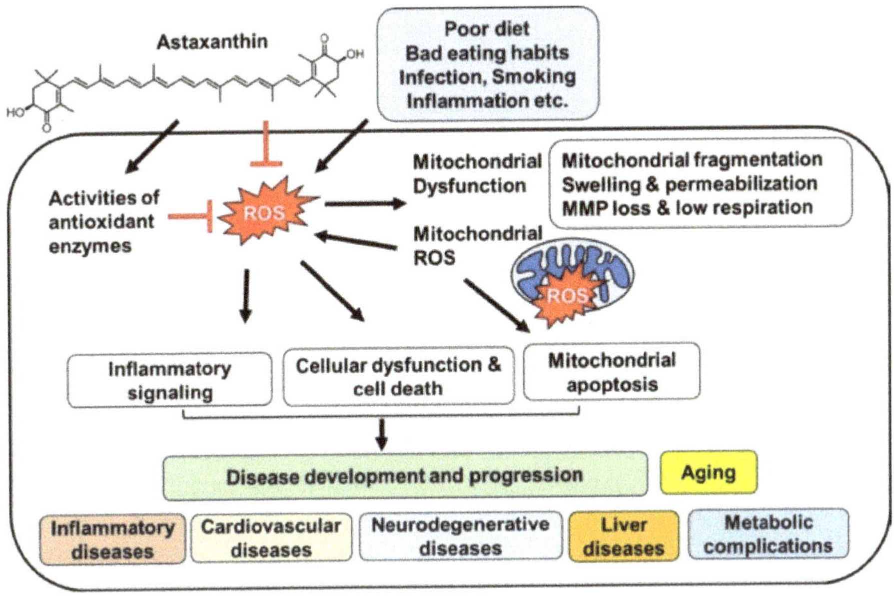

Figure 4.17 The proposed mechanism by which astaxanthin inhibits oxidative stress-induced mitochondrial dysfunction, and development and progression of diseases [211].

Astaxanthin exerts significant antioxidant activities not only via direct radical scavenging, but also by activating the cellular antioxidant defense system through modulation of the nuclear factor erythroid 2-related factor (Nrf2) pathway. Fang et.al, 2017 demonstrated that astaxanthin protected against early burn-wound progression by attenuating ROS-induced oxidative stress in a rat deep-burn model [201]. In vitro, astaxanthin effectively suppresses cell damage caused by free radicals and induction of MMP-1 in skin after UV irradiation [202]. Chou et.al, 2016 reported that an enriched astaxanthin extract from *H. pluvialis* increased collagen content through inhibition of MMP-1 and MMP-3 expression in human dermal fibroblasts [203]. Meephansan et.al, 2017 reported that astaxanthin-treated wounds in mice showed significantly increased expression of wound healing biological markers such as collagen type I α 1 (Col1A1) and basic fibroblast growth factor (bFGF) [204]. The immunomodulatory action of astaxanthin has been also reported in dogs and cats, enhancing both cell-mediated and humoral immune responses. In these studies, astaxanthin increased natural killer (NK) cell cytotoxic activity, suggesting that astaxanthin may regulate NK cells that serve as an immunosurveillance system against tumors and virus-infected cells [206,207]. Astaxanthin is reported to improve the DNA repair capacity of cells exposed to

UV radiation. In particular, astaxanthin was capable of minimizing DNA damage and influencing the kinetics of DNA repair [208]. Human cells possess multiple protection mechanisms against UV-induced ROS, either by preventing damage or by damage repair. Camera et.al, 2009 reported that astaxanthin inhibits the UV-induced DNA damage and increases the expression of oxidative stress-responsive enzymes [209]. Tominaga et.al, 2017 suggested that long-term prophylactic astaxanthin supplementation may inhibit age-related skin deterioration and maintain skin conditions associated with environmentally induced damage via its anti-inflammatory effect [210].

D. Colostrum

Colostrum is the initial milk or "first milk" that is produced by mammals (including humans) immediately following parturition. As expected, colostrum was more effective than milk with the total lipid, linoleic acid, linolenic acid, ganglioside, and glycolipid contents were higher in colostrum when compared to milk. In addition, with further analysis, the fat globule fraction provided the strongest stimulation for wound repair that contained Epidermal Growth Factors. The milk fluid produced by all female mammalian species after birth has the function to meet the complete nutritional requirements of the neonate and, at the same time, provide all of the biochemical needs and support the many biological functions of the immature newborn to help the newborn survive and develop. Starting in the 1980s and through the mid-1990s, supplemented cell culture medium with milk or colostrum was reported to improve the growth rate of many cell types including skin (fibroblasts). Peptides from milk protein hydrolysates improved the growth of human keratinocytes in culture. Medium supplemented with 300 μg/mL for 12 days where the average molecular weight of 800 Da containing a high concentration of amino acids promoted the growth of the keratinocytes by 108% [174]. Colostrum is the only known natural source of the enzyme, telomerase, which may help to slow down the aging of DNA. There is evidence that short telomeres and a lack of telomerase can exert a longevity-promoting effect via the prevention of cancer [212]. Colostrum also includes EGF and IGF-1, which are known to assist in the repair and regeneration of cells. EGF and IGF-1 play essential roles in wound healing, which makes colostrum an important potential adjunct to the skin's repair following a surgical cosmetic procedure. Let's not forget about the lactoferrin in colostrum, either. Lactoferrin helps manage the immune response in the skin cells, which means supplementing with lactoferrin may potentially help a person increase his or her skin's anti-inflammatory response [213].

E. Selenium

Selenium (Se) is an essential trace element in the human body and plays an important role in the body via selenoprotein, which contains selenium. Selenoproteins (glutathione peroxidase, thioredoxin reductase, methionine sulfoxide reductase-1 and endoplasmic reticulum-selenoproteins, etc.) have antioxidant effects and are involved in regulating antioxidant activities [217]. Se and the selenoproteins are essential for keratinocyte function and skin development. A lack of selenoenzymes in the mouse epidermis leads to abnormalities in the skin and hair follicles, premature skin aging, and premature death. Additionally, several studies have shown that Se pretreatment can drastically protect keratinocytes, melanocytes, and fibroblasts from UV-induced cytotoxicity. Low doses of Se were very potently protective against UVA-induced cytotoxicity in young keratinocytes, whereas the aged keratinocytes require four times more Se than the young keratinocytes to be protected from UVA-induced cytotoxicity [218,219]. Se protects keratinocyte stem cells (KSCs) against senescence via preservation of their stemness phenotype through adhesion to the basement membrane [219]. Wang et. al, 2017 showed that Vitamin C (250 mg/kg), vitamin E (250 mg/kg) and Se (0.2 mg/kg) exerted antioxidant effects and consequently may prevent skin damage caused by streptozotocin-induced diabetes (65 mg/kg) in Swiss albino rats [220].

F. Hyaluronic Acid

Hyaluronic acid (HA) is part of the body's connective tissues, and is known to cushion and lubricate. Aging destroys HA. Diet and smoking can also affect your body's level of HA over time. Skin care products with HA are most frequently used to treat wrinkled skin although they don't replace anything the body has naturally lost. These are very effective moisturizers [119]. UV radiation damage causes initially a mild form of wound healing and is associated at first with an increase of dermal HA. As little as 5 min of UV exposure in nude mice caused enhanced deposition of HA, indicating that UV radiation induced skin damage is an extremely rapid event. The initial redness of the skin following exposure to UV radiation may be due to a mild edematous reaction induced by the enhanced HA deposition and histamine release. Repeated and extensive exposures to UV ultimately simulate a typical wound healing response with deposition of scarlike type I collagen, rather than the usual types I and III collagen mixture that gives skin resilience and pliability [120]. HA based formulations (i.e., gels, creams, intra-dermal filler injections, dermal fillers, facial fillers, autologous fat gels, lotion, serum, and implants, etc.) exhibit remarkable anti-wrinkle, anti-nasolabial fold, anti-aging, space-filling, and face rejuvenating properties. This has been achieved via soft tissue augmentation, improved skin hydration, collagen and elastin stimulation, and face volume restoration. HA, alone or in combination with lidocaine and other co-agents, showed promising efficacy in skin tightness and elasticity, face rejuvenation, improving aesthetic scores, reducing the wrinkle scars, longevity, and tear trough rejuvenation [125]. Sparavigna et.al, 2019 reported significant improvement of wrinkles' grade around the eyes, vertical lip lines and wrinkles' severity of nasolabial folds after the first injection and the effect increased after the second injection. Aging/photoaging grade and surface microrelief improved

2 months after the first injection procedure. The treatments were very well tolerated by the volunteers as determined by the self-grading score [121]. Lee et.al, 2019 reported that Cross-linked hyaluronic acid (CLHA) patches were not an irritant, whereas a clinical study showed that application of single CLHA patches significantly improved skin hydration at the periorbital region for 3 days and at the nasolabial fold for 6 days. Patch application also improved superficial wrinkles at the periorbital region for 3 days and at the nasolabial fold for 1 day. The absence of side effects indicated that application of these CLHA microstructure patches is both safe and convenient for moisturization and anti-wrinkle effects [122]. Jeon et.al, 2019 reported that CTP-EGF has a superior ability, compared with natural EGF, to permeate skin and induce HA synthesis and collagen formation. Thus, it has great potential to be used in cosmetics and therapeutic agents to improve wrinkles and the health of the skin [123]. There exist many different types of HA gel fillers that differ in their HA concentration, particle size, cross-linking density, duration, and presence of lidocaine. High-density, large-particle fillers are recommended for deep dermal injections while the low-density, small-particle fillers are recommended for fine lines. HA gel is used by several healthcare professionals include the plastic surgeon, primary care provider, dermatologist, nurse practitioner and internist to enhance cosmesis. HA fillers are injected to restore volume lost due to age or disease, provide facial contour, and help maintain a youthful appearance. Filler injection has become one of the most commonly performed procedures in a dermatology cosmetic practice [124].

G. Poly-L-lactic acid

Poly-L-lactic acid (PLLA) is an injectable filler used for restoring facial fat volume loss. Polydioxanone Cog thread and poly-L-lactic acid (PLLA) thread have been used clinically for lifting and antiaging purposes [221]. PLLA is an effective treatment for patients seeking to correct volume loss due to aging. Although the US FDA has approved PLLA for use in people with HIV in 2004, it is well-suited for patients seeking cosmetic treatment. By 2009 PLLA was FDA-approved for the correction of nasolabial fold contour deficiencies and other lines and wrinkles. There have since been limited but promising results with off-label use of PLLA for non-facial volumization as well, including the hands, neck/décolleté, abdomen, and gluteal area [222]. PLLA is a safe, biodegradable volumizer used to reverse the signs of aging by gradually correcting volume loss. Patients should be aware of possible adverse reactions during the course of treatment [221]. Injection of PLLA in the deep dermis or subcutaneous tissue may cause an immediate augmentation of the treated tissue. This is a temporary but immediate response that is due to tissue edema and fluid from the reconstitution of the product. It will resolve within 2 to 3 days after injection. Once the carrier substance is absorbed, the poly-L-lactic acid particles induce an inflammatory response through phagocytosis by tissue macrophages. This is a similar process to suture reabsorption in the skin. The inflammatory response breaks down the poly-L-lactic acid into lactic acid monomers and is then metabolized to carbon dioxide and water while stimulating the production of new collagen type-I fibers in the skin. Approximately half of the product is digested within 6 months. The duration of action is 12 to 24 months [223]. Kapicioğlu et.al, 2019 reported that PLLA and Cog sutures were effective in facial rejuvenation (studied in female rats); both increased dermis thickness and stimulated collagen production [110]. Repeated PLLA treatments may improve skin quality in a time-dependent manner. Pigmentation, erythema, and pore size were significantly decreased, whereas radiance and smoothness were significantly increased at 12 months. No treatment-related adverse events occurred. Repeated PLLA treatments may improve skin quality in a time-dependent manner [111]. The process of hydration, loss of cohesion and molecular weight, and solubilization and phagocytosis of PLA by the host's macrophages, degrades PLA into lactic acid microspheres and eliminates CO2 by way of respiratory excretion. Crystals are left behind to stimulate collagen and a granulomatous reaction. This inflammatory reaction elicits resorption and the formation of fibrous connective tissue about the foreign body, causing dermal fibroplasia that leads to the desired cosmetic effect [2]. Kim et.al, 2019 reported that powdered polydioxanone injection induces collagen formation more effectively than PLLA injection [223].

H. Hormone Replacement Therapy

In postmenopausal women, dermal collagen decreases, and skin becomes thinner [241]. Hormone replacement therapy (HRT) is shown tobe effective in alleviating menopausal symptoms. However, its use is controversial owing to potential health risks, such as thromboembolism and cancer. Bioidentical hormone therapy has also been used by dermatologists for its anti-aging effects on the skin, but little is known about efficacy and side effects of bioidentical hormones in this field [236]. Women's Health Initiative (WHI) study showed a higher risk for breast cancer, stroke, cardiovascular disease, and thromboembolic events with combined treatment of estrogens and progestin. Synthetic progestins mostly used worldwide include medroxyprogesterone acetate (most frequently used in the US), norethidrone acetate, cyproteron acetate, norgestimate, norgestrel, and dydrogesterone [238]. The HRT impact on skin thickness and dermal density was demonstrated early when estrogens were initially administered to postmenopausal women. Such replenishment therapy was therefore considered as an attempt at alleviating in part skin atrophy and xerosis in postmenopausal women. Indeed, HRT controls in part the dermal thickness and laxity, and the collagen content and density, as well as the tissue mechanical reactivity to stress [237]. Physicians and patients have become extremely reluctant concerning HRT following the WHI study. Numbers of HRT prescriptions in the US rose from 58 million in 1995 to 90 million in 1999, corresponding to 15 million women per year. Numbers remained stable through to 2002. Within 3 months after publication of the results of the WHI study, prescriptions of various formulations of combined estrogens and progesterone dropped by 33% to 66% [238]. Vinogradova et.al, 2019 reported association between risk of venous thromboembolism and different types of HRT. Transdermal treatment was the safest type of hormone replacement therapy when risk of venous thromboembolism was assessed. Transdermal treatment appears to be underused, with the overwhelming preference still for oral preparations [239]. Both oral and transdermal estradiol caused a significant decrease in FSH while only transdermal resulted in a significant decrease in LH.The oral estradiol, though not transdermal estradiol, increased serum high density lipoprotein, thyroxine binding protein and growth hormone binding protein [240]. Applying estrogen cream to the skin after menopause improves the external appearance of facial skin [241]. There is strong evidence that transdermal estradiol has a cardioprotective effect [243]. Due to their lack of first-pass hepatic metabolism, transdermal products achieve clinical benefits while minimizing patient exposure to estrogens, which is consistent with the most recent clinical guidelines [244]. Also, by increasing skin collagen content, and increasing acid mucopolysaccharides and HA, estrogen therapy encourages the growth and development of vaginal epithelial cells which make up the thick layers of the vaginal wall, and condone a moist, supple and elastic environment [242]. Botelho et.al, 2014 reported that nanostructured formulation of progesterone (10%) combined with estriol (0.1%) + estradiol (0.25%) is safe and effective in re-establishing optimal serum levels of estradiol and follicle-stimulating hormone and relieving the symptoms of menopause [243]. Abdi et.al, 2017 also concluded that the use of transdermal nano-formulations in hormone therapy can relieve climacteric symptoms and prevent other postmenopausal symptoms [245].

EPILOGUE

As more and more anti-ageing and antioxidant skin care products flood the market, there is growing concern about definitions and experimental proof of effectiveness. The physician has an important role in understanding which treatment options are appropriate for mild, moderate, and severe photoaging, and in educating patients on the risks and benefits of each. The choice of the right active compounds, the verification of their activity inside a cosmetic formulation, their stability and synergistic effects should be the first step toward the creation of modern and effective products. To be active inside the skin, the antioxidants have to penetrate into the living layers of the skin, where free radicals are generated and should be effective against ROS. This is possible only if the topical applied formulation holds the potential to be effective. Moisturizing and emollient products are gaining increasing importance in dry skin treatment, maintenance of daily care of normal skin as well as ancillary therapy of many skin diseases.

Consumers are nowadays more focused on their health and appearance. As a result, there has been an increasing demand in topical antiaging formulations with natural and nutraceutical ingredients. Novel and innovative delivery systems are transforming the new product development in the cosmetic field because of consumer perceivable benefits and optimized sensory attributes. The applications of novel drug delivery systems can be found in many cosmetic products. Nanomaterials are nowadays used in almost all the major cosmetic industries. The truth is, there is no magic pill at present that will retard aging. But that is not to say there are not simple lifestyle and dietary adjustments that can make people live longer. A cosmetic product that produces clinically objective effects on the most-reported signs of aging is an attractive option for those unable to avoid extrinsic aging factors but wishing to improve their appearance without resorting to more invasive measures.

SUMMARY

Skin care products with antioxidative and anti-aging claims are one of the most fast-growing markets for cosmetics worldwide. Anti-aging in dermatology primarily focuses on the prevention of skin aging with UV protection (clothing and sunscreens), free radical scavengers (synthetic or botanic), and cell-protecting agents. Many synthetic and natural products have been reported to enhance levels of antioxidant enzymes, which make them therapeutic candidates to mitigate UV-mediated damage and to prevent the health consequences of UV exposure. Topical hormonal prescriptions are also an option if UV damage has not been the leading culprit for aging. Chemical peeling leads to a marked increase in collagen formation, the deeper the better. Ingredients in cream preparations can reduce superficial skin folds (polyphenols, amino acid peptides). Modulators of regular pigmentation are important for anti-aging preparations. New approaches are being designed to exploit the signaling pathways to delay or even prevent free-radical induced symptoms of aging. There are too many products on the market, from so many brands, with more and more ingredients, and at various price points. Selecting the right anti-aging product is a daunting task, but this guide is meant to simplify the process and help to choose the right anti-aging skin care products for an individual skin.

ABBREVIATIONS

luteinizing hormone (LH); follicle stimulating hormone (FSH); adrenocorticotropic hormone (ACTH); growth hormone (GH); Transforming growth factor beta (TGF-β); matrix metalloproteinases (MMPs); activator protein-1 (AP-1); glycosaminoglycan (GAG); Reactive oxygen species (ROS); 4-hydroxy-2-nonenal (HNE); particulate matter (PM2.5); transepidermal water loss (TEWL); glycation end products (AGEs); National Health and Nutrition Examination Surveys (NHANES); Dutch Healthy Diet Index (DHDI); principal component analysis (PCA); carboxymethyl lysine (CML); dermal White Adipose Tissue (dWAT); Peroxisome Proliferator-Activated Receptor γ (PPARγ); hypothalamic-pituitary-adrenal (HPA);Glucocorticoid receptors (GRs); nuclear receptor subfamily 3 group C member 1 (NR3C1); Pulsed electromagnetic fields (PEMFs); Multipolar Magnetic Pulse (MP)2; sun protection factor (SPF); Epidermal growth factor (EGF); cytoplasmic transduction peptide (CTP); ferric-reducing activity of plasma (FRAP); sodium-dependent vitamin C transporters (SVCTs); matrix metalloproteinase-1 (MMP-1); epithelial/epidermal growth factor (EGF); insulin-like growth factor (IGF-1); nuclear factor erythroid 2-related factor (Nrf2); collagen type I α 1 (Col1A1); basic fibroblast growth factor (bFGF)

BIBLIOGRAPHY AND WEBLIOGRAPHY

1. Quiroga RM. Chapter 1. Anti-Aging Medicine As It Relates to Dermatology. In: Cheryl M. Burgess. Cosmetic Dermatology, published by Springer Science & Business Media, 2005 ISBN 3540230645, 9783540230649
2. Ganceviciene R, Liakou AI, Theodoridis A, Makrantonaki E, Zouboulis CC. Skin anti-aging strategies. Dermatoendocrinol. 2012 Jul 1;4(3):308-19. doi: 10.4161/derm.22804. PubMed PMID: 23467476; PubMed Central PMCID: PMC3583892.
3. Bhatt N, Agrawal S, Mehta K. Risk factors and self-perception for facial aging among Nepalese population. J Cosmet Dermatol. 2019 Feb 17. doi: 10.1111/jocd.12885. [Epub ahead of print] PubMed PMID: 30772949.
4. Addor FAS. Beyond photoaging: additional factors involved in the process of skin aging. Clin CosmetInvestig Dermatol. 2018 Sep 20;11:437-443. doi: 10.2147/CCID.S177448. eCollection 2018. Review. PubMed PMID: 30288075; PubMed Central PMCID: PMC6159789.
5. Asakura K, Nishiwaki Y, Milojevic A, Michikawa T, Kikuchi Y, Nakano M, Iwasawa S, Hillebrand G, Miyamoto K, Ono M, Kinjo Y, Akiba S, Takebayashi T. Lifestyle factors and visible skin aging in a population of Japanese elders. J Epidemiol. 2009;19(5):251-9. Epub 2009 Aug 22. PubMed PMID: 19700917; PubMed Central PMCID: PMC3924128.
6. Tito A, Barbulova A, Zappelli C, Leone M, Ruvo M, Mercurio FA, Chambery A, Russo R, Colucci MG, Apone F. The Growth Differentiation Factor 11 is Involved in Skin Fibroblast Ageing and is Induced by a Preparation of Peptides and Sugars Derived from Plant Cell Cultures. Mol Biotechnol. 2019 Mar;61(3):209-220. doi: 10.1007/s12033-019-00154-w. PubMed PMID: 30661170.
7. Barone F, Bashey S, Woodin Jr. FW. Clinical Evidence of Dermal and Epidermal Restructuring from a Biologically Active Growth Factor Serum for Skin Rejuvenation. J Drugs Dermatol. 2019 Mar 1;18(3):290-295. PubMed PMID: 30909351.
8. Clarys P, Barel AO. Chapter 27. New Trends in Antiaging Cosmetic Ingredients and Treatments: An Overview. In: André O. Barel, Marc Paye, Howard I. Maibach. Handbook of Cosmetic Science and Technology, 3rd Edition, published by CRC Press, 2014. ISBN 9781842145647
9. LecciaMT, Lebbe C, Claudel JP, Narda M, Basset-Seguin N. New Vision in Photoprotection and Photorepair. Dermatol Ther (Heidelb). 2019 Mar;9(1):103-

115. doi: 10.1007/s13555-019-0282-5. Epub 2019 Jan 23. Review. PubMed PMID: 30674003; PubMed Central PMCID: PMC6380982.

10. KarapetsasA, Voulgaridou GP, Konialis M, Tsochantaridis I, Kynigopoulos S, Lambropoulou M, Stavropoulou MI, Stathopoulou K, Aligiannis N, Bozidis P, Goussia A, Gardikis K, Panayiotidis MI, Pappa A. Propolis Extracts Inhibit UV-Induced Photodamage in Human Experimental In Vitro Skin Models. Antioxidants (Basel). 2019 May 9;8(5). pii: E125. doi: 10.3390/antiox8050125. PubMed PMID: 31075866.
11. Zhang S, Duan E. Fighting against Skin Aging: The Way from Bench to Bedside. Cell Transplant. 2018 May;27(5):729-738. doi: 10.1177/0963689717725755. Epub 2018 Apr 25. Review. PubMed PMID: 29692196; PubMed Central PMCID: PMC6047276.
12. Krutmann J, Bouloc A, Sore G, Bernard BA, Passeron T. The skin aging exposome. J Dermatol Sci. 2017 Mar;85(3):152-161. doi: 10.1016/j.jdermsci.2016.09.015. Epub 2016 Sep 28. Review. PubMed PMID: 27720464.
13. Cho S, Shin MH, Kim YK, Seo JE, Lee YM, Park CH, Chung JH. Effects of infrared radiation and heat on human skin aging in vivo. J Investig Dermatol Symp Proc. 2009 Aug;14(1):15-9. doi: 10.1038/jidsymp.2009.7. Review. PubMed PMID: 19675547.
14. Kettelhut EA, Traylor J, Roach JP. Erythema Ab Igne. [Updated 2019 Feb 10]. In: StatPearls [Internet]. Treasure Island (FL): StatPearls Publishing; 2019 Jan-. Available from: https://www.ncbi.nlm.nih.gov/books/NBK538250/
15. PecorelliA, Woodby B, Prieux R, Valacchi G. Involvement of 4-hydroxy-2-nonenal in pollution-induced skin damage. Biofactors. 2019 May 14. doi: 10.1002/biof.1513. [Epub ahead of print] Review. PubMed PMID: 31087730.
16. Burke KE, Wei H. Synergistic damage by UVA radiation and pollutants. Toxicol Ind Health. 2009 May-Jun;25(4-5):219-24. doi: 10.1177/0748233709106067. Review. PubMed PMID: 19651790.
17. Ding A, Yang Y, Zhao Z, Hüls A, Vierkötter A, Yuan Z, Cai J, Zhang J, Gao W, Li J, Zhang M, Matsui M, Krutmann J, Kan H, Schikowski T, Jin L, Wang S. Indoor PM(2.5) exposure affects skin aging manifestation in a Chinese population. Sci Rep. 2017 Nov 10;7(1):15329. doi: 10.1038/s41598-017-15295-8. PubMed PMID: 29127390; PubMed Central PMCID: PMC5681690.
18. Schikowski T, Krutmann J. [Air pollution (particulate matter and nitrogen dioxide) and skin aging]. Hautarzt. 2019 Mar;70(3):158-162. doi: 10.1007/s00105-018-4338-8. Review. German. PubMed PMID: 30627745.
19. Park SY, Byun EJ, Lee JD, Kim S, Kim HS. Air Pollution, Autophagy, and Skin Aging: Impact of Particulate Matter (PM(10)) on Human Dermal Fibroblasts. Int J Mol Sci. 2018 Sep 12;19(9). pii: E2727. doi: 10.3390/ijms19092727. PubMed PMID: 30213068; PubMed Central PMCID: PMC6163910.
20. Urbańska M, Nowak G, Florek E. [Cigarette smoking and its influence on skin aging]. Przegl Lek. 2012;69(10):1111-4. Review. Polish. PubMed PMID: 23421102.

21. Wang AS, Dreesen O. Biomarkers of Cellular Senescence and Skin Aging. Front Genet. 2018 Aug 23;9:247. doi: 10.3389/fgene.2018.00247. eCollection 2018. Review. PubMed PMID: 30190724; PubMed Central PMCID: PMC6115505.
22. Sundelin T, Lekander M, Sorjonen K, Axelsson J. Negative effects of restricted sleep on facial appearance and social appeal. R Soc Open Sci. 2017 May 17;4(5):160918. doi: 10.1098/rsos.160918. eCollection 2017 May. PubMed PMID: 28572989; PubMed Central PMCID: PMC5451790.
23. Walia HK, Mehra R. Overview of Common Sleep Disorders and Intersection with Dermatologic Conditions. Int J Mol Sci. 2016 Apr 30;17(5). pii: E654. doi: 10.3390/ijms17050654. Review. PubMed PMID: 27144559; PubMed Central PMCID: PMC4881480.
24. Oyetakin-White P, Suggs A, Koo B, Matsui MS, Yarosh D, Cooper KD, Baron ED. Does poor sleep quality affect skin ageing? Clin Exp Dermatol. 2015 Jan;40(1):17-22. doi: 10.1111/ced.12455. Epub 2014 Sep 30. PubMed PMID: 25266053.
25. Clatici VG, Racoceanu D, Dalle C, Voicu C, Tomas-Aragones L, Marron SE, Wollina U, Fica S. Perceived Age and Life Style. The Specific Contributions of Seven Factors Involved in Health and Beauty. Maedica (Buchar). 2017 Sep;12(3):191-201. PubMed PMID: 29218067; PubMed Central PMCID: PMC5706759.
26. Anson G, Kane MA, Lambros V. Sleep Wrinkles: Facial Aging and Facial Distortion During Sleep. Aesthet Surg J. 2016 Sep;36(8):931-40. doi: 10.1093/asj/sjw074. Epub 2016 Jun 21. Review. PubMed PMID: 27329660.
27. Katta R, Desai SP. Diet and dermatology: the role of dietary intervention in skin disease. J Clin Aesthet Dermatol. 2014 Jul;7(7):46-51. Review. PubMed PMID: 25053983; PubMed Central PMCID: PMC4106357.
28. Schagen SK, Zampeli VA, Makrantonaki E, Zouboulis CC. Discovering the link between nutrition and skin aging. Dermatoendocrinol. 2012 Jul 1;4(3):298-307. doi: 10.4161/derm.22876. PubMed PMID: 23467449; PubMed Central PMCID: PMC3583891.
29. Pem D, Jeewon R. Fruit and Vegetable Intake: Benefits and Progress of Nutrition Education Interventions- Narrative Review Article. Iran J Public Health. 2015 Oct;44(10):1309-21. Review. PubMed PMID: 26576343; PubMed Central PMCID: PMC4644575.
30. Moore LV, Thompson FE, Demissie Z. Percentage of Youth Meeting Federal Fruit and Vegetable Intake Recommendations, Youth Risk Behavior Surveillance System, United States and 33 States, 2013. J AcadNutr Diet. 2017 Apr;117(4):545-553.e3. doi: 10.1016/j.jand.2016.10.012. Epub 2016 Dec 15. PubMed PMID: 27988220; PubMed Central PMCID: PMC5367980.
31. Bragazzi NL, Sellami M, Salem I, Conic R, Kimak M, Pigatto PDM, Damiani G. Fasting and Its Impact on Skin Anatomy, Physiology, and Physiopathology: A Comprehensive Review of the Literature. Nutrients. 2019 Jan 23;11(2). pii: E249. doi: 10.3390/nu11020249. Review. PubMed PMID: 30678053; PubMed Central PMCID: PMC6413166.

32. MekićS, Jacobs LC, Hamer MA, Ikram MA, Schoufour JD, Gunn DA, Kiefte-de Jong JC, Nijsten T. A healthy diet in women is associated with less facial wrinkles in a large Dutch population-based cohort. J Am Acad Dermatol. 2019 May;80(5):1358-1363.e2. doi: 10.1016/j.jaad.2018.03.033. Epub 2018 Mar 27. PubMed PMID: 29601935.
33. Cosgrove MC, Franco OH, Granger SP, Murray PG, Mayes AE. Dietary nutrient intakes and skin-aging appearance among middle-aged American women. Am J Clin Nutr. 2007 Oct;86(4):1225-31. Erratum in: Am J Clin Nutr. 2008 Aug;88(2):480. PubMed PMID: 17921406.
34. Mukhopadhyay P. Cleansers and their role in various dermatological disorders. Indian J Dermatol. 2011 Jan;56(1):2-6. doi: 10.4103/0019-5154.77542. PubMed PMID: 21572782; PubMed Central PMCID: PMC3088928.
35. Gfatter R, Hackl P, Braun F. Effects of soap and detergents on skin surface pH, stratum corneum hydration and fat content in infants. Dermatology. 1997;195(3):258-62. PubMed PMID: 9407174.
36. Kulthanan K, Maneeprasopchoke P, Varothai S, Nuchkull P. The pH of antiseptic cleansers. Asia Pac Allergy. 2014 Jan;4(1):32-6. doi: 10.5415/apallergy.2014.4.1.32. Epub 2014 Jan 31. PubMed PMID: 24527408; PubMed Central PMCID: PMC3921871.
37. Rosen J, Yosipovitch G. Skin Manifestations of Diabetes Mellitus. [Updated 2018 Jan 4]. In: Feingold KR, Anawalt B, Boyce A, et al., editors. Endotext [Internet]. South Dartmouth (MA): MDText.com, Inc.; 2000-. Available from: https://www.ncbi.nlm.nih.gov/books/NBK481900/
38. Waller JM, Maibach HI. Chapter 23. A Quantitative Approach to Age and Skin Structure and Function: Protein, Glycosaminoglycan, Water, and Lipid Content and Structure. In: André O. Barel, Marc Paye, Howard I. Maibach. Handbook of Cosmetic Science and Technology, 3rd Edition, published by CRC Press, 2014. ISBN 9781842145647
39. UruskaA, Gandecka A, Araszkiewicz A, Zozulinska-Ziolkiewicz D. Accumulation of advanced glycation end products in the skin is accelerated in relation to insulin resistance in people with Type 1 diabetes mellitus. Diabet Med. 2019 May;36(5):620-625. doi: 10.1111/dme.13921. Epub 2019 Feb 15. PubMed PMID: 30706538.
40. Pageon H, Zucchi H, Rousset F, Monnier VM, Asselineau D. Skin aging by glycation: lessons from the reconstructed skin model. Clin Chem Lab Med. 2014 Jan 1;52(1):169-74. doi: 10.1515/cclm-2013-0091. PubMed PMID: 23770560.
41. Kong JG, Park JB, Lee D, Park EY. Effect of high glucose on stress-induced senescence of nucleus pulposus cells of adult rats. Asian Spine J. 2015 Apr;9(2):155-61. doi: 10.4184/asj.2015.9.2.155. Epub 2015 Apr 15. PubMed PMID: 25901224; PubMed Central PMCID: PMC4404527.
42. Davalli P, Mitic T, Caporali A, Lauriola A, D'Arca D. ROS, Cell Senescence, and Novel Molecular Mechanisms in Aging and Age-Related Diseases. Oxid Med Cell Longev. 2016;2016:3565127. doi: 10.1155/2016/3565127. Epub 2016 May 10. Review. PubMed PMID: 27247702; PubMed Central PMCID: PMC4877482.

43. NoordamR, Gunn DA, Tomlin CC, Maier AB, Mooijaart SP, Slagboom PE, Westendorp RG, de Craen AJ, van Heemst D; Leiden Longevity Study Group. High serum glucose levels are associated with a higher perceived age. Age (Dordr). 2013 Feb;35(1):189-95. doi: 10.1007/s11357-011-9339-9. Epub 2011 Nov 20. PubMed PMID: 22102339; PubMed Central PMCID: PMC3543736.
44. Yoon HS, Baik SH, Oh CH. Quantitative measurement of desquamation and skin elasticity in diabetic patients. Skin Res Technol. 2002 Nov;8(4):250-4. PubMed PMID: 12423544.
45. Lyons TJ, Bailie KE, Dyer DG, Dunn JA, Baynes JW. Decrease in skin collagen glycation with improved glycemic control in patients with insulin-dependent diabetes mellitus. J Clin Invest. 1991 Jun;87(6):1910-5. PubMed PMID: 1904067; PubMed Central PMCID: PMC296942.
46. Sami K, Elshahat A, Moussa M, Abbas A, Mahmoud A. Image analyzer study of the skin in patients with morbid obesity and massive weight loss. Eplasty. 2015 Jan 23;15:e4. eCollection 2015. PubMed PMID: 25671051; PubMed Central PMCID: PMC4311578.
47. Kyrou I, Randeva HS, Tsigos C, et al. Clinical Problems Caused by Obesity. [Updated 2018 Jan 11]. In: Feingold KR, Anawalt B, Boyce A, et al., editors. Endotext [Internet]. South Dartmouth (MA): MDText.com, Inc.; 2000-. Available from: https://www.ncbi.nlm.nih.gov/books/NBK278973/
48. IbukiA, Kuriyama S, Toyosaki Y, Aiba M, Hidaka M, Horie Y, Fujimoto C, Isami F, Shibata E, Terauchi Y, Akase T. Aging-like physiological changes in the skin of Japanese obese diabetic patients. SAGE Open Med. 2018 Feb 6;6:2050312118756662. doi: 10.1177/2050312118756662. eCollection 2018. PubMed PMID: 29449943; PubMed Central PMCID: PMC5808963.
49. Rzepecki AK, Murase JE, Juran R, Fabi SG, McLellan BN. Estrogen-deficient skin: The role of topical therapy. Int J Womens Dermatol. 2019 Mar 15;5(2):85-90. doi: 10.1016/j.ijwd.2019.01.001. eCollection 2019 Jun. Review. PubMed PMID: 30997378; PubMed Central PMCID: PMC6451761.
50. Thornton MJ. Estrogens and aging skin. Dermatoendocrinol. 2013 Apr 1;5(2):264-70. doi: 10.4161/derm.23872. Review. PubMed PMID: 24194966; PubMed Central PMCID: PMC3772914.
51. Raine-Fenning NJ, Brincat MP, Muscat-Baron Y. Skin aging and menopause : implications for treatment. Am J Clin Dermatol. 2003;4(6):371-8. Review. PubMed PMID: 12762829.
52. O'Daniel TG. Multimodal management of atrophic acne scarring in the aging face. Aesthetic Plast Surg. 2011 Dec;35(6):1143-50. doi: 10.1007/s00266-011-9715-y. Epub 2011 Apr 14. Review. PubMed PMID: 21491169; PubMed Central PMCID: PMC3236289.
53. Dunn JH, Koo J. Psychological Stress and skin aging: a review of possible mechanisms and potential therapies. Dermatol Online J. 2013 Jun 15;19(6):18561. Review. PubMed PMID: 24011311.
54. MaaroufM, Maarouf CL, Yosipovitch G, Shi VY. The impact of stress on epidermal barrier function: an evidence-based review. Br J Dermatol. 2019 Jan 7. doi: 10.1111/bjd.17605. [Epub ahead of print] Review. PubMed PMID: 30614527.

55. Liu PZ, Nusslock R. How Stress Gets Under the Skin: Early Life Adversity and Glucocorticoid Receptor Epigenetic Regulation. Curr Genomics. 2018 Dec;19(8):653-664. doi: 10.2174/1389202919666171228164350. Review. PubMed PMID: 30532645; PubMed Central PMCID: PMC6225447.
56. Pie´rard GE, Pie´rard-Franchimont C, Quatresooz P. Chapter 22. Skin Ageprint: The Causative Factors. In: André O. Barel, Marc Paye, Howard I. Maibach. Handbook of Cosmetic Science and Technology, 3rd Edition, published by CRC Press, 2014. ISBN 9781842145647
57. Umar M, Sastry KS, Chouchane AI. Role of Vitamin D Beyond the Skeletal Function: A Review of the Molecular and Clinical Studies. Int J Mol Sci. 2018 May 30;19(6). pii: E1618. doi: 10.3390/ijms19061618. Review. PubMed PMID: 29849001; PubMed Central PMCID: PMC6032242.
58. Bartke A. Growth Hormone and Aging: Updated Review. World J Mens Health. 2019 Jan;37(1):19-30. doi: 10.5534/wjmh.180018. Epub 2018 May 11. Review. PubMed PMID: 29756419; PubMed Central PMCID: PMC6305861.
59. Ito N, Seki S, Ueda F. Effects of Composite Supplement Containing Collagen Peptide and Ornithine on Skin Conditions and Plasma IGF-1 Levels-A Randomized, Double-Blind, Placebo-Controlled Trial. Mar Drugs. 2018 Dec 3;16(12). pii: E482. doi: 10.3390/md16120482. PubMed PMID: 30513923; PubMed Central PMCID: PMC6315531.
60. Carroll PV, Christ ER, Bengtsson BA, Carlsson L, Christiansen JS, Clemmons D, Hintz R, Ho K, Laron Z, Sizonenko P, Sönksen PH, Tanaka T, Thorne M. Growth hormone deficiency in adulthood and the effects of growth hormone replacement: a review. Growth Hormone Research Society Scientific Committee. J Clin Endocrinol Metab. 1998 Feb;83(2):382-95. Review. PubMed PMID: 9467546.
61. Arlt W. Dehydroepiandrosterone and ageing. Best Pract Res Clin Endocrinol Metab. 2004 Sep;18(3):363-80. Review. PubMed PMID: 15261843.
62. Lee KS, Oh KY, Kim BC. Effects of dehydroepiandrosterone on collagen and collagenase gene expression by skin fibroblasts in culture. J Dermatol Sci. 2000 Jun;23(2):103-10. PubMed PMID: 10808127.
63. Calvo E, Luu-The V, Morissette J, Martel C, Labrie C, Bernard B, Bernerd F, Deloche C, Chaussade V, Leclaire J, Labrie F. Pangenomic changes induced by DHEA in the skin of postmenopausal women. J Steroid Biochem Mol Biol. 2008 Dec;112(4-5):186-93. doi: 10.1016/j.jsbmb.2008.10.008. Epub 2008 Nov 1. PubMed PMID: 19013239.
64. Kanda N, Watanabe S. Regulatory roles of sex hormones in cutaneous biology and immunology. J Dermatol Sci. 2005 Apr;38(1):1-7. Epub 2004 Dec 9. Review. PubMed PMID: 15795118.
65. Lephart ED. A review of the role of estrogen in dermal aging and facial attractiveness in women. J Cosmet Dermatol. 2018 Jun;17(3):282-288. doi: 10.1111/jocd.12508. Epub 2018 Feb 13. Review. PubMed PMID: 29436770.
66. Dyer JM, Miller RA. Chronic Skin Fragility of Aging: Current Concepts in the Pathogenesis, Recognition, and Management of Dermatoporosis. J Clin Aesthet Dermatol. 2018 Jan;11(1):13-18. Epub 2018 Jan 1. Review. PubMed PMID: 29410724; PubMed Central PMCID: PMC5788262.

67. Alexis AF, Obioha JO. Ethnicity and Aging Skin. J Drugs Dermatol. 2017 Jun 1;16(6):s77-s80. Review. PubMed PMID: 29028856.
68. Vashi NA, de Castro Maymone MB, Kundu RV. Aging Differences in Ethnic Skin. J ClinAesthet Dermatol. 2016 Jan;9(1):31-8. Review. PubMed PMID: 26962390; PubMed Central PMCID: PMC4756870.
69. Chan IL, Cohen S, da Cunha MG, Maluf LC. Characteristics and management of Asian skin. Int J Dermatol. 2019 Feb;58(2):131-143. doi: 10.1111/ijd.14153. Epub 2018 Jul 24. Review. PubMed PMID: 30039861.
70. CampicheR, Trevisan S, Séroul P, Rawlings AV, Adnet C, Imfeld D, Voegeli R. Appearance of aging signs in differently pigmented facial skin by a novel imaging system. J Cosmet Dermatol. 2019 Apr;18(2):614-627. doi: 10.1111/jocd.12806. Epub 2018 Oct 31. PubMed PMID: 30381859.
71. Alexis AF, Alam M. Racial and ethnic differences in skin aging: implications for treatment with soft tissue fillers. J Drugs Dermatol. 2012 Aug;11(8):s30-2; discussion s32. PubMed PMID: 22859226.
72. Vierkötter A, Krutmann J. Environmental influences on skin aging and ethnic-specific manifestations. Dermatoendocrinol. 2012 Jul 1;4(3):227-31. doi: 10.4161/derm.19858. PubMed PMID: 23467702; PubMed Central PMCID: PMC3583881.
73. Sugawara T, Nakagawa N, Shimizu N, Hirai N, Saijo Y, Sakai S. Gender- and age-related differences in facial sebaceous glands in Asian skin, as observed by non-invasive analysis using three-dimensional ultrasound microscopy. Skin Res Technol. 2019 May;25(3):347-354. doi: 10.1111/srt.12657. Epub 2019 Jan 4. PubMed PMID: 30609153.
74. Kim BY, Choi JW, Park KC, Youn SW. Sebum, acne, skin elasticity, and gender difference - which is the major influencing factor for facial pores? Skin Res Technol. 2013 Feb;19(1):e45-53. doi: 10.1111/j.1600-0846.2011.00605.x.Epub 2011 Dec 28. PubMed PMID: 22211382.
75. Rahrovan S, Fanian F, Mehryan P, Humbert P, Firooz A. Male versus female skin: What dermatologists and cosmeticians should know. Int J Womens Dermatol. 2018 Jun 22;4(3):122-130. doi: 10.1016/j.ijwd.2018.03.002. eCollection 2018 Sep. Review. PubMed PMID: 30175213; PubMed Central PMCID: PMC6116811.
76. TrojahnC, Dobos G, Lichterfeld A, Blume-Peytavi U, Kottner J. Characterizing facial skin ageing in humans: disentangling extrinsic from intrinsic biological phenomena. Biomed Res Int. 2015;2015:318586. doi: 10.1155/2015/318586. Epub2015 Feb 12. PubMed PMID: 25767806; PubMed Central PMCID: PMC4341846.
77. Xiong ZM, O'Donovan M, Sun L, Choi JY, Ren M, Cao K. Anti-Aging Potentials of Methylene Blue for Human Skin Longevity. Sci Rep. 2017 May 30;7(1):2475. doi: 10.1038/s41598-017-02419-3. PubMed PMID: 28559565; PubMed Central PMCID: PMC5449383.
78. Kruglikov IL, Scherer PE. Skin aging: are adipocytes the next target? Aging (Albany NY). 2016 Jul;8(7):1457-69. doi: 10.18632/aging.100999. Review. PubMed PMID: 27434510; PubMed Central PMCID: PMC4993342.

79. Bayerl C. [Skin aging and evidence-based topical strategies]. Hautarzt. 2016 Feb;67(2):140-7. doi: 10.1007/s00105-015-3737-3. German. PubMed PMID: 26683808.
80. Rodan K, Fields K, Majewski G, Falla T. Skincare Bootcamp: The Evolving Role of Skincare. PlastReconstr Surg Glob Open. 2016 Dec 14;4(12 Suppl Anatomy and Safety in Cosmetic Medicine: Cosmetic Bootcamp):e1152. doi: 10.1097/GOX.0000000000001152. eCollection 2016 Dec. PubMed PMID: 28018771; PubMed Central PMCID: PMC5172479.
81. Singer S, Karrer S, Berneburg M. Modern sun protection. CurrOpinPharmacol. 2019 Feb 4;46:24-28. doi: 10.1016/j.coph.2018.12.006. [Epub ahead of print] Review. PubMed PMID: 30731327.
82. AK Mohiuddin , (2019). Sunscreen and Suntan Preparations . ARC Journal of Pharmaceutical Sciences (AJPS), 5(2), pp.8 - 4 4 . DOI: http://dx.doi.org/ 10.20431/2455 - 1538 .0502002
83. Gabros S, Zito PM. Sunscreens And Photoprotection. [Updated 2019 Jan 13]. In: StatPearls [Internet]. Treasure Island (FL): StatPearls Publishing; 2019 Jan-. Available from: https://www.ncbi.nlm.nih.gov/books/NBK537164/
84. The American Society for Aesthetic Plastic Surgery (ASAPS) The American Society for Aesthetic Plastic Surgery Reports Americans Spent More Than 12 Billion in 2014: Procedures for Men Up 43% Over Five Year Period.
85. de Oliveira TC, Rocha SF, Ramos DG, Ramos CG, Carvalho MV, Ramos MG. Effects of Multipolar Radiofrequency and Pulsed Electromagnetic Field Treatment for Face and Neck Rejuvenation. Dermatol Res Pract. 2017;2017:4146391. doi: 10.1155/2017/4146391. Epub 2017 Mar 8. PubMed PMID: 28373880; PubMed Central PMCID: PMC5360959.
86. Gold MH. Noninvasive Skin Tightening Treatment. J Clin Aesthet Dermatol. 2015 Jun;8(6):14-8. PubMed PMID: 26155322; PubMed Central PMCID: PMC4479364.
87. Venus Legacy Body Shaping Featured on KTLA 5 News. Available From: https://www.venusconcept.com/en-us/news/venus-legacy-body-shaping-treatments-featured-on-ktla-5-news/
88. Lee YB, Eun YS, Lee JH, Cheon MS, Cho BK, Park HJ. Effects of multi-polar radiofrequency and pulsed electromagnetic field treatment in Koreans: case series and survey study. J Dermatolog Treat. 2014 Aug;25(4):310-3. doi: 10.3109/09546634.2012.714454. Epub 2012 Sep 19. PubMed PMID: 22812649.
89. Nassab R. The evidence behind noninvasive body contouring devices. Aesthet Surg J. 2015 Mar;35(3):279-93. doi: 10.1093/asj/sju063. Epub 2015 Feb 17. Review. PubMed PMID: 25691381.
90. Bissett DL Chapter 11. Anti-aging Skin Care Formulations. In: Zoe Diana Draelos, Lauren A. Thaman. Cosmetic Formulation of Skin Care Products Cosmetic Science and Technology, published by Taylor & Francis, 2005 ISBN 0849339685, 9780849339684
91. Mukherjee S, Date A, Patravale V, Korting HC, Roeder A, Weindl G. Retinoids in the treatment of skin aging: an overview of clinical efficacy and safety. Clin Interv

Aging. 2006;1(4):327-48. Review. PubMed PMID: 18046911; PubMed Central PMCID: PMC2699641.

92. Zito PM, Mazzoni T. Acitretin. [Updated 2018 Dec 2]. In: StatPearls [Internet]. Treasure Island (FL): StatPearls Publishing; 2019 Jan-. Available from: https://www.ncbi.nlm.nih.gov/books/NBK519571/
93. Kim MS, Lee S, Rho HS, Kim DH, Chang IS, Chung JH. The effects of a novel synthetic retinoid, seletinoid G, on the expression of extracellular matrix proteins in aged human skin in vivo. Clin Chim Acta. 2005 Dec;362(1-2):161-9. Epub 2005 Aug 1. PubMed PMID: 16055107.
94. Shao Y, He T, Fisher GJ, Voorhees JJ, Quan T. Molecular basis of retinol anti-ageing properties in naturally aged human skin in vivo. Int J Cosmet Sci. 2017 Feb;39(1):56-65. doi: 10.1111/ics.12348. Epub 2016 Jul 4. PubMed PMID: 27261203; PubMed Central PMCID: PMC5136519.
95. Graf J. Chapter 2. Anti-Aging Skin Care Ingredient. In: Technologies Anti-Aging Medicine As It Relates to Dermatology. In: Cheryl M. Burgess. Cosmetic Dermatology, published by Springer Science & Business Media, 2005 ISBN 3540230645, 9783540230649
96. Kong R, Cui Y, Fisher GJ, Wang X, Chen Y, Schneider LM, Majmudar G. A comparative study of the effects of retinol and retinoic acid on histological, molecular, and clinical properties of human skin. J Cosmet Dermatol. 2016 Mar;15(1):49-57. doi: 10.1111/jocd.12193. Epub 2015 Nov 18. PubMed PMID: 26578346.
97. BagatinE, Gonçalves HS, Sato M, Almeida LMC, Miot HA. Comparable efficacy of adapalene 0.3% gel and tretinoin 0.05% cream as treatment for cutaneous photoaging. Eur J Dermatol. 2018 Jun 1;28(3):343-350. doi: 10.1684/ejd.2018.3320. PubMed PMID: 30105991.
98. Fu JJ, Hillebrand GG, Raleigh P, Li J, Marmor MJ, Bertucci V, Grimes PE, Mandy SH, Perez MI, Weinkle SH, Kaczvinsky JR. A randomized, controlled comparative study of the wrinkle reduction benefits of a cosmetic niacinamide/peptide/retinyl propionate product regimen vs. a prescription 0.02% tretinoin product regimen. Br J Dermatol. 2010 Mar;162(3):647-54. doi: 10.1111/j.1365-2133.2009.09436.x. PubMed PMID: 20374604; PubMed Central PMCID: PMC2841824.
99. Kwon HS, Lee JH, Kim GM, Bae JM. Efficacy and safety of retinaldehyde 0.1% and 0.05% creams used to treat photoaged skin: A randomized double-blind controlled trial. J Cosmet Dermatol. 2018 Jun;17(3):471-476. doi: 10.1111/jocd.12551. Epub 2018 Apr 16. PubMed PMID: 29663701.
100. Sorg O, Saurat JH. Topical retinoids in skin ageing: a focused update with reference to sun-induced epidermal vitamin A deficiency. Dermatology. 2014;228(4):314-25. doi: 10.1159/000360527. Epub 2014 May 9. Review. PubMed PMID: 24821234.
101. Chaudhuri RK, Bojanowski K. Bakuchiol: a retinol-like functional compound revealed by gene expression profiling and clinically proven to have anti-aging effects. Int J Cosmet Sci. 2014 Jun;36(3):221-30. doi: 10.1111/ics.12117. Epub 2014 Mar 6. PubMed PMID: 24471735.

102. Dhaliwal S, Rybak I, Ellis SR, Notay M, Trivedi M, Burney W, Vaughn AR, Nguyen M, Reiter P, Bosanac S, Yan H, Foolad N, Sivamani RK. Prospective, randomized, double-blind assessment of topical bakuchiol and retinol for facial photoageing. Br J Dermatol. 2019 Feb;180(2):289-296. doi: 10.1111/bjd.16918. Epub 2018 Sep 21. PubMed PMID: 29947134.

103. Moghimipour E. Hydroxy Acids, the Most Widely Used Anti-aging Agents. Jundishapur J Nat Pharm Prod. 2012 Winter;7(1):9-10. Epub 2012 Jan 4. PubMed PMID: 24624144; PubMed Central PMCID: PMC3941867.

104. Tang SC, Tang LC, Liu CH, Liao PY, Lai JC, Yang JH. Glycolic acid attenuates UVB-induced aquaporin-3, matrix metalloproteinase-9 expression, and collagen degradation in keratinocytes and mouse skin. Biochem J. 2019 May 21;476(10):1387-1400. doi: 10.1042/BCJ20180974. PubMed PMID: 31036716.

105. Tran D, Townley JP, Barnes TM, Greive KA. An antiaging skin care system containing alpha hydroxy acids and vitamins improves the biomechanical parameters of facial skin. Clin CosmetInvestig Dermatol. 2014 Dec 19;8:9-17. doi: 10.2147/CCID.S75439. eCollection 2015. PubMed PMID: 25552908; PubMed Central PMCID: PMC4277239.

106. Sharad J. Glycolic acid peel therapy - a current review. Clin CosmetInvestig Dermatol. 2013 Nov 11;6:281-8. doi: 10.2147/CCID.S34029. Review. PubMed PMID: 24399880; PubMed Central PMCID: PMC3875240.

107. Tang SC, Yang JH. Dual Effects of Alpha-Hydroxy Acids on the Skin. Molecules. 2018 Apr 10;23(4). pii: E863. doi: 10.3390/molecules23040863. Review. PubMed PMID: 29642579; PubMed Central PMCID: PMC6017965.

108. Smith WP. Epidermal and dermal effects of topical lactic acid. J Am Acad Dermatol. 1996 Sep;35(3 Pt 1):388-91. PubMed PMID: 8784274.

109. Prestes PS, Oliveira MM, Leonardi GR. Randomized clinical efficacy of superficial peeling with 85% lactic acid versus 70% glycolic acid. An Bras Dermatol. 2013 Nov-Dec;88(6):900-5. doi: 10.1590/abd1806-4841.20131888. PubMed PMID: 24474097; PubMed Central PMCID: PMC3900339.

110. KapicioğluY, Gül M, Saraç G, Yiğitcan B, Gözükara H. Comparison of Antiaging Effects on Rat Skin of Coq Thread and Poly-L-Lactic Acid Thread. Dermatol Surg. 2019 Mar;45(3):438-445. doi: 10.1097/DSS.0000000000001717. PubMed PMID: 30608294.

111. Bohnert K, Dorizas A, Lorenc P, Sadick NS. Randomized, Controlled, Multicentered, Double-Blind Investigation of Injectable Poly-L-Lactic Acid for Improving Skin Quality. Dermatol Surg. 2019 May;45(5):718-724. doi: 10.1097/DSS.0000000000001772. PubMed PMID: 30741790.

112. Algiert-ZielińskaB, Mucha P, Rotsztejn H. Lactic and lactobionic acids as typically moisturizing compounds. Int J Dermatol. 2019 Mar;58(3):374-379. doi: 10.1111/ijd.14202. Epub 2018 Sep 30. PubMed PMID: 30270529.

113. Lew LC, Liong MT. Bioactives from probiotics for dermal health: functions and benefits. J Appl Microbiol. 2013 May;114(5):1241-53. doi: 10.1111/jam.12137. Epub 2013 Feb 1. Review. PubMed PMID: 23311666.

114. Yamamoto Y, Uede K, Yonei N, Kishioka A, Ohtani T, Furukawa F. Effects of alpha-hydroxy acids on the human skin of Japanese subjects: the rationale for chemical peeling. J Dermatol. 2006 Jan;33(1):16-22. PubMed PMID: 16469079.
115. Vender RB, Andriessen A, Barankin B, Freiman A, Kyritsis D, Mistos LM, Salsberg J, Amar L. Cohort Using a Ceramides Containing Cleanser and Cream With Salicylic Acid for Dry, Flaking, and Scaling Skin Conditions. J Drugs Dermatol. 2019 Jan 1;18(1):80-85. PubMed PMID: 30681802.
116. Kantikosum K, Chongpison Y, Chottawornsak N, Asawanonda P. The efficacy of glycolic acid, salicylic acid, gluconolactone, and licochalcone A combined with 0.1% adapalene vs adapalene monotherapy in mild-to-moderate acne vulgaris: a double-blinded within-person comparative study. Clin CosmetInvestig Dermatol. 2019 Feb 19;12:151-161. doi: 10.2147/CCID.S193730. eCollection 2019. PubMed PMID: 30858720; PubMed Central PMCID: PMC6386354.
117. ShamalnasabM, Gravel SP, St-Pierre J, Breton L, Jäger S, Aguilaniu H. A salicylic acid derivative extends the lifespan of Caenorhabditis elegans by activating autophagy and the mitochondrial unfolded protein response. Aging Cell. 2018 Dec;17(6):e12830. doi: 10.1111/acel.12830. Epub 2018 Sep 7. Erratum in: Aging Cell. 2019 Apr;18(2):e12917. PubMed PMID: 30192051; PubMed Central PMCID: PMC6260907.
118. Zheng Y, Yin S, Xia Y, Chen J, Ye C, Zeng Q, Lai W. Efficacy and safety of 2% supramolecular salicylic acid compared with 5% benzoyl peroxide/0.1% adapalene in the acne treatment: a randomized, split-face, open-label, single-center study. CutanOculToxicol. 2019 Mar;38(1):48-54. doi: 10.1080/15569527.2018.1518329. Epub 2018 Dec 20. PubMed PMID: 30173582.
119. Understanding Skin Care Products. Available From: https://www.webmd.com/beauty/skin-care-products#3-8
120. Papakonstantinou E, Roth M, Karakiulakis G. Hyaluronic acid: A key molecule in skin aging. Dermatoendocrinol. 2012 Jul 1;4(3):253-8. doi: 10.4161/derm.21923. PubMed PMID: 23467280; PubMed Central PMCID: PMC3583886.
121. SparavignaA, Tenconi B, Giori AM, Bellia G, La Penna L. Evaluation of the efficacy of a new hyaluronic acid gel on dynamic and static wrinkles in volunteers with moderate aging/photoaging. Clin CosmetInvestig Dermatol. 2019 Jan 17;12:81-90. doi: 10.2147/CCID.S191935. eCollection 2019. PubMed PMID: 30697060; PubMed Central PMCID: PMC6340359.
122. Lee YJ, Kim HT, Lee WJ, Chang SE, Lee MW, Choi JH, Won CH. Anti-aging and hydration efficacy of a cross-linked hyaluronic acid microstructure patch. Dermatol Ther. 2019 Apr 3:e12888. doi: 10.1111/dth.12888. [Epub ahead of print] PubMed PMID: 30942947.
123. Jeon YJ, Kim YH, Jeon YJ, Lee WW, Bae IG, Yi KW, Hong SH. Increased synthesis of hyaluronic acid by enhanced penetration of CTP-EGF recombinant in human keratinocytes. J Cosmet Dermatol. 2019 Jan 20. doi: 10.1111/jocd.12855. [Epub ahead of print] PubMed PMID: 30661271.
124. Walker K, Zito PM. Hyaluronic Acid. [Updated 2019 May 1]. In: StatPearls [Internet]. Treasure Island (FL): StatPearls Publishing; 2019 Jan-. Available from: https://www.ncbi.nlm.nih.gov/books/NBK482440/

125. Bukhari SNA, Roswandi NL, Waqas M, Habib H, Hussain F, Khan S, Sohail M, Ramli NA, Thu HE, Hussain Z. Hyaluronic acid, a promising skin rejuvenating biomedicine: A review of recent updates and pre-clinical and clinical investigations on cosmetic and nutricosmetic effects. Int J Biol Macromol. 2018 Dec;120(Pt B):1682-1695. doi: 10.1016/j.ijbiomac.2018.09.188. Epub 2018 Oct 1. Review. PubMed PMID: 30287361.

126. GarreA, Narda M, Valderas-Martinez P, Piquero J, Granger C. Antiaging effects of a novel facial serum containing L-Ascorbic acid, proteoglycans, and proteoglycan-stimulating tripeptide: ex vivo skin explant studies and in vivo clinical studies in women. Clin CosmetInvestig Dermatol. 2018 May 29;11:253-263. doi: 10.2147/CCID.S161352. eCollection 2018. PubMed PMID: 29881301; PubMed Central PMCID: PMC5985795.

127. Zasada M, Markiewicz A, Drożdż Z, Mosińska P, Erkiert-Polguj A, Budzisz E. Preliminary randomized controlled trial of antiaging effects of l-ascorbic acid applied in combination with no-needle and microneedle mesotherapy. J Cosmet Dermatol. 2019 Jun;18(3):843-849. doi: 10.1111/jocd.12727. Epub 2018 Aug 2. PubMed PMID: 30070034.

128. Wang SF, Liu X, Ding MY, Ma S, Zhao J, Wang Y, Li S. 2-O-β-d-glucopyranosyl-(l)-ascorbic acid, a novel vitamin C derivative from Lyciumbarbarum, prevents oxidative stress. Redox Biol. 2019 Mar 18;24:101173. doi: 10.1016/j.redox.2019.101173. [Epub ahead of print] PubMed PMID: 30903981; PubMed Central PMCID: PMC6430735.

129. GęgotekA, Ambrożewicz E, Jastrząb A, Jarocka-Karpowicz I, Skrzydlewska E. Rutin and ascorbic acid cooperation in antioxidant and antiapoptotic effect on human skin keratinocytes and fibroblasts exposed to UVA and UVB radiation. Arch Dermatol Res. 2019 Apr;311(3):203-219. doi: 10.1007/s00403-019-01898-w. Epub 2019 Feb 19. PubMed PMID: 30783768.

130. Abdullah M, Attia FN. Vitamin C (Ascorbic Acid) [Updated 2019 Feb 19]. In: StatPearls [Internet]. Treasure Island (FL): StatPearls Publishing; 2019 Jan-. Available from: https://www.ncbi.nlm.nih.gov/books/NBK499877/

131 Pullar JM, Carr AC, Vissers MCM. The Roles of Vitamin C in Skin Health. Nutrients. 2017 Aug 12;9(8). pii: E866. doi: 10.3390/nu9080866. Review. PubMed PMID: 28805671; PubMed Central PMCID: PMC5579659.

132. CrisanD, Roman I, Crisan M, Scharffetter-Kochanek K, Badea R. The role of vitamin C in pushing back the boundaries of skin aging: an ultrasonographic approach. Clin CosmetInvestig Dermatol. 2015 Sep 2;8:463-70. doi: 10.2147/CCID.S84903. eCollection 2015. PubMed PMID: 26366101; PubMed Central PMCID: PMC4562654.

133. Zhai H, Behnam S, Villarama CD, Arens-Corell M, Choi MJ, Maibach HI. Evaluation of the antioxidant capacity and preventive effects of a topical emulsion and its vehicle control on the skin response to UV exposure. Skin Pharmacol Physiol. 2005 Nov-Dec;18(6):288-93. Epub 2005 Sep 5. PubMed PMID: 16145283.

134. Keen MA, Hassan I. Vitamin E in dermatology. Indian Dermatol Online J. 2016 Jul-Aug;7(4):311-5. doi: 10.4103/2229-5178.185494. PubMed PMID: 27559512; PubMed Central PMCID: PMC4976416.

135. Traber MG, Stevens JF. Vitamins C and E: beneficial effects from a mechanistic perspective. Free Radic Biol Med. 2011 Sep 1;51(5):1000-13. doi: 10.1016/j.freeradbiomed.2011.05.017. Epub 2011 May 25. Review. PubMed PMID: 21664268; PubMed Central PMCID: PMC3156342.

136. Cho S. The Role of Functional Foods in Cutaneous Anti-aging. J Lifestyle Med. 2014 Mar;4(1):8-16. doi: 10.15280/jlm.2014.4.1.8. Epub 2014 Mar 31. Review. PubMed PMID: 26064850; PubMed Central PMCID: PMC4390761.

137. Rahman S, Bhatia K, Khan AQ, Kaur M, Ahmad F, Rashid H, Athar M, Islam F, Raisuddin S. Topically applied vitamin E prevents massive cutaneous inflammatory and oxidative stress responses induced by double application of 12-O-tetradecanoylphorbol-13-acetate (TPA) in mice. Chem Biol Interact. 2008 Apr 15;172(3):195-205. doi: 10.1016/j.cbi.2007.11.017. Epub 2008 Jan 4. PubMed PMID: 18262176.

138. Thiele JJ, Hsieh SN, Ekanayake-Mudiyanselage S. Vitamin E: critical review of its current use in cosmetic and clinical dermatology. Dermatol Surg. 2005 Jul;31(7 Pt 2):805-13; discussion 813. Review. PubMed PMID: 16029671.

139. Farris P, Yatskayer M, Chen N, Krol Y, Oresajo C. Evaluation of efficacy and tolerance of a nighttime topical antioxidant containing resveratrol, baicalin, and vitamin e for treatment of mild to moderately photodamaged skin. J Drugs Dermatol. 2014 Dec;13(12):1467-72. PubMed PMID: 25607790.

140. Wang K, Jiang H, Li W, Qiang M, Dong T, Li H. Role of Vitamin C in Skin Diseases. Front Physiol. 2018 Jul 4;9:819. doi: 10.3389/fphys.2018.00819. eCollection 2018. Review. PubMed PMID: 30022952; PubMed Central PMCID: PMC6040229.

141. Burns EM, Tober KL, Riggenbach JA, Kusewitt DF, Young GS, Oberyszyn TM. Differential effects of topical vitamin E and C E Ferulic® treatments on ultraviolet light B-induced cutaneous tumor development in Skh-1 mice. PLoS One. 2013 May 14;8(5):e63809. doi: 10.1371/journal.pone.0063809. Print 2013. PubMed PMID: 23691100; PubMed Central PMCID: PMC3653797.

142. Watson RE, Long SP, Bowden JJ, Bastrilles JY, Barton SP, Griffiths CE. Repair of photoaged dermal matrix by topical application of a cosmetic 'antiageing' product. Br J Dermatol. 2008 Mar;158(3):472-7. Epub 2007 Dec 6. PubMed PMID: 18070204.

143. Knott A, Achterberg V, Smuda C, Mielke H, Sperling G, Dunckelmann K, Vogelsang A, Krüger A, Schwengler H, Behtash M, Kristof S, Diekmann H, Eisenberg T, Berroth A, Hildebrand J, Siegner R, Winnefeld M, Teuber F, Fey S, Möbius J, Retzer D, Burkhardt T, Lüttke J, Blatt T. Topical treatment with coenzyme Q10-containing formulas improves skin's Q10 level and provides antioxidative effects. Biofactors. 2015 Nov-Dec;41(6):383-90. doi: 10.1002/biof.1239. Epub 2015 Dec 9. PubMed PMID: 26648450; PubMed Central PMCID: PMC4737275.

144. Yue Y, Zhou H, Liu G, Li Y, Yan Z, Duan M. The advantages of a novel CoQ10 delivery system in skin photo-protection. Int J Pharm. 2010 Jun 15;392(1-2):57-63. doi: 10.1016/j.ijpharm.2010.03.032. Epub 2010 Mar 17. PubMed PMID: 20302925.

145. Passi S, De Pità O, Grandinetti M, Simotti C, Littarru GP. The combined use of oral and topical lipophilic antioxidants increases their levels both in sebum and stratum corneum. Biofactors. 2003;18(1-4):289-97. PubMed PMID: 14695946.

146. El-LeithyES, Makky AM, Khattab AM, Hussein DG. Optimization of nutraceutical coenzyme Q10 nanoemulsion with improved skin permeability and anti-wrinkle efficiency. Drug Dev Ind Pharm. 2018 Feb;44(2):316-328. doi: 10.1080/03639045.2017.1391836. Epub 2017 Nov 2. PubMed PMID: 29096550.

147. Choi BS, Song HS, Kim HR, Park TW, Kim TD, Cho BJ, Kim CJ, Sim SS. Effect of coenzyme Q10 on cutaneous healing in skin-incised mice. Arch Pharm Res. 2009 Jun;32(6):907-13. doi: 10.1007/s12272-009-1613-3. Epub 2009 Jun 26. PubMed PMID: 19557369.

148. ŽmitekK, Pogačnik T, Mervic L, Žmitek J, Pravst I. The effect of dietary intake of coenzyme Q10 on skin parameters and condition: Results of a randomised, placebo-controlled, double-blind study. Biofactors. 2017 Jan 2;43(1):132-140. doi: 10.1002/biof.1316. Epub 2016 Aug 22. PubMed PMID: 27548886.

149. Zhao Q, Ma YM, Jing L, Zheng TX, Jiang HF, Li PA, Zhang JZ. Coenzyme Q10 Protects Astrocytes from Ultraviolet B-Induced Damage Through Inhibition of ERK 1/2 Pathway Overexpression. Neurochem Res. 2019 May 15. doi: 10.1007/s11064-019-02812-6. [Epub ahead of print] PubMed PMID: 31093903.

150. Barcelos IP, Haas RH. CoQ10 and Aging. Biology (Basel). 2019 May 11;8(2). pii: E28. doi: 10.3390/biology8020028. Review. PubMed PMID: 31083534.

151. Kubota Y, Musashi M, Nagasawa T, Shimura N, Igarashi R, Yamaguchi Y. Novel nanocapsule of α-lipoic acid reveals pigmentation improvement: α-Lipoic acid stimulates the proliferation and differentiation of keratinocyte in murine skin by topical application. Exp Dermatol. 2019 Feb;28 Suppl 1:55-63. doi: 10.1111/exd.13828. Review. PubMed PMID: 30698882.

152. SherifS, Bendas ER, Badawy S. The clinical efficacy of cosmeceutical application of liquid crystalline nanostructured dispersions of alpha lipoic acid as anti-wrinkle. Eur J Pharm Biopharm. 2014 Feb;86(2):251-9. doi: 10.1016/j.ejpb.2013.09.008. Epub 2013 Sep 18. PubMed PMID: 24056055.

153. Lin JY, Lin FH, Burch JA, Selim MA, Monteiro-Riviere NA, Grichnik JM, Pinnell SR. Alpha-lipoic acid is ineffective as a topical antioxidant for photoprotection of skin. J Invest Dermatol. 2004 Nov;123(5):996-8. PubMed PMID: 15482491.

154. El-Komy M, Shalaby S, Hegazy R, Abdel Hay R, Sherif S, Bendas E. Assessment of cubosomal alpha lipoic acid gel efficacy for the aging face: a single-blinded, placebo-controlled, right-left comparative clinical study. J Cosmet Dermatol. 2017 Sep;16(3):358-363. doi: 10.1111/jocd.12298. Epub 2016 Nov 22. PubMed PMID: 27873449.

155. Kim GD, Kim TH, Jang AH, Ahn HJ, Park YS, Park CS. α-Lipoic acid suppresses the development of DNFB-induced atopic dermatitis-like symptoms in NC/Nga

mice. Exp Dermatol. 2011 Feb;20(2):97-101. doi: 10.1111/j.1600-0625.2010.01165.x.Epub 2010 Dec 17. PubMed PMID: 21166725.

156. Isaac VL, Chiari-Andréo BG, Marto JM, Moraes JD, Leone BA, Corrêa MA, Ribeiro HM. Rheology as a Tool to Predict the Release of Alpha-Lipoic Acid from Emulsions Used for the Prevention of Skin Aging. Biomed Res Int. 2015;2015:818656. doi: 10.1155/2015/818656. Epub 2015 Dec 16. PubMed PMID: 26788510; PubMed Central PMCID: PMC4695648.

157. Majtan J, Jesenak M. β-Glucans: Multi-Functional Modulator of Wound Healing. Molecules. 2018 Apr 1;23(4). pii: E806. doi: 10.3390/molecules23040806. Review. PubMed PMID: 29614757; PubMed Central PMCID: PMC6017669.

158. Vetvicka V, Vannucci L, Sima P, Richter J. Beta Glucan: Supplement or Grug? From Laboratory to Clinical Trials. Molecules. 2019 Mar 30;24(7). pii: E1251. doi: 10.3390/molecules24071251. Review. PubMed PMID: 30935016; PubMed Central PMCID: PMC6479769.

159. Hong YH, Lee HS, Jung EY, Han SH, Park Y, Suh HJ. Photoprotective effects of topical ginseng leaf extract using Ultraflo L against UVB-induced skin damage in hairless mice. J Ginseng Res. 2017 Oct;41(4):456-462. doi: 10.1016/j.jgr.2016.07.007. Epub 2016 Aug 6. PubMed PMID: 29021691; PubMed Central PMCID: PMC5628359.

160. Bacha U, Nasir M, Iqbal S, Anjum AA. Nutraceutical, Anti-Inflammatory, and Immune Modulatory Effects of β-Glucan Isolated from Yeast. Biomed Res Int. 2017;2017:8972678. doi: 10.1155/2017/8972678. Epub 2017 Aug 23. PubMed PMID: 28913359; PubMed Central PMCID: PMC5587958.

161. JesenakM, Urbancek S, Majtan J, Banovcin P, Hercogova J. β-Glucan-based cream (containing pleuran isolated from pleurotusostreatus) in supportive treatment of mild-to-moderate atopic dermatitis. J Dermatolog Treat. 2016 Aug;27(4):351-4. doi: 10.3109/09546634.2015.1117565. Epub 2015 Dec 10. PubMed PMID: 26654776.

162. Bashir KMI, Choi JS. Clinical and Physiological Perspectives of β-Glucans: The Past, Present, and Future. Int J Mol Sci. 2017 Sep 5;18(9). pii: E1906. doi: 10.3390/ijms18091906. Review. PubMed PMID: 28872611; PubMed Central PMCID: PMC5618555.

163. Wang Y, Viennet C, Jeudy A, Fanian F, He L, Humbert P. Assessment of the efficacy of a new complex antisensitive skin cream. J Cosmet Dermatol. 2018 Dec;17(6):1101-1107. doi: 10.1111/jocd.12486. Epub 2018 Jan 22. PubMed PMID: 29356277.

164. Choi FD, Sung CT, Juhasz ML, Mesinkovsk NA. Oral Collagen Supplementation: A Systematic Review of Dermatological Applications. J Drugs Dermatol. 2019 Jan 1;18(1):9-16. PubMed PMID: 30681787.

165. Maia Campos PMBG, Melo MO, Siqueira César FC. Topical application and oral supplementation of peptides in the improvement of skin viscoelasticity and density. J Cosmet Dermatol. 2019 Mar 4. doi: 10.1111/jocd.12893. [Epub ahead of print] PubMed PMID: 30834689.

166. ProkschE, Segger D, Degwert J, Schunck M, Zague V, Oesser S. Oral supplementation of specific collagen peptides has beneficial effects on human

skin physiology: a double-blind, placebo-controlled study. Skin Pharmacol Physiol. 2014;27(1):47-55. doi: 10.1159/000351376. Epub 2013 Aug 14. PubMed PMID: 23949208.

167. Pyun HB, Kim M, Park J, Sakai Y, Numata N, Shin JY, Shin HJ, Kim DU, Hwang JK. Effects of Collagen Tripeptide Supplement on Photoaging and Epidermal Skin Barrier in UVB-exposed Hairless Mice. PrevNutr Food Sci. 2012 Dec;17(4):245-53. doi: 10.3746/pnf.2012.17.4.245. PubMed PMID: 24471092; PubMed Central PMCID: PMC3866733.

168. Kim DU, Chung HC, Choi J, Sakai Y, Lee BY. Oral Intake of Low-Molecular-Weight Collagen Peptide Improves Hydration, Elasticity, and Wrinkling in Human Skin: A Randomized, Double-Blind, Placebo-Controlled Study. Nutrients. 2018 Jun 26;10(7). pii: E826. doi: 10.3390/nu10070826. PubMed PMID: 29949889; PubMed Central PMCID: PMC6073484.

169. Czajka A, Kania EM, Genovese L, Corbo A, Merone G, Luci C, Sibilla S. Daily oral supplementation with collagen peptides combined with vitamins and other bioactive compounds improves skin elasticity and has a beneficial effect on joint and general wellbeing. Nutr Res. 2018 Sep;57:97-108. doi: 10.1016/j.nutres.2018.06.001. Epub 2018 Jun 9. PubMed PMID: 30122200.

170. Lee HJ, Jang HL, Ahn DK, Kim HJ, Jeon HY, Seo DB, Lee JH, Choi JK, Kang SS. Orally administered collagen peptide protects against UVB-induced skin aging through the absorption of dipeptide forms, Gly-Pro and Pro-Hyp. BiosciBiotechnolBiochem. 2019 Jun;83(6):1146-1156. doi: 10.1080/09168451.2019.1580559. Epub2019 Feb 11. PubMed PMID: 30739561.

171. Addor FAS, Cotta Vieira J, Abreu Melo CS. Improvement of dermal parameters in aged skin after oral use of a nutrient supplement. Clin CosmetInvestig Dermatol. 2018 Apr 30;11:195-201. doi: 10.2147/CCID.S150269. eCollection 2018. PubMed PMID: 29750046; PubMed Central PMCID: PMC5933363.

172. Zague V, do Amaral JB, Rezende Teixeira P, de Oliveira Niero EL, Lauand C, Machado-Santelli GM. Collagen peptides modulate the metabolism of extracellular matrix by human dermal fibroblasts derived from sun-protected and sun exposed body sites. Cell Biol Int. 2018 Jan;42(1):95-104. doi: 10.1002/cbin.10872. Epub 2017 Oct 9. PubMed PMID: 28906033.

173. Song H, Meng M, Cheng X, Li B, Wang C. The effect of collagen hydrolysates from silver carp (Hypophthalmichthys molitrix) skin on UV-induced photoaging in mice: molecular weight affects skin repair. Food Funct. 2017 Apr 19;8(4):1538-1546. doi: 10.1039/c6fo01397j. PubMed PMID: 28266663.

174. Vollmer DL, West VA, Lephart ED. Enhancing Skin Health: By Oral Administration of Natural Compounds and Minerals with Implications to the Dermal Microbiome. Int J Mol Sci. 2018 Oct 7;19(10). pii: E3059. doi: 10.3390/ijms19103059. Review. PubMed PMID: 30301271; PubMed Central PMCID: PMC6213755.

175. Kimoto-Nira H. New lactic acid bacteria for skin health via oral intake of heat-killed or live cells. Anim Sci J. 2018 Jun;89(6):835-842. doi: 10.1111/asj.13017. Epub 2018 Apr 26. Review. PubMed PMID: 29696746; PubMed Central PMCID: PMC6001785.

176. Fabbrocini G, Bertona M, Picazo Ó, Pareja-Galeano H, Monfrecola G, Emanuele E. Supplementation with Lactobacillus rhamnosus SP1 normalises skin expression of genes implicated in insulin signalling and improves adult acne. Benef Microbes. 2016 Nov 30;7(5):625-630. Epub 2016 Sep 6. PubMed PMID: 27596801.
177. Isawa K, Noma T, Yamamoto M et al. Verifying the ability of yogurt prepared with LB81 lactic acid bacteria to improve skin function. J Int Microbiol 2008;22: 1–5.
178. Mori N, Kano M, Masuoka N, Konno T, Suzuki Y, Miyazaki K, Ueki Y. Effect of probiotic and prebiotic fermented milk on skin and intestinal conditions in healthy young female students. Biosci Microbiota Food Health. 2016;35(3):105-12. doi: 10.12938/bmfh.2015-022. Epub 2016 Apr 1. PubMed PMID: 27508111; PubMed Central PMCID: PMC4965514.
179. Spada F, Barnes TM, Greive KA. Skin hydration is significantly increased by a cream formulated to mimic the skin's own natural moisturizing systems. Clin CosmetInvestig Dermatol. 2018 Oct 15;11:491-497. doi: 10.2147/CCID.S177697. eCollection 2018. PubMed PMID: 30410378; PubMed Central PMCID: PMC6197824.
180. Di Marzio L, Cinque B, Cupelli F, De Simone C, Cifone MG, Giuliani M. Increase of skin-ceramide levels in aged subjects following a short-term topical application of bacterial sphingomyelinase from Streptococcus thermophilus. Int J ImmunopatholPharmacol. 2008 Jan-Mar;21(1):137-43. PubMed PMID: 18336739.
181. MutanuJungersted J, Hellgren LI, Høgh JK, Drachmann T, Jemec GB, Agner T. Ceramides and barrier function in healthy skin. Acta DermVenereol. 2010 Jul;90(4):350-3. doi: 10.2340/00015555-0894. PubMed PMID: 20574598.
182. Jensen JM, Förl M, Winoto-Morbach S, Seite S, Schunck M, Proksch E, Schütze S. Acid and neutral sphingomyelinase, ceramide synthase, and acid ceramidase activities in cutaneous aging. Exp Dermatol. 2005 Aug;14(8):609-18. PubMed PMID: 16026583.
183. VozellaV, Basit A, Piras F, Realini N, Armirotti A, Bossù P, Assogna F, Sensi SL, Spalletta G, Piomelli D. Elevated plasma ceramide levels in post-menopausal women: a cross-sectional study. Aging (Albany NY). 2019 Jan 8;11(1):73-88. doi: 10.18632/aging.101719. PubMed PMID: 30620722; PubMed Central PMCID: PMC6339790.
184. DraelosZD, Raymond I. The Efficacy of a Ceramide-based Cream in Mild-to-moderate Atopic Dermatitis. J Clin Aesthet Dermatol. 2018 May;11(5):30-32. Epub 2018 May 1. PubMed PMID: 29785236; PubMed Central PMCID: PMC5955631.
185. YazdanparastT, Nasrollahi SA, Firouzabadi LI, Firooz A. A Phase II Trial to Assess the Safety and Efficacy of a Topical Repair Cream Containing Skin-identical Ceramide Complex in Patients with Contact Dermatitis. J Clin Aesthet Dermatol. 2018 Nov;11(11):40-44. Epub 2018 Nov 1. PubMed PMID: 30588273; PubMed Central PMCID: PMC6303115.
186. Zeichner JA, Del Rosso JQ. Multivesicular Emulsion Ceramide-containing Moisturizers: An Evaluation of Their Role in the Management of Common Skin

Disorders. J Clin Aesthet Dermatol. 2016 Dec;9(12):26-32. Epub 2016 Dec 1. Review. PubMed PMID: 28210396; PubMed Central PMCID: PMC5300724.

187. Zhang Q, Flach CR, Mendelsohn R, Mao G, Pappas A, Mack MC, Walters RM, Southall MD. Topically applied ceramide accumulates in skin glyphs. Clin CosmetInvestig Dermatol. 2015 Jul 1;8:329-37. doi: 10.2147/CCID.S83857. eCollection 2015. PubMed PMID: 26170709; PubMed Central PMCID: PMC4493983.

188. Soma Y, Kashima M, Imaizumi A, Takahama H, Kawakami T, Mizoguchi M. Moisturizing effects of topical nicotinamide on atopic dry skin. Int J Dermatol. 2005 Mar;44(3):197-202. PubMed PMID: 15807725.

189. AshkaniEsfahani S, Khoshneviszadeh M, Namazi MR, Noorafshan A, Geramizadeh B, Nadimi E, Razavipour ST. Topical Nicotinamide Improves Tissue Regeneration in Excisional Full-Thickness Skin Wounds: A Stereological and Pathological Study. Trauma Mon. 2015 Nov;20(4):e18193. doi: 10.5812/traumamon.18193. Epub 2015 Nov 23. PubMed PMID: 26839851; PubMed Central PMCID: PMC4727459.

190. Shalita AR, Smith JG, Parish LC, Sofman MS, Chalker DK. Topical nicotinamide compared with clindamycin gel in the treatment of inflammatory acne vulgaris. Int J Dermatol. 1995 Jun;34(6):434-7. PubMed PMID: 7657446.

191. Navarrete-Solís J, Castanedo-Cázares JP, Torres-Álvarez B, Oros-Ovalle C, Fuentes-Ahumada C, González FJ, Martínez-Ramírez JD, Moncada B. A Double-Blind, Randomized Clinical Trial of Niacinamide 4% versus Hydroquinone 4% in the Treatment of Melasma. Dermatol Res Pract. 2011;2011:379173. doi: 10.1155/2011/379173. Epub 2011 Jul 21. PubMed PMID: 21822427; PubMed Central PMCID: PMC3142702.

192. Gehring W. Nicotinic acid/niacinamide and the skin. J Cosmet Dermatol. 2004 Apr;3(2):88-93. PubMed PMID: 17147561.

193. Levin J, Momin SB. How much do we really know about our favorite cosmeceutical ingredients? J Clin Aesthet Dermatol. 2010 Feb;3(2):22-41. PubMed PMID: 20725560; PubMed Central PMCID: PMC2921764.

194. Oblong JE, Bissett DL, Ritter JL, Kurtz KK, Schnicker MS. Effect of niacinamide on collagen synthesis and markers of keratinocyte differentiation. Presented at: The 60th Annual Meeting of the American Academy of Dermatology. 2002; New Orleans.

195. Kawada A, Konishi N, Momma T, Oiso N, Kawara S. Evaluation of anti-wrinkle effects of a novel cosmetic containing retinol using the guideline of the Japan Cosmetic Industry Association. J Dermatol. 2009 Nov;36(11):583-6. doi: 10.1111/j.1346-8138.2009.00716.x. PubMed PMID: 19878390.

196. Khodaeiani E, Fouladi RF, Amirnia M, Saeidi M, Karimi ER. Topical 4% nicotinamide vs. 1% clindamycin in moderate inflammatory acne vulgaris. Int J Dermatol. 2013 Aug;52(8):999-1004. doi: 10.1111/ijd.12002. Epub 2013 Jun 20. PubMed PMID: 23786503.

197. Eren B, TuncayTanrıverdi S, AydınKöse F, Özer Ö. Antioxidant properties evaluation of topical astaxanthin formulations as anti-aging products. J Cosmet

Dermatol. 2019 Feb;18(1):242-250. doi: 10.1111/jocd.12665. Epub 2018 May 10. PubMed PMID: 29745467.

198. Davinelli S, Nielsen ME, Scapagnini G. Astaxanthin in Skin Health, Repair, and Disease: A Comprehensive Review. Nutrients. 2018 Apr 22;10(4). pii: E522. doi: 10.3390/nu10040522. Review. PubMed PMID: 29690549; PubMed Central PMCID: PMC5946307.
199. Eren B, TuncayTanrıverdi S, AydınKöse F, Özer Ö. Antioxidant properties evaluation of topical astaxanthin formulations as anti-aging products. J Cosmet Dermatol. 2019 Feb;18(1):242-250. doi: 10.1111/jocd.12665. Epub 2018 May 10. PubMed PMID: 29745467.
200. Fang Q, Guo S, Zhou H, Han R, Wu P, Han C. Astaxanthin protects against early burn-wound progression in rats by attenuating oxidative stress-induced inflammation and mitochondria-related apoptosis. Sci Rep. 2017 Jan 27;7:41440. doi: 10.1038/srep41440. PubMed PMID: 28128352; PubMed Central PMCID: PMC5269753.
201. Davinelli S, Nielsen ME, Scapagnini G. Astaxanthin in Skin Health, Repair, and Disease: A Comprehensive Review. Nutrients. 2018 Apr 22;10(4). pii: E522. doi: 10.3390/nu10040522. Review. PubMed PMID: 29690549; PubMed Central PMCID: PMC5946307.
202. Suganuma K, Nakajima H, Ohtsuki M, Imokawa G. Astaxanthin attenuates the UVA-induced up-regulation of matrix-metalloproteinase-1 and skin fibroblast elastase in human dermal fibroblasts. J Dermatol Sci. 2010 May;58(2):136-42. doi: 10.1016/j.jdermsci.2010.02.009. Epub 2010 Feb 18. PubMed PMID: 20219323.
203. Chou HY, Lee C, Pan JL, Wen ZH, Huang SH, Lan CW, Liu WT, Hour TC, Hseu YC, Hwang BH, Cheng KC, Wang HM. Enriched Astaxanthin Extract from Haematococcuspluvialis Augments Growth Factor Secretions to Increase Cell Proliferation and Induces MMP1 Degradation to Enhance Collagen Production in Human Dermal Fibroblasts. Int J Mol Sci. 2016 Jun 16;17(6). pii: E955. doi: 10.3390/ijms17060955. PubMed PMID: 27322248; PubMed Central PMCID: PMC4926488.
204. MeephansanJ, Rungjang A, Yingmema W, Deenonpoe R, Ponnikorn S. Effect of astaxanthin on cutaneous wound healing. Clin CosmetInvestig Dermatol. 2017 Jul 13;10:259-265. doi: 10.2147/CCID.S142795. eCollection 2017. PubMed PMID: 28761364; PubMed Central PMCID: PMC5516620.
205. Camera E, Mastrofrancesco A, Fabbri C, Daubrawa F, Picardo M, Sies H, Stahl W. Astaxanthin, canthaxanthin and beta-carotene differently affect UVA-induced oxidative damage and expression of oxidative stress-responsive enzymes. Exp Dermatol. 2009 Mar;18(3):222-31. doi: 10.1111/j.1600-0625.2008.00790.x.Epub 2008 Sep 18. PubMed PMID: 18803658.
206. Chew BP, Mathison BD, Hayek MG, Massimino S, Reinhart GA, Park JS. Dietary astaxanthin enhances immune response in dogs. Vet Immunol Immunopathol. 2011 Apr 15;140(3-4):199-206. doi: 10.1016/j.vetimm.2010.12.004. Epub 2010 Dec 14. PubMed PMID: 21208664.

207. Park JS, Mathison BD, Hayek MG, Massimino S, Reinhart GA, Chew BP. Astaxanthin stimulates cell-mediated and humoral immune responses in cats. Vet Immunol Immunopathol. 2011 Dec 15;144(3-4):455-61. doi: 10.1016/j.vetimm.2011.08.019. Epub 2011 Sep 3. PubMed PMID: 21930306.
208. Santocono M, Zurria M, Berrettini M, Fedeli D, Falcioni G. Influence of astaxanthin, zeaxanthin and lutein on DNA damage and repair in UVA-irradiated cells. J PhotochemPhotobiol B. 2006 Dec 1;85(3):205-15. Epub 2006 Sep 8. PubMed PMID: 16962787.
209. Camera E, Mastrofrancesco A, Fabbri C, Daubrawa F, Picardo M, Sies H, Stahl W. Astaxanthin, canthaxanthin and beta-carotene differently affect UVA-induced oxidative damage and expression of oxidative stress-responsive enzymes. Exp Dermatol. 2009 Mar;18(3):222-31. doi: 10.1111/j.1600-0625.2008.00790.x.Epub 2008 Sep 18. PubMed PMID: 18803658.
210. Tominaga K, Hongo N, Fujishita M, Takahashi Y, Adachi Y. Protective effects of astaxanthin on skin deterioration. J Clin BiochemNutr. 2017 Jul;61(1):33-39. doi: 10.3164/jcbn.17-35. Epub 2017 Jun 20. PubMed PMID: 28751807; PubMed Central PMCID: PMC5525019.
211. Kim SH, Kim H. Inhibitory Effect of Astaxanthin on Oxidative Stress-Induced Mitochondrial Dysfunction-A Mini-Review. Nutrients. 2018 Aug 21;10(9). pii: E1137. doi: 10.3390/nu10091137. Review. PubMed PMID: 30134611; PubMed Central PMCID: PMC6165470.
212. Hornsby PJ. Telomerase and the aging process. Exp Gerontol. 2007 Jul;42(7):575-81. Epub 2007 Mar 30. Review. PubMed PMID: 17482404; PubMed Central PMCID: PMC1933587.
213. Anti-Aging Skin Care Benefits of Colostrum. Available From: https://www.sovereignlaboratories.com/blog/anti-aging-skin-care-benefits-colostrum/
214. Cabrera ÁJ. Zinc, aging, and immunosenescence: an overview. Pathobiol Aging Age Relat Dis. 2015 Feb 5;5:25592. doi: 10.3402/pba.v5.25592. eCollection 2015. PubMed PMID: 25661703; PubMed Central PMCID: PMC4321209.
215. Ogawa Y, Kinoshita M, Shimada S, Kawamura T. Zinc and Skin Disorders. Nutrients. 2018 Feb 11;10(2). pii: E199. doi: 10.3390/nu10020199. Review. PubMed PMID: 29439479; PubMed Central PMCID: PMC5852775.
216. Gupta M, Mahajan VK, Mehta KS, Chauhan PS. Zinc therapy in dermatology: a review. Dermatol Res Pract. 2014;2014:709152. doi: 10.1155/2014/709152. Epub 2014 Jul 10. Review. PubMed PMID: 25120566; PubMed Central PMCID: PMC4120804.
217. Cai Z, Zhang J, Li H. Selenium, aging and aging-related diseases. Aging Clin Exp Res. 2018 Dec 3. doi: 10.1007/s40520-018-1086-7. [Epub ahead of print] Review. PubMed PMID: 30511318.
218. Favrot C, Beal D, Blouin E, Leccia MT, Roussel AM, Rachidi W. Age-Dependent Protective Effect of Selenium against UVA Irradiation in Primary Human Keratinocytes and the Associated DNA Repair Signature. Oxid Med Cell Longev. 2018 Feb 22;2018:5895439. doi: 10.1155/2018/5895439. eCollection 2018. PubMed PMID: 29682159; PubMed Central PMCID: PMC5842700.

219. Jobeili L, Rousselle P, Béal D, Blouin E, Roussel AM, Damour O, Rachidi W. Selenium preserves keratinocyte stemness and delays senescence by maintaining epidermal adhesion. Aging (Albany NY). 2017 Nov 25;9(11):2302-2315. doi: 10.18632/aging.101322. PubMed PMID: 29176034; PubMed Central PMCID: PMC5723688.
220. Wang N, Tan HY, Li S, Xu Y, Guo W, Feng Y. Supplementation of Micronutrient Selenium in Metabolic Diseases: Its Role as an Antioxidant. Oxid Med Cell Longev. 2017;2017:7478523. doi: 10.1155/2017/7478523. Epub 2017 Dec 26. Review. PubMed PMID: 29441149; PubMed Central PMCID: PMC5758946.
221. Palm MD, Woodhall KE, Butterwick KJ, Goldman MP. Cosmetic use of poly-l-lactic acid: a retrospective study of 130 patients. Dermatol Surg. 2010 Feb;36(2):161-70. doi: 10.1111/j.1524-4725.2009.01419.x.Epub 2009 Dec 21. PubMed PMID: 20039924.
222. Jabbar A, Arruda S, Sadick N. Off Face Usage of Poly-L-Lactic Acid for Body Rejuvenation. J Drugs Dermatol. 2017 May 1;16(5):489-494. Review. PubMed PMID: 28628686.
223. Sickles CK, Gross GP. Poly-L-Lactic Acid. [Updated 2019 Jan 23]. In: StatPearls [Internet]. Treasure Island (FL): StatPearls Publishing; 2019 Jan-. Available from: https://www.ncbi.nlm.nih.gov/books/NBK507871/
224. Kim CM, Kim BY, Hye Suh D, Lee SJ, Moon HR, Ryu HJ. The efficacy of powdered polydioxanone in terms of collagen production compared with poly-L-lactic acid in a murine model. J Cosmet Dermatol. 2019 Feb 27. doi: 10.1111/jocd.12894. [Epub ahead of print] PubMed PMID: 30809959.
225. de Jager MW, Gooris GS, Dolbnya IP, Bras W, Ponec M, Bouwstra JA. Novel lipid mixtures based on synthetic ceramides reproduce the unique stratum corneum lipid organization. J Lipid Res. 2004 May;45(5):923-32. Epub 2004 Feb 16. PubMed PMID: 14967818.
226. Kim M, Park HJ. Molecular Mechanisms of Skin Aging and Rejuvenation. IntechOpen August 31st 2016, DOI: 10.5772/62983.
227. Goenka S. Monica Belluci's Makeup, Beauty And Fitness Secrets Revealed. STYLECRAZE, November 1, 2017.
228. Monica Bellucci Beauty Secrets. Available From: https://monicabellucci.net/monica-bellucci-beauty-secrets/
229. Zahr AS, Kononov T, Sensing W, Biron JA, Gold MH. An open-label, single-site study to evaluate the tolerability, safety, and efficacy of using a novel facial moisturizer for preparation and accelerated healing pre and post a single full-face radiofrequency microneedling treatment. J Cosmet Dermatol. 2019 Feb;18(1):94-106. doi: 10.1111/jocd.12817. Epub 2018 Nov 19. PubMed PMID: 30456804.
230. Portugal-Cohen M, Oron M, Cohen D, Ma'or Z. Antipollution skin protection - a new paradigm and its demonstration on two active compounds. Clin CosmetInvestig Dermatol. 2017 May 17;10:185-193. doi: 10.2147/CCID.S129437. eCollection 2017. PubMed PMID: 28553131; PubMed Central PMCID: PMC5439538.
231. Mistry N. Guidelines for Formulating Anti-Pollution Products. Cosmetics 2017, 4(4), 57; https://doi.org/10.3390/cosmetics4040057

232. Fernández JR, Webb C, Rouzard K, Voronkov M, Huber KL, Stock JB, Healy J, Tamura M, Stock M, Armbrister W, Gordon JS, Pérez E. SIG-1273 protects skin against urban air pollution and when formulated in AgeIQ™ Night Cream anti-aging benefits clinically demonstrated. J Cosmet Dermatol. 2018 Nov 19. doi: 10.1111/jocd.12825. [Epub ahead of print] PubMed PMID: 30456862.
233. AddorFAS. Topical effects of SCA(®) (Cryptomphalusaspersa secretion) associated with regenerative and antioxidant ingredients on aged skin: evaluation by confocal and clinical microscopy. Clin CosmetInvestig Dermatol. 2019 Feb 14;12:133-140. doi: 10.2147/CCID.S191153. eCollection 2019. PubMed PMID: 30858719; PubMed Central PMCID: PMC6386352.
234. Narda M, Bauza G, Valderas P, Granger C. Protective effects of a novel facial cream against environmental pollution: in vivo and in vitro assessment. Clin CosmetInvestig Dermatol. 2018 Nov 12;11:571-578. doi: 10.2147/CCID.S180575. eCollection 2018. PubMed PMID: 30519068; PubMed Central PMCID: PMC6237134.
235. GiacomelliL, Togni S, Meneghin M, Eggenhöffner R, Maramaldi G. In vivo validation of the multicomponent powder (Vitachelox(®)) against the deposition of polluting ions. Clin CosmetInvestig Dermatol. 2018 Mar 8;11:109-113. doi: 10.2147/CCID.S156324. eCollection 2018. PubMed PMID: 29563824; PubMed Central PMCID: PMC5846751.
236. Borda LJ, Wong LL, Tosti A. Bioidentical hormone therapy in menopause: relevance in dermatology. Dermatol Online J. 2019 Jan 15;25(1). pii: 13030/qt4c20m28z. Review. PubMed PMID: 30710894.
237. Piérard GE, Humbert P, Berardesca E, Gaspard U, Hermanns-Lê T, Piérard-Franchimont C. Revisiting the cutaneous impact of oral hormone replacement therapy. Biomed Res Int. 2013;2013:971760. doi: 10.1155/2013/971760. Epub 2013 Dec 21. Review. PubMed PMID: 24455744; PubMed Central PMCID: PMC3881660.
238. Samaras N, Papadopoulou MA, Samaras D, Ongaro F. Off-label use of hormones as an antiaging strategy: a review. Clin Interv Aging. 2014 Jul 23;9:1175-86. doi: 10.2147/CIA.S48918. eCollection 2014. Review. PubMed PMID: 25092967; PubMed Central PMCID: PMC4116364.
239. Vinogradova Y, Coupland C, Hippisley-Cox J. Use of hormone replacement therapy and risk of venous thromboembolism: nested case-control studies using the QResearch and CPRD databases. BMJ. 2019 Jan 9;364:k4810. doi: 10.1136/bmj.k4810. Erratum in: BMJ. 2019 Jan 15;364:l162. PubMed PMID: 30626577; PubMed Central PMCID: PMC6326068.
240. Jospe N, Orlowski CC, Furlanetto RW. Comparison of transdermal and oral estrogen therapy in girls with Turner's syndrome. J Pediatr Endocrinol Metab. 1995 Apr-Jun;8(2):111-6. PubMed PMID: 7584704.
241. Warren MP, Shu AR, Dominguez JE. Menopause and Hormone Replacement. [Updated 2015 Feb 25]. In: Feingold KR, Anawalt B, Boyce A, et al., editors. Endotext [Internet]. South Dartmouth (MA): MDText.com, Inc.; 2000-. Available from: https://www.ncbi.nlm.nih.gov/books/NBK279050/

242. Jenifer Sassarini, Mary Ann Lumsden, Oestrogen replacement in postmenopausal women, Age and Ageing, Volume 44, Issue 4, July 2015, Pages 551–558, https://doi.org/10.1093/ageing/afv069
243. Botelho MA, Queiroz DB, Barros G, Guerreiro S, Fechine P, Umbelino S, Lyra A, Borges B, Freitas A, Queiroz DC, Ruela R, Almeida JG, Quintans L Jr. Nanostructured transdermal hormone replacement therapy for relieving menopausal symptoms: a confocal Raman spectroscopy study. Clinics (Sao Paulo). 2014 Feb;69(2):75-82. doi: 10.6061/clinics/2014(02)01. PubMed PMID: 24519196; PubMed Central PMCID: PMC3912337.
244. Kopper NW, Gudeman J, Thompson DJ. Transdermal hormone therapy in postmenopausal women: a review of metabolic effects and drug delivery technologies. Drug Des DevelTher. 2009 Feb 6;2:193-202. PubMed PMID: 19920906; PubMed Central PMCID: PMC2761184.
245. Abdi F, Darooneh T, Ghorbani M, Banihashemi F, Roozbeh N. Transdermal hormone replacement therapy with nanostructured medicines. Ginekol Pol. 2017;88(2):103-108. doi: 10.5603/GP.a2017.0018. Review. PubMed PMID: 28326520.

CHAPTER 5

SUNSCREEN AND SUNTAN PREPARATIONS

5.1 BACKGROUND

Ra (Re) was the primary name of the sun god of Ancient Egypt. According to Osiris myth, Nut, the mother of Osiris swallowed the setting sun (Ra) each evening and gave birth to him each morning. The Ancient Egyptians were well aware of the dangers of the sun. Their lands were scorched with heat. Women protected their skin, preferring light skin to dark in their cultural hierarchy of beauty. Recent discoveries written on papyri and the walls of several tombs unearthed ingredients and formulations in use in Ancient Egypt specifically addressing issues of sun damage to the hair and skin. Also, a brief historical review manifests the following interesting things indeed:

- Jasmin was used to heal the sun-damaged skin. Recent evidence reveals that Jasmin aids in DNA repair at the cellular level.
- Aloe was used to heal sun-damaged skin.
- Olive oil was used as a hydrating oil for both skin and hair damaged by overexposure to the sunlight.
- Almond oil was applied before and after sun exposure to hydrate the sun-damaged skin, improving elasticity and texture.
- Rice bran extracts were used in sunscreen preparations. Today, gamma oryzanol extracted from rice bran has UV absorbing properties.
- kohl (to darken eyes in order to combat sunlight impairment to the retina in the glare of the desert sun), red ochre (to redden and impart a rosy glow in women's makeup mimicking the effect of the sun on the skin), and henna oil (to dye the lips and nails, darken the color of the hair and skin, and protect light skin from the sun). Today, henna is one of the most widely used natural sunscreen with both UVA and UVB protection.

- Lupin extract was used to block the rays of the sun and is still used to date to lighten the color of the skin.
- Calcite powder and clay were used as UV filters similar to the modern-day inorganic particulates zinc oxide and titanium dioxide.
- Aquatic lotus oil was used for protection of the skin from the sun.

5.2 ABSTRACT

The sunscreen industry is achieving remarkable worldwide prominence by responding to the growing need for skin protection with fast-paced innovation. Increased consumer awareness of the harmful effects of sunlight has fueled the demand for improved photo protection. The need for broad-spectrum protection from both UVA and UVB rays has inspired scientists worldwide to research new cosmetic formulations and delivery systems. More effective sunscreen actives, emollients and novel cosmetic and functional ingredients have been regularly added to the formulator's repertoire. Creativity in innovation has been hindered only by regulatory agencies and patent restrictions worldwide. Familiarity with the current restrictive regulations and patent law infringements has become integral to any research effort attempting to provide improved protection to individuals affected by the sun's damaging effects. The increasing incidence of skin cancers and photo damaging effects caused by ultraviolet radiation has increased the use of sun screening agents, which have shown beneficial effects in reducing the symptoms and reoccurrence of these problems. Unlike the situation in Europe where sunscreen ingredients are considered under cosmetics guidelines, the FDA is required to define sunscreens as drugs since they are advertised to prevent sunburn and, more recently, the risk of skin cancer. In the USA, the FDA has been regulating this industry since August 25, 1978, with the publication of the Advance Notice of Proposed Rulemaking. Sunscreens are considered drugs and cosmetics and therefore must be governed by the FDA-OTC monograph. With the variety of sunscreen agents used in cosmetic and UV protection products, Australia, Canada, and the European Union (EU) have also developed regulatory protocols on safe sunscreen product use. Unlike the USA though, Australia has approved 34 active sunscreen ingredients and the EU has approved 28 of these ingredients. Current FDA regulations allow labeling of sunscreen products to a maximum of 30þ, despite the many products currently available with numbers as high as 100. From a cosmetic formulation point of view, increasing the SPF number in a product is governed by simple chemical principles.

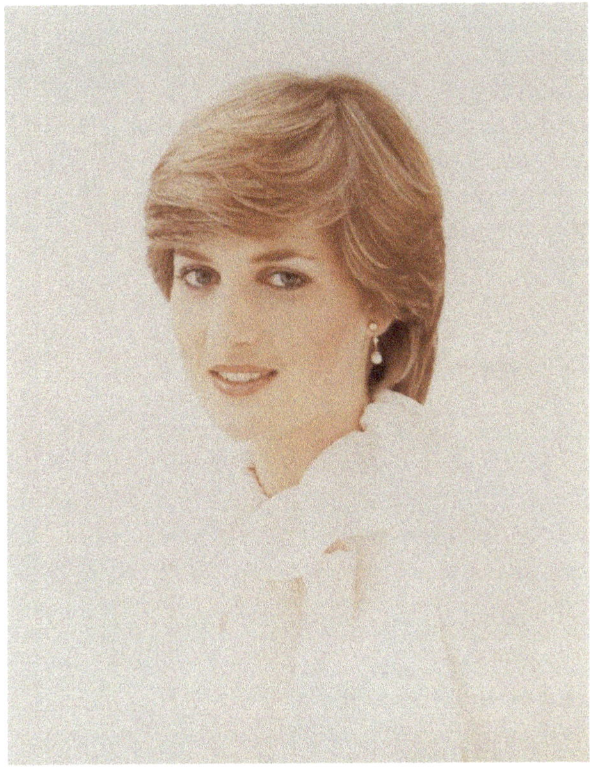

Figure 5.1 Diana, Princess of Wales, Vogue 1981. According to the magazine Longevity, Princess Diana was "scrupulous about using an SPF-8 sunblock." While the American Academy of Dermatology recommends applying at least SPF 30, protection against UV rays can prevent both sunburn and dangerous skin cancers Courtacy: GoodHousekeeping.com,).

5.3 INTRODUCTION

Protection from sunlight is often equated with the use of sunscreens, but this approach is too narrow, and protection should consist of a package of measures: avoiding overexposure to sunlight, using sunscreens, and wearing protective clothing. Solar ultraviolet (UV) radiation significantly influences the skin, causing aging, sunburns, precancerous and cancerous lesions, and immunosuppression. UV radiation has an immunosuppressive effect on the antigen-presenting cells within the epidermis and contributes to the likelihood of skin cancer. If solar radiation is a primary risk factor for malignant melanoma, it is reasonable to conclude that reducing sun exposure via topical sunscreen use would be associated with reduced disease risk. Melanoma is more common in Whites than in Blacks and Asians. The incidence of non-melanoma skin cancer (NMSC) is dramatically increasing worldwide, despite the increased use of improved sunscreens. In 2014, the Surgeon General estimated that 2.2-

5.0 million people were treated annually for NMSC. As the number of newly diagnosed skin cancers continues to rise, there is a need for additional preventative measures beyond sunscreens. UV radiation is the second most prevalent carcinogenic exposure in Canada, fifth in Switzerland and is similarly important in other countries with large Caucasian populations. Within the UK, Wales has among the highest rates of skin cancer annually and skin cancer diagnosis rates have increased 63% in 10 years. Australia and New Zealand have the world's highest skin cancer cases. People living in Australia and New Zealand are now advised to apply sunscreen every day when the UV index is predicted to reach 3 or above. Denmark has one of the highest incidences of melanoma in the world, although it is a relatively northern country. Implications for public health: Increased use of sunscreen as part of the daily routine to reduce incidental sun exposure will lead to decreased incidence of skin cancer in the future. There are 3 kinds of UV radiation: UVC, UVB, and UVA. The ozone layer ingests 100% of UVC, 90% of UVB, and a negligible measure of UVA. Therefore, exhaustion of the ozone layer expands UV transmission. UVA is related with aging and pigmentation. It enters profound into the skin layer and creates free extreme oxygen species, in a roundabout way damaging DNA. UVA expands the number of incendiary cells in the dermis and diminishes the quantity of antigens introducing cells. UVB causes sunburn and DNA strand breaks. It causes pyrimidine dimer changes which are related with non-melanoma skin malignancies. Photoprotection includes both essential and secondary protective variables. Essential variables are sunscreens; these incorporate physical barriers which reflect and dissipate light, and substance barriers which ingest light. Secondary components incorporate cancer prevention agents, osmolytes, and DNA repair enzymes which help to constrain skin harm by exasperating the photochemical cascade that happens by UV sunlight. People with black skin are much less susceptible to sunburn than white-skinned individuals. Black people living in the UK were more likely to use sunscreen as a form of sun protection, whereas sunscreen was the least popular modality in the two African countries with shade being the most common form of limiting sun exposure. A significant benefit from regular sunscreen use has not yet been demonstrated for primary prevention of basal cell carcinoma and melanoma. Concerning the prevention of actinic keratoses, squamous cell carcinomas, and skin aging, the effect of sunscreens is significant, but it remains incomplete. Some organic UV filters (PABA derivatives, cinnamates, benzophenones, and octocrylene) have been described to cause photo allergy. Percutaneous absorption and endocrine disrupting activity of small-sized organic and nano-sized inorganic UV filters have been reported.

5.4 POSITIVE EFFECTS OF UVR

Exposure to UVR is not always considered bad. In fact, UVR has been found to be particularly helpful in treating vitamin D deficiency, seasonal affective disorders, psoriasis, sarcoidosis, mycosis fungoides, and numerous other cutaneous conditions. Within the epidermis, 7-dehydrocholesterol is converted to vitamin D (cholecalciferol) by UVB light. The elderly and young children are the ones who are particularly susceptible to vitamin D deficiency. Vitamin D deficiency can lead to rickets in children, osteomalacia in adults, osteopenia/osteoporosis, and fractures in the elderly. The Institute of Medicine recommends the following vitamin D allowances: 400 IU for 0 to 12 months, 600 IU for 1 to 70 years, and 800 IU for greater than 70 years. Light therapy is an inexpensive treatment and can be beneficial in treating certain diseases. Although it has been known for the last 100 years that UV light (particularly UVC with a wavelength range of 240–280 nm) is highly germicidal, its use to treat wound or other localized infections remains at an early stage of development. *Candida auris* is a globally emerging yeast, causing severe infections in patients with underlying diseases. This yeast is responsible for several outbreaks within healthcare facilities, where it can be found on hospital surfaces and patient care devices. Spread from these fomites may be prevented by improving the decontamination of hospital surfaces. UV-C decontamination may constitute an effective adjunct to routine room cleaning. Additionally, difficult-to-treat psoriasis patients sometimes find relief with UVR. It is thought that UVR has both antiproliferative and anti-inflammatory effects through the downregulation of T-cell response to antigens. Studies have also shown improvement of the cutaneous effects of sarcoidosis with UVA-1 light and topical psoralen plus UVA (PUVA) therapy. PUVA and narrowband UVB has been shown to induce and maintain remissions of mycosis fungoides. Phototherapy is the use of light for reducing the concentration of bilirubin in the body of infants. However, the exposure to UV in childhood has been established as an important contributing factor for melanoma risk in adults and considering the high susceptibility to UV-induced skin damage of the newborn, related to his pigmentary traits, the UV exposure of the infant during phototherapy should be "as low as reasonably achievable," considering that it is unnecessary to the therapy. Protective eyewear can be necessary during newborn assistance activities carried out in proximity of some sources. Most people judge sun exposure in non-erythemic doses as pleasant. Exposure to sunlight has been linked to improved energy and elevated mood. Seasonal affective disorder (SAD) is a seasonal pattern of recurrent major depressive episodes that most commonly occurs during autumn or winter and remits in spring. The prevalence of SAD ranges from 1.5% to 9%, depending on latitude. Evidence on light therapy as a preventive treatment for patients with a history of SAD is limited, preventive treatment of SAD and the treatment selected should be strongly based on patient preferences Light therapy, an effective treatment for seasonal affective disorder (SAD), may also be appropriate for MDD which is the second-ranked cause of disability worldwide. Bright light treatment, both as monotherapy and in combination with fluoxetine, was efficacious and well-tolerated in the treatment of adults with nonseasonal MDD. The combination treatment had the most consistent effects [77-83].

5.5 SUNBURN

5.5.1 SUNBURN AND SUNSCREEN FACTS

- Sunburn and sun poisoning are forms of skin damage due to UV ray exposure. The symptoms can range from mild to severe and may require treatment.
- Sunburn might be sun poisoning if there is blisters, hives or rash, fever and chills, nausea, dehydration, headache, pain and tingling, vision problems [1].
- UV rays are most intense at noon and the hours immediately before and after (between 10AM and 4PM) [2], [10].
- Immediate symptoms of sunburn are hot, red, tender skin; pain when the skin is touched or rubbed; and dehydration; several days after exposure the skin may swell, blister, and peel [3].
- Most sunburns are mild and can be treated with home remedies such as applying damp cloths or compresses to reduce the pain, soaking in a tepid bath (with no soap), gently patting the skin dry, applying soothing creams or lotions, OTC pain relievers such as Tylenol or others, and moisturizing the skin [4].
- Sunburn may cause permanent skin damage and skin cancer (malignant melanoma, basal cell carcinoma, squamous cell carcinoma) [5].
- Persons with certain pigment disorders and individuals with fair skin are at most risk of sunburn [6].
- Certain diseases and conditions pose a higher risk of sunburn (for example, albinism, lupus, porphyria, vitiligo, and xeroderma pigmentosum) [7].
- Some medications may increase sensitivity to sunburn (photosensitivity) [8], [10].
- Sun poisoning is caused by severe sunburn; its symptoms include fever, nausea, chills, dizziness, rapid pulse, rapid breathing, dehydration, and shock [9].
- UVA and UVB are mainly responsible for skin pathologies such as sunburns, cutaneous degeneration, photosensitivity, phototoxicity, photo-aging, immunosuppression and skin cancer [27].
- Snow reflects up to 80% of the sun's rays, sand reflects 15%, and grass, soil, and water reflect 10%. Due to these factors, an individual sitting under a solitary standard beach umbrella can be exposed to up to 84% of the total

UV radiation despite feeling adequately covered. For these reasons, it is best to seek deep shade [28].

- Less than 50% of the SPF number claimed on the label is spread on the consumer's skin, meaning that a sunscreen with an SPF 30 will give the real protection of an SPF of 15. Therefore, SPF 60 should be recommended if real protection of 30 is desired. Significant injury, DNA damage, mutations, and carcinogenesis can and do occur also with cumulative sub-erythemal UV exposure [29].
- The SPF was created in 1956 by Schulze and it reflects the ratio between the lower amount of UV energy required to produce a minimal erythema on sunscreen protected skin and the amount of energy required to produce the same erythema on unprotected skin [31].
- Since many of UV filters were shown to cross the blood-brain barrier (BBB), the risk for neurotoxicity also occurs [37].
- Sunscreen compounds might block vitamin D synthesis or act as endocrine disruptor and lead to developmental toxicity. The effects of sunscreen on cutaneous synthesis of vitamin D induced by sunlight have been a subject of debate for recent years; however the newest analysis suggests, that normal usage of sunscreen by adults do not decrease cutaneous synthesis of vitamin D [38].
- The FDA is notoriously slow in approving sunscreen compounds, requiring exhaustive evidence of their safety. Indeed, FDA has approved only 16 sunscreen ingredients (14 organic filters and two nonorganic filters, including zinc oxide and titanium dioxide), while other areas of the world, like the European Union and Australia, have approved nearly twice as many [39].
- FDA approved sunscreen ingredients are Aminobenzoic acid, Avobenzone, Cinoxate, Dioxybenzone, Homosalate, Meradimate, Octocrylene, Octinoxate, Octisalate, Oxybenzone, Padimate O, Ensulizole, Sulisobenzone, Titanium dioxide, Trolamine salicylate, Zinc oxide [44].
- Two of the 16 main ingredients used in OTC sunblock products are safe, the FDA said. Moreover, the FDA is requesting more information on 12 ingredients among the 16 [45].
- The FDA has changed its guidelines to address broad-spectrum sunscreen use, which involves UVA and UVB coverage; water resistance, to indicate the time duration the sunscreen is effective; and sun protection factor (SPF). SPF-15 or higher is recommended and can be labeled as reducing the risk of skin cancer and early skin aging [40].
- PABA and trolamine salicylate — are not GRASE for use in sunscreens, are no longer permitted for use in OTC sunscreen products. No sunscreens sold in the United States contain PABA or trolamine salicylate [41,42].

- For a decade, Environmental Working Group (EWG) has worked to raise concerns about sunscreens with oxybenzone, which is found in nearly all Americans, detected in breast milk and potentially causing endocrine disruption [43].
- Hawaii recently enacted legislation that will ban the use of two major ingredients -oxybenzone and octinoxate-that have also been implicated in coral toxicity and will be banned. This creates a healthcare dilemma: Will the protection of coral reefs result in an increase in human skin cancers? [51].

5.5.2 SUNBURN: PATHOPHYSIOLOGY

Sunburn is a radiation burn to the skin caused by too much exposure to the sun's UV rays or artificial sources such as tanning beds. Chronic sun exposure creates premature cutaneous aging, decreases immune response to environmental pathogens, and increases the risk for developing premalignant and malignant neoplasms [77]. The biggest risk factors for sunburn is the amount of time the skin is exposed to UV rays, plus the intensity. Many factors such as time of day, medications, ozone depletion, high altitude, clear skies, and skin phototypes influence sunburns [11]. Exposure to solar radiation has the beneficial effects of stimulating the cutaneous synthesis of vitamin D and providing radiant warmth. Unfortunately, when the skin is subjected to excessive radiation in the ultraviolet range, deleterious effects may occur. The most conspicuous is acute sunburn or solar erythema. Initially, UVR causes vasodilation of cutaneous blood vessels, resulting in the characteristic erythema. Within 1 hour of UVR exposure, mast cells release preformed mediators including histamine, serotonin, and tumor necrosis factor, leading to prostaglandin and leukotriene synthesis. Within 2 hours after UV exposure, damage to epidermal skin cells is seen. Erythema usually occurs 3-4 hours after exposure, with peak levels at 24 hours [12]. Sunburns are graded as pink, red, and blistering. In contrast, thermal burns are graded by degree (first, second, and third), but this classification should not be applied to sunburns because thermal burns have quite different sequelae, such as scarring and death, which are extremely rare consequences of sunburn. Keratoconjunctivitis or ocular sunburn can also be caused by UV radiation, and it follows a similar time course [13]. Studies have shown that UVA impairs the antigen presenting cell (APC) activity of the epidermal cells and thereby causes immune suppression, thus contributing to the growth of skin cancer [30]. In summary, UVA radiation can cause nuclear and mitochondrial DNA damage, gene mutations and skin cancer, dysregulation of enzymatic chain reactions, immune suppression, lipid peroxidation (membrane damage), and photoallergic and phototoxic effects.

On the molecular level, exposure to UV radiation can result in a covalent joining of pyrimidine (usually thymine) dimers. DNA repair mechanisms, such as nucleotide excision repair, base excision repair, or mismatch repair genes, do not recognize dimers, the mutations go uncorrected to the cell cycle. When mutated genes reach the cell cycle, if not repaired by the induction of the p53 pathway, a series of changes can result in malignant transformation and immunosupression. UV-induced immunosuppression contributes to skin cancer due to damage to DNA and inhibition of protective mechanisms within the skin (**Figure 5.2**). A common type of sun-related skin damage is actinic keratosis (AK). Age, Fitzpatrick skin type 1 or 2 (**See exhibit 1**), and UV light are the major risk factors for developing AK. Most AKs do not progress into invasive squamous cell carcinoma (SCC), but the risk is still present. The risk of malignant transformation of an AK to SCC within one year is approximately 1 in 1,000. However, approximately 60% of invasive SCCs of the skin probably arise from AKs. If not treated or protected against additional sun damage, AKs may eventually progress to invasive SCC. Avoiding sun exposure and daily application of sunscreen statistically decreases the number of AKs [77].

Exhibit 1. Fitzpatrick's Skin Phototypes [14]

- **Type I:** Pale white skin, burns easily, does not tan
- **Type II:** White skin, burns easily, tans with difficulty
- **Type III:** White skin, may burn but tans easily
- **Type IV:** Light brown/olive skin, hardly burns, tans easily
- **Type V:** Brown skin, usually does not burn, tans easily
- **Type VI:** Black skin, very unlikely to burn, becomes darker with UV radiation exposure

* Individuals with Type I to III Fitzpatrick skin phototypes were at increased risk for sunburn.

The diagnosis of SCC has increased over the past 30 years. The most important risk factor for SCC is cumulative sun damage and age, the risk was greatest in those with more than 30,000 hours of cumulative lifetime sun exposure. UVA, UVB, PUVA, and tanning beds have been shown to increase the incidence of cutaneous SCC. Prevention of SCC includes protection from the sun, including the use of protective clothing and the application of sunscreen. Basal cell carcinoma (BCC) is the most common skin cancer and occurs most frequently on the face and head. In Caucasians, the incidence of BCC has steadily increased and the lifetime risk of developing BCC is 30% [86]. BCC arises from the basal layer of epidermis and its appendages. The most important risk factor is chronic UVR. Other known risk factors include fair skin, light eyes, red hair, chronic arsenic exposure, therapeutic radiation, immunosuppression, basal cell nevus syndrome, and various other genetic predispositions. Primary prevention is protection from sun exposure beginning at an early age [77]. Other than UVR, exposure to arsenic, radiation, chronic inflammatory conditions in skin, and burns, scars, infections complications or even tattoos are also the contributing factors for BCC [96].

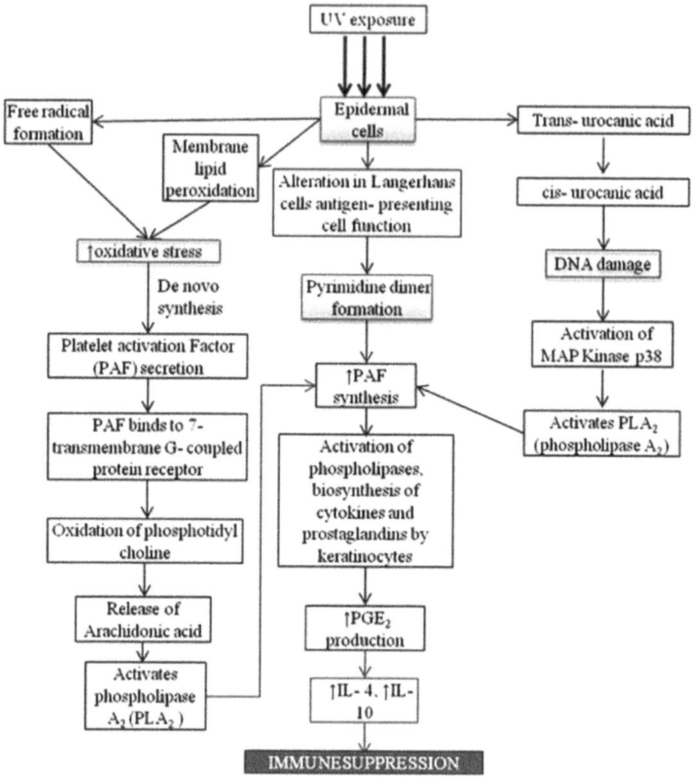

Figure 5.2 Mechanism of UV induced immunosuppression [130], [139-141]. UVR, in particular the UVB range, suppresses the immune system in several ways. UVB inhibits antigen presentation, induces the release of immunosuppressive cytokines and causes apoptosis of leukocytes. UVB, however, does not cause general immunosuppression but rather inhibits immune reactions in an antigen-specific fashion. Application of contact allergens onto UV-exposed skin does not cause sensitization but induces antigen-specific tolerance since such an individual cannot be sensitized against the very same allergen later, although sensitization against other allergens is not impaired. This specific immunosuppression is mediated by antigen-specific suppressor/ regulatory T cells. UVB-induced DNA damage is a major molecular trigger of UV-mediated immunosuppression. Reduction of DNA damage mitigates UV-induced immunosuppression. Likewise, interleukin-12 which exhibits the capacity to reduce DNA damage can prevent UV-induced immunosuppression and even break tolerance. Presentation of the antigen by UV-damaged Langerhans cells in the lymph nodes appears to be an essential requirement for the development of regulatory T cells. Studies addressing the molecular mechanisms underlying UV-induced immunosuppression will contribute to a better understanding of how UV acts as a pathogen but on the other hand can be also used as a therapeutic tool.

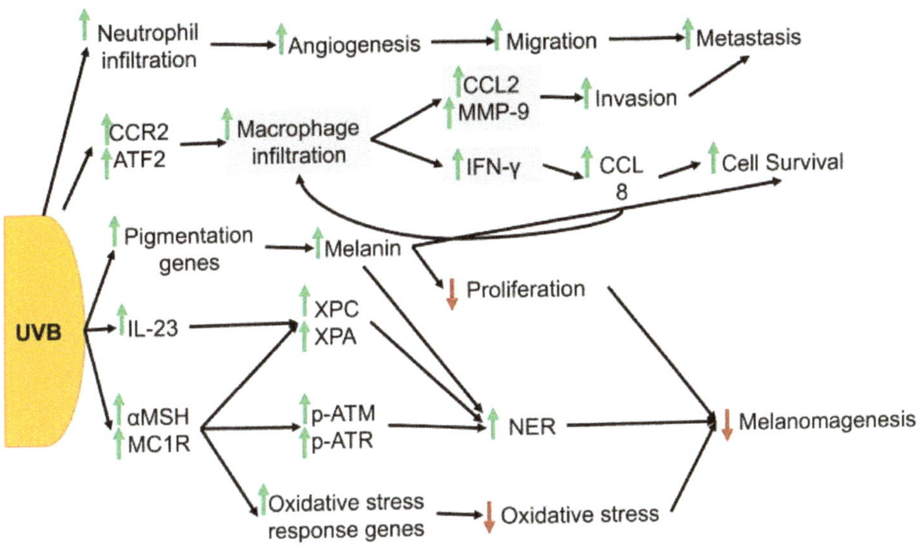

Figure 5.3 UVB response in melanoma [85]. UVB exposure triggers macrophage and neutrophil infiltration into the skin. Upregulation of CCR2 and ATF2 in melanocytes promotes recruitment of macrophages into the skin, which in turn stimulates production of CCL2, MMP-9, and IFN-γ in macrophages. IFN-γ signaling from macrophages promotes a positive feedback loop between melanocytes and macrophages, in which melanocytes upregulate CCL8, a CCR2 ligand, and promote further recruitment of macrophages. The inflammatory response created by macrophage and neutrophil recruitment promotes angiogenesis, as well as melanoma cell invasion, survival, and metastasis. UVB also independently regulates melanin production and MC1R signaling. Induction of pigmentation genes and subsequent increase in melanin production following UVB increases cell survival and NER, but decreases proliferation and ultimately, melanomagenesis. Signaling through MC1R is induced by UVB and activates DNA damage response. Signaling through αMSH and MC1R promotes phosphorylation of ATM and ATR, upregulates XPC, and promotes XPA recruitment to stimulate NER. αMSH also activates oxidative stress response genes to reduce oxidative stress in melanocytes/melanoma. UVB-induced expression of IL-23 also activates XPC and XPA to induce NER. IL-23 signaling, melanin production, and MC1R signaling can all inhibit melanomagenesis induced by UVB. Abbreviation: Activating Transcription Factor 2 (ATF2); Chemokine (C-C motif) Receptor 2 (CCR2); Chemokine (C-C motif) Ligand 2 (CCL2); Matrix Metalloproteinase-9 (MMP-9); type II Interferon (IFN-γ); Interleukin-23 (IL-23); Nucleotide Excision Repair (NER); Melanocortin 1 Receptor (MC1R); Ataxia-Telangiectasia Mutated gene (ATM); α-Melanocyte-Stimulating Hormone (αMSH); Ataxia Telangiectasia and Rad3-related (ATR); Xeroderma Pigmentosum Group C (XPC); Xeroderma Pigmentosum group A (XPA).

Epidemiological analysis reveals that annually in the United States alone, ~5 million skin cancer patients are treated and that between 40 and 50% of Americans are susceptible to develop skin cancer at least once by the age of 65 [96]. More than 90% of melanoma cases in the United States are attributed to skin cell damage from UV radiation exposure. Skin cancer is the most common form of cancer, representing 40–50% of all cancers diagnosed in the US.

Melanoma is the most serious form of skin cancer. Melanoma is responsible for the most skin cancer deaths, with about 9,000 persons dying from it each year [84]. Despite early screening and detection programs, the overall mortality rate from melanoma has remained stable or continues to rise. The incidence of melanoma has more than tripled in the Caucasian population in the United States over the past 30 years. An estimated 60–70% of cutaneous malignant melanomas are thought to be caused by UV radiation exposure. Two types of UV radiation are primarily responsible for causing carcinogenic skin damage: UVA (315 nm-400 nm) and UVB (280 nm-315 nm) [85]. Intense and intermittent sun exposure at a young age increases a patient's risk of melanoma. Individuals with five or more severe sunburns in childhood or adolescence have an estimated twofold greater risk of developing melanoma. Melanoma is commonly found in areas sporadically exposed to UVR, such as the back of the legs in women and the backs of men. UVB, UVA, and PUVA therapy all have been proven to increase the risk of melanoma. Appropriate UVR protection decreases the risk of developing a melanoma or having a secondary melanoma. Studies indicate that decreasing recreational sun exposure following the diagnosis of primary melanoma can significantly decrease the chance of developing a second melanoma [77].

Exhibit 2. Environmental Factors That Influence Ultraviolet Radiation [32-36]

- **Ozone layer:** The main absorber of UVR, is produced for the most part in the terrestrial stratosphere of the equatorial region of the planet. Ozone layer is the name given to the region with high concentration of this gas in the Earth's atmosphere, located at a height between 15 and 30 km. This layer contains between 80 and 90% of the total ozone in the terrestrial atmosphere and is responsible for the intensive absorption of UVB radiation and part of the extinction of UVC radiation.
- **Altitude**: The higher the altitude of a location, the thinner is the atmosphere above it and, consequently, the larger the quantity of UVR reaching the surface. In situations of clear and cloudless skies, the UVR flux may increase between 5 and 10% for each 1000 m altitude. Nevertheless, this altitude-related increase in URV may vary to values close to 20% per kilometer, as it depends on a series of other factors, such as the quantity of ozone in the lower layers of the atmosphere, the type of surface that reflects UV radiation, the particulates present in the atmosphere and even the position of the sun.
- **The time of day**: In a clear sky situation, the "higher" the Sun is in the sky, the higher the levels of UV radiation are. This means that the farther the Sun is from the horizon, the shorter the optical pathway the radiation has to cross in the atmosphere.

Contd...

- **The season of the year**: In the summer, the Sun reaches higher positions in relation to the horizon than in the winter and, consequently, the UVR flux is more intense. The differences between the seasons of the year become more relevant as the latitude becomes higher.
- **Clouds**: Clouds can both attenuate and enhance UVB radiation, although attenuation is generally the case. Completely overcast clouds always attenuate UVB rays, even up to 99% of UVB radiation in extreme cases. Up to 50% enhancement of UVB radiation can occur from broken clouds [39] or at elevated sites above clouds.
- **Suspended Particles:** Polluted environments or those with suspended dust may show UVR attenuation in relation to clear sky situations. Some studies demonstrate that polluted locations, such as São Paulo or Mexico City, may present situations with around 20% of the incident UVR.
- **Surface reflection (albedo):** The term 'albedo' is used to express the relationship between the radiation reflected by a surface and the radiation such surface receives from the Sun. Very light colored surfaces, such as freshly fallen snow, may reflect up to 90% of the incident radiation; therefore, wearing adequate protection for the eyes and skin is required in environments like mountains and ski tracks.
- **Outdoor Vs Indoor Working:** Outdoor workers can get three to nine times as much solar UVR exposure as indoor workers. Paradoxically, outdoor workers have a lower incidence of cutaneous malignant melanoma compared to indoor workers. It is supposed that indoor solar UVA exposure, which causes mutations, depletes vitamin D3 in the skin. Behavior includes the time spent outdoors and the use of photoprotective agents. In adult life, a British indoor worker in the UK might typically receive 30% of his or her annual UV exposure from sun-seeking holidays, 40% from summer weekends, 20% from casual weekday exposure between April and September and just 10% from sun exposure during the 6 months period October to March.

5.5.3 PHOTOAGING

Every organ experience aging in various ways. Skin aging can be categorized into three groups, intrinsic, photo, and hormonal aging. The consequences of photo-aging are usually characterized by morphological changes including wrinkle formation or by histological changes in connective tissues. In order to generate more wrinkles, vasculature structures are needed to develop. Numerous reports suggested that angiogenesis plays a significant role in inducing wrinkle formation in photo-damaged skin [142]. Among harmful environmental factors that contribute to extrinsic aging, long-term effects of repeated exposure to ultraviolet light are the most significant and are referred to as photoaging. Premature skin aging and development of malignant cutaneous tumors, melanoma and non-melanoma, are interrelated issues that are increasingly important problems in the field of dermatology. Skin aging is important aesthetically, whereas skin cancer is a direct threat to the health of the patient [143]. Photoaging is a multisystem degenerative process that involves the skin and skin support system. It is a cumulative process and depends primarily on the degree of sun exposure and skin pigment. The epidermis and dermis are both affected by UVB, but the dermis is also affected to a significant extent by UVA. It has long been thought that the majority of human photo-lesions due to UVB rays, now it is believed that UVA play a substantial role in photoaging. Photoaging affects the sun-exposed areas and is characterized clinically by fine and coarse wrinkling, roughness, dryness, laxity, teleangiectasia, loss of tensile strength and pigmentary changes [144]. These changes are more severe in individuals with fair skin and are further influenced by individual ethnicity and genetics. Photoaging may be prevented and treated with a variety of modalities, including topical retinoids, cosmeceuticals, chemical peels, injectable neuromodulators, soft tissue fillers, and light sources [145]. There is also an increase in the development of benign and malignant neoplasms on photoaged skin. During the years the progress has been made in understanding the photoaging in human skin. UV irradiation invokes a complex sequence of specific molecular responses that damage skin connective tissue [146]. In severely damaged skin, there is loss of epidermal polarity (orderly maturation) and individual keratinocytes may show atypia, especially the lower epidermal layers. More profound changes occur in the dermis, where photodamage is characterized by degeneration of collagen and deposition of abnormal elastotic material, reflected by wrinkles, furrows, and yellow discoloration of the skin. The greater the photodamage, the more the accumulation of thickened, tangled and degraded elastic fibers [153]. The application of topical growth factors after microneedling can be useful to reduce visual signs of facial photoaging by improving skin texture and minimizing the appearance of fine lines and wrinkles [151]. Amongst retinoids, tretinoin is the most potent and best-studied retinoid. However, its irritation potential has prompted dermatologists to switch over to less irritating but comparably effective retinoids like adapalene and to some extent retinol and retinaldehyde [154]. Bakuchiol (functional analogue of topical retinoids, as both compounds have been shown to induce similar gene expression in the skin) is a phytochemical that has demonstrated cutaneous antiageing effects when applied topically. Bakuchiol is promising as a more tolerable alternative to retinol [152].

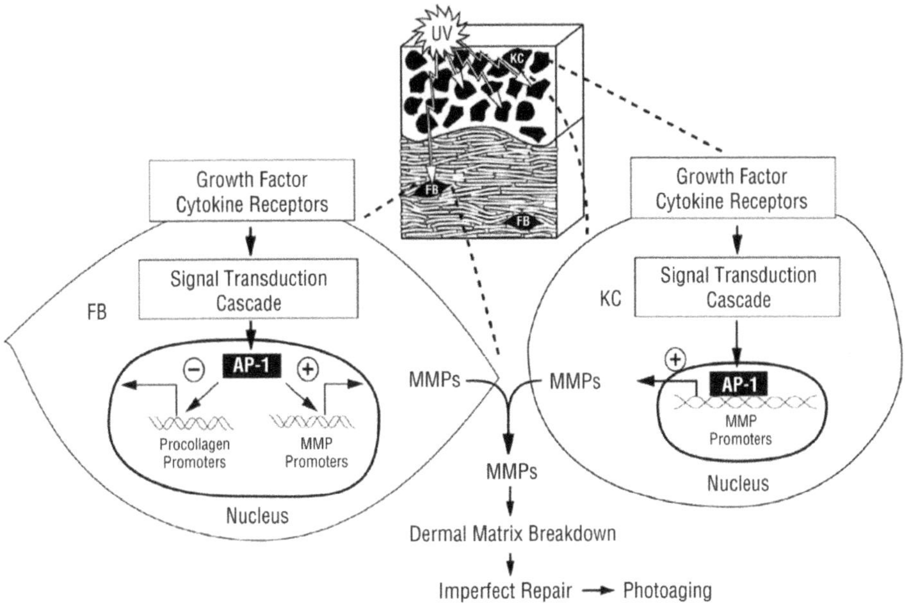

Figure 5.4 Mechanisms of Photoaging and Chronological Skin Aging [143], [147-150]. Photodamaged skin displays variable epidermal thickness, dermal elastosis, decreased/fragmented collagen, increased matrix-degrading metalloproteinases, inflammatory infiltrates and vessel ectasia. The main effects of acute and chronic exposure to UV radiation are DNA damage, inflammation and immunosuppression. These effects are direct as well as indirect due to ROS production. The ROS are particularly harmful in that they destabilize other molecules and promote chain reactions that damage biomolecules rapidly, such as telomere shortening and deterioration, mitochondrial damage, membrane degradation and oxidation of structural and enzymatic proteins. Collagen and elastin are the structural proteins of the ECM. The deterioration/remodeling of the collagen and elastin fibers facilitates angiogenesis and metastasis, and the damaged collagen and elastin proteins serve as additional sensitizers of photooxidative stress. Accumulation of collagen fragments, which occurs with chronic UV exposure and the passage of time, impairs the mechanical and functional properties of the dermal extracellular matrix. Elastic fibres, such as oxytalan fibres in papillary dermis, are associated with not only skin resilience, but also skin surface texture, and elastic fibre formation by fibroblasts is facilitated by increased expression of fibulin-5. Thus, induction of fibulin-5 expression is a damage-repair mechanism, and fibulin-5 is an early marker of photoaged skin.

Exhibit 3. Comparison between photoaging and intrinsic aging [130]

Particular	Photoaging	Intrinsic aging
Epidermal changes	Thickness increases, acanthropic in early phase and atrophy in later stages	Thin epidermis
	Proliferative rate is higher than normal	Proliferative rate is lower than normal

Contd...

Particular	Photoaging	Intrinsic aging
	Non-uniform and random distribution of keratinocytes, polarity of cells is lost, frequent enlargement	Uniform and defined distribution of keratinocytes, polarity is maintained, usually atrophied
	Diversifi ed melanosomes	Uniformly distributed melanosomes
	Increased number of stratum corneum (SC) cell layer	Normal cell layer
	Vitamin A content is destroyed by sun exposure	Plasma content of retinol increases
Dermal changes	Marked elastogenesis followed by massive degeneration	Elastogenesis followed by elastolysis
	Massive increase in elastic fibers	Gradual decline in production of dermal matrix
	Increased lysozyme deposition on elastic fibers	Modest lysozyme deposition on elastic fibers
	Decrease in amounts of mature collagen	Mature collagen more stable in degradation
	Increased mast cells	Decreased mast cells
	Vessels become dilated	Micro vessels decrease
	Pronounced inflammation	No inflammatory response
	Marked increase in glycosaminoglycans	Slight decrease in glycosaminoglycans
Common signs and symptoms	Mild (age 28–35 years): Few wrinkles, no keratoses Moderate (age 35–50 years): Early wrinkling, sallow complexion with early actinic keratoses	Fine wrinkles, thin and transparent skin Loss of underlying fat leading to hollowed cheeks and eye sockets with noticeable loss of firmness on the hands and neck
	Advanced (age 50–60 years): Persistent wrinkling, discoloration of the skin with telangiectases and actinic keratoses	Bones shrink away from the skin as a result of bone loss, which causes sagging of skin, dry skin with pruritus
	Severe (age 65–70 years): Severe wrinkling, photo aging, gravitational and dynamic forces affecting the skin, actinic keratoses with or without skin cancer	Inability to sweat sufficiently to cool the skin, faster graying of hair

Exhibit 4. Exogenous antioxidants with photoprotective or damage protective effects [154]

Antioxidants	Outcome of the study
Ascorbic acid	Topical vitamin C 5% cream applied for six months led to clinical improvement in the appearance of photoaged skin
	Topical vitamin C stimulates the collagen-producing activity of the dermis
	Magnesium ascorbyl phosphate administration immediately after exposure in hairless mice significantly delayed skin tumor formation and hyperplasia induced by chronic exposure to UV radiation
	Ascorbic acid was a photoprotectant when applied to mice and pig skin before exposure to ultraviolet (UV) radiation
Vitamin E	UV-induced vitamin E depletion
	The interaction of vitamin E with the eicosanoid system may result in an anti-inflammatory effect and thereby complement the photoprotective effects of other antioxidants in the skin
	Vitamin E has skin barrier-stabilizing properties
Lycopene	UV light decreased skin lycopene concentrations more so than skin β-carotene concentrations
	Lycopene protects against UV-induced erythema in humans
Carotenoids (carotene, β-carotene, and carotenoid mix)	Carotenoids are efficient in photoprotection, scavenging singlet oxygen, and peroxyl radicals. Supplements or a carotenoid-rich diet decreased sensitivity against UV-induced erythema
	Supplementation with carotenoids contributes to basal protection of the skin but is not sufficient to obtain complete protection against severe UV irradiation
	Dietary beta-carotene has effect on wrinkles and elasticity, procollagen gene expression, and ultraviolet (UV)-induced DNA damage in human skin
	Erythema-protective effect of a carotenoid mix inhibited serum lipid peroxidation
	Presupplementation with β-carotene before and during sunlight exposure provides protection against sunburn
	Inhibition of UV-induced epidermal damage and tumor formation in mouse models
Tretinoin	Topical tretinoin ameliorates the clinical signs of photoaging
	The treatment of photodamaged skin with tretinoin increased collagen I formation.

Contd...

	Topical tretinoin is safe and effective in the treatment of photodamage
	Improvement in photodamaged skin
	Topical tretinoin reduced the effects of photoaging
	Topical tretinoin in combination with sun protection as a useful approach to the treatment of sun-damaged skin
Coenzyme Q10 (CoQ10)	Topical application of CoQ10 has the beneficial effect of preventing photoaging
	Coenzyme Q10 protects against oxidative stress-induced cell death and enhances the synthesis of basement membrane components in dermal and epidermal cells
	CoQ10 was shown to reduce UVA-induced MMPs in cultured human dermal fibroblasts
Glutathione	Glutathione is a photoprotective agent in skin cells
Zinc	Zn-treated fibroblasts were more resistant to UVR than cells grown in normal medium
	Zn can positively influence the effects of oxidative stress on cultured human retinal pigment epithelial (RPE) cells
Resveratrol	Application of resveratrol to the skin of hairless mice effectively prevented the UVB-induced increase in skin thickness and the development of the skin edema
Green tea	Green tea polyphenols were shown to reduce UV light-induced oxidative stress and immunosuppression
	Topical treatment or oral consumption of green tea polyphenols (GTP) inhibits chemical carcinogen- or UV radiation-induced skin carcinogenesis in different laboratory animal models
Green tea or caffeine	Oral administration of green tea or caffeine in amounts equivalent to three or five cups of coffee per day to UVB-exposed mice increased levels of p53, slowed cell cycling, and increased apoptotic sun burn cells in the epidermis
Sylimarin	Silymarin strongly prevents both photocarcinogenesis and skin tumor promotion in mice
	Skin cancer chemopreventive effects
Genistein	Antioxidant and anticarcinogenic effects on skin
Cocoa	Dietary flavanols from cocoa contribute to endogenous photoprotection, improve dermal blood circulation, and affect cosmetically relevant skin surface and hydration variables
	Photoprotection against UV-induced erythema

5.5.4 SUNBURN HOME REMEDIES AND TREATMENT

Certain medical treatments have been tried and studied to treat sunburn. However, in general, most remedies have not shown any clinically proven benefit as far as speeding the recovery or reversing the damage. Therefore, most of the treatments available are only used to treat symptoms.

- **Nonsteroidal anti-inflammatory drugs** (NSAIDs): Systemic and topical nonsteroidal anti-inflammatory drugs, when used at dosages to achieve optimal serum levels for anti-inflammatory effect, only result in an early and mild reduction of ultraviolet B-induced erythema [15]. In oral (ibuprofen, Motrin, Naprosyn, Advil etc.) or topical diclofenac 0.1% gel (Solaraze) forms have shown to reduce redness if applied before or immediately after UVB exposure. This benefit may be diminished after 24 hours. These medications may also help relieve the symptoms of sunburn such as pain and discomfort [4].
- **Topical steroid creams** have not shown any significant improvement in sunburn symptoms. Oral steroids such as prednisone have not proven to be beneficial and have been associated with some significant side effects. Treatment with topical moderate-potency or high-potency corticosteroids does not provide a clinically useful decrease in the acute sunburn reaction when applied 6 or 23 hours after UV exposure [16].
- **Applying Aloe Vera gel**: The topical application of Aloe Vera is not an effective prevention for radiation-induced injuries and has no sunburn or suntan protection [17]. The Aloe Vera cream was continuing applied at the test sites twice daily for the next three weeks. The results showed no sunburn or suntan protection and no efficacy in sunburn treatment when compared to placebo. The Aloe Vera cream has no bleaching effect too. However, this may be beneficial in treating the symptoms [18].
- **Topical anesthetics:** Advertised remedies such as topical anesthetics (benzocaine) may help with symptoms of sunburn, however, very little clinical data is available to substantiate their effectiveness. LMX is a topical liposomal formulation containing 4% or 5% lidocaine. LMX 4% is available OTC and is FDA-approved for temporary relief of pain and itching associated with minor cuts, minor burns, sunburn, and insect bites [19].
- **Vitamin D Preparations:** Vitamin D enables anti-inflammation to promote tissue repair in response to injury. Mechanistically, vitamin D signaling activated M2-autophagy regulators Kruppel like factor 4 (KLF4), peroxisome proliferator activated receptor gamma (PPARG), and arginase 1. Analysis of UV-exposed human skin biopsies detected a similar increase in macrophage autophagy following vitamin D intervention, identifying an essential role for autophagy in vitamin D-mediated protection of skin from UV damage [25].

- **Sunscreens:** Sunscreens represent a practical approach to photoprotection for the skin. The importance of beginning sun protection at a young age cannot be overstated. In humans, the regular use of sunscreens has been shown to reduce AKs, solar elastosis, UV-induced immunosupression, and photosensitivities. Sunscreens also prevent the formation of SCCs in animals. A thorough understanding of the mechanism of action of sunscreens, different sunscreen vehicle choices, and adverse effects can help educate patients on their choice of sunscreens [77].

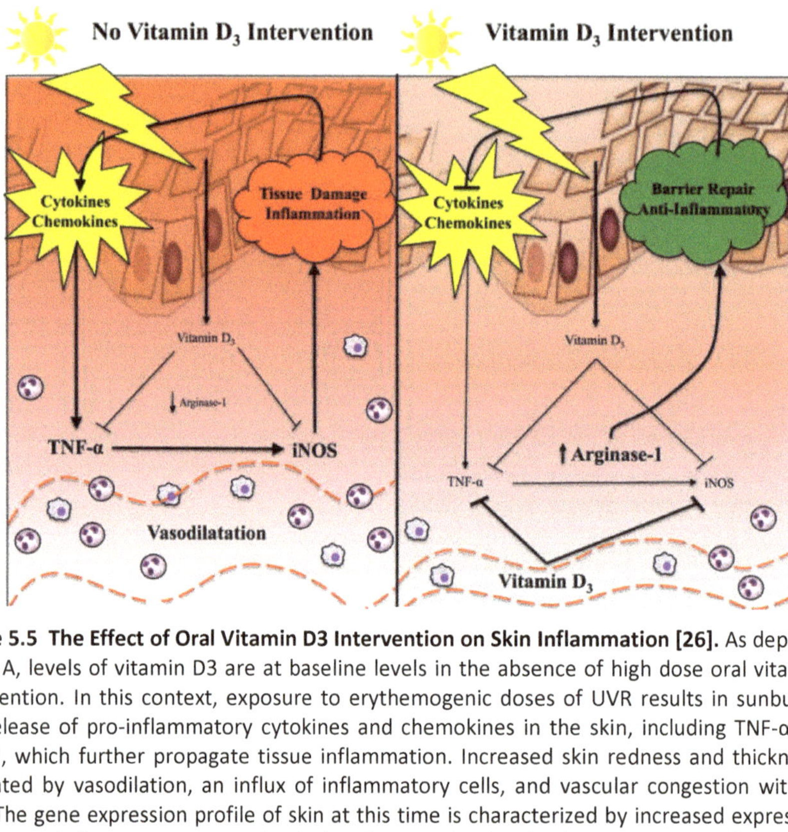

Figure 5.5 The Effect of Oral Vitamin D3 Intervention on Skin Inflammation [26]. As depicted in panel A, levels of vitamin D3 are at baseline levels in the absence of high dose oral vitamin D3 intervention. In this context, exposure to erythemogenic doses of UVR results in sunburn and the release of pro-inflammatory cytokines and chemokines in the skin, including TNF-α** and iNOS*, which further propagate tissue inflammation. Increased skin redness and thickness are mediated by vasodilation, an influx of inflammatory cells, and vascular congestion within the skin. The gene expression profile of skin at this time is characterized by increased expression of various pro-inflammatory genes. As depicted in panel B, levels of vitamin D3 rapidly rise within the serum after high dose oral vitamin D3 intervention. Arginase-1 is up- regulated within the skin, and production of the pro-inflammatory mediator's TNF-α and iNOS are attenuated after sunburn. Reduced skin erythema and thickness are observed clinically. The gene expression profile of skin at this time is characterized by increased expression of skin barrier genes, which help to repair the epidermal barrier and attenuate the inflammatory insult. *iNOS is the synthase isoform most commonly associated with malignant disease.** TNF-α is a primary cytokine that can be induced in keratinocytes and in dermal fibroblasts by UVB, synthesized in adipose tissue by adipocytes and other cells in the tissue matrix. TNF-α is mainly secreted by activated macrophages immediately postburn. The host immune response is activated by TNF-α, as is the subsequent release of cytokines following trauma and infection.

5.5.5 MEDICATION RESPONSIBLE FOR INCREASE SKIN SENSITIVITY TO SUNLIGHT

A large number of medications are known to increase skin sensitivity to sunlight and are called photosensitive drugs or medications. Photo-sensitizing chemicals usually have a low molecular weight (200 to 500 Daltons) and are planar, tricyclic, or polycyclic configurations, often with heteroatoms in their structures enabling resonance stabilization. All absorb UV and/or visible radiation, a characteristic that is essential for the chemical to be regarded as a photosensitizer. Some of the common ones include:

- **NSAIDs** (nonsteroidal anti-inflammatory drugs)
- **Antibiotics:** Tetracyclines (tetracycline, doxycycline [Vibramycin]), Quinolone (ciprofloxacin [Cipro], levofloxacin [Levaquin]), Sulfonamides (sulfamethoxazole and trimethoprim; cotrimoxazole [Bactrim, Septra], sulfamethoxazole [Gantanol]).
- **Diuretics (water pills):** thiazides (hydrochlorothiazide [Hydrodiuril], furosemide [Lasix])
- **Cardiac medications:** amiodarone (Cordarone), quinidine
- **Diabetes drugs:** sulfonylureas such as chlorpropamide (Diabinese), glyburide (Micronase, DiaBeta, Glynase)
- **Psychiatric drugs:** chlorpromazine (Thorazine), tricyclic antidepressants such as desipramine (Norpramin) and imipramine (Tofranil)
- **Acne medications:** isotretinoin (Accutane) [20-24], [34].

Exhibit 5. Cosmetic ingredients and cancer risk [34]

Cosmetic substance	Risk
DEA (diethanolamine) TEA (triethanolamine)	Can result in the formation of carcinogenic nitrosamines
Bronopol (2-bromo-2-nitropropane-1,3-diol)	May break down into formaldehyde and also cause the formation of nitrosamines
1,2-Dioxane in surfactants/detergents	Contaminated with carcinogenic 1,4-dioxane
Artificial colors (as Blue 1 and Green 3)	Carcinogenic
Hair dyes	Dark colors ingredients are carcinogenic
Cosmetic lanolin	Can be contaminated with carcinogenic pesticides such as DDT, dieldrin, and lindane, in addition to other neurotoxic pesticides
Talc	Carcinogenic
Silica	May be contaminated with carcinogenic crystalline quartz

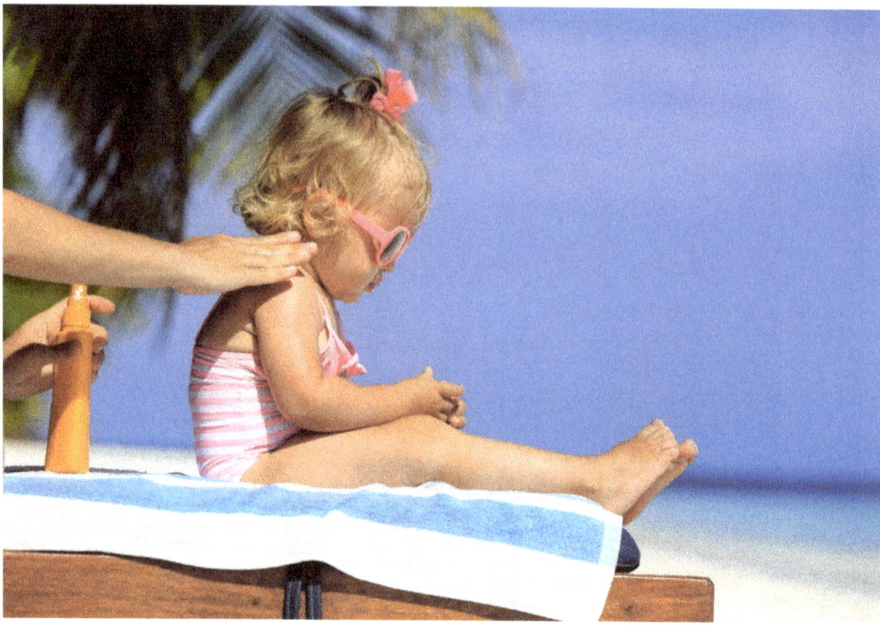

Figure 5.6 Use of Sun Protective [178]. Public guidelines for sun protection have been updated as stakeholders warn that Australians are using sunscreen as a "suit of armour". Heather Walker, chair of Cancer Council Australia's National Skin Cancer Committee, said that recent research shows 85% of people do not apply sunscreen correctly. The Australasian College of Dermatologists and Cancer Council updated the guidelines following concerns that many Australians only use sunscreen to protect their skin. By not using clothing, a broad-brimmed hat, shade, sunglasses and sunscreen correctly when the ultraviolet index reaches three or above, they are putting themselves at risk, the organizations say (Courtacy: imfarmacias.es).

Exhibit 6. Endocrine disrupting effects of the commonly used UV filters [74]		
UV Filters	**Endocrine Disrupting Effects**	
Benzophenones	**Estrogenic disrupting effects**	Activation of ERα, ERβ; Inhibition of the activity of 17β-Estradiol; Induction of proliferation of MCF-7 cell; Induction of VTG in fathead minnows; Reduce of the uterine weight in immature Long-Evans rats
	Androgenic disrupting effects	Antagonists of human AR transactivation; Repression of 4,5-dihydrotestosterone-induced transactivational activity; Inhibition of testosterone formation in mice and rats
	Disrupting effects toward other nuclear receptors	Inhibition of human recombinant TPO; Interference with THR; Inhibition of TPO activity in rats; Antagonists of PR

Contd...

Camphor derivatives	**Disrupting effects toward estrogen receptor**	Activation of ERα, ERβ; Inhibition of the activity of 17β-Estradiol; Induction of proliferation of MCF-7 cell; Induction of pS2 protein in MCF-7 cells; Reduce of the uterine weight in rats; Induction of VTG in fish
	Disrupting effects toward androgen receptor	Repression of 4,5-dihydrotestosterone-induced transactivational activity; Inhibition of testosterone formation in HEK-293 cells; Antagonists of Human AR
	Disrupting effects toward progesterone receptor	Antagonists of PR; Increase of PR mRNA levels in rats; Inhibition of the expression of PR protein in rats; Disturbance of the expression of membrane-associate PR in insects
Cinnamate derivatives	**Disrupting effects toward estrogen receptor**	Activation of ERα; Inhibition of the activity of 17β-Estradiol; Induction of proliferation of MCF-7 cell; Reduce of the uterine weight in rats; Induction of VTG in fish
	Disrupting effects toward thyroid hormone receptor	Decrease of T4 level; Inhibition of the conversion of T4 to triiodothyronine in rats
	Disrupting effects toward other nuclear receptors	Antagonists of PR and AR; Inhibition of 4,5-dihydrotestosterone activity; Reduce of the prostate and testicular weight in rats

*AR: androgen receptor; ER: estrogen receptor alpha; PR: progesterone receptor; T4: thyroxine; THR: thyroid hormone receptor; TPO: thyroid peroxidase; VTG: vitellogenin

5.5.6 TANNING/PIGMENTATION WITH OR WITHOUT SUN EXPOSURE

Some Africans and Asians avoid the Sun and use bleaching products to lighten skin, while many Caucasians seek the sun for tanning to achieve a bronze skin to "look good." UV radiation from the sun or from artificial sources increases skin pigmentation. Sunlight and indoor UV induced tanning is a common behavior, especially among adolescents, young adults, and individuals with lighter skin. Several health benefit claims such as improved appearance, enhanced mood, and increased vitamin D levels have been attributed to tanning. The Indoor Tanning Association claims that a base tan can act as "the body's natural protection against sunburn. Sunless tanning products may serve as a sensible, safer alternative for those who desire tanned skin [155]. There are three phases of tanning: immediate pigment darkening (IPD), persistent pigment darkening (PPD) and delayed tanning (DT). IPD occurs during the first minutes of exposure to UVA, and then fades within few hours. PPD appears within hours of higher doses of UVA exposure and persist up to several days or weeks. DT develops over 3–7 days after UVB exposure, and then remains for weeks. The mechanisms of UVA- and UVB-induced pigmentation are different. UVA induces IPD and PPD through oxidation of pre-existing melanin or melanogenic precursors. IPD is oxygen dependent, and reactive oxygen radicals are considered to be responsible for this process. PPD is also due to the upward movement of melanosomes toward the surface of the skin. Persons with lightest skin (skin type I) do almost not tan, while IPD and PPD are strongest in moderately and darkly pigmented skin. DT results from synthesis of melanin in the melanocytes, followed by melanin distribution to neighboring keratinocytes [156]. UVA (320–400 nm) causes immediate pigment darkening (IPD) as well as persistent pigment darkening (PPD) of skin within hours via photooxidation and/or polymerization of existing melanin or melanogenic precursors due to the generation of reactive oxygen species(ROS).In contrast, UVB (280–320 nm) induces a slower but more stable type of pigmentation termed delayed tanning (DT) which requires the increased synthesis of melanin following the stimulation of tyrosinase activity and the entire melanogenic cascade [157]. UVB-induced DT is photoprotective (it is estimated to have a SPF of 3)- while DT induced by UVA is not considered to be photoprotective. DT is maximal from 10 days to 3-4 weeks, depending on the UV dose and the individual's skin color. It may take several weeks or months for the skin to return to its base constitutive color. UVA-induced DT is 2-3 orders of magnitude less efficient per unit dose than UVB and has an earlier onset, often directly after IPD [158]. The IPD method can also be used as an appropriate endpoint in the determination of UVA protection. It is time saving, and thus considerably lowers the risk of UV exposure, particularly when testing sunscreen products with higher UVAPF [159]. IPD typically appears gray to black while PPD is brown. Both IPD and PPD do not require any new pigment synthesis and are thought to result from oxidation and/or polymerization of pre-existing melanin or melanogenic precursors and metabolites. Melanosomes have also been shown to redistribute within both keratinocytes and melanocytes during the IPD/PPD response. PPD is not protective against neither UVB-induced erythema nor UVB-induced DNA lesions [160]. Exposure to ultraviolet radiation from indoor tanning device use is associated with an increased risk of skin cancer, including risk of malignant melanoma, and is an urgent public health problem. By reducing indoor tanning, future cases of skin cancer could be prevented, along with the associated morbidity, mortality, and healthcare costs [175].

Exhibit 7. Common Tanning Methods [171-174]

1. *UV Tanning*: Tanning salons offer an indoor method of UVR with tanning beds and booths. These salons expose people to man-made UV light. Tanning beds were introduced in North America in 1978 and gained considerable popularity in the 1980s. Indoor tanning salons are a common choice among those who tan as they do not require people to spend hours outside in the sunlight. At any given tanning salon, there are typically three to five different types of beds. They are classified as level 1 through 6. In general, increasing levels correspond to increasing concentrations of UVA relative to UVB. Increasing the bed level also increases the pressure and number of lamps, resulting in a deeper tan that appears faster and fades slower than lower level beds. In tanning salons, the user has the option to stand (e.g., in a booth) or lie supine (e.g., in a bed). The time spent in a bed is limited by the strength of lamps used and ranges from 8 to 20 minutes. One of the most important differences between beds is the percent of UVA versus UVB light.
2. *Tanners for Topical Use*: Topical sunless tanners are products that are applied to the skin to give the appearance of a tan. These products come in many forms including lotions, gels, mousses, sprays, wipes, creams, and powders. Temporary bronzers are one type of topical self-tanner. Bronzers come in creams, lotions, and powders. When a bronzer is applied to the skin, it coats the outer layers of the epidermis. Bronzers are considered temporary because they only last until they are washed off by normal soap and water use. The use of a bronzer is similar to putting on make-up every day. Commonly used ingredients for temporary bronzers include caramel, walnut oil extract, and jojoba extract. DHA formulations have become popular among the public due to their relative ease of application and longer lasting tan when compared to temporary color bronzers, which wash off readily with soap and water. The temporary color bronzers also have a higher tendency to cause blotchiness, an uneven tan, and a less natural looking color. DHA is not approved for use on non-skin areas, such as the eyes, lips, and mucous membranes. As a result, DHA has not been approved in the use of spray tanning booths due to the potential exposure to non-FDA approved sites, even when taking precautions, such as wearing nose plugs, goggles, or applying petroleum jelly to the lips.
3. *Tanning Pills*: The FDA has banned canthaxanthin-containing tanning pills due to their significant adverse effects when ingested in large quantities. Some of the side effects include gastrointestinal disturbance, urticaria, hepatitis, retinopathy, and potentially fatal aplastic anemia. Tanning pills are non-prescription formulations that are readily available to customers for purchase over the Internet. The most common active ingredient is canthaxanthin. Another common ingredient in tanning pills is beta-carotene, a different carotenoid. Beta-carotene is obtained through the dietary consumption of fruits and vegetables, and it contributes to the yellow pigment found in human skin. Its deposition in the skin is thought to contribute to photoprotection,

Contd...

guarding against the deleterious effects of both natural and artificial UV light exposure, and raising the minimum amount of UVR exposure required to cause a sunburn.

4. *Alpha-Melanocyte Stimulating Hormone Analogues*: Afamelanotide is a subcutaneous implant administered once a month. It has been approved for erythropoietic protoporphyria in Europe. Other analogues of alpha-MSH, Melanotan I and II, are available and unregulated to enhance skin pigmentation for cosmetic tanning. They are not equivalent to afamelanotide. They have been reported to cause side effects, such as satiety, hypertension, and penile erections. Other risks include the potential to transmit blood-borne infections, rhabdomyolysis, encephalopathy, and renal dysfunction. These side effects have not been reported with the controlled-release subcutaneous afamelanotide implant that is undergoing clinical trials.

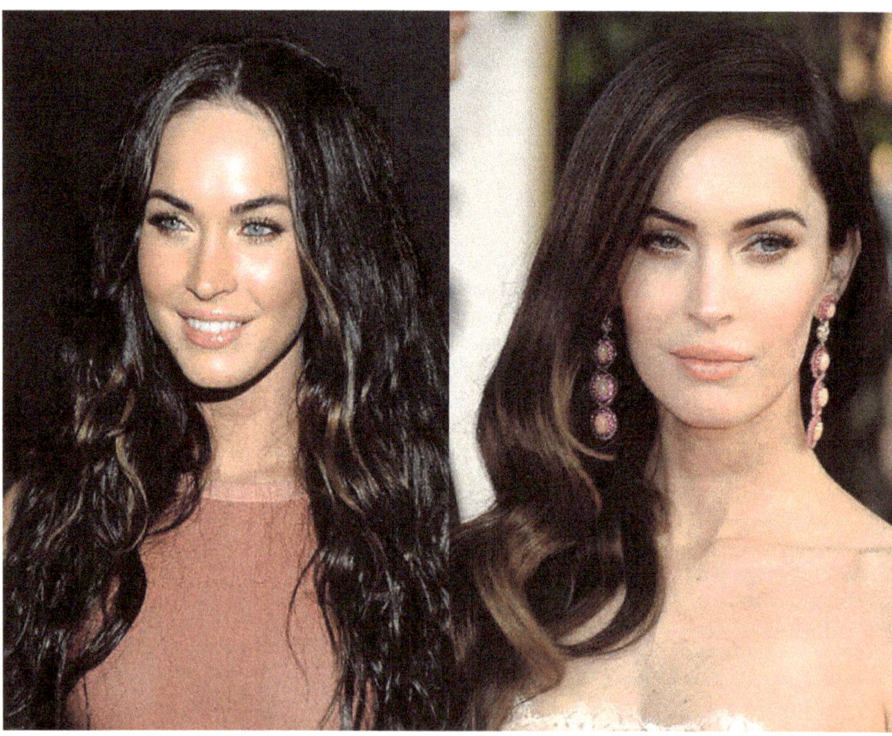

Figure 5.7 Give me a tan! - Megan Fox [176,177]. Megan Fox comes up the most when searching online for pale vs. tan photos. She demanded a sun bed be delivered to the set of Transformers: Revenge of the Fallen, because she was feeling self-conscious about her pale skin, according to Fox News. But they didn't have one available so offered to send an expert to give Megan a customized spray tan. However, Megan turned down the offer, saying she wanted a sun bed instead (Courtacy: Cosmopolitan).

Exhibit 8. Future research opportunities to inform efforts to reduce indoor tanning in the US [175]

Individual-level strategies

- Continue to develop and evaluate tailored and targeted messaging strategies.
- Evaluate the long-term impact that messages have on indoor tanning behaviors.
- Test the efficacy of behavioral counseling among groups other than female undergraduate tanners.

The roles of parents, clinicians, and schools

- Assess parents' perceptions of the risks associated with indoor tanning.
- Assess parents' awareness of their children's use of indoor tanning devices.
- Examine the prevalence of the practice of parents doing indoor tanning with their children.
- Evaluate strategies for engaging parents in prevention efforts targeting children.
- Identify ways to disseminate information about and tools for behavioral counseling to clinicians.
- Monitor clinicians' behavioral counseling practices.
- Develop and evaluate educational, systems, and environmental interventions in school settings.

Mass media campaigns

- Develop and evaluate the efficacy of mass media campaigns.
- Engage celebrities and other public figures in mass media campaign efforts.

Legislation

- Track the development and implementation of new indoor tanning legislation.
- Compare the effects of various types of indoor tanning legislation on behaviors.
- Develop informational resources for decision makers.
- Monitor public support for indoor tanning legislation.

Assessment, monitoring, and evaluation

- Continue surveillance efforts at the national level to track indoor tanning device use.
- Increase surveillance efforts at the state and local levels to track indoor tanning device use.
- Collect data on the prevalence and use of unsupervised indoor tanning devices.
- Monitor indoor tanning attitudes and beliefs among the U.S. population and among indoor tanners.
- Monitor trends in outdoor tanning (i.e., sunbathing).

Contd...

- Conduct economic analyses to quantify the impact on morbidity, mortality, productivity, and health care costs.
- Monitor trends within the indoor tanning industry over time (e.g., industry size and pricing).
- Continue surveillance of melanoma incidence and mortality rates.
- Collect data on basal and squamous cell carcinomas using electronic medical records.
- Conduct modeling studies to estimate trends in the incidence of basal and squamous cell carcinomas.

5.5.7 THE SUN CARE INDUSTRY

The U.S. sun care market size was estimated at USD 1.95 billion in 2016. The growing consumer awareness regarding the ill-effects of over exposure to ultraviolet (UV) rays on the undefended skin is expected to propel growth. Furthermore, rising utilization of organic sun care products owing to absence of synthetic chemicals in the formulation is expected to drive growth over the forecast period. The sunscreen manufacturers are actively using these formulations as it increases the endurance of skin cells against UV rays and enhances the self-defense mechanism. Enhanced standard of living coupled with increasing disposable income of the middle-class working population in economies of North America, including the U.S., is expected to propel sun care market growth over the forecast period. The industry players including L'Oréal are using nanotechnology by manipulating the materials at an atomic or molecular in order to enhance the efficiency of the product. Over the past five years, the Sunscreen Manufacturing industry has grown by 1.6% to reach revenue of $407m in 2018. In the same timeframe, the number of businesses has grown by 3.9% and the number of employees has grown by 1.5% [179,180].

5.6 CLASSIFICATION OF SUNSCREENS

Sunscreens are classically divided into physical or chemical sunscreens. Chemical sunscreen absorbs into the skin and then absorbs UV rays, converts the rays into heat, and releases them from the body. Physical blockers are inorganic and reflect, scatter, and/or absorb UVR. Physical UV absorbers like titanium dioxide and zinc oxide have been considered as highly protective agents against UVR. ZnO and TiO_2 combinations are particularly valuable because of their ability to filter both UVA and UVB radiations, providing broader UVR protection than that observed with individual component [95]. They are used in sunscreens as nanoparticles, which denotes a size <100 nm. The smaller size of these mineral particles increases their cosmetic acceptability by users as they are much less visible after application. ZnO has a broad UVA-UVB absorption curve, while TiO_2 provides better UVB protection. Overall, the human health risks with inorganic filters are extremely low given a lack of percutaneous absorption; however, there is potential risk when exposed via inhalation, prompting recommendations against spray sunscreen products with nanoparticles [111]. UV-A rays heavily contribute to both premature skin aging and skin cancer, while UV-B rays cause sunburn. Hence, the use of sunscreen is strongly encouraged by many healthcare practitioners in order to minimize or possibly eradicate the harmful effects of UV rays on our skin, keeping in mind, that about 90% of all skin cancers are associated with exposure to the sun's harmful radiation. Protection against both UVB and UVA radiation is advocated. Most sunscreens combine chemical UV absorbing sunscreens and physical inorganic sunscreens, which reflect UV, to provide broad-spectrum protection. The correct use of sunscreens should be combined with the avoidance of midday sun and the wearing of protective clothing and glasses, as part of an overall sun protection regimen [94,95]. Unfortunately, inaccurate information is currently roaming the media and the Internet regarding the safety, toxicity, and acute side effects of the active ingredients currently used in sunscreens, therefore discouraging people from using sunscreens [92]. Chemical sunscreens are organic and generally aromatic compounds conjugated with a carbonyl group. They are designed to absorb high-intensity UVR, produce excitation to a higher energy state, and, with the return to the ground state, result in conversion of the absorbed energy into a longer, lower energy wavelength. Chemical sunscreens can be classified based on their portion of UV coverage. Commonly known ingredients for UVB sunscreen protection are Padimate O, octinoxate, octisalate, octocrylene, and ensulizole. Commonly known Studies reveal that Persistent Pigment Darkening (PPD) to be a stable end point inducible by all the UVA wavelengths, not affected by fluence rate, i.e. a reliable endogenous UVA dosimeter in the skin [89]. Problems associated with chemical sunscreens are: (i) Requires about 20 minutes after application before it starts to work (ii) Chemical sunscreens may cause side effects, such as erythema, edema, and irritation (especially for those who have dry skin with a damaged moisture barrier) due to the multiple ingredients combined in order to achieve broad spectrum UVA and UVB protection (iii) The higher the SPF (such as formulas of SPF 50 or greater), the higher the risk of irritation for sensitive skin types (iv) The protection it offers gets used up more quickly when in direct UV light, so re-application must be more frequent. (v) Increased chance of redness for rosacea-prone skin types because it changes UV rays into heat which can exacerbate flushing (vi) May clog pores for oily skin types [93]. The importance of adequate UVA protection has become apparent in recent years. The United States and Europe have different standards for assessing UVA protection in sunscreen products. The majority of tested sunscreens offered adequate UVA protection according to US Food and Drug Administration guidelines for broad-spectrum status, but almost half of the sunscreens tested did not pass standards set in the European Union. UVA sunscreen ingredients are oxybenzone, meradimate, avobenzene, and tetraphthalydine dicamphor sulfonic acid [90,91]. Broad spectrum is a term designed to mean protection from both UVA and UVB. Problems associated with physical sunscreens are: (i) Can rub off, sweat off and rinse off easily, meaning more frequent re-application when outdoors as needed (ii) The physical sunscreen agents impart high opacity to the topical preparation, which makes the formulated creams cosmetically unacceptable and leave a whitish layer on the skin, making some formulas incompatible for medium to dark skin tones (iii) Can be less protective if not applied and re-applied generously and accurately since UV light can get between the sunscreen molecules and get into the skin [93]. There are few reports available on the application of Polymeric Nanoparticles (NPs) of physical and chemical sunscreen ingredients (titanium dioxide, zinc oxide, octyl methoxycinnamate, oxybenzone, octocrylene, and luteolinon) to improve sun protection efficacy. UV-absorbing agents must accumulate within the upper skin layers in order to provide a dense light-absorbing layer and guarantee water resistance. Incorporation of antioxidants could provide additional benefit by scavenging free radicals. Natural polyphenols are attractive in this respect, due to their potential activity as photoprotectans and antioxidants [95].

5.6.1 FDA APPROVED SUNSCREEN INGREDIENTS: LITERATURE REVIEW

A. **Aminobenzoic acid:** Aminobenzoic acid is a Vitamin B Complex Member. The chemical classification of aminobenzoic acid is Vitamin B Complex Compounds. In 1943, p-aminobenzoic acid (PABA) was patented. Red petrolatum was used by the United States military as a sunblock during World War II. The initial compounds were primarily ultraviolet B radiation (UVB) blockers as it was to blame for the most observable effect, sunburn [48]. When exposed to light, aminobenzoic acid (para-aminobenzoic acid or PABA) absorbs UV light and emits excess energy via a photochemical reaction that may cause damage to DNA. Because DNA defects contribute to skin cancer, aminobenzoic acid is no longer widely used in sunscreen formulations. Aminobenzoic acid may also increase oxygen uptake at the tissue level and may enhance monoamine oxidase (MAO) activity to promote the degradation of serotonin, which in excess, may lead to fibrotic changes [46]. Aminobenzoates are the most potent UVB absorber but do not absorb UVA. Their use has declined due to para-aminobenzoic acid (PABA) sensitivity. PABA is a very effective UVB filter; however, it was reportedly the most common photoallergen and contact allergen [47]. (**See also 5.1. Sunburn and Sunscreen Facts**)

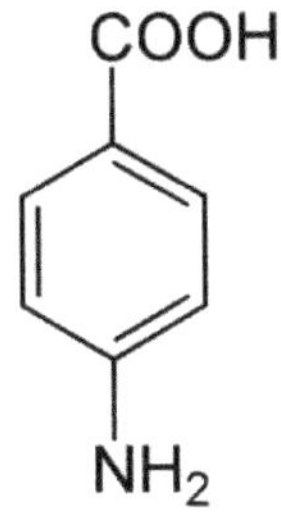

Figure 5.8 p-aminobenzoic acid (PABA)

B. **Avobenzone**: UVA blockers, considered broad spectrum and have a high efficacy against UVA I (>380 nm); however, they are very photounstable and lose from 50% to 90% of their particles after 1 hour of UV exposure. It is also reported that they degrade the UV filter octinoxate [40], [59]. Avobenzone is the most widely used UVA filter in sunscreen lotion and it is prone to degradation in the presence of sunlight/UV radiation, they show a significant skin penetration [56]. 30% HPCD-Avobenzone system was the most photostable following UVA exposure at various regimens and also enabled photoprotective efficiency in vivo, evidenced by lower levels of sunburn cells and skin edema induction [60]. To overcome the photo-instability of avobenzone, various photostabilizers have been used as additives, including antioxidants such as vitamin C, vitamin E, and ubiquinone. The dual role of glutathione as a skin whitening agent and a photostabilizer of avobenzone may be useful for the development of multipurpose cosmetic lotions [49]. Avobenzone is dibenzoyl methane derivative. It is oil soluble crystalline solid [50], [58]. Mesoporous silicas (MSs) containing avobenzone or oxybenzone effectively ameliorated UVA-induced skin disruption and reduced the possible toxicity elicited by percutaneous penetration [56]. Photosensitization by drugs is a problem of increasing importance in modern life. This phenomenon occurs when a chemical substance in the skin is exposed to sunlight. Photosensitizing drugs are reported to cause severe skin dermatitis, and indeed, it is generally advised to avoid sunbathing and to apply sunscreen. In this context, the NSAID diclofenac is a photosensitive drug, especially when administered in topical form. avobenzone provides partial photoprotection to diclofenac from photocyclization to carbazole derivatives [52]. Avobenzone is widely used in various personal care products, is present in swimming pools, and is toxic to aquatic organisms. Avobenzone induces mitochondrial dysfunction-mediated apoptosis leading to abnormal placentation during early pregnancy [53]. Avobenzone was more unstable/toxic than octyl p-methoxycinnamate (an organic UV-B filter originally developed in the 1950s, has been one of the most widely used sunscreens for decades) [54,55]. Octocrylene helps stabilize avobenzone, which is good, but it is a known endocrine disruptor that also releases free radicals [57].

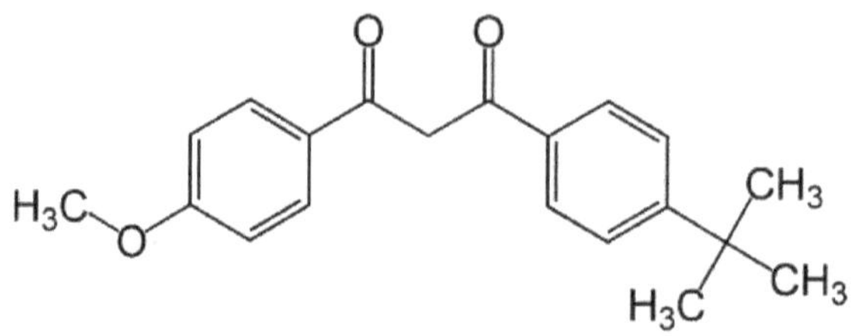

Figure 5.9 Avobenzone

C. Oxybenzone: Oxybenzone is a benzophenone derivative used as a sunscreen agent. Oxybenzone absorbs UVB and UVA II rays, resulting in a photochemical excitation and absorption of energy [116]. Oxybenzone (Benzophenone-3) is an emerging human and environmental contaminant used in sunscreens and personal care products to help minimize the damaging effects of ultraviolet radiation. The Center for Disease Control (CDC) fourth national report on human exposure to environmental chemicals demonstrated that approximately 97% of the people tested have oxybenzone present in their urine, and independent scientists have reported various concentrations in waterways and fish worldwide. Oxybenzone can also react with chlorine, producing hazardous by-products that can concentrate in swimming pools and wastewater treatment plants. Moreover, adverse reactions could very well be increased by the closed loop of ingesting fish contaminated with oxybenzone and/or washing the ingredient off our bodies and having it return in drinking water as treatment plants do not effectively remove the chemical as part of their processing protocols. In humans, oxybenzone has been reported to produce contact and photocontact allergy reactions, implemented as a possible endocrine disruptor and has been linked to Hirschsprung's disease. Environmentally, oxybenzone has been shown to produce a variety of toxic reactions in coral and fish ranging from reef bleaching to mortality [117]. (**See also 5.1. Sunburn and Sunscreen Facts**)

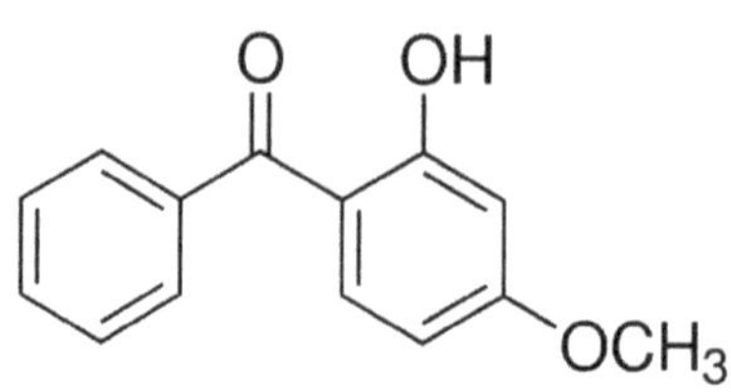

Figure 5.10 Oxybenzone

D. **Dioxybenzone**: Dioxybenzone is an approved sunscreen ingredient in concentrations up to 3% [67]. The benzophenone sunscreens, octabenzone (UV-1) and dioxybenzone (UV-2) were found to exhibit significant chemopreventive activity against mouse skin carcinogenesis which correlated with their antioxidant potency [63]. In a study aimed to qualify photo-safety screening, benzophenone derivatives and ketoprofen exhibited significant reactive oxygen species (ROS) generation upon exposure to simulated sunlight, however ROS generation from sulisobenzone and dioxybenzone was negligible [68]. Polymerization with natural polymer pullulan not only provides a long polymer backbone to dioxybenzone, but also keeps the distance between benzene rings of the dioxybenzone and prevents reduction of photoabsorption intensity. UV/vis spectrophotometry confirmed that dioxybenzone-pullulan polymer and dioxybenzone demonstrated similar UV absorption. Dioxybenzone showed higher plasma concentration after multiple applications compared to that of dioxybenzone-pullulan polymer [64]. Chlorine is used as a chemical disinfectant in swimming pools. Its reactivity suggests sunscreen components might be chlorinated, altering their absorptive and/or cytotoxic properties. Chlorinated oxybenzone and dioxybenzone (caused significantly more cell death than unchlorinated controls. In contrast, chlorination of sulisobenzone reduced cytotoxicity of the parent compound. Exposing a commercially available sunscreen product to chlorine also resulted in decreased UV absorbance, loss of UV protection, and enhanced cytotoxicity [65]. Bromal hydrate was also detected as one of the byproducts generated by oxybenzone and dioxybenzone, which is highly toxic, the "positive halogen" properties of bromal hydrate are responsible for its high toxicity [66]. In addition to allergic reactions, concerns have been raised about the relative ease of which benzophenone is absorbed into the skin and may promote generation of potentially harmful free radicals [69].

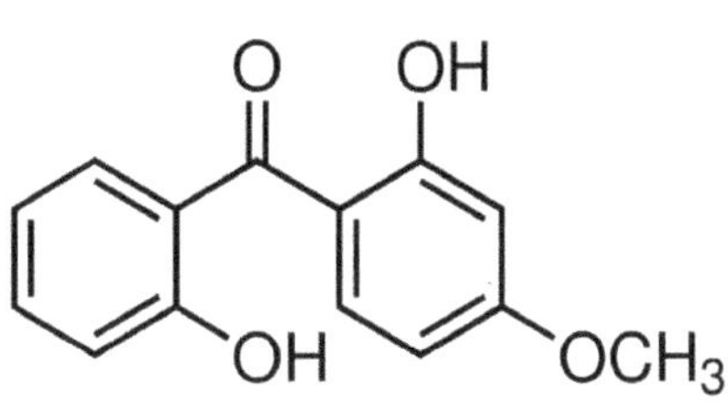

Figure 5.11 Dioxybenzone

E. **Cinoxate:** Ester derivatives such as ethylhexyl methoxycinnamate (octinoxate), isoamyl p-methoxycinnamte (amiloxiate), octocrylene and cinoxate are used in cosmetics all over the world as UV filters. However, their maximum concentrations in cosmetic products are restricted due to their adverse effects, which include contact and photo contact allergies, phototoxic contact dermatitis, contact dermatitis, estrogenic modulation and generation of reactive oxygen species. 4-hydroxycinnamic acid, which is currently indexed as a skin-conditioning cosmetics ingredient, has been widely tested in vitro and in vivo as a new drug candidate for the treatment of hyperpigmentation [61]. Cinnamates have replaced PABA as the next most potent UVB absorber and include octinoxate (OMC) and cinoxate (2-ethoxyethyl-methoxycinnamate). Cinoxate is less commonly used [62]. Major Key players with cinoxate are Major Key Players are Parchem(US), Carbosynth Limited(UK), Synchem UG & Co. KG(DE) [110].

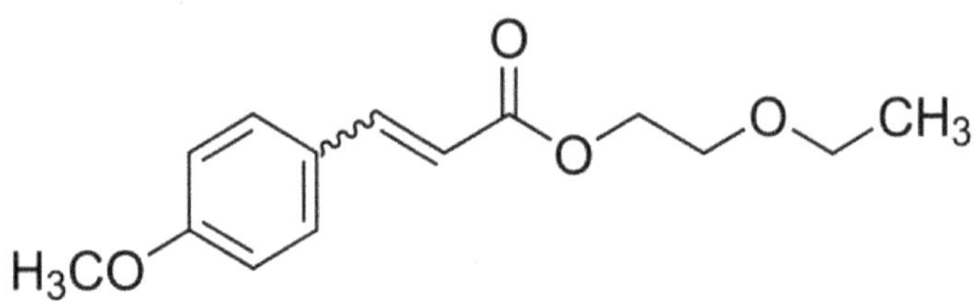

Figure 5.12 Cinoxate

F. Octinoxate: Octinoxate (Octyl Methoxycinnamate, OMC) is a cinnamate ester and common ingredient in sunscreen and other skin care products to minimize DNA photodamage. It was originally developed in 1950's as an organic UV-B filter that absorbs UV-B rays from sun. It is often combined with nanoparticles or other water-resistant liposomes in formulations to increase the localization at the epidermis and decrease the risk of percutaneous absorption [105]. OMC is the most commonly used UVB filter in the US. It is not as potent a UVB absorber as padimate O; for this reason, other UVB absorbers are used in combination to increase the SPF. OMC is not very photostable and degrades in the presence of sunlight after a short period.. OMC is a potent UVB absorber and is the most frequently used sunscreen ingredient. The efficacy of OMC can be further increased when encapsulated in polymethyl methacrylate microsphere [62]. Due to low water solubility (<1 mg/L), OMC is suitable for most waterproof sunscreen formulations [106]. Hawaii legislature passed a bill that outlaws products that contain Oxybenzone and OMC, effective January 2021. The bill is based on studies that show that oxybenzone may harm coral larvae and that both compounds may "bleach" coral, causing it to lose symbiotic algae [107-109]. OMC has been detected in human urine, blood and breast milk, which indicates that humans are systemically exposed to this compound. OMC is an endocrine disruptor that mimics estrogen and can disrupt thyroid function [112,113].

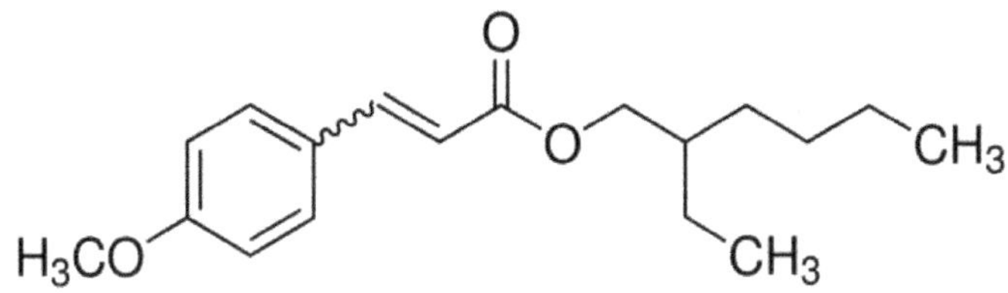

Figure 5.13 Octinoxate

G. **Homosalate:** Homomenthyl salicylate or 3,3,5-Trimethylcyclohexyl Salicylate. After topical application of gel, the bioavailability of HMS was 5.4 ± 1.1 and 4.2 ± 0.6% for high and low doses (10 and 20 mg), respectively. Homosalate (HMS) is an UV filtering agent used in sunscreens and other cosmetics for skin protection purposes. It is a viscous or light yellow to slightly tan liquid or oil, derives from salicylic acid [70,71]. Salicylates are weak UVB absorbers and they are generally used in combination with other UV filters. Both octisalate and homosalate are water insoluble that leads to their high substantivity, which is the ability to retain its effectiveness after exposure to water and perspiration [72]. HMS does not have endocrine disruptor effects on thyroid function and the pubertal development of female and male rats [73]. Another study says HMS is a potential endocrine disruptor and studies in cells suggest it may impact hormones. In addition to direct health concerns following homosalate exposure, the chemical may also enhance the absorption of pesticides in the body [75]. Homosalate suppressed the ear edema response to dinitrobenzene, a possible mechanism of action of the salicylates is suppression of COX [114].

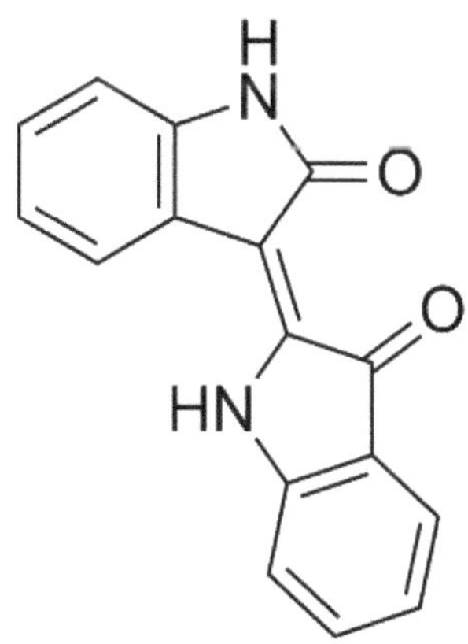

Figure 5.14 Homosalate (Homomenthyl salicylate)

H. Octisalate: Also, Ethylhexyl salicylate, a benzoate ester and a member of phenols. It derives from a salicylic acid. Salicylates are weaker UVB absorbers. It has an approved usage level of 3 to 5% in both the US and EU and is a good solubilizer for benzophenone 3. In suntan lotions, it is used as a preservative and antimicrobial. This salicylate salt is found in wintergreen leaves [115]. They have a long history of use but were supplanted by the more efficient PABA and cinnamate derivatives. They are generally used to augment other UVB absorbers. With the trend to higher SPFs, more octisalate or octyl salicylate (ethylhexyl salicylate) is being used followed by homosalate or homomenthyl salicylate. Both materials can solubilize oxybenzone and avobenzone [97]. Both homosalate and octisalate were found to suppress experimental autoimmune encephalomyelitis (EAE), a widely used animal model of Multiple sclerosis (MS). Thus, salates may be useful new insight into mechanisms of controlling autoimmune disease [114].

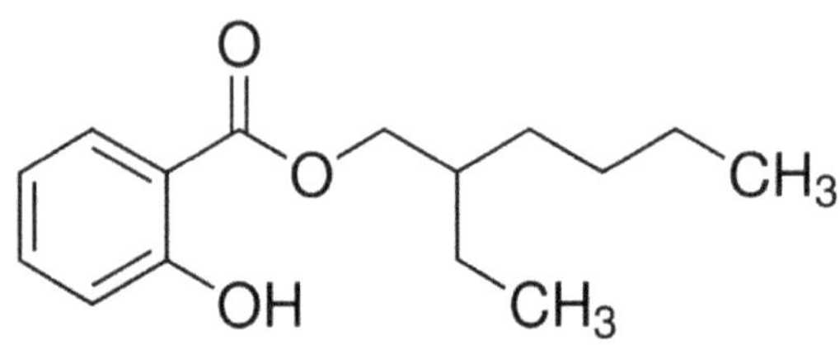

Figure 5.15 Octisalate (Ethylhexyl salicylate)

I. Meradimate (Menthyl Anthranilate)**:** Meradimate, before known as menthyl anthranilate, is used in a maximal concentration of 5% in different products as a UV filter. It is currently required to be named as meradimate in all FDA approved OTC products. Meradimate is approved by the FDA and Health Canada to be used as an ingredient in sunblocking products Meradimate is a monoterpenoid, a broad-spectrum ultraviolet absorber used as a chemical filter in commercial sunscreens [76]. A moderately effective UVA protector not permitted for use in Europe or Japan. Its protective effective action does not cover completely the UVA rays as it only reaches 336 nm. This has been proven even though meradimate has a theoretical protective coverage range between 200-380 nm. Its function is related to the intrinsic structure of meradimate which is an ortho-disubstituted aminobenzoate. This structure allows easy electron delocalization and shifts in the maximum absorption. Poor photoprotection reported by Rodrigues et.al, 2018 makes it a poor choice for an efficient, efficacious sunscreen chemical filter [76], [87,88].

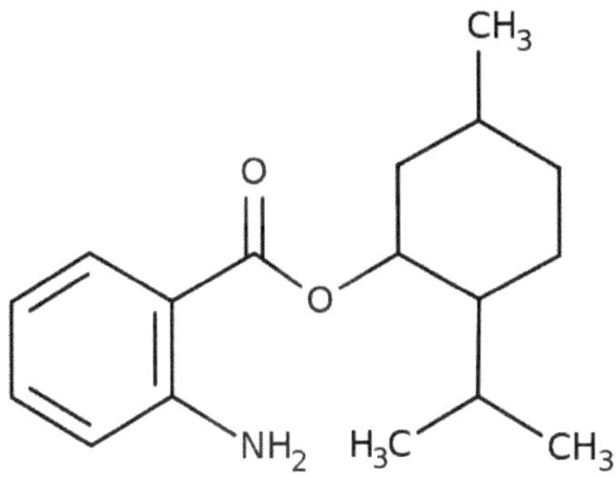

Figure 5.16 Meradimate (Menthyl Anthranilate)

J. Octocrylene: 2-Ethylhexyl-2-cyano-3,3 diphenylacrylate or octocrylene is chemically related to cinnamates. It can be used to boost SPF and improve water resistance in a given formulation. Octocrylene is photostable and can improve the photostability of other sunscreens. It is expensive and can present difficulties in the formulation [97]. The absorption profile of octocrylene spans from 290 to 360 nm with peak absorption at 307 nm. The compound has an excellent safety profile with low irritation, phototoxicity, and photoallergic potential. Octocrylene may be used in combination with other UV absorbers to achieve higher SPF formulas and to add stability. [62]. Photostability refers to the ability of a molecule to remain intact with irradiation. Photostability is potentially a problem with all UV filters. This issue has been raised specifically with avobenzone. This effect may degrade other sunscreens in a formulation, including octyl methoxycinnamate. Octocrylene and some of the newer suncreens, including BEMT, stabilized avobenzone [97]. Chlorination reactions showed that only octocrylene was stable in chlorinated seawater [66]. UVA and UVB screening potentials of octocrylene and zinc oxide formulations were compared in the 290-400 nm wavelength region. Zinc oxide loaded SLN suspensions were found to be more effective in the UVA region while octocrylene loaded ones performed better in the UVB region [98]. Octocrylene appears to be a strong allergen leading to contact dermatitis in children and mostly photoallergic contact dermatitis in adults with an often-associated history of photoallergy from ketoprofen. Patients with photoallergy from ketoprofen frequently have positive photopatch test reactions to octocrylene. These patients need to be informed of sunscreen products not containing octocrylene, benzophenone-3, or fragrances [99,100]. The clinical studies show that octocrylene is both a photocontact allergen and a contact allergen [103]. Octocrylene's ability to cause contact allergy is probably attributable to its reactivity towards lysine [101]. A reduction of the UV filter in the formulation packed in HDPE/LDPE material can occur over time, reducing the protective effect of the product when applied to the skin [102]. Wide application in cosmetics leads to contamination of the aquatic environment, mainly affects transcription of genes related to developmental processes in the brain and liver as well as metabolic processes in the liver (bioaccumulation study in male zebrafish) [104].

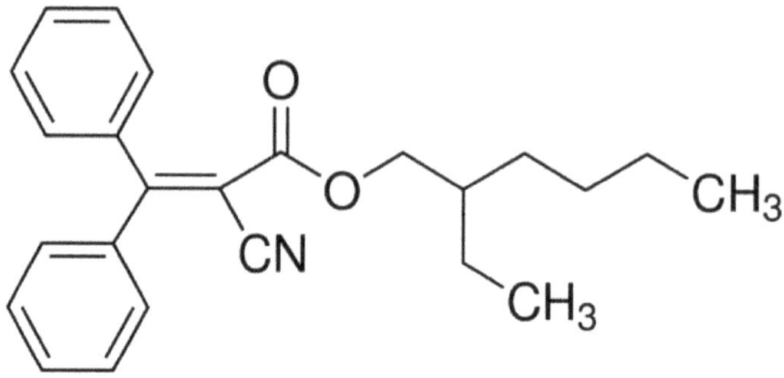

Figure 5.17 Octocrylene (2-Ethylhexyl-2-cyano-3,3 diphenylacrylate)

K. Padimate O: Padimate A and Padimate O were introduced as substitutes for PABA to reduce the number of reactions seen with PABA. Ethylhexyl dimethyl PABA is also known as padimate O, OD-PABA, or octyl dimethyl p-aminobenzoate. It is a viscous liquid tends to retain on the surface of the stratum corneum with little penetration. It has a very low potential for sensitization. Ester derivatives of PABA became more popular with greater compatibility in a variety of more substantive vehicles and a lower potential for staining or adverse reactions. Padimate O is an active sunscreen agent in cosmetics and over-the-counter sunscreen drug products in concentrations up to 8%, as regulated by the FDA. No irritation was reported when both eyes are washed and left unattended. 5% ethylhexyl dimethyl PABA mixed with mineral oil applied to rabbit skin did not cause irritation and no skin sensitization in guinea pigs with the same. High concentrations of padimate O may be toxic to the epididymis and caution should be exercised when administering this substance to infants younger than six months of age due to lack of understanding of its metabolism and absorption. It is widely used as an ingredient in many cosmetics at an average concentration of 1.25% (0.5–2.0%) in Korea. It is toxic to the following four organs: testis, epididymis, spleen, and liver. In addition, experiments using human keratinocytes found that ethylhexyl dimethyl PABA inhibits cell growth and DNA synthesis at low concentrations, and halted the cell cycle of malignant melanoma cell line (MM96L) at the G1 phase. According to the EWG database, it is used in many products including lipstick, conditioner, shampoo, anti-aging agents, hair spray, and sunscreen. No significant reproductive toxicity, genotoxicity, carcinogenicity, skin sensitization, skin irritation, or phototoxicity was observed in response to Padimate O administration (limited studies there, requires further investigations) [97], [118,119].

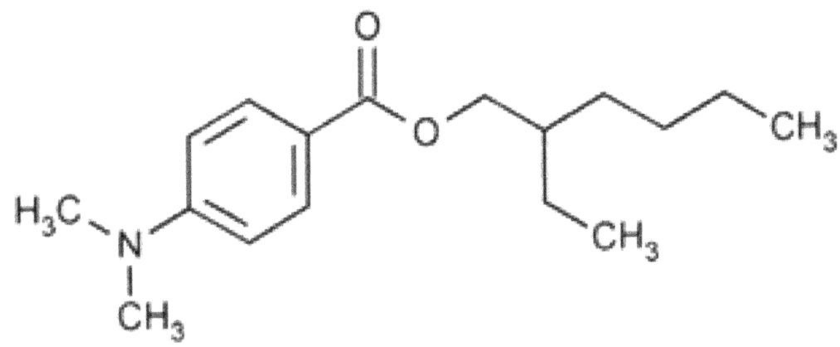

Figure 5.18 Padimate O (Ethylhexyl dimethyl PABA)

L. **Ensulizole:** 2-phenylbenzimidazole-5-sulfonic acid/ Phenylbenzimada-zole sulfonic acid or ensulizole is a water-soluble UVB absorber that can be used in the water phase of emulsion systems. It is commonly found in cosmetic products and sunscreen formulas in combination with other UV filter compounds due to its minimal protection against UV-A wavelengths indicated to be used as an UV-B-absorbing molecule in sunscreen formulations. in contrast to most oil-soluble sunscreen ingredients, allowing for a less-greasy, more aesthetically pleasing formulation such as a daily use moisturizer containing sunscreen. Phenybenzimidazole sulfonic acid boosts the SPF of organic and inorganic sunscreens. It can also be used in clear gels owing to its water solubility. Due to its water solubility, ensulizole is commonly used in products formulated to feel light and less oily. It was demonstrated by studies that ensulizole treatment provided protection against cyclobutane pyrimidine dimers and photosensitized the formation of oxidized guanine bases after UV-A or UV-B exposure. According to the FDA, the maximal approved concentration of ensulizole is 148 mM although concentrations ranging between 74 and 148mM can be found in commercial sunscreen products. Ensulizole is capable of generating reactive oxygen species, including singlet oxygen upon photoexcitation. Based on the findings in vitro and in cellulo, ensulizole induces damage on the DNA, causes DNA strand breaks and photosensitizes the formation of oxidized guanines via type I and II photosensitization mechanisms following UV-A or UV-B irradiation [87], [120-125].

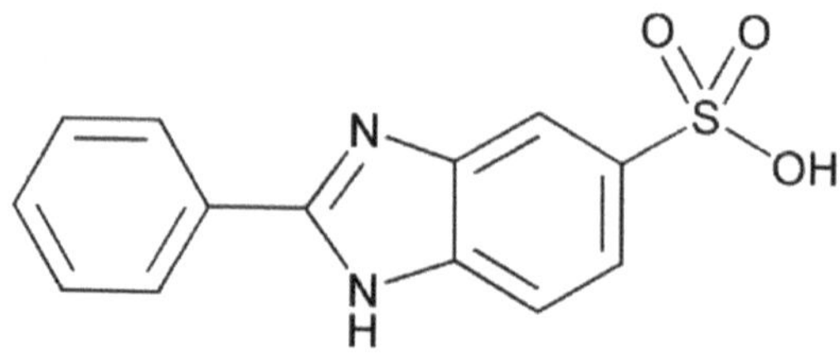

Figure 5.19 Ensulizole (Phenylbenzimadazole sulfonic acid)

M. Sulisobenzone: A benzophenone does not undergo decomposition to an inactive form if it does not couple to target molecules. Instead, it degrades from the photo-excited state back to its initial state, so it can be once again photolyzed to an active state. This process increases the likelihood that the benzophenone will couple to a target molecule during the photoreaction. Benzophenones are used as photoinitiators, fragrance enhancers, ultraviolet curing agents, and, occasionally, as flavor ingredients; they are also used in the manufacture of insecticides, agricultural chemicals, and pharmaceuticals and as an additive for plastics, coatings, and adhesives. The UV-filter substance Sulisobenzone (BP-4) is widely employed in sunscreens and other personal care products. Sulisobenzone is approved by the FDA in concentrations of up to 10% and in Canada, is approved by Health Canada at the same concentrations. It works to filter out both UVA and UVB rays, protecting the skin from sun UV damage. The benzophenones are a group of aromatic ketones that have both pharmaceutical and industrial applications. Benzophenones may be found organically in fruits such as grapes, used primarily as a UVA absorber, but boosts SPF values in combination with other UVB absorbers. Sulisobenzone water soluble, somewhat unstable, and used with less frequency. It can cause skin and eye irritation. It does not penetrate the skin to a large degree, but enhances the ability of other chemicals to penetrate. safety use in sunscreen is questionable [88], [126-130].

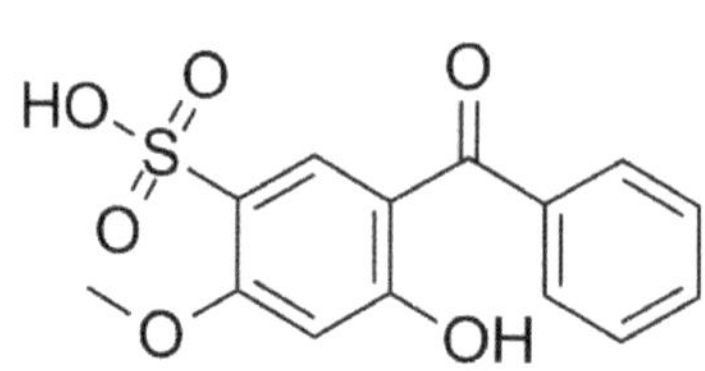

Figure 5.20 Sulisobenzone (benzophenone-4/BP-4)

N. Trolamine salicylate: Trolamine salicylate is an organic compound or a salt formed between triethanolamine and salicylic acid. Triethanolamine neutralizes the acidity of the salicylic acid. It is a topical analgesic used for temporary relief of minor pain associated with arthritis, simple backache, muscle strains, sprains, and bruises. Unlike other topical analgesics, trolamine salicylate has no distinct odor which improves patient acceptability. Trolamine or triethanolamine salicylate has good water solubility. It is mostly used for water soluble sunscreens to help increase the SPF of a cosmetics owing to their substantivity to the skin. It also displays low systemic absorption upon dermal or topical administration and has low skin irritant properties. Approved in both the US and Canada, trolamine salicylate is used in concentrations of up to 12%. It filters UVB rays, but has no effect on UVA rays, which means it can't be relied on alone as a sunscreen. It has found to cause photocontact dermatitis [106], [131,132]. **(See also 5.1. Sunburn and Sunscreen Facts)**

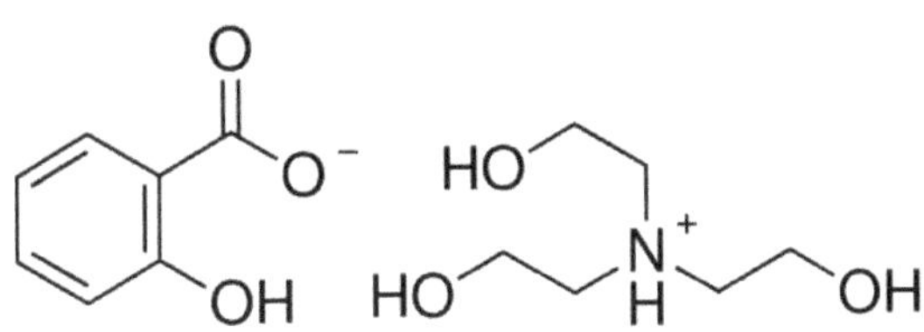

Figure 5.21 Trolamine salicylate

O. Titanium dioxide: TiO_2 occurs naturally in three crystalline structures: rutile, anatase, and brokite. Rutile is the most common and stable form of this pigment. Important optical properties of this birefringent crystal are its refractive indices in the UV and visible wavelength range. The USP classifies it as a topical protective. The protection is primarily for its opacity due to high refractive index (2.7). However, the high refractive index is not the only property that determines how well a substance blocks light. The film thickness in which the substance is suspended as well as the size of the individual particles also affects the efficacy of the sunscreen. Advantages offered by sunscreens based on inorganic compounds comprise absence of skin irritation and sensitization, inertness of the ingredients, limited skin penetration, and a broad-spectrum protection. As a solar ray protective, it is used in a conc. 5% to 25% in ointments and lotions. Since it is not absorbed into the skin, this effect may not be an issue in topical use on unbroken skin. It is also used as a white pigment in cosmetics and paints. According to the US FDA, the protection factor against UVA should be at least one-third of the overall sun protection factor. Previously, TiO_2 had a suboptimal cosmetic profile, appearing thick and white on application. Current formulations are micronized or nanoparticle formulations, which blend in with the skin tone and attain better cosmesis. As micro-sized TiO2 is the most effective in UVB and micro-sized ZnO in the UVA range, the combination of the two oxides assures the required broad band UV protection. The particle sizes that result, within human SC, in higher UV absorption and scattering and lower UV transmission improve the UV attenuation. Emulsions are generally unstable, often change from water–oil to oil–water or break down during application on the skin, and may increase the cutaneous permeability. It has been demonstrated that sunscreen TiO_2 particles penetrate deeper into human skin from an oily than from an aqueous dispersion. The International Agency for Research on Cancer (IARC) has recently classified TiO_2 as an IARC group 2B carcinogen, possibly carcinogenic to humans. The IARC conclusions are based on evidence showing that high concentrations of pigment-grade and ultrafine TiO_2 dust cause respiratory tract cancer in rats. Intrinsic cyto- and genotoxicity of both TiO2 and ZnO NPs (<100 nm) has been frequently reported. Coating the NPs does reduce the toxic effects, especially when silica-based coatings are used, but cannot completely prevent these effects. TiO2, however, has currently attracted more scientific attention than ZnO [40], [133,134].

P. Zinc oxide: Sunscreens containing metal oxide nanoparticles appear transparent on the skin and provide excellent protection against sunburn caused by UV radiation. Zinc oxide is a widely used broad-spectrum sunscreen, repeated application of ZnO-NPs to the skin, as used in global sunscreen products, appears to be safe, with no evidence of ZnO-NP penetration into the viable epidermis nor toxicity in the underlying viable epidermis. It was associated with the release and penetration of zinc ions into the skin, but this did not appear to cause local toxicity. In the past two decades, ZnO NPs have become one of the most popular metal oxide nanoparticles in biological applications due to their excellent biocompatibility, economic, and low toxicity. ZnO NPs have emerged a promising potential in biomedicine, especially in the fields of anticancer and antibacterial fields, which are involved with their potent ability to trigger excess ROS production, release zinc ions, and induce cell apoptosis. In addition, ZnO NPs have superior antibacterial, antimicrobial, and excellent UV-blocking properties. ZnO NPs-exposed HepG2 cells presented higher cytotoxicity and genotoxicity, which were associated with cell apoptosis mediated by the ROS triggered mitochondrial pathway. In the brain, the oxidative stress and inflammation reaction were found after ZnO NP exposure and more remarkable changes were identified in aged individual.

These kinds of neurotoxicity might due to the destruction of the BBB integrity caused partly by ZnO NPs-induced systemic inflammation [135-138].

5.7 SUNSCREEN FORMULATION

On the surface, sunscreen products are pretty simple. They consist of a delivery vehicle containing one or more sunscreen active ingredients. When applied to the skin, these sunscreen actives intercept solar UV rays before they can damage the underlying skin. However, while conceptually simple, a detailed analysis reveals that sunscreen formulations are quite complex, requiring careful selection of sunscreen active and vehicle components to control multiple performance and in-use parameters [164].

Exhibit 9. Aqueous, Non- Aqueous and Clear Sunscreen Lotion Formulation

Aqueous Lotion		Non- Aqueous Lotion		Clear Lotion	
Ingredients	**(%)**	**Ingredients**	**(%)**	**Ingredients**	**(%)**
Filtrosol B	7	Giv-Tan F/Cinoxate	1.5	Isobutyl PABA	5
Methyl Cellulose	0.5	Denatured ethyl alcohol	65	Tween 20	9
Glycerin	2	Oleyl alcohol	10	Alcohol SD 40	45
Ethyl alcohol	10	Water	23	Water	41
Water	80.5	Perfume	q.s.		
Perfume	q.s.				

Alpha-Tocopherol (Filtrosol) has many protective actions, such as decreasing immunosuppression, erythema, photoaging, and photocarcinogenesis [40]. Naturally occurring vitamin E is not a single compound; instead, vitamin E is a group of molecules with related structures, some of which may have unique properties in skin. After topical application, vitamin E accumulates not only in cell membranes but also in the extracellular lipid matrix of the stratum corneum, where vitamin E contributes to antioxidant defenses. However, much of a topically applied dose of vitamin E alone will be destroyed in the skin following exposure to UV light. This suggests that although vitamin E is working as an antioxidant, it is unstable on its own and easily lost from the skin. Thus, improving the stability of topical applications with vitamin E is important [165]. Methyl Cellulose (Methylester of cellulose) is used as an emulsifying, suspending and thickening agent in cosmetics, pharmaceutics and the chemical industry. It's a non-ionic polymer, is highly hydrophilic and thus easily dissolves in cold and hot water [166]. Ethyl alcohol is an antimicrobial preservative; disinfectant; skin penetrant; solvent. Cetyl and cetearyl are both derived from coconut and are fatty alcohols. Typically, fatty alcohols are used as emollients and thickeners in skin-care products. Fatty alcohols are not irritating and, in fact, can be beneficial for dry skin. If LMW alcohols are high up on the ingredients list on a bottle of sunscreen then they are going to dry out skin. However, the topical application of 10% ethanol stimulates the proliferation of peritoneal tissue explants – a semi in-vivo wound model – which can be interpreted as positive influence for stimulation of wound healing by ethanol [167,168]. Oleyl alcohol is mainly used in topical pharmaceutical formulations and is generally regarded as a nontoxic and nonirritant material at the levels employed as an excipient. However, contact dermatitis due to oleyl alcohol has been reported. It's an antifoaming agent; dissolution enhancer; emollient; emulsifying agent; skin penetrant; sustained-release agent. SD alcohol 40 is a type of denatured alcohol used in cosmetics and personal care products as an anti-foaming agent, astringent, antimicrobial agent, and a solvent. In addition to SD alcohol 40, the specially denatured alcohols acceptable for use in cosmetics are SD Alcohol 23-A and SD Alcohol 40-B. As an astringent, SD alcohol 40 causes biological tissue to contract or draw together. After topical application, astringents work on proteins called keratins, which function to hold skin cells together to form a barrier. The bonds between keratins are affected by temperature and pH, forming only when skin is slightly acidic or cool. If the bonds break, the keratin molecules will separate, causing the outer layer of skin to swell. Astringents cool the skin and cause the bonds to reform. It is this process that produces the temporary toning effect associated with astringents [169]. 2-Ethoxyethyl-p-Methoxycinnamate (Giv Tan® F/Cinoxate) used as sunscreen. The most common moisturizing ingredients are occlusive agents which create a barrier that blocks water from escaping the skin. Ingredients like Petrolatum, Mineral Oil and Dimethicone can all be used as occlusive agents. Humectants, which are ingredients that attract water, are also added to lotions. Glycerin is the most commonly used humectant. Finally, emollients are added to improve the feel of the lotion on the skin. They can reduce the tackiness and greasiness caused by the other moisturizing ingredients. Common emollients include coconut oil, cetyl esters, and certain silicones. Sunscreen formulations are typically thinner in viscosity than standard skin lotions [170].

Exhibit 10. Sunscreen formulations with Avobenzone, TiO_2 and ZnO NPs [95]

Ingredients	Quantity (% w/w)							
	SC1	SC2	SC3	SC4	SC5	SC6	SC7	SC8
Oil phase	25.05	25.05	25.05	25.05	25.05	25.05	25.05	25.05
Preservative	0.03	0.03	0.03	0.03	0.03	0.03	0.03	0.03
Aqueous phase	1.8	1.8	1.8	1.8	1.8	1.8	1.8	1.8
Plain morin	–	–	0.05	–	–	–	0.05	–
Avobenzone	–	–	–	–	–	2.66	2.66	2.66
Nano titanium dioxide	–	4.55	4.43	4.55	4.55	4.43	4.43	4.43
Nano zinc oxide	–	4.55	4.43	4.55	4.55	4.43	4.43	4.43
Morin nanoparticles	–	–	–	–	0.05	–	–	0.05
Plain nanoparticles	–	–	–	0.05	–	–	–	–
Water (solvent)	to 100	to 100	to 100	to 100	to 100	to 100	to 100	to 100

Morin is a yellow chemical compound that can be isolated from *Maclura pomifera* (Osage orange), *Maclura tinctoria* (old fustic) and from leaves of *Psidium guajava* (common guava) [161]. Morin is a pentahydroxyflavone that is 7-hydroxyflavonol bearing three additional hydroxy substituents at positions 2' 4' and 5. It has a role as an antioxidant, a metabolite, an antihypertensive agent, a hepatoprotective agent, a neuroprotective agent, an anti-inflammatory agent, an antineoplastic agent, an antibacterial agent, an EC 5.99.1.2 (DNA topoisomerase) inhibitor and an angiogenesis modulating agent. It is a pentahydroxyflavone and a 7-hydroxyflavonol [162]. ZnO and TiO_2 combinations are particularly valuable because of their ability to filter both UVA and UVB radiations, providing broader UVR protection than that observed with individual component [95]. In 2018, the EWG reported that a large increase in these inorganic filters with ~41% of sunscreens in the United States designated as mineral only. This figure has more than doubled (from 17%) since 2007 [111]. Only two sunscreen active ingredients approved in the US, avobenzone (butylmethoxydibenzoylmethane) and zinc oxide (ZnO), provide true broad-spectrum protection against UVA wavelengths >360 nm. Although effective against shorter UVR wavelengths <360 nm, titanium dioxide TiO_2 is also often believed to confer broad-spectrum protection and is substituted for ZnO or avobenzone. The use of proper formulation strategies can ensure that avobenzone losses are minimized to the extent that they have no impact on a product's ability to deliver sustained protection, even over periods of prolonged exposure to UVR [163].

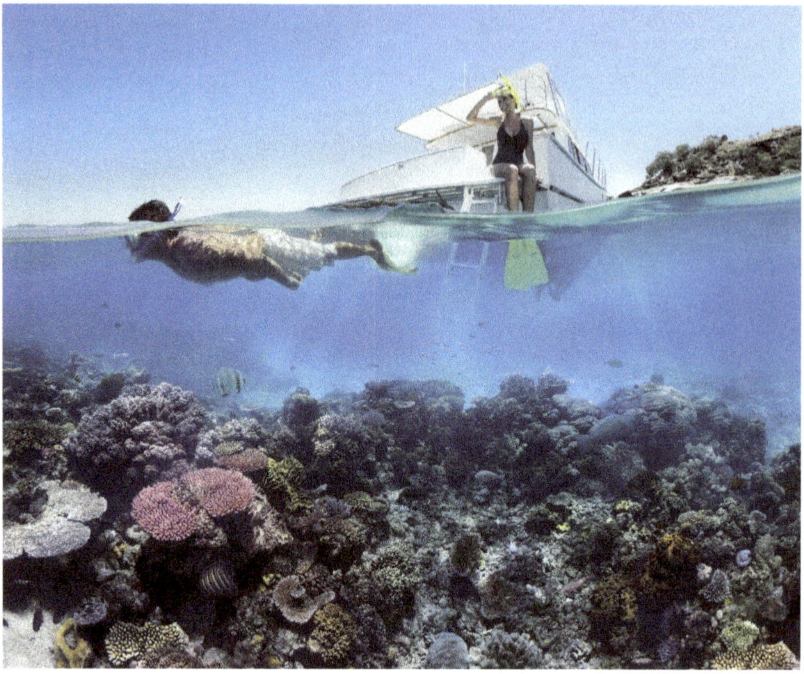

Figure 5.22 Colorful reefs are a major draw for tourists. But chemicals in sunscreen and ocean warming pose serious threats to them [183]. Studies have shown that oxybenzone and octinoxate are found in over 3,500 sunscreen products, including household names like Tropicana, Banana Boat, and Coppertone. When corals absorb these chemicals, they have a similar reaction as they would if surrounding water temperatures were to get too warm. In addition, the presence of these chemicals in sea water allows viruses to thrive, putting corals at high risk of catching an infection that could lead to bleaching and death (Courtacy: Observador).

5.8 SUNSCREEN VS CORAL REEF

While covering less than 1% of the ocean surface, coral reefs provide habitat for nearly one third of marine fish species as well as 10% of all fish captured for human consumption. Coral reefs also provide major essential benefits to people, like food production, tourism, biotechnology development, and coastal protection. There is strong evidence that some sunscreen ingredients, especially oxybenzone, are harmful to corals if the concentration in water is high. In some situations, primarily related to the number of swimmers and the geography of the shoreline, concentrations of oxybenzone far exceed the levels shown to be harmful to corals [181]. In 2015, the nonprofit Haereticus Environmental Laboratory surveyed Trunk Bay beach on St. John, where visitors ranged from 2,000 to 5,000 swimmers daily, and estimated over 6,000 pounds of sunscreen was deposited on the reef annually. The same year, it found an average of 412 pounds of sunscreen was deposited daily on the reef at Hanauma Bay, a popular snorkeling destination in Oahu (Hawaii) that draws an average of 2,600 swimmers each day. Over the past three years, one-fifth of the world's coral reefs have died off — and there is a growing awareness that sunscreen is playing a role. From 6,000 to 14,000 tons of sunscreen slide off of humans into coral reef areas each year, exposing the gorgeous underwater ecosystems to chemicals that can kill them. Global warming is the main reason that coral reefs are dying — but sunscreens play a role, too [182]. Danovaro et.al, 2008 revealed that sunscreens, by promoting viral infection, potentially play an important role in coral bleaching in areas prone to high levels of recreational use by humans. Coral bleaching has negative impacts on biodiversity and functioning of reef ecosystems and their production of goods and services. This increasing world-wide phenomenon is associated with temperature anomalies, high irradiance, pollution, and bacterial diseases. Hard-coral bleaching and the increase in viral abundance in seawater were also seen after coral treatment with mitomycin C, an antibiotic commonly used to induce the lytic cycle in latent viral infections [184]. Unfortunately, the World Conservation Institute estimates that 20% of coral reefs are already destroyed, another 25% are in great immediate threat, and another 25% will be threatened by 2050 [185].

EPILOGUE

The skin stratum corneum acts as a barrier that isolates the organism from the environment and avoids water loss from tissues. Such a sealed sheath is essential for the physiological processes of the skin and of the entire body but poses problems for the topical delivery of substances to the tissues. This kind of hindrance has been known since ancient times and has been empirically approached, e.g., by the use of greasy or oily materials in skin care applications. Technological achievements in the topical administrations of medicaments and in skin care products have led to the development of vehicles and penetration enhancer and to the design of technologically advanced formulations. While synthetic chemical structures have been used extensively in this field, traditional practices and scientific studies have shown over the years that botanical sources can provide all kinds of elements for vehiculating drugs and active compounds and improving their permeation through the skin. . There is wide variability in price, SPF protection, and product claims among commercially available sunscreens. Cosmetic elegance is one of the most important positive features, followed by product performance. Dermatologists should counsel patients that sunscreen products come with numerous marketing claims and varying cosmetic applicability, all of which must be balanced with adequate photoprotection. In addition, consumers should be advised to select a product with broad-spectrum coverage, an SPF of 30 or higher, and water and/or sweat resistance in the setting of water activities or high ambient temperatures. UV filters are analyzed in their pure form by ingredient suppliers and also by cosmetic companies that purchase those filters for incorporation into their finished products. Once these UV filters are included into cosmetic finished products, they also need to be analyzed for both quality control and regulatory compliance. Use of sun screening agents is beneficial in minimizing the occurrence of skin cancers in people with fair skin. However, the same effect on Asian skin is debatable, as this skin type is considered to be resistant to skin cancers. Sunscreen use is advisable in young adults to prevent and minimize other photodamaging effects. Affordability and proper application techniques are the challenges that must be addressed in order to achieve regular sunscreen usage.

SUMMARY

Promoting sunscreen use is an integral part of prevention programs aimed at reducing UV radiation-induced skin damage and skin cancers. Protection against both UVB and UVA radiation is advocated. Despite the efforts of physicians and regulatory authorities to spread awareness regarding sunburn, skin cancer, and the benefits of regularly using sun screening agents, treatment adherence is low. Providing cosmetically acceptable preparations and educating people about following the application instructions, is a challenge often faced by treating physicians. Pricing sunscreens reasonably and making them water resistant and non-sticky are a few of the challenges faced by manufacturers. Manufacturers must also consider sensitization reactions, especially in those having eczema or photo dermatoses. Sun protection factor (SPF) is affected by application density, water resistance, and other factors. An adequate SPF for an individual should be balanced to skin phenotype and exposure habits. The correct use of sunscreens should be combined with the avoidance of midday sun and the wearing of protective clothing and glasses, as part of an overall sun protection regimen. The FDA approved sunscreen ingredients are extensively reviewed. A clear and straightforward recommendation on their safety and efficacy still remains a big challenge.

ABBREVIATIONS

Non-Melanoma Skin Cancer (NMSC); Kruppel Like Factor 4 (KLF4); Peroxisome Proliferator Activated Receptor Gamma (PPARG); Antigen Presenting Cell (APC); Blood-Brain Barrier (BBB); Environmental Working Group (EWG); Generally Recognized As Safe And Effective (GRASE); P-Aminobenzoic Acid (PABA); Mesoporous Silicas (MSs); hydroxypropyl-beta-cyclodextrin (HPCD); octyl methoxycinnamate (OMC); reactive oxygen species (ROS); Psoralen plus UVA (PUVA); Seasonal Affective Disorder (SAD); Major Depressive Disorder (MDD); Actinic Keratosis (AK); Squamous Cell Carcinoma (SCC); Basal Cell Carcinoma (BCC); Polymeric Nanoparticles (NPs); Bisethylhexyloxyphenol Methoxyphenyl Triazine (BEMT); Solid Lipid Nanoparticle (SLN); high-density polyethylene/low-density polyethylene (HDPE/LDPE); autoimmune encephalomyelitis (EAE); Multiple sclerosis (MS); Inducible Nitric Oxide Synthase (iNOS); Tumor Necrosis Factor Alpha (TNF-α); International Agency for Research on Cancer (IARC); Ultraviolet (UV) A Protection Factor (UVAPF)

BIBLIOGRAPHY AND WEBLIOGRAPHY

1. Budzowski A. Sunburn vs Sun Poisoning, Web UPMC MyHealth Matters
2. Moan J, Grigalavicius M, Dahlback A, Baturaite Z, Juzeniene A. Ultraviolet-radiation and health: optimal time for sun exposure. Adv Exp Med Biol. 2014;810:423-8. PubMed PMID: 25207380.
3. MedicineNet. Sunburn (Sun Poisoning) Symptoms, Pain Relief, and Healing Time, medically Reviewed on 4/10/2018.
4. MedicineNet. Get Rid of Sunburn Fast: Pain Relief, Blisters,Peeling, Home Remedies, May 11, 2012.
5. Koh D, Wang H, Lee J, Chia KS, Lee HP, Goh CL. Basal cell carcinoma, squamous cell carcinoma and melanoma of the skin: analysis of the Singapore Cancer Registry data 1968-97. Br J Dermatol. 2003 Jun;148(6):1161-6. PubMed PMID: 12828744.
6. Amaro-Ortiz A, Yan B, D'Orazio JA. Ultraviolet radiation, aging and the skin: prevention of damage by topical cAMP manipulation. Molecules. 2014 May 15;19(5):6202-19. doi: 10.3390/molecules19056202. Review. PubMed PMID: 24838074; PubMed Central PMCID: PMC4344124.
7. Amblard P, Leccia MT. [Skin diseases with photosensitivity]. Rev Prat. 1992 Jun 1;42(11):1365-8. Review. French. PubMed PMID: 1529248.
8. Zuba EB, Koronowska S, Osmola-Mańkowska A, Jenerowicz D. Drug-induced Photosensitivity. Acta Dermatovenerol Croat. 2016 Apr;24(1):55-64. Review. PubMed PMID: 27149132.
9. WebMD. Sun Poisoning. Available From: https://www.webmd.com/skin-problems-and-treatments/sun-poisoning#1
10. Guerra KC, Crane JS. Skin Cancer Prevention. 2019 Jan 19. StatPearls [Internet]. Treasure Island (FL): StatPearls Publishing; 2019 Jan-. Available from http://www.ncbi.nlm.nih.gov/books/NBK519527/ PubMed PMID: 30137812.
11. Guerra KC, Crane JS. Sunburn. [Updated 2018 Nov 23]. In: StatPearls [Internet]. Treasure Island (FL): StatPearls Publishing; 2019 Jan-. Available from: https://www.ncbi.nlm.nih.gov/books/NBK534837/
12. McStay CM. What is the pathophysiology of sunburn? Medscape, Nov 08, 2018.
13. Chapter 14 Diseases of the skin. In: Rick D. Kellerman, David Rakel. Conn's Current Therapy 2019, published by Elsevier Health Sciences, 2018 ISBN 0323596509, 9780323596503, Page 1031.
14. Azevedo M, Bandeira L, Luza C, Lemos A, Bandeira F. Vitamin D Deficiency, Skin Phototype, Sun Index, and Metabolic Risk Among Patients with High Rates of Sun Exposure Living in the Tropics. J Clin Aesthet Dermatol. 2018 Aug;11(8):15-18. Epub 2018 Aug 1. PubMed PMID: 30214662; PubMed Central PMCID: PMC6122513.
15. Driscoll MS, Wagner RF Jr. Clinical management of the acute sunburn reaction. Cutis. 2000 Jul;66(1):53-8. Review. PubMed PMID: 10916693.

16. Faurschou A, Wulf HC. Topical corticosteroids in the treatment of acute sunburn: a randomized, double-blind clinical trial. Arch Dermatol. 2008 May;144(5):620-4. doi: 10.1001/archderm.144.5.620. PubMed PMID: 18490588.
17. Feily A, Namazi MR. Aloe vera in dermatology: a brief review. G Ital Dermatol Venereol. 2009 Feb;144(1):85-91. Review. PubMed PMID: 19218914.
18. Puvabanditsin P, Vongtongsri R. Efficacy of aloe vera cream in prevention and treatment of sunburn and suntan. J Med Assoc Thai. 2005 Sep;88 Suppl 4:S173-6. PubMed PMID: 16623024.
19. Tadicherla S, Berman B. Percutaneous dermal drug delivery for local pain control. Ther Clin Risk Manag. 2006 Mar;2(1):99-113. PubMed PMID: 18360585; PubMed Central PMCID: PMC1661648.
20. Moore DE. Drug-induced cutaneous photosensitivity: incidence, mechanism, prevention and management. Drug Saf. 2002;25(5):345-72. Review. PubMed PMID: 12020173.
21. Drucker AM, Rosen CF. Drug-induced photosensitivity: culprit drugs, management and prevention. Drug Saf. 2011 Oct 1;34(10):821-37. doi: 10.2165/11592780-000000000-00000. Review. PubMed PMID: 21879777.
22. Harth Y, Rapoport M. Photosensitivity associated with antipsychotics, antidepressants and anxiolytics. Drug Saf. 1996 Apr;14(4):252-9. Review. PubMed PMID: 8713693.
23. Pile HD, Nicolas D. Isotretinoin. [Updated 2019 Feb 21]. In: StatPearls [Internet]. Treasure Island (FL): StatPearls Publishing; 2019 Jan-. Available from: https://www.ncbi.nlm.nih.gov/books/NBK525949/
24. Hodgkiss-Harlow CJ, Eichenfield LF, Dohil MA. Effective monitoring of isotretinoin safety in a pediatric dermatology population: a novel "patient symptom survey" approach. J Am Acad Dermatol. 2011 Sep;65(3):517-524. doi: 10.1016/j.jaad.2010.06.040. Epub 2011 May 31. PubMed PMID: 21632153; PubMed Central PMCID: PMC4336191.
25. Das LM, Binko AM, Traylor ZP, Peng H, Lu KQ. Vitamin D improves sunburns by increasing autophagy in M2 macrophages. Autophagy. 2019 May;15(5):813-826. doi: 10.1080/15548627.2019.1569298. Epub 2019 Jan 24. PubMed PMID: 30661440.
26. Scott JF, Das LM, Ahsanuddin S, Qiu Y, Binko AM, Traylor ZP, Debanne SM, Cooper KD, Boxer R, Lu KQ. Oral Vitamin D Rapidly Attenuates Inflammation from Sunburn: An Interventional Study. J Invest Dermatol. 2017 Oct;137(10):2078-2086. doi: 10.1016/j.jid.2017.04.040. Epub 2017 May 30. PubMed PMID: 28576736; PubMed Central PMCID: PMC5610950.
27. Golmohammadzadeh S, Imani F, Hosseinzadeh H, Jaafari MR. Preparation, characterization and evaluation of sun protective and moisturizing effects of nanoliposomes containing safranal. Iran J Basic Med Sci. 2011 Nov;14(6):521-33. PubMed PMID: 23493792; PubMed Central PMCID: PMC3586861.
28. Opene C, Chren MM, Linos E. Types of Shade Vary in Protection Just Like Sunscreens. JAMA Dermatol. 2017 Oct 1;153(10):1070-1071. doi: 10.1001/jamadermatol.2017.1718. Erratum in: JAMA Dermatol. 2017 Oct

1;153(10):1072. PubMed PMID: 28636687; PubMed Central PMCID: PMC5908476.

29. Wolf R, Matz H, Orion E, Lipozencić J. Sunscreens--the ultimate cosmetic. Acta Dermatovenerol Croat. 2003;11(3):158-62. Review. PubMed PMID: 12967508.
30. Latha MS, Martis J, Shobha V, Sham Shinde R, Bangera S, Krishnankutty B, Bellary S, Varughese S, Rao P, Naveen Kumar BR. Sunscreening agents: a review. J ClinAesthet Dermatol. 2013 Jan;6(1):16-26. PubMed PMID: 23320122; PubMed Central PMCID: PMC3543289.
31. Rego D, Fernandes L, Nascimento T, Grenha A. Evaluation of a sunscreen during a typical beach period. J Pharm Bioallied Sci. 2010 Jan;2(1):47-50. doi: 10.4103/0975-7406.62711. PubMed PMID: 21814431; PubMed Central PMCID: PMC3146092.
32. Schalka S, Steiner D, Ravelli FN, Steiner T, Terena AC, Marçon CR, Ayres EL, Addor FA, Miot HA, Ponzio H, Duarte I, Neffá J, Cunha JA, Boza JC, SamoranoLde P, CorrêaMde P, Maia M, Nasser N, Leite OM, Lopes OS, Oliveira PD, Meyer RL, Cestari T, Reis VM, Rego VR; Brazilian Society of Dermatology. Brazilian consensus on photoprotection. An Bras Dermatol. 2014 Nov-Dec;89(6 Suppl 1):1-74. doi: 10.1590/abd1806-4841.20143971. PubMed PMID: 25761256; PubMed Central PMCID: PMC4365470.
33. Web WHO. Ultraviolet radiation (UV). Available From: https://www.who.int/uv/uv_and_health/en/
34. Volkovova K, Bilanicova D, Bartonova A, Letašiová S, Dusinska M. Associations between environmental factors and incidence of cutaneous melanoma. Review. Environ Health. 2012 Jun 28;11 Suppl 1:S12. doi: 10.1186/1476-069X-11-S1-S12. Review. PubMed PMID: 22759494; PubMed Central PMCID: PMC3388446.
35. Engelsen O. The relationship between ultraviolet radiation exposure and vitamin D status. Nutrients. 2010 May;2(5):482-95. doi: 10.3390/nu2050482. Epub 2010 May 4. Review. PubMed PMID: 22254036; PubMed Central PMCID: PMC3257661.
36. Diffey BL. Human exposure to solar ultraviolet radiation. J Cosmet Dermatol. 2002 Oct;1(3):124-30. Review. PubMed PMID: 17147711.
37. Ruszkiewicz JA, Pinkas A, Ferrer B, Peres TV, Tsatsakis A, Aschner M. Neurotoxic effect of active ingredients in sunscreen products, a contemporary review. Toxicol Rep. 2017 May 27;4:245-259. doi: 10.1016/j.toxrep.2017.05.006. eCollection 2017. Review. PubMed PMID: 28959646; PubMed Central PMCID: PMC5615097.
38. Kannan S, Lim HW. Photoprotection and vitamin D: a review. PhotodermatolPhotoimmunolPhotomed. 2014 Apr-Jun;30(2-3):137-45. doi: 10.1111/phpp.12096. Epub 2014 Jan 9. Review. PubMed PMID: 24313629.
39. Pandika M. Looking to Nature for New Sunscreens. ACS Cent Sci. 2018 Jul 25;4(7):788-790. doi: 10.1021/acscentsci.8b00433. Epub 2018 Jul 16. PubMed PMID: 30062106; PubMed Central PMCID: PMC6062824.
40. Gabros S, Zito PM. Sunscreens And Photoprotection. [Updated 2019 Jan 13]. In: StatPearls [Internet]. Treasure Island (FL): StatPearls Publishing; 2019 Jan-. Available from: https://www.ncbi.nlm.nih.gov/books/NBK537164/

41. FDA aims to strengthen sunscreen rules. Medical Press (Health), February 21, 2019.
42. Maddipatla M. U.S. FDA proposes new regulations for over-the-counter sunscreens. Reuters, February 22, 2019.
43. Ripamonti E, Allifranchini E, Todeschi S and Bocchietto E. Endocrine Disruption by Mixtures in Topical Consumer Products. Cosmetics 2018, 5, 61; doi:10.3390/cosmetics5040061
44. Sunscreen: How to Help Protect Your Skin from the Sun. Web US FDA, February 21, 2019.
45. Only TWO of the 16 ingredients in sunscreen are definitely safe, FDA declares: Two other chemicals will be banned as the agency demands more research on the other 12. Available From: https://www.dailymail.co.uk/health/article-6731267/U-S-FDA-proposes-new-regulations-counter-sunscreens.html
46. National Center for Biotechnology Information. PubChem Database. 4-Aminobenzoic acid, CID=978, https://pubchem.ncbi.nlm.nih.gov/compound/978 (accessed on Apr. 25, 2019)
47. Kullavanijaya P, Lim HW. Photoprotection. J Am Acad Dermatol. 2005 Jun;52(6):937-58; quiz 959-62. Review. PubMed PMID: 15928611.
48. Tahiliani S, Shirolikar M. Viva voce on sunscreens. Indian J Drugs Dermatol 2018;4:92-6
49. Govindu PCV, Hosamani B, Moi S, Venkatachalam D, Asha S, John VN, Sandeep V, Gowd KH. Glutathione as a photo-stabilizer of avobenzone: an evaluation under glass-filtered sunlight using UV-spectroscopy. PhotochemPhotobiol Sci. 2019 Jan 1;18(1):198-207. doi: 10.1039/c8pp00343b. Epub 2018 Nov 13. PubMed PMID: 30421772.
50. National Center for Biotechnology Information. PubChem Database. Avobenzone, CID=51040, https://pubchem.ncbi.nlm.nih.gov/compound/51040 (accessed on Apr. 25, 2019)
51. Raffa RB, Pergolizzi JV Jr, Taylor R Jr, Kitzen JM; NEMA Research Group. Sunscreen bans: Coral reefs and skin cancer. J Clin Pharm Ther. 2019 Feb;44(1):134-139. doi: 10.1111/jcpt.12778. Epub 2018 Nov 28. PubMed PMID: 30484882.
52. Aparici-Espert I, Miranda MA, Lhiaubet-Vallet V. Sunscreen-Based Photocages for Topical Drugs: A Photophysical and Photochemical Study of A Diclofenac-Avobenzone Dyad. Molecules. 2018 Mar 16;23(3). pii: E673. doi: 10.3390/molecules23030673. PubMed PMID: 29547525; PubMed Central PMCID: PMC6017856.
53. Yang C, Lim W, Bazer FW, Song G. Avobenzone suppresses proliferative activity of human trophoblast cells and induces apoptosis mediated by mitochondrial disruption. ReprodToxicol. 2018 Oct;81:50-57. doi: 10.1016/j.reprotox.2018.07.003. Epub 2018 Jul 4. PubMed PMID: 29981360.
54. Uco DP, Leite-Silva VR, Silva HDT, Duque MD, Grice J, Mathor MB, Andréo-Filho N, Lopes PS. UVA and UVB formulation phototoxicity in a three-dimensional human skin model: Photodegradation effect. Toxicol In Vitro. 2018 Dec;53:37-44. doi: 10.1016/j.tiv.2018.07.009. Epub 2018 Jul 26. PubMed PMID: 30055310.

55. Monteiro MS, Ozzetti RA, Vergnanini AL, de Brito-Gitirana L, Volpato NM, de Freitas ZM, Ricci-Júnior E, dos Santos EP. Evaluation of octyl p-methoxycinnamate included in liposomes and cyclodextrins in anti-solar preparations: preparations, characterizations and in vitro penetration studies. Int J Nanomedicine. 2012;7:3045-58. doi: 10.2147/IJN.S28550. Epub 2012 Jun 20. PubMed PMID: 22787399; PubMed Central PMCID: PMC3391002.
56. Lin YC, Lin CF, Alalaiwe A, Wang PW, Fang YP, Fang JY. UV filter entrapment in mesoporous silica hydrogel for skin protection against UVA with minimization of percutaneous absorption. Eur J Pharm Sci. 2018 Sep 15;122:185-194. doi: 10.1016/j.ejps.2018.07.013. Epub 2018 Jul 4. PubMed PMID: 29981405.
57. De Coster S, van Larebeke N. Endocrine-disrupting chemicals: associated disorders and mechanisms of action. J Environ Public Health. 2012;2012:713696. Epub 2012 Sep 6. Review. PubMed PMID: 22991565; PubMed Central PMCID: PMC3443608.
58. Nash JF, Tanner PR. Chapter 9. Sunscreens. In: Zoe Diana Draelos, Lauren A. Thaman. Cosmetic Formulation of Skin Care Products Cosmetic Science and Technology, published by Taylor & Francis, 2005 ISBN 0849339685, 9780849339684, Page 139.
59. Chapter 4. Sun Sense, Page 132, Avobenzone Under Fire. In: Paula Begoun. The Complete Beauty Bible: The Ultimate Guide to Smart Beauty, published by Rodale, 2004 ISBN 1579549993, 9781579549992.
60. Ainbinder D, Touitou E. Chapter 44. Skin Photodamage Prevention: State-of-the-art and new prospects. In: Miranda A. Farage, Kenneth W. Miller, Howard I. Maibach. Textbook of Aging Skin, published by Springer Science & Business Media, 2009 ISBN 3540896554, 9783540896555, Page 436
61. Gunia-Krzyżak A, Słoczyńska K, Popiół J, Koczurkiewicz P, Marona H, Pękala E. Cinnamic acid derivatives in cosmetics: current use and future prospects. Int J Cosmet Sci. 2018 Aug;40(4):356-366. doi: 10.1111/ics.12471. Epub 2018 Aug 24. Review. PubMed PMID: 29870052.
62. Rai R, Shanmuga SC, Srinivas C. Update on photoprotection. Indian J Dermatol. 2012 Sep;57(5):335-42. doi: 10.4103/0019-5154.100472. PubMed PMID: 23112351; PubMed Central PMCID: PMC3482794.
63. Rao GS, Tokuda H, Ichiishi E, Takasaki M, Iida A, Suzuki N, Konoshima T, Kapadia GJ. Oral chemoprevention of skin cancer in mice by benzophenone sunscreens dioxybenzone and octabenzone in drinking water. Anticancer Res. 2013 Jun;33(6):2535-40. PubMed PMID: 23749905.
64. Heo S, Hwang HS, Jeong Y, Na K. Skin protection efficacy from UV irradiation and skin penetration property of polysaccharide-benzophenone conjugates as a sunscreen agent. CarbohydrPolym. 2018 Sep 1;195:534-541. doi: 10.1016/j.carbpol.2018.05.010. Epub 2018 May 4. PubMed PMID: 29805009.
65. Sherwood VF, Kennedy S, Zhang H, Purser GH, Sheaff RJ. Altered UV absorbance and cytotoxicity of chlorinated sunscreen agents. CutanOculToxicol. 2012 Dec;31(4):273-9. doi: 10.3109/15569527.2011.647181. Epub 2012 Jan 18. PubMed PMID: 22257218.

66. Butler TC. Bromal Hydrate And Chloral Hydrate: A Pharmacological Contrast And Its Chemical Basis. ournal of Pharmacology and Experimental Therapeutics December 1948, 94 (4) 401-411.
67. Fediuk DJ. Pharmacokinetic and Toxicological Characterization of Repellent DEET and Sunscreen Oxybenzone (Thesis Submitted for PhD). Available From:https://mspace.lib.umanitoba.ca/bitstream/handle/1993/8112/fediuk_daryl.pdf?sequence=1
68. Seto Y, Ohtake H, Kato M, Onoue S. Phototoxic Risk Assessments on Benzophenone Derivatives: Photobiochemical Assessments and Dermal Cassette-Dosing Pharmacokinetic Study. J Pharmacol Exp Ther. 2015 Aug;354(2):195-202. doi: 10.1124/jpet.115.223644. Epub 2015 May 27. PubMed PMID: 26016852.
69. Ngan V. Allergy to benzophenone. Web DermNet NZ, 2012.
70. National Center for Biotechnology Information. PubChem Database. Homosalate, CID=8362, https://pubchem.ncbi.nlm.nih.gov/compound/8362 (accessed on Apr. 26, 2019)
71. Kim TH, Shin BS, Kim KB, Shin SW, Seok SH, Kim MK, Kim EJ, Kim D, Kim MG, Park ES, Kim JY, Yoo SD. Percutaneous absorption, disposition, and exposure assessment of homosalate, a UV filtering agent, in rats. J Toxicol Environ Health A. 2014;77(4):202-13. doi: 10.1080/15287394.2013.861376. PubMed PMID: 24555679.
72. Kullavanijaya P, Lim HW. Photoprotection. J Am Acad Dermatol. 2005 Jun;52(6):937-58; quiz 959-62. Review. PubMed PMID: 15928611.
73. Erol M, Çok I, BostanGayret Ö, Günes P, Yigit Ö, Sayman E, Günes A, Çelik DS, Hamilçikan S, Altinay S, Ercan O. Evaluation of the endocrine-disrupting effects of homosalate (HMS) and 2-ethylhexyl 4-dimethylaminobenzoate (OD-PABA) in rat pups during the prenatal, lactation, and early postnatal periods. Toxicol Ind Health. 2017 Oct;33(10):775-791. doi: 10.1177/0748233717718974. Epub 2017 Sep 7. PubMed PMID: 28879804.
74. Wang J, Pan L, Wu S, Lu L, Xu Y, Zhu Y, Guo M, Zhuang S. Recent Advances on Endocrine Disrupting Effects of UV Filters. Int J Environ Res Public Health. 2016 Aug 3;13(8). pii: E782. doi: 10.3390/ijerph13080782. Review. PubMed PMID: 27527194; PubMed Central PMCID: PMC4997468.
75. Homosalate. Available From: http://www.safecosmetics.org/get-the-facts/chemicals-of-concern/homosalate/
76. Rodrigues NDN, Cole-Filipiak NC, Blodgett KN, Abeysekera C, Zwier TS, Stavros VG. Wavepacket insights into the photoprotection mechanism of the UV filter methyl anthranilate. Nat Commun. 2018 Dec 5;9(1):5188. doi: 10.1038/s41467-018-07681-1. PubMed PMID: 30518753; PubMed Central PMCID: PMC6281654.
77. Dale Wilson B, Moon S, Armstrong F. Comprehensive review of ultraviolet radiation and the current status on sunscreens. J Clin Aesthet Dermatol. 2012 Sep;5(9):18-23. PubMed PMID: 23050030; PubMed Central PMCID: PMC3460660.
78. Sivamani RK, Crane LA, Dellavalle RP. The benefits and risks of ultraviolet tanning and its alternatives: the role of prudent sun exposure. Dermatol Clin.

2009 Apr;27(2):149-54, vi. doi: 10.1016/j.det.2008.11.008. Review. PubMed PMID: 19254658; PubMed Central PMCID: PMC2692214.

79. Pinto I, Bogi A, Picciolo F, Stacchini N, Buonocore G, Bellieni CV. Blue Light and Ultraviolet Radiation Exposure from Infant Phototherapy Equipment. J Occup Environ Hyg. 2015;12(9):603-10. doi: 10.1080/15459624.2015.1029611. PubMed PMID: 25894632.

80. de Groot T, Chowdhary A, Meis JF, Voss A. Killing of Candida auris by UV-C: Importance of exposure time and distance. Mycoses. 2019 May;62(5):408-412. doi: 10.1111/myc.12903. Epub 2019 Mar 12. PubMed PMID: 30748018.

81. Dai T, Kharkwal GB, Zhao J, St Denis TG, Wu Q, Xia Y, Huang L, Sharma SK, d'Enfert C, Hamblin MR. Ultraviolet-C light for treatment of Candida albicans burn infection in mice. PhotochemPhotobiol. 2011 Mar-Apr;87(2):342-9. doi: 10.1111/j.1751-1097.2011.00886.x.Epub 2011 Feb 10. PubMed PMID: 21208209; PubMed Central PMCID: PMC3048910.

82. Nussbaumer B, Kaminski-Hartenthaler A, Forneris CA, Morgan LC, Sonis JH, Gaynes BN, Greenblatt A, Wipplinger J, Lux LJ, Winkler D, Van Noord MG, Hofmann J, Gartlehner G. Light therapy for preventing seasonal affective disorder. Cochrane Database Syst Rev. 2015 Nov 8;(11):CD011269. doi: 10.1002/14651858.CD011269.pub2. Review. Update in: Cochrane Database Syst Rev. 2019 Mar 18;3:CD011269. PubMed PMID: 26558494.

83. Lam RW, Levitt AJ, Levitan RD, Michalak EE, Cheung AH, Morehouse R, Ramasubbu R, Yatham LN, Tam EM. Efficacy of Bright Light Treatment, Fluoxetine, and the Combination in Patients With Nonseasonal Major Depressive Disorder: A Randomized Clinical Trial. JAMA Psychiatry. 2016 Jan;73(1):56-63. doi: 10.1001/jamapsychiatry.2015.2235. Erratum in: JAMA Psychiatry. 2016 Jan;73(1):90. PubMed PMID: 26580307.

84. Guy GP Jr, Thomas CC, Thompson T, Watson M, Massetti GM, Richardson LC; Centers for Disease Control and Prevention (CDC). Vital signs: melanoma incidence and mortality trends and projections - United States, 1982-2030. MMWR Morb Mortal Wkly Rep. 2015 Jun 5;64(21):591-6. PubMed PMID: 26042651; PubMed Central PMCID: PMC4584771.

85. Sample A, He YY. Mechanisms and prevention of UV-induced melanoma. PhotodermatolPhotoimmunolPhotomed. 2018 Jan;34(1):13-24. doi: 10.1111/phpp.12329. Epub 2017 Aug 2. Review. PubMed PMID: 28703311; PubMed Central PMCID: PMC5760354.

86. Mackiewicz-Wysocka M, Bowszyc-Dmochowska M, Strzelecka-Węklar D, Dańczak-Pazdrowska A, Adamski Z. Basal cell carcinoma - diagnosis. ContempOncol (Pozn). 2013;17(4):337-42. doi: 10.5114/wo.2013.35684. Epub 2013 Oct 7. Review. PubMed PMID: 24592119; PubMed Central PMCID: PMC3934050.

87. Sunscreen Options. In: Stephen E. Wolverton. Comprehensive Dermatologic Drug Therapy, Edition 2, published by Elsevier Health Sciences, 2007 ISBN 1437720706, 9781437720709

88. Chapter 9. Photoallergens. In: James G Marks Jr, Bryan E Anderson, Vincent A DeLeo. Contact & Occupational Dermatology, published by JP Medical Ltd, 2016 ISBN 9351529363, 9789351529361
89. Moyal D, Chardon A, Kollias N. UVA protection efficacy of sunscreens can be determined by the persistent pigment darkening (PPD) method. (Part 2). PhotodermatolPhotoimmunolPhotomed. 2000 Dec;16(6):250-5. PubMed PMID: 11132127.
90. Wang SQ, Xu H, Stanfield JW, Osterwalder U, Herzog B. Comparison of ultraviolet A light protection standards in the United States and European Union through in vitro measurements of commercially available sunscreens. J Am Acad Dermatol. 2017 Jul;77(1):42-47. doi: 10.1016/j.jaad.2017.01.017. Epub 2017 Feb 24. PubMed PMID: 28238452.
91. Schalka S., Naranjo Ravelli F., Perim N., Vasconcelos R. (2017) Chemical and Physical Sunscreens. DOI https://doi.org/10.1007/978-3-319-12589-3_7 In: Issa M., Tamura B. (eds) Daily Routine in Cosmetic Dermatology. Clinical Approaches and Procedures in Cosmetic Dermatology, vol 1. Springer, Cham. ISBN 978-3-319-12588-6, 978-3-319-12589-3
92. Jallad KN. Chemical characterization of sunscreens composition and its related potential adverse health effects. J Cosmet Dermatol. 2017 Sep;16(3):353-357. doi: 10.1111/jocd.12282. Epub 2016 Sep 5. Review. PubMed PMID: 27596093.
93. Protecting Your Skin. Chemical vs Physical (Mineral) Sunscreens: Pros and Cons. Blog Dr. Desjarlais, June 2, 2016.
94. Moloney FJ, Collins S, Murphy GM. Sunscreens: safety, efficacy and appropriate use. Am J Clin Dermatol. 2002;3(3):185-91. Review. PubMed PMID: 11978139.
95. Shetty PK, Venuvanka V, Jagani HV, Chethan GH, Ligade VS, Musmade PB, Nayak UY, Reddy MS, Kalthur G, Udupa N, Rao CM, Mutalik S. Development and evaluation of sunscreen creams containing morin-encapsulated nanoparticles for enhanced UV radiation protection and antioxidant activity. Int J Nanomedicine. 2015 Oct 13;10:6477-91. doi: 10.2147/IJN.S90964. eCollection 2015. PubMed PMID: 26508854; PubMed Central PMCID: PMC4610788.
96. Kumar R, Deep G, Agarwal R. An Overview of Ultraviolet B Radiation-Induced Skin Cancer Chemoprevention by Silibinin. CurrPharmacol Rep. 2015 Jun 1;1(3):206-215. PubMed PMID: 26097804; PubMed Central PMCID: PMC4471873.
97. Levy SB. Chapter 29. UV Filters. In: André O. Barel, Marc Paye, Howard I. Maibach. Handbook of Cosmetic Science and Technology, published by CRC Press, 2009 ISBN 1420069683, 9781420069686
98. Avenel-Audran M, Dutartre H, Goossens A, Jeanmougin M, Comte C, Bernier C, Benkalfate L, Michel M, Ferrier-Lebouëdec MC, Vigan M, Bourrain JL, Outtas O, Peyron JL, Martin L. Octocrylene, an emerging photoallergen. Arch Dermatol. 2010 Jul;146(7):753-7. doi: 10.1001/archdermatol.2010.132. PubMed PMID: 20644036.
99. de Groot AC, Roberts DW. Contact and photocontact allergy to octocrylene: a review. Contact Dermatitis. 2014 Apr;70(4):193-204. doi: 10.1111/cod.12205. Review. PubMed PMID: 24628344.

100. Berkman MS, Yazan Y. Solid lipid nanoparticles: a possible vehicle for zinc oxide and octocrylene. Pharmazie. 2012 Mar;67(3):202-8. PubMed PMID: 22530300.

101. Karlsson I, Vanden Broecke K, Mårtensson J, Goossens A, Börje A. Clinical and experimental studies of octocrylene's allergenic potency. Contact Dermatitis. 2011 Jun;64(6):343-52. doi: 10.1111/j.1600-0536.2011.01899.x.Epub 2011 Apr 19. PubMed PMID: 21504434.

102. Briasco B, Capra P, Mannucci B, Perugini P. Stability Study of Sunscreens with Free and Encapsulated UV Filters Contained in Plastic Packaging. Pharmaceutics. 2017 May 31;9(2). pii: E19. doi: 10.3390/pharmaceutics9020019. PubMed PMID: 28561775; PubMed Central PMCID: PMC5489936.

103. Manová E, von Goetz N, Hungerbühler K. Ultraviolet filter contact and photocontact allergy: consumer exposure and risk assessment for octocrylene from personal care products and sunscreens. Br J Dermatol. 2014 Dec;171(6):1368-74. doi: 10.1111/bjd.13372. Epub 2014 Nov 3. PubMed PMID: 25154366.

104. Blüthgen N, Meili N, Chew G, Odermatt A, Fent K. Accumulation and effects of the UV-filter octocrylene in adult and embryonic zebrafish (Danio rerio). Sci Total Environ. 2014 Apr 1;476-477:207-17. doi: 10.1016/j.scitotenv.2014.01.015. Epub 2014 Jan 24. PubMed PMID: 24463256.

105. National Center for Biotechnology Information. PubChem Database. Octinoxate, CID=5355130, https://pubchem.ncbi.nlm.nih.gov/compound/5355130 (accessed on Apr. 27, 2019)

106. Lim HW, Thomas L, Rigel DS. Chapter 6. Photoprotection. In: Darrell S. Rigel, Robert A. Weiss, Henry W. Lim, Jeffrey S. Dover. Photoaging Basic and Clinical Dermatology, published by CRC Press, 2004 ISBN 0824752090, 9780824752095

107. Molecule of the Week Archive. In a few years, coral in Hawaiian waters will no longer have to put up with us. What molecules are we? Web ACS, July 16, 2018.

108. Siller A, Blaszak SC, Lazar M, Olasz Harken E. Update About the Effects of the Sunscreen Ingredients Oxybenzone and Octinoxate on Humans and the Environment. Plast Surg Nurs. 2018 Oct/Dec;38(4):158-161. doi: 10.1097/PSN.0000000000000244. PubMed PMID: 30507815.

109. Raffa RB, Pergolizzi JV Jr, Taylor R Jr, Kitzen JM; NEMA Research Group. Sunscreen bans: Coral reefs and skin cancer. J Clin Pharm Ther. 2019 Feb;44(1):134-139. doi: 10.1111/jcpt.12778. Epub 2018 Nov 28. PubMed PMID: 30484882.

110. Cinoxate Market is Likely to Witness huge Growth – Major Key Players are Parchem(US), Carbosynth Limited(UK), Synchem UG & Co. KG(DE). Market Research Gazette, April 17, 2019.

111. Schneider SL, Lim HW. A review of inorganic UV filters zinc oxide and titanium dioxide. PhotodermatolPhotoimmunolPhotomed. 2018 Nov 16. doi: 10.1111/phpp.12439. [Epub ahead of print] Review. PubMed PMID: 30444533.

112. Axelstad M, Boberg J, Hougaard KS, Christiansen S, Jacobsen PR, Mandrup KR, Nellemann C, Lund SP, Hass U. Effects of pre- and postnatal exposure to the UV-filter octyl methoxycinnamate (OMC) on the reproductive, auditory and

neurological development of rat offspring. Toxicol Appl Pharmacol. 2011 Feb 1;250(3):278-90. doi: 10.1016/j.taap.2010.10.031. Epub 2010 Nov 6. PubMed PMID: 21059369.

113. Darbre PD. Environmental oestrogens, cosmetics and breast cancer. Best Pract Res Clin Endocrinol Metab. 2006 Mar;20(1):121-43. Review. PubMed PMID: 16522524.

114. Wang Y, Marling SJ, Plum LA, DeLuca HF. Salate derivatives found in sunscreens block experimental autoimmune encephalomyelitis in mice. Proc Natl Acad Sci U S A. 2017 Aug 8;114(32):8528-8531. doi: 10.1073/pnas.1703995114. Epub 2017 Jul 24. PubMed PMID: 28739922; PubMed Central PMCID: PMC5559021.

115. M. VariniaMichalun, Joseph C. DiNardo. Skin Care and Cosmetic Ingredients Dictionary, published by Cengage Learning, 2014 ISBN 1305178211, 9781305178212

116. National Center for Biotechnology Information. PubChem Database. Oxybenzone, CID=4632, https://pubchem.ncbi.nlm.nih.gov/compound/4632 (accessed on Apr. 27, 2019)

117. DiNardo JC, Downs CA. Dermatological and environmental toxicological impact of the sunscreen ingredient oxybenzone/benzophenone-3. J Cosmet Dermatol. 2018 Feb;17(1):15-19. doi: 10.1111/jocd.12449. Epub 2017 Oct 31. Review. PubMed PMID: 29086472.

118. Sung CR, Kim KB, Lee JY, Lee BM, Kwack SJ. Risk Assessment of Ethylhexyl Dimethyl PABA in Cosmetics. Toxicol Res. 2019 Apr;35(2):131-136. doi: 10.5487/TR.2019.35.2.131. Epub 2019 Apr 15. Review. PubMed PMID: 31015895; PubMed Central PMCID: PMC6467356.

119. Zoe Diana Draelos. Procedures in Cosmetic Dermatology Edition 2, published by Elsevier Health Sciences, 2008 ISBN 1437720943, 9781437720945

120. Bastien N, Millau JF, Rouabhia M, Davies RJ, Drouin R. The sunscreen agent 2-phenylbenzimidazole-5-sulfonic acid photosensitizes the formation of oxidized guanines in cellulo after UV-A or UV-B exposure. J Invest Dermatol. 2010 Oct;130(10):2463-71. doi: 10.1038/jid.2010.150. Epub 2010 Jun 24. PubMed PMID: 20574440.

121. Inbaraj JJ, Bilski P, Chignell CF. Photophysical and photochemical studies of 2-phenylbenzimidazole and UVB sunscreen 2-phenylbenzimidazole-5-sulfonic acid. PhotochemPhotobiol. 2002 Feb;75(2):107-16. PubMed PMID: 11883597.

122. Rai R, Shanmuga SC, Srinivas C. Update on photoprotection. Indian J Dermatol. 2012 Sep;57(5):335-42. doi: 10.4103/0019-5154.100472. PubMed PMID: 23112351; PubMed Central PMCID: PMC3482794.

123. Darrell S. Rigel, Robert Friedman, June K. Robinson, Merrick I. Ross, Clay J Cockerell, Henry Lim, Eggert Stockfleth, John M Kirkwood. Cancer of the Skin E-Book: Expert Consult Edition 2, published by Elsevier Health Sciences, 2011 ISBN 1437736149, 9781437736144

124. Approved Drug Products and Legal Requirements Volume 3 of USP DI: V. 3 of USP, United States Pharmacopeial Convention, Inc, published by Thomson Micromedex, 2006 ISBN 1563635763, 9781563635762

125. USP DI: Approved Drug Products and Legal Requirement USP DI VOL 3, published by Thomson/MICROMEDEX, 2005, ISBN 156363516X, 9781563635168

126. Lin EW, Boehnke N, Maynard HD. Protein-polymer conjugation via ligand affinity and photoactivation of glutathione S-transferase. Bioconjug Chem. 2014 Oct 15;25(10):1902-9. doi: 10.1021/bc500380r. Epub 2014 Sep 27. PubMed PMID: 25315970; PubMed Central PMCID: PMC4205000.

127. Hermanson GT. Chapter 18 - PEGylation and Synthetic Polymer Modification. In: Greg Hermanson. Bioconjugate Techniques (Third edition) 2013, Pages 787-838. DOI: https://doi.org/10.1016/B978-0-12-382239-0.00018-2, ISBN: 9780123822390, 9780123822406

128. US FDA Database. CFR - Code of Federal Regulations Title 21

129. Nicholas J. Lowe. Sunscreens: Development: Evaluation, and Regulatory Aspects: Second Edition, Cosmetic science and technology series, published by CRC Press, 1996 ISBN 0824793064, 9780824793067

130. Kaur A, Thatai P, Sapra B. Need of UV protection and evaluation of efficacy of sunscreens. J Cosmet Sci. 2014 Sep-Oct;65(5):315-45. PubMed PMID: 25682622.

131. National Center for Biotechnology Information. PubChem Database. Trolamine salicylate, CID=25213, https://pubchem.ncbi.nlm.nih.gov/compound/25213 (accessed on Apr. 27, 2019)

132. Trolamine salicylate. Available From: http://dermapproved.com/active-ingredients/trolamine-salicylate

133. Smijs TG, Pavel S. Titanium dioxide and zinc oxide nanoparticles in sunscreens: focus on their safety and effectiveness. Nanotechnol Sci Appl. 2011 Oct 13;4:95-112. doi: 10.2147/NSA.S19419. Review. PubMed PMID: 24198489; PubMed Central PMCID: PMC3781714.

134. Trivedi M, Murase J. Chapter 4. Titanium Dioxide in Sunscreen. In: Magdalena Janus. Application of Titanium Dioxide, published by Intech Open, 2017 ISBN 9535134299, 9789535134299

135. Mohammed YH, Holmes A, Haridass IN, Sanchez WY, Studier H, Grice JE, Benson HAE, Roberts MS. Support for the Safe Use of Zinc Oxido Nanoparticle Sunscreens: Lack of Skin Penetration or Cellular Toxicity after Repeated Application in Volunteers. J Invest Dermatol. 2019 Feb;139(2):308-315. doi: 10.1016/j.jid.2018.08.024. Epub 2018 Nov 15. PubMed PMID: 30448212.

136. Wright PFA. Realistic Exposure Study Assists Risk Assessments of ZnO Nanoparticle Sunscreens and Allays Safety Concerns. J Invest Dermatol. 2019 Feb;139(2):277-278. doi: 10.1016/j.jid.2018.09.014. Epub 2018 Nov 15. PubMed PMID: 30448211.

137. Jiang J, Pi J, Cai J. The Advancing of Zinc Oxide Nanoparticles for Biomedical Applications. Bioinorg Chem Appl. 2018 Jul 5;2018:1062562. doi: 10.1155/2018/1062562. eCollection 2018. Review. PubMed PMID: 30073019; PubMed Central PMCID: PMC6057429.

138. Tian L, Lin B, Wu L, Li K, Liu H, Yan J, Liu X, Xi Z. Neurotoxicity induced by zinc oxide nanoparticles: age-related differences and interaction. Sci Rep. 2015 Nov

3;5:16117. doi: 10.1038/srep16117. PubMed PMID: 26527454; PubMed Central PMCID: PMC4630782.

139. Schwarz T. Mechanisms of UV-induced immunosuppression. Keio J Med. 2005 Dec;54(4):165-71. Review. PubMed PMID: 16452825.
140. Ullrich SE. Mechanisms underlying UV-induced immune suppression. Mutat Res. 2005 Apr 1;571(1-2):185-205. Epub 2005 Jan 21. Review. PubMed PMID: 15748647.
141. Katiyar SK. UV-induced immune suppression and photocarcinogenesis: chemoprevention by dietary botanical agents. Cancer Lett. 2007 Sep 18;255(1):1-11. Epub 2007 Mar 26. Review. PubMed PMID: 17382466; PubMed Central PMCID: PMC1995595.
142. Cho BA, Yoo SK, Seo JS. Signatures of photo-aging and intrinsic aging in skin were revealed by transcriptome network analysis. Aging (Albany NY). 2018 Jul 18;10(7):1609-1626. doi: 10.18632/aging.101496. PubMed PMID: 30021930; PubMed Central PMCID: PMC6075446.
143. Bosch R, Philips N, Suárez-Pérez JA, Juarranz A, Devmurari A, Chalensouk-Khaosaat J, González S. Mechanisms of Photoaging and Cutaneous Photocarcinogenesis, and Photoprotective Strategies with Phytochemicals. Antioxidants (Basel). 2015 Mar 26;4(2):248-68. doi: 10.3390/antiox4020248. Review. PubMed PMID: 26783703; PubMed Central PMCID: PMC4665475.
144. Kang S, Fisher GJ, Voorhees JJ. Photoaging: pathogenesis, prevention, and treatment. Clin Geriatr Med. 2001 Nov;17(4):643-59, v-vi. Review. PubMed PMID: 11535421.
145. Han A, Chien AL, Kang S. Photoaging. Dermatol Clin. 2014 Jul;32(3):291-9, vii. doi: 10.1016/j.det.2014.03.015. Review. PubMed PMID: 24891052.
146. SjerobabskiMasnec I, Poduje S. Photoaging. Coll Antropol. 2008 Oct;32 Suppl 2:177-80. Review. PubMed PMID: 19140280.
147. Fisher GJ, Kang S, Varani J, et al. Mechanisms of Photoaging and Chronological Skin Aging. Arch Dermatol. 2002;138(11):1462–1470. doi:10.1001/archderm.138.11.1462
148. Rabe JH, Mamelak AJ, McElgunn PJ, Morison WL, Sauder DN. Photoaging: mechanisms and repair. J Am Acad Dermatol. 2006 Jul;55(1):1-19. Review. PubMed PMID: 16781287.
149. Rittié L, Fisher GJ. Natural and sun-induced aging of human skin. Cold Spring HarbPerspect Med. 2015 Jan 5;5(1):a015370. doi: 10.1101/cshperspect.a015370. Review. PubMed PMID: 25561721; PubMed Central PMCID: PMC4292080.
150. Amano S. Characterization and mechanisms of photoageing-related changes in skin. Damages of basement membrane and dermal structures. Exp Dermatol. 2016 Aug;25 Suppl 3:14-9. doi: 10.1111/exd.13085. Review. PubMed PMID: 27539897.
151. Pamela RD. Topical Growth Factors for the Treatment of Facial Photoaging: A Clinical Experience of Eight Cases. J Clin Aesthet Dermatol. 2018 Dec;11(12):28-29. Epub 2018 Dec 1. PubMed PMID: 30666276; PubMed Central PMCID: PMC6334836.

152. Dhaliwal S, Rybak I, Ellis SR, Notay M, Trivedi M, Burney W, Vaughn AR, Nguyen M, Reiter P, Bosanac S, Yan H, Foolad N, Sivamani RK. Prospective, randomized, double-blind assessment of topical bakuchiol and retinol for facial photoageing. Br J Dermatol. 2019 Feb;180(2):289-296. doi: 10.1111/bjd.16918. Epub 2018 Sep 21. PubMed PMID: 29947134.
153. Mukherjee S, Date A, Patravale V, Korting HC, Roeder A, Weindl G. Retinoids in the treatment of skin aging: an overview of clinical efficacy and safety. Clin Interv Aging. 2006;1(4):327-48. Review. PubMed PMID: 18046911; PubMed Central PMCID: PMC2699641.
154. Pandel R, Poljšak B, Godic A, Dahmane R. Skin photoaging and the role of antioxidants in its prevention. ISRN Dermatol. 2013 Sep 12;2013:930164. doi: 10.1155/2013/930164. Review. PubMed PMID: 24159392; PubMed Central PMCID: PMC3789494.
155. Sivamani RK, Crane LA, Dellavalle RP. The benefits and risks of ultraviolet tanning and its alternatives: the role of prudent sun exposure. Dermatol Clin. 2009 Apr;27(2):149-54, vi. doi: 10.1016/j.det.2008.11.008. Review. PubMed PMID: 19254658; PubMed Central PMCID: PMC2692214.
156. Juzeniene A, Moan J. Beneficial effects of UV radiation other than via vitamin D production. Dermatoendocrinol. 2012 Apr 1;4(2):109-17. doi: 10.4161/derm.20013. PubMed PMID: 22928066; PubMed Central PMCID: PMC3427189.
157. Choi W, Miyamura Y, Wolber R, Smuda C, Reinhold W, Liu H, Kolbe L, Hearing VJ. Regulation of human skin pigmentation in situ by repetitive UV exposure: molecular characterization of responses to UVA and/or UVB. J Invest Dermatol. 2010 Jun;130(6):1685-96. doi: 10.1038/jid.2010.5. Epub 2010 Feb 11. PubMed PMID: 20147966; PubMed Central PMCID: PMC3478754.
158. Brenner M, Hearing VJ. The protective role of melanin against UV damage in human skin. PhotochemPhotobiol. 2008 May-Jun;84(3):539-49. doi: 10.1111/j.1751-1097.2007.00226.x. Review. PubMed PMID: 18435612; PubMed Central PMCID: PMC2671032.
159. Hwang YJ, Park HJ, Hahn HJ, Kim JY, Ko JH, Lee YW, Choe YB, Ahn KJ. Immediate pigment darkening and persistent pigment darkening as means of measuring the ultraviolet A protection factor in vivo: a comparative study. Br J Dermatol. 2011 Jun;164(6):1356-61. doi: 10.1111/j.1365-2133.2011.10225.x.Epub 2011 May 9. PubMed PMID: 21250967.
160. Del Bino S, Duval C, Bernerd F. Clinical and Biological Characterization of Skin Pigmentation Diversity and Its Consequences on UV Impact. Int J Mol Sci. 2018 Sep 8;19(9). pii: E2668. doi: 10.3390/ijms19092668. Review. PubMed PMID: 30205563; PubMed Central PMCID: PMC6163216.
161. Rattanachaikunsopon P, Phumkhachorn P. Bacteriostatic effect of flavonoids isolated from leaves of Psidium guajava on fish pathogens. Fitoterapia. 2007 Sep;78(6):434-6. Epub 2007 May 5. PubMed PMID: 17553634.
162. National Center for Biotechnology Information. PubChem Database. Morin, CID=5281670, https://pubchem.ncbi.nlm.nih.gov/compound/5281670 (accessed on Apr. 28, 2019)

163. Beasley DG, Meyer TA. Characterization of the UVA protection provided by avobenzone, zinc oxide, and titanium dioxide in broad-spectrum sunscreen products. Am J Clin Dermatol. 2010 Dec 1;11(6):413-21. doi: 10.2165/11537050-000000000-00000. PubMed PMID: 20806994.
164. Tanner PR. Sunscreen product formulation. Dermatol Clin. 2006 Jan;24(1):53-62. Review. PubMed PMID: 16311167.
165. Weber C, Podda M, Rallis M, Thiele JJ, Traber MG, Packer L. Efficacy of topically applied tocopherols and tocotrienols in protection of murine skin from oxidative damage induced by UV-irradiation. Free Radic Biol Med. 1997;22(5):761-9. PubMed PMID: 9119243.
166. Chapter 2. Raw materials of cosmetics. In: Hiroshi Iwata, Kunio Shimada. Formulas, Ingredients and Production of Cosmetics: Technology of Skin- and Hair-Care Products in Japan, published by Springer Science & Business Media, 2012 ISBN 4431540601, 9784431540601
167. Alcohol (Page 17). In: Raymond C. Rowe, Paul J. Sheskey, Marian E. Quinn. Handbook of Pharmaceutical Excipients, edition 6, published by Pharmaceutical Press, 2009 ISBN 1582121354, 9781582121352
168. Lachenmeier DW. Safety evaluation of topical applications of ethanol on the skin and inside the oral cavity. J Occup Med Toxicol. 2008 Nov 13;3:26. doi: 10.1186/1745-6673-3-26. PubMed PMID: 19014531; PubMed Central PMCID: PMC2596158.
169. SD Alcohol 40. Available From: https://thedermreview.com/sd-alcohol-40/
170. Romanowski P. Cosmetic formulation basics – Sunscreens. Available From: https://chemistscorner.com/cosmetic-formulation-basics-sunscreens/
171. Habbema L, Halk AB, Neumann M, Bergman W. Risks of unregulated use of alpha-melanocyte-stimulating hormone analogues: a review. Int J Dermatol. 2017 Oct;56(10):975-980. doi: 10.1111/ijd.13585. Epub 2017 Mar 7. Review. PubMed PMID: 28266027.
172. Garone M, Howard J, Fabrikant J. A review of common tanning methods. J Clin Aesthet Dermatol. 2015 Feb;8(2):43-7. Review. PubMed PMID: 25741402; PubMed Central PMCID: PMC4345932.
173. Ciriminna R, Fidalgo A, Ilharco LM, Pagliaro M. Dihydroxyacetone: An Updated Insight into an Important Bioproduct. ChemistryOpen. 2018 Mar 6;7(3):233-236. doi: 10.1002/open.201700201. eCollection 2018 Mar. Review. PubMed PMID: 29531886; PubMed Central PMCID: PMC5838383.
174. Martini MC. [Self-tanning and sunless tanning products]. Ann Dermatol Venereol. 2017 Oct;144(10):638-644. doi: 10.1016/j.annder.2017.03.021. Epub2017 Aug 18. French. PubMed PMID: 28823805.
175. Holman DM, Fox KA, Glenn JD, Guy GP Jr, Watson M, Baker K, Cokkinides V, Gottlieb M, Lazovich D, Perna FM, Sampson BP, Seidenberg AB, Sinclair C, Geller AC. Strategies to reduce indoor tanning: current research gaps and future opportunities for prevention. Am J Prev Med. 2013 Jun;44(6):672-81. doi: 10.1016/j.amepre.2013.02.014. PubMed PMID: 23683986; PubMed Central PMCID: PMC4413462.
176. Give me a tan! - Megan Fox. News24.com Archives, 2008-11-07

177. March B. 10 celebs who look better tan-free. COSMOPOLITAN, July 14, 2014.
178. Haggan M.Warning on incorrect sunscreen use. Australian Journal of Pharmacy, 16/01/2018.
179. Grand View Research. U.S. Sun Care Market Size, Share, Industry Trends Report, 2018-2025.
180. Sunscreen Manufacturing Industry in the US. IBISWorld, September, 2018
181. Zirwas MJ, Andrasik W. Can Sunscreens Harm Coral Reefs? Addressing Environmental Concerns and Offering Practical Recommendations. Skinmed. 2018 Jul 1;16(4):223-229. eCollection 2018. PubMed PMID: 30207523.
182. Belluz J. Hawaii is banning sunscreens that kill coral reefs. Vox, July 2, 2018.
183. Reef-safe Sunscreen: What You Need To Know. Blog CHASING CORAL.
184. Danovaro R, Bongiorni L, Corinaldesi C, Giovannelli D, Damiani E, Astolfi P, Greci L, Pusceddu A. Sunscreens cause coral bleaching by promoting viral infections. Environ Health Perspect. 2008 Apr;116(4):441-7. doi: 10.1289/ehp.10966. PubMed PMID: 18414624; PubMed Central PMCID: PMC2291018.
185. Leonardo DiCaprio Foundation. Replenishing Coral Reefs in the Pacific Ocean.

CHAPTER 6

FACE POWDERS: FUNCTIONAL USES AND FORMULATIONS

6.1 BACKGROUND

First made popular in the 1930s, until recently, it's arguably lacked the finesse of modern makeup (like foundation) which, over the last decade, has been fine-tuned, finely milled and given a twenty-first century makeover. The use of 'paint' was criticized in Victorian times but pale, flawless skins were fashionable so many women resorted to face powders to cover blemishes like sunburn, spots and freckles. Perspiration and oily secretions could also be rectified with powder, making it useful in places where summers were warm and women were more likely to 'glow'. As a cosmetic care product, face powder appeared in ancient Egypt when the Queen Cleopatra applied powder before applying makeup. White skin was the sign of high status in the society since wealthy women did not have to work in the open air under the heavy sun light and their face never got tanned. When tanned for any reason, the Egyptians concealed the bronze under the layers of powder. The ingredients used for powder were various substances, even very exotic. So, Cleopatra who was ready for everything scarifying for her beauty used the powder made from crocodile excrements. In Roman times (A.D. 100s), "chalk and vinegar face creams lightened the complexion, and finely ground orris root was used in face powder," reports Gabriella Hernandez's "Classic Beauty: The History of Makeup". The women would use the powder presented as the mixture of crushed chalk and lead extremely toxic and harmful for the health, though immediately concealing all defects and drawbacks of the skin under the layer of dangerous makeup. In spite of the obvious harmfulness for the skin, such mixture was highly appreciated, and only the most rich and wealthy Romans could afford it. The other, less wealthy Roman women were satisfied with application of mixture from wheat flour. And in Ancient China, rice powder was used to whiten and smooth out the complexion. Also, Japanese women and men commonly used the face powder made from rice flour, while in Europe such flour appeared a little bit later, in the 16th century, when rice was marketed in some of European countries including main cores of fashion and noble life, as France, Spain and England. The powder made from grinded rice was used to apply onto the face skin and wigs that became more massive. During the reign of Louis 15th, the powder was made a cosmetic means by the favorite of the King, marquise de Pompadour. The court ladies applied the thick layer of powder onto the face, hands, and shoulders making them aristocratically pale and hiding the skin defects. The colorful powder became fashionable when the tender pink powder was used to accentuate the beauty of cheeks and the blue powder was applied under eyes. Later on, the powder disappeared from practice since in the end of the 17th century a plenty of wheat and rice flour was spent to make the powder to the extent that powder pro was officially forbidden in France first and then in other countries to produce powder to save the assets. And the powder sank into oblivion for almost a hundred years and a healthy and tanned look came in fashion. The Queen Victoria of Great Britain was the one who prohibited using the makeup for the reason that it seemed vulgar. The face powder returned its fame in the beginning of the 20th century when theater actresses concealed skin defects under the layer of powder not only on the stage but in everyday life also. In the early 20th century Anthony Overton launched his first powder for Afro-Americans under High Brown Brand. Then in France the powder was invented similar to the face powder we use now. The base for the powder was the talk without harmful lead admixtures not irritating the skin. For several decades the cosmetic industry underwent sea changes and revolutions. And in 1923 the English Company Laughton & Sons proceeded to manufacture the comfortable compact powder-cases with sponges, and in the fifties, the legendary Hollywood stylist Max Factor launched affordable to actresses and ordinary woman a version of foundation powder for everyday use called "Pan Cake", that effectively conceal drawbacks.

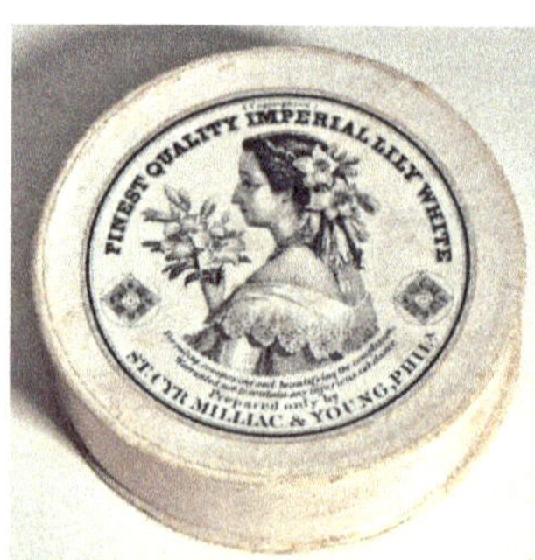

(a) 1871 Milliac & Young powder box (Courtacy: perfumebottles.org)

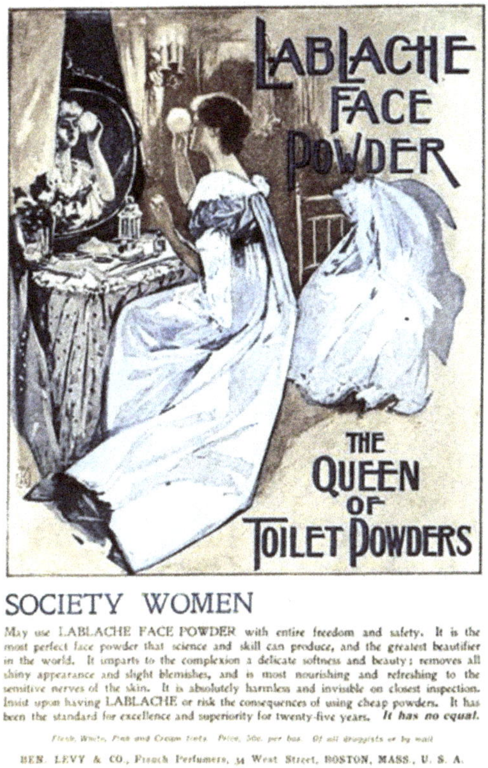

(b) 1896 LaBlache Face Powder.(Courtacy: thebuddingherbalist.com)

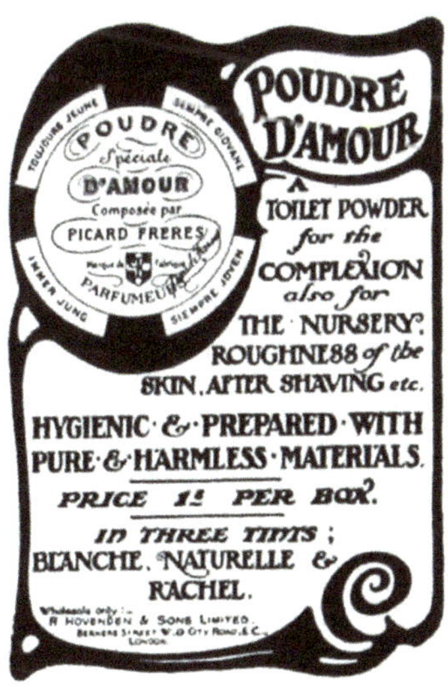

(c) 1903 Poudre D'Amour (Courtacy: Graces Guide)

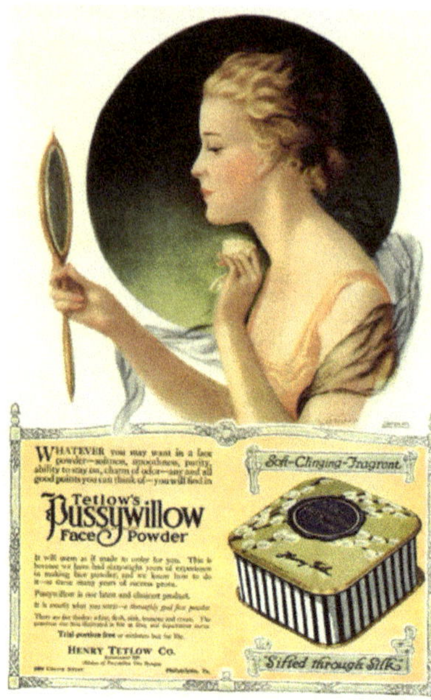

(d) 1917 Tetlow Pussywillow Face Powder.(Courtacy: Collecting Vintage Compacts)

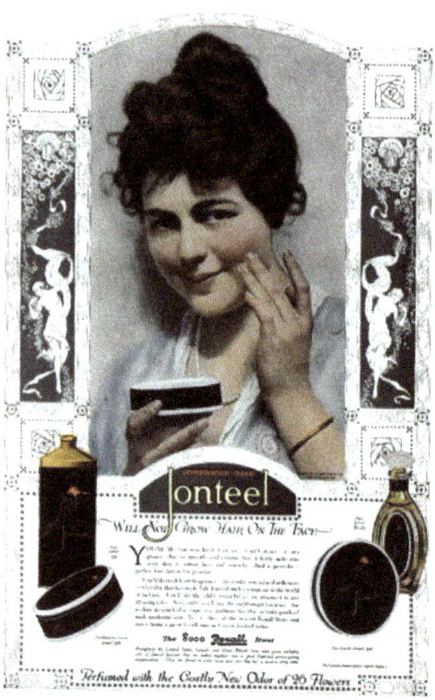

(e) 1919 Jonteel Face Powder.
(Courtacy: Rexall)

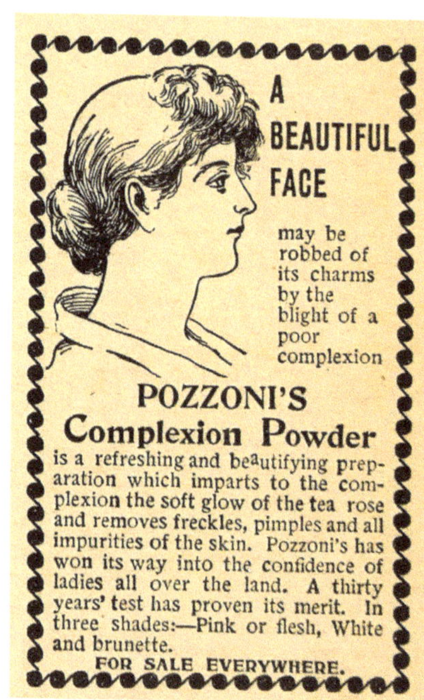

(f) 1894 Ad POZZONI'S Complexion Powder of Victorian era (Courtacy: periodpaper.com)

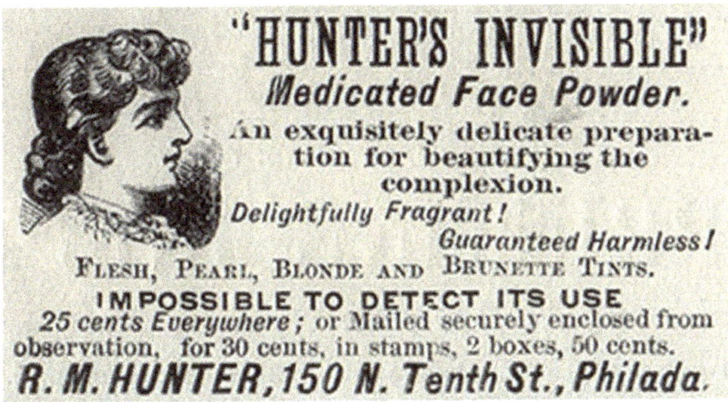

(g) Hunter's Invisible of Victorian Era.Like several other Victorian beauty techniques, lead cosmetics often caused problems it was meant to remedy. Combining lead face powders and paints with corrosive washes resulted in wounds and scars. Women tried to hide the blemishes beneath heavier layers of lead makeup, which made the problem worse. These thick layers of make-up cracked like porcelain if a woman was too expressive. Since women were expected to be naturally beautiful during the era, appearing at a social event with cracking face paste would have been extremely mortifying. Though face powders like this one claimed to be harmless, women rarely knew the ingredients. To cover unsightly blemishes and scars, women turned to face paints and powders. Some of these concoctions were rather mild, containing ingredients like rice powder, zinc oxide, or the extremely expensive blend of chloride of bismuth and talc. Others were made of lead flakes. Not only is lead highly toxic, it is easily absorbed through the skin. Side effects of lead poisoning include headache, constipation, memory loss, pain and numbness, and if ingested in large enough quantities, will cause paralysis and death (Courtacy: RSSing.com).

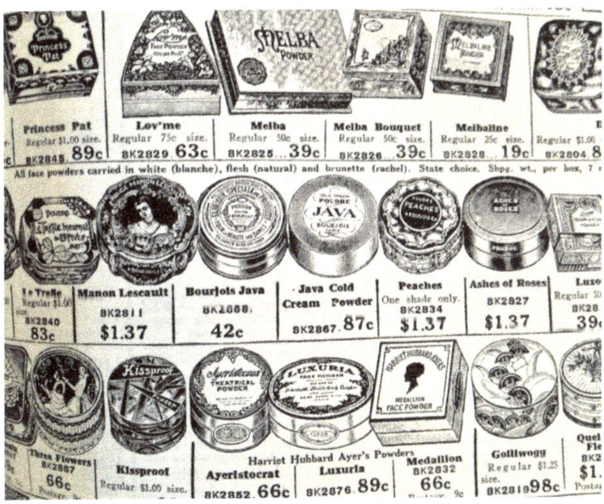
Princess Pat
89c
Lov'me
63c
Melba
39c
Melba Bouquet
39c
Melbaline
19c
All face powders carried in white (blanche), flesh (natural) and brunette (rachel). State choice.
Manon Lescault
$1.37
Bourjois Java
42c
Java Cold Cream Powder
87c
Peaches
$1.37
Ashes of Roses
$1.37
Three Flowers
66c
Kissproof
Harriet Hubbard Ayer's Powders
Ayeristocrat
66c
Luxuria
89c
Medallion
66c
Golliwogg
98c

(h) 1927 Selection of Face Powders for Sale. Most makeup in the 1920s was limited to just a few shades that never matched natural skin tone. The initial look of women in makeup was ghastly! With limited colors, chalky foundations, and no previous generations of women to teach them how to apply makeup, the first attempts were anything but glamorous. Women didn't seem to mind. As the decade progressed, the quality of makeup improved. The number of products went from a few dozen to 450 by 1924. By the end of the twenties, there were 1300 brands and shades of face powder, 350 rouges, and a hundred red lipsticks. It was a 52 million-dollar industry. Poor women used home remedies such as ivory face powder, although the tanned look was in and many women shunned the pale skin of the past (Courtacy: Vintage Dancer).

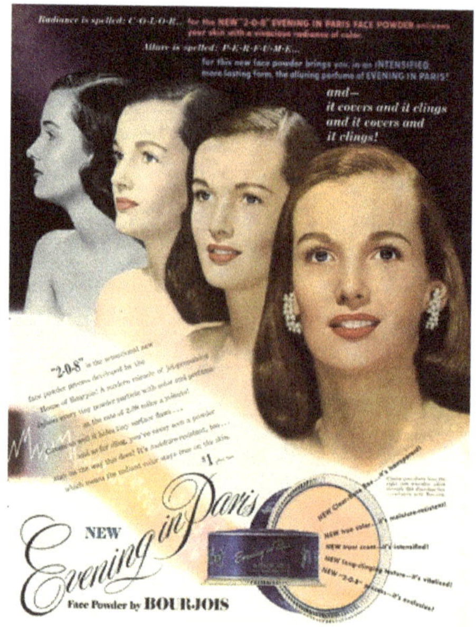

(i) 1947 Bourjois Face Powder (Courtacy: Cosmetics and Skin)

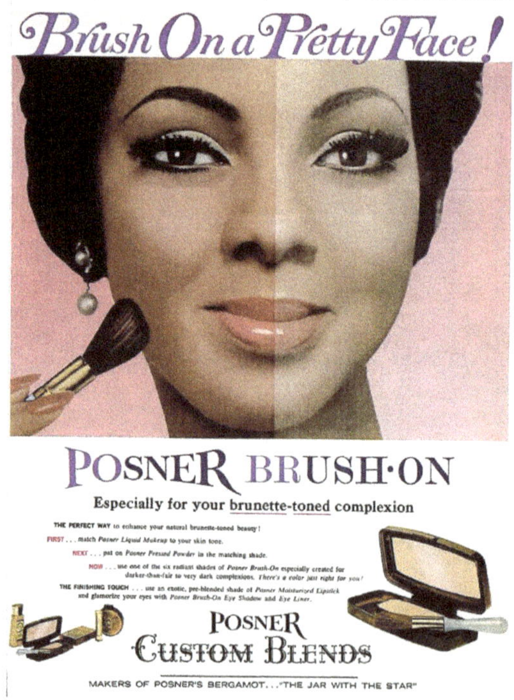

(j) 1960s Posner Makeup Adrange of cosmetics all scented with Evening in Paris perfume (*Courtacy:* Bustle 32 Black)

Figure 6.1 Historical Face Powders

6.2 ABSTRACT

The face powder was demanded by many nations in the world in the beginning AD and in Asia white skin was believed to be the sign of aristocratism, membership of the elite, and yet, white color is the pure symbol of the internal beauty and nobility. In addition, some face powders are sold in varying specialty shades to suit different skin needs; for example, a face powder with a greenish tinge will minimize the appearance of redness, while a purple-tinted powder may help the appearance of sallow or yellow skin. There is a legitimate reason to use face powder, and the pharmacopeias prescribe them in the treatment of many skin affections. At all events the proper use of powder is beneficial, it lightly covers and unifies a complexion, hiding the ravages of time, improving even the beautiful face. Face powder comes in different shades to match varying skin tones, and it is a good idea to choose the skin tone that most closely matches the natural skin. This will help the makeup appear more natural; it should be virtually unnoticeable. It may be necessary to use different face powders for summer and winter, as the skin may become tanner in the summer, or drier and in need of extra moisture in the winter. They are of benefit in acne, freckles, sunburn and red nose. Beneath their attractive aspect and odor, face powders should be made by the perfumer to combine the qualities of an elegant cosmetic and therapeutic agent; they must primarily possess adherence, lightness and be transparent; secondly, they should be detergent and delicately absorbent to aid the natural functions of the skin, taking up the fatty matters not easily dislodged by water; they should also tend to increase the natural elasticity and regular functions of the skin.

Keywords: Absorbency; adhesion; covering power; pressed powder; moisture absorption

6.3 INTRODUCTION

Face powders provide coverage of complexion imperfections, oil control, a matte finish, and tactile smoothness to the skin. Powders give a good lasting effect to foundation makeup and possess oil-absorbing properties that are very useful for oily-skin types. Free powders are used to fix the foundation and compact powders to retouch one's face during the day. Certain face powders are readily made, but it is not easy to produce a really good face powder, i.e., one that spreads well and smoothly on the skin, has the right matt look and degree of opacity, wears well in hot weather and blustery weather, is available in a variety of color shades, is attractively perfumed; and is at all times uniform and consistent in quality. Face powder is more complicated and made by a mixture of products: Talc and sericite (to help to spread), chalk or kaolin (to give moisture-absorbing qualities), magnesium stearate (gives adherence), zinc oxide and titanium oxide (to help cover the skin thoroughly), and pigments (for color). The use of mica in powder formulations improves skin feel, product application,

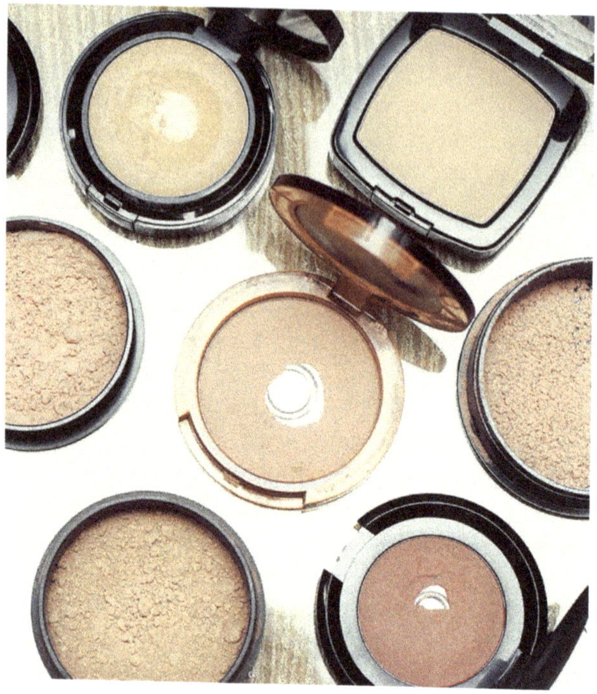

(a) Compact Collection (*Courtacy:* Stylecraze)

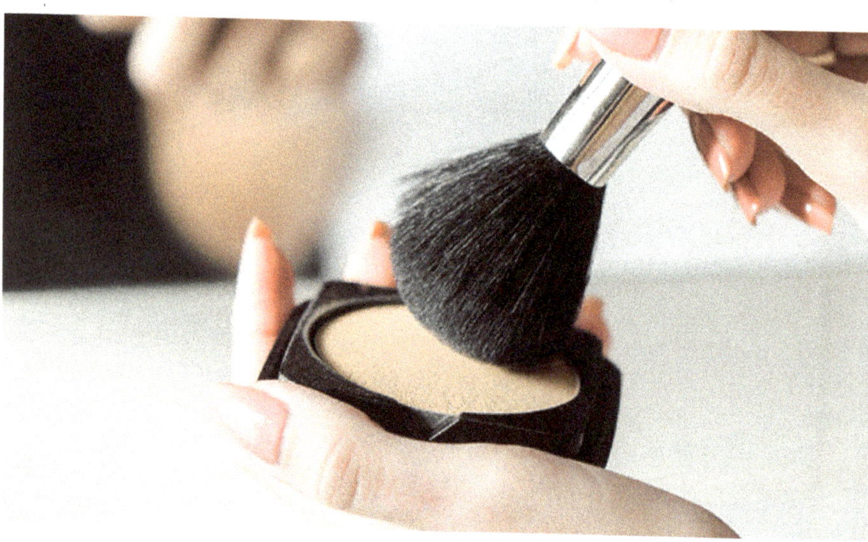

(b) Powder for Oily Skin (*Courtacy:* femalenetwork.com)

Figure 6.2 Modern day Face Setting Powders and Compacts

and skin adhesion. The favorable effects are obtained with wet ground micas that have a particle size of <15 mm. Mica can also be modified by coating with inorganic or organic materials to produce another large group of fillers (spherical, special, and surface modified). Spherical fillers are widely used to improve skin feel. There are a variety of materials available, the organic types consisting mainly of polyamides, nylon spheres and inorganic types consisting mainly of silica, both as solid or hollow spheres. The improvement of skin feel is attributed to the ball bearing–like action of the spheres between other powder ingredients in the formulation and the spherical filler. When spherical materials are used, there is also an increase in the viscosity of the emulsion, allowing for a reduction of viscosity modifiers in the final formulation. These early commercial face powders were generally simple mixtures of three or more substances. Common ingredients included talc, natural starches like potato and rice, calcium carbonate (chalk), magnesium carbonate, kieselguhr (diatomite), washed china clay (kaolin), bismuth subchloride and subnitrate, zinc and magnesium stearate, ground orris root and zinc oxide. A very important constituent of powder is oxide of zinc, owing to its great covering power, also because of its adhesive properties, as an addition to the lighter kinds of starch and also of carbonate of magnesia. It forms an important component of all kinds of powders, aside from the fact that from a hygienic point of view it is very desirable. Some of these, such as orris root and bismuth compounds, fell out of favor, while others, like zinc oxide, that were initially treated with suspicion, became staple ingredients. Nowadays, BiOCl is much more stable to UV light. Special fillers are a group of fillers that are made up of several components, which combine their individual advantages when they are processed together into a composite material. For surface-modified fillers, most coating materials are organic polymers (collagen, elastin, and vitamin E). Powders also contain between 10% and 20% of organic texture agents (polymers) or mineral agents (boron nitride and silica), preservatives, anti-oxidants, and perfumes (neutral or more sophisticated) can also be added there

6.3.1 FUNCTIONAL USE OF FACE POWDER

New uses for 'face powders' have been established, such as the correction of heightened color where there is too much red coloration or too much yellow in the case of sallow complexions. The borderline between what constitutes a face powder and a foundation has become very blurred with the development of dual-function products. The main function of early face powders was to visually cover the skin, so that shine was reduced and imperfections were hidden. The amount of concealment needed varied from woman to woman, so powders were produced in various grades loosely referred to as light, medium and heavy. However, the main functional uses are:

- Its prime function goes with the ability to complement skin color by imparting a velvet like finish.

- It is opaque enough to make minor blemishes, masking minor imperfections but it must not impart a mask like effect.
- Whatever the finish it must possess some reasonable lasting properties to avoid need for re-powdering i.e. it must adhere to the skin.
- It must be reasonably resistant to the mixed secretions of the skin.
- Finally, it should serve as a vehicle for a pleasing odor to be disseminated by intimate contact of perfume laden particles over a warm and relatively large area.

Also, there are some other interesting uses of face powders such as:

- *As an eyeshadow primer*: Using an eye primer helps eyeshadow look more vibrant and fresher for longer, powdering eyelids can be an emergency solution. Not only will this mattify oily eyelids, it'll also make blending easier since powders blend over other powders better than over bare eyelids.
- *As a lipstick mattifier*: First thing is to settle a thin layer of tissue on lips, then with a brush, and then taping some loose powder over the area to seal that color in.
- *As a mascara primer*: In between applying thin layers of mascara, some translucent loose powder over lashes to be brushed before mascara is completely dried.
- *As emergency dry shampoo*: The majority of dry shampoos consists of highly absorbent powder like ingredients such as starch and clay etc., which acts to soak up the oil and grease at the roots of hair. However, to absorb the bulk of oils, a pre-blot with a piece of tissue or blotting paper is necessary to prevent the powder from clumping up and taping of some colorless loose powder on top of those oily areas afterwards [1-7].

Table 6.1 Formulation: Face Powder Vs Make-Up Cream

Fatty powder for rough/dry skin		Matt effect or shimmer		Make-Up Cream	
Ingredients	**Parts**	**Ingredients**	**(%)**	**Ingredients**	**(%)**
Talc	1000	Talc	77	Glyceryl mono & di-stearate	2
Vaseline	50	Zn-stearate	5	PEG 400 monostearate	1
White Beeswax	40	ZnO	2	Stearic acid	11.5
Petroleum Jelly	40	Kaolin	5	Cetyl alcohol	0.5
Stearin	20	Mica	10	Isopropyl palmitate	2
Glyceryl monostearate	75	Red Iron Oxide	0.36	PG	12

Contd...

Fatty powder for rough/dry skin		Matt effect or shimmer		Make-Up Cream	
Ingredients	**Parts**	**Ingredients**	**(%)**	**Ingredients**	**(%)**
		Black Iron Oxide	0.03	Preservative	0.1
		Perfume	0.25	TiO_2	2.2
				Talc	8
				Color Pigments	1
				Water	57.4

Exhibit 1. Powdered Make-up Vs Cream [111]

Powder pros	Powder cons	Cream pros	Cream Cons
Gives a matte, velvety finish to the skin for an 'airbrush' effect	Can be ageing as it settles into fine lines and wrinkles	Easy to blend into skin as they 'melt' into it	Not as long-lasting as powder
Very long-lasting, especially if applied on top of foundation	Requires brushes generally and a bit of technique	No brushes are required	Tends to crease more easily (especially on the eyes), can turn shiny and move around.
Helps absorb natural skin oils so doesn't crease easily, best option for oily skin	Looks slightly less natural as it sits on top of skin	Highly pigmented in general, a small amount is needed	Not the best option for oily skins (although matt-finish cream-to-powder formulas can work well)
Can be layered on top of each other as well as on top of cream products	Can make skin feel dry or dehydrated	Good for drier or more mature skins	Only works on top of other creams, can't applied on top of powder
Blending different powder colors and textures is easy	Can cause 'powder fallout' under the eyes and too-matt powders can make skin look flat and dull	Leaves skin with a dewy glow and a hydrated feel	Blending cream colors together not as easy as powders

6.3.2 ESSENTIAL PROPERTIES OF A GOOD FACE POWDER

In recent times the fashion has changed from a 'painted clown' look to one that appears to be as natural as if the skin had no product applied but without the imperfections. Modern products are also required to be 'long-lasting', preferably all day, and consequently avoid repeated application; they should not rub off onto clothing (either that of the wearer or of anybody else).

- *Covering Power* - ability to mask skin defects such as skin shine, enlarged pores and minor blemishes.
- *Slip*- faculty of spreading over the skin without dragging and giving the characteristic smooth feeling. There must be sufficient slip to enable the powder to be applied to the skin with a suitable applicator, such as a puff or brush, without dragging or producing a blotchy effect.
- *Adhesiveness* - ability to cling to the face. It should adhere to the skin and must not be completely dissipated in a short time, so avoiding frequent re-powdering.
- *Absorbency* - capable of absorbing skin secretions (perspiration and oiliness) without showing evidence of such absorption.
- *Bloom*- ability to impart a velvety peach like finish to the skin. Shine on or around the nose must be completely eliminated. The powder must be absorbent without changing its appearance on the skin [6-10].

6.3.3 CHOOSING RIGHT FACE POWDER

Face powder is hardly exciting, but it can play a big role in adding polish to finished look, not to mention helping makeup last longer. Prior choosing a face powder one should focus the actual need or objective.

- *A long-lasting make-up* needs improved staying power and it is suggested to look for products labeled as "setting" or "finishing" powders. These all-purpose powders can keep foundation from separating and, to some degree, protect it from the effects of heat and humidity.
- *For oily or combination skin*, a powder that's described as "mattifying," "oil control," "shine control," or "blotting." Should be considered. A powder with these qualities generally has additional absorbent ingredients to help with oily skin concerns. However, this is not the powder for those with dry to very dry skin because the extra absorbency will likely make dry skin feel tighter and uncomfortable.
- Using powder is still a good idea *in case of dry skin* because it can keep makeup from creasing. Its best to seek out formulas that go a bit lighter on the absorbent ingredients, like starches and clays. If someone want to enliven dull, dry skin, choose products that have words like "glow," "luminous," or "brightening" in their descriptions. These types generally include mineral pigments that reflect light off the face, and have a softer texture.

- Once the *role play of the powder* is selected, there are a couple of other factors to consider, which are mainly a matter of personal preference. Tinted powders can enhance the color of foundation, but translucent is the way to go if the color of base makeup is found ok.
- There's also the *consideration of pressed or loose powder*. Loose powder is easier to pick up on a brush and it's easier to tell how much it's in use, but for touching up on the go, pressed powder is a relatively good option [3,4].

6.3.4 TYPES OF FACE POWDER

The marketplace offers a profusion of powders. There are two main forms of face powder. Loose face powder comes in a sealed tambourine inside a decorative plastic container. It is either applied directly from this by a puff or large brush, or is transferred to a special compact in which it can be carried in a handbag and is applied with a sponge or small puff that also fits in the compact. To prevent leakage a nylon mesh covers the surface of the powder. In its second form the powder is compacted or pressed and a binding agent is used in its manufacture. There are matte face powders, in loose or pressed form, that are designed for dry, normal or oily skin; translucent powders that allow the natural skin color to show through; opalescent powders that give the skin a slight shimmer; tinted powders that tone down ruddiness; body powders that are suffused with fragrance or with glitter for nighttime sparkle; baby powders that are made from either talc or cornstarch; medicated powders that fight body odor and troublesome microorganisms or soothe irritations, and even perfumed liquid body "coolers" - powder suspended in an alcohol base - that dry on the skin to a powder finish. However, in various books and articles, face powders are classified in the following way:

- *Loose Powder*: Leaves the skin with a refined texture and soft glow. Loose powder is the original type of face powder. It has light and soft texture. The talc powder makes the formula easily absorbed on the skin and make face free from oil. That is why, loose powder is suitable for oily skin. Typically, loose powder is packaged in a jar equipped with a puff. The disadvantages of this powder are not durable and easily smudged by sweat. It also helps to prevent makeup transfer or runoff one may experience in the middle of the day. For people with oily skin, wearing loose powder is a must because it helps to control oil, keeping the face free from shine. Loose powder seals the moist consistency of foundation and makes it last longer.
- *Pressed Powder*: Compact powder or pressed powder is a loose powder that was compacted. The main difference between loose and pressed powders is the way the product is packaged. Pressed powders are pressed into a compact, loose powders are often packaged in jars or tubs. Typically, compact powder has been formulated with a moisturizer and oil. It makes the texture heavier than loose powder. It also makes face look greasy in 2-3

hours after wear this powder. Therefore, compact powder is recommended for dry skin. Beside brighten the face, it also moisturizes the skin.

- *Two Way Cake Powder*: This multitasking pressed powder glides easily over skin to provide a flawless, natural-looking matte finish. The coverage of this powder is very perfect, because it contains a foundation formula. This powder very recommended to cover blemishes, dark spot, with durable results.
- *Setting Powder*: Designed to "set" or hold foundation in place, setting powders prevent base makeup from rubbing off and reduce shine for a long-lasting, flawless complexion. Available in two common forms – loose and pressed – setting powders can be translucent or slightly tinted to match skin tone. Setting powder serves to eliminate oil and keeping makeup to be more durable, and also give it that extra wow factor by combatting shine and maintaining an even, matte finish. Typically, setting powder comes with the type of translucent or transparent powder.
- *Finishing powder*: It is used to lock the finished makeup. It can be used to maximize the bright makeup that looks uneven, and fading the fine lines or pores in the face. Typically, finishing powder is the white powder. The fine line between finishing powder and setting powder is frustratingly blurry. Most commonly sold in loose form, finishing powders blur fine lines, conceal pores and leave a flawless, camera-ready finish [8,9].

Table 6.2 Compact Face Powder

	Formula 1		**Formula 2**	
	Ingredients	**%**	**Ingredients**	**%**
Part A	Stearic Acid (Triple Pressed)	1.35	Stearic Acid (Triple Pressed)	3.1
	Propylene Glycol Monostearate	3.95	Propylene Glycol Monostearate	3.55
	Lanolin	1.05	Lanolin	1
	Mineral Oil 80-90	12.2	Mineral Oil 65-75	9.2
	Propyl *p*-hydroxybenzoate	0.05	Propyl p-hydroxybenzoate	0.05
	Amerchol L-101	2.65	Ceraphyl 31	4.7
			Ceraphyl 140	3.1
Part B	Water	56.8	Water	53
	Triethanolamine	0.2	Triethanolamine	2.15
	Propylene glycol	5.3		
	Na-CMC	0.25		
	Veegum	1.1	Veegum	0.55
	Methyl *p*-hydroxybenzoate	0.1	Methyl *p*-hydroxybenzoate	0.1

Contd...

	Formula 1		Formula 2	
	Ingredients	%	Ingredients	%
Part C	Titanium dioxide 3328	8.3	Titanium dioxide	8
	Kaolin Colloidal	5.1	Kaolin Colloidal	4.1
	Na-Lauryl sulfate	0.8	Na-Lauryl sulfate	0.7
	Talc Alabama #141	0.35	Talc	1.6
	Iron oxide	0.45		
Perfume		q.s.		q.s.

Procedure: Part B is to be heated and agitated at 70^{0}C. It requires at least 3 hours for the Veegum to absorb all the water. Then balance of B added and heated to 80^{0}C. Part A is to be heated at 75^{0}C. Then Part B is to be added to Part A with rapid agitation. Part C is to be added at 60^{0}C. The whole formulation should be passed through colloid mill. The whole mixture is to be agitated until room temperature is reached. *Function of Ingredients*: In topical formulations, stearic acid is used as an emulsifying and solubilizing agent. It is highly soluble in structurally diverse solvents. Stearic acid is a hard, white or faintly yellow-colored, somewhat glossy, crystalline solid or a white or yellowish white powder. Propylene Glycol Monostearate is a lipophilic emulsifier that is a propylene glycol ester. It is a colorless, viscous liquid. It has a wide range of applications including industrial solvents, paint and coating solvents, polyester and alkyd resins, antifreeze coolants, heat transfer fluids, deicing fluids, plasticizers, detergents and surfactants, and bactericide. USP grade is used in foods, pharmaceutical, and personal care products. Propylene glycol monostearate is not approved in Germany. It is only slightly water dispersible, but completely soluble in fats and oils, therefore it is used only in combination with oils and fats as an emulsifier and emulsion stabilizer. In cosmetic industry it is used as an emulsifier for lotions, soft cream, makeup, humectant in dry skin products. Hydrous lanolin should be stored in a well-filled, well-closed container protected from light, in a cool, dry place. Normal storage life is 2 years. Lanolin is widely used in topical pharmaceutical formulations and cosmetics. Lanolin may be used as a hydrophobic vehicle and in the preparation of water-in-oil creams and ointments. When mixed with suitable vegetable oils or with soft paraffin, it produces emollient creams that penetrate the skin and hence facilitate the absorption of drugs. Lanolin mixes with about twice its own weight of water, without separation, to produce stable emulsions that do not readily become rancid on storage. Amerchol L-101 is a mixture of mineral oil and lanolin alcohols. It is an oily liquid used in topical pharmaceutical formulations and cosmetics as an emulsifying agent with emollient properties. A pale yellow-colored, oily liquid with a faint characteristic sterol odor. It is generally regarded as an essentially nontoxic and nonirritant material. However, lanolin alcohols may be irritant to the skin and causes hypersensitivity in some individuals. Veegum® (Magnesium aluminum silicate) is smectite clay that forms a colloidal structure in water that is well suited for suspension stabilization. It exhibits synergistic interaction with thickening agents. It occurs as off-white to creamy white, odorless, tasteless, soft, slippery small flakes, or as a fine, micronized powder. It is used as a stabilizing agent at 0.5% to 2.5% concentration and topical suspending agent at 1% to 10% concentration. Sodium Lauryl sulfate is widely used surfactant in shampoos, bath products, hair colorings, facial makeup, deodorants and perfumes. It is infused into skincare emulsifying products to function as an effective cleansing agent.

6.3.5 INGREDIENTS USED IN FACE POWDERS

The highly purified powders of the present are a far cry from the crude cosmetics of the past. From the dawn of history, vanity led women to sometimes life-threatening lengths to whiten their skin. The earliest powders were concocted from ingredients such as bean flour, chalk and ceruse, a highly toxic white lead. Today, most powders are a blend of several ingredients, including talc, zinc oxide, titanium dioxide, kaolin and magnesium carbonate, each of which imparts specific benefits. Face powder is more complicated and made by a mixture of products: According to cosmetic chemists, the ideal powders should have five characteristics: covering power, absorbency, adhesiveness, slip and bloom. Transparent powders have the same formulation as full-coverage powders except they contain less talc, titanium dioxide, or zinc oxide, since coverage is not a priority. Transparent facial powders commonly have a light shine, produced by nacreous pigments, such as bismuth oxychloride, mica, titanium-dioxide-coated mica, or crystalline calcium carbonate. Facial powder usually uses iron oxides as the main pigment, but other inorganic pigments such as ultramarines, chrome oxide, and chrome hydrate may also be used [10-12].

6.3.6 COVERING POWER

Covering power is the quality that enables a powder to conceal blemishes, skin imperfections and shine. Ingredients such as titanium dioxide, zinc oxide, kaolin and magnesium oxide are used for their covering power. Titanium dioxide is the most potent covering agent. Zinc oxide is somewhat astringent and antiseptic, and has a soothing effect. It also acts as a sunscreen agent [13,14].

A. Talc

Talc is a kind of soft and smooth stone which is called Katuseki in Japanese. Talc is the sole component of face powders; in some products, it could comprise up to 70% or 75% of the formulation. Chemically it is a hydrated magnesium silicate with the assigned formula $3MgO_2.4SiO_2.H_2O$, and is found in Italy, France, Norway, India, Spain, the USA, Australia, China, Egypt and Japan. Of these the Italian, French, American, Australian and some Indian and Chinese grades can be used for cosmetic powders [12], [15]. Grades of talc should be judged on slip, smoothness, fineness, grit, density, color and odor [16]. In addition, a check should be made for impurities such as carbonates and water-soluble iron and the talc must be free from asbestos impurities, such as actinolite and tremolite, chrysotile and anthophyllite (found responsible for mesothelioma in women) [17,18]. The particle size of the talc can significantly affect the appearance and feel of the finished formulation; the smaller the particle sizes the smoother it will feel. However, very fine talc can start to feel gritty. It is also important to note that the finer the talc the opaquer it becomes, and it therefore, becomes a question of balance to give the desired feel and opacity [16]. Care must be taken to ensure that the talc has been adequately treated to overcome any possible microbial contamination, the major concern being tetanus spores. In an older study, 17% of the talc preparations were examined contained coliforms in the range of 230-500 c.f.u./g. *Staphylococcus* spp., more than 80% of the talcum powders examined were contaminated with fungi (100 fungal cells/g.) [19]. Talc is used mainly because of outstanding spreadability (slip) and low covering power (translucency) [16]. Talc is not genotoxic. Mechanistic, pathology and animal model studies have not found evidence for a carcinogenic effect except studies reported strong association of epithelial ovarian cancer from perineal talc use [20-25]. Talc is a translucent mineral with a pearly luster. Talc is the softest known mineral and is assigned a hardness of 1 (as compared to a diamond's hardness of 10) on the Mohs Hardness scale. Generally, talc is a semi-free flowing powder, talc smears and tends to fluidize, meaning the fine talc particles take on characteristics of a liquid. Talc powder is best kept as dry as possible. Once it is wet, talc in powder form becomes very slimy and is extremely hard to handle as a heavy precipitate [26].

Table 6.3 Talc-Based Face Powder Formulations

Transparent "Light" Type		Opaque Matt Finish		Medium Weight & Opacity		Other Variation	
Ingredient	**%**	**Ingredient**	**%**	**Ingredient**	**%**	**Ingredient**	**%**
Talc	80	Talc	30	Talc	65	Talc	50
Zinc Oxide	5	Zinc Oxide	24	Zinc Oxide	20	Zinc Oxide	15
Zinc Stearate	5	Zinc Stearate	6	Zinc Stearate	5	Zinc Stearate	5
Rice Starch	10	Precipitated Chalk	40	Precipitated Chalk	10	Rice Starch	15
Perfume	q.s.	Perfume	q.s.	Perfume	q.s.	Precipitated Chalk	15
Color	q.s.	Color	q.s.	Color	q.s.	-	-

B. Titanium dioxide

It is naturally opaque and bright, which makes it useful for use in paper, ceramics, rubber, textiles, paints and cosmetics. It is also UV-resistant, and is used widely in sunscreens and pigments that are likely to be exposed to light. It is used in a wide variety of personal care products, including color cosmetics such as eye shadow and blush, loose and pressed powders and in sunscreens [27]. TiO_2 was the first micro-pigment extensively used. Advantages include a broad spectrum of protection and inability to cause contact dermatitis. Particle size and uniformity of dispersion is key to achieving SPF. Primary particle size may be 10 to 15 nm with secondary particle assembly to 100 nm. Particle size needs to be less than 200 nm to achieve transparency [28]. Its high technological attractiveness originates from its light-scattering properties and very high refractive index, which mean that relatively low levels of the pigment are required to achieve a white, opaque coating. The range of light that is scattered depends on the particle size. The increasing production of nano-sized TiO_2 powder has led to growing concerns about the consequences of exposure of humans and the environment. The natural opaqueness of these micro-sized sunscreen components is eliminated without reducing their UV blocking efficacy by utilizing nanosized ZnO and TiO_2 particles [29]. Crystalline TiO_2 occurs naturally in three polymorphs – anatase, rutile and brookite – among which rutile is the most stable [30]. anatase is 100 times more toxic than rutile in the nanoparticular form [31]. Prior to coating, titanium dioxide-rutile pigments that are produced by chlorination contain about 1% alumina, which is concentrated at the surface of the particles, but not titanium dioxide-anatase [32]. The use of rutile as opposed to anatase crystal forms of TiO_2 lessens photoactivity [30]. Titanium accumulates in the liver, muscle, and brain and decreased muscular AChE activity after acute exposure, showing neurotoxic potential [33]. However, the lack of penetration through the epidermis is also the main reason for the absence of skin carcinogenesis-promoting effects [34,35]. Its covering power of TiO_2 is 1.6 times more than the ZnO on dry skin and 2.5 times more on moist and greasy skin [36]. Under similar experimental conditions, presence of 5% TiO_2 increased the refractive index approximately seven times compared with that of ZnO alone [29]. Currently, the annual consumption volume of TiO_2 particles reaches four million tons, which makes it the most widely used pigment globally [37].

C. Zinc Oxide

Zinc oxide, with its unique physical and chemical properties, such as high chemical stability, high electrochemical coupling coefficient, broad range of radiation absorption and high photostability, is a multifunctional material. Its low toxicity, biocompatibility and biodegradability make it a material of interest for biomedicine and in pro-ecological systems [38,39]. Zinc also possesses antioxidant property and has been found useful in preventing UV-induced damage and reducing the incidence of malignancies. Its use has also expanded manifold over the years for a number of dermatological conditions including infections (warts, leishmaniasis), inflammatory dermatoses (acne vulgaris, rosacea), pigmentary disorders (melasma), and neoplasias (basal cell carcinoma) [40] and thanks to its non-toxicity, biocompatibility and antimicrobial activity [41]. ZnO exhibits three crystal structures named wurtzite, zinc-blend, and an occasionally noticed rock-salt [42]. It has been developed in different nanostructures to enhance its interaction with the skin and to improve the existing products. Zinc oxide is the broadest spectrum UVA and UVB reflector approved for use as a sunscreen by the FDA and is allowed in concentrations up to 25% [43]. Nano-ZnO, due to its extremely small size, gives paper coating pigment a high covering power apart from antifungal and UV-protecting properties [44]. It helps with skin repair by keeping the area surrounding the wound moist and clean and supplying the added zinc that the skin needs to facilitate repair. Additionally, ZnO increases collagen degradation in necrotic wounds [45]. It works as a skin astringent that prevents oil formation on the surface of the skin. It is a substance that effectively works in drying excess oil in skin [46]. Unlike chemical sunscreens that can cause hormonal disturbance, using products with zinc oxide as one of the main ingredients are a great choice even for those with sensitive skin. Only nanosized ZnO was able to reach into the deep layers of the allergic skin, but bulk-sized ZnO stayed in the upper layers of both damaged and allergic skin [47]. If zinc oxide nanoparticles produce ROS, they can damage the skin and cannot be used as sunscreen. The efficiency of zinc oxide nanoparticles depends mainly on the medium of reaction to form Zn2+ and their penetration into the cell [48].

D. Kaolin

Natural clays have been used to heal skin infections since the earliest recorded history. The high adsorption and absorption capacities, cation exchange capacity, as well as the extremely fine particle size of certain clays, e.g. smectites (expandable clay minerals) and kaolin group minerals are important reasons why these minerals are used to remove oils, secretions, toxins, and contaminants from the skin. By adsorbing and absorbing moisture and impurities from the skin, the clays also serve to cleanse and refresh the skin surface and to aid in the healing of topical blemishes, the major selling point for many cosmetics [49]. Kaolin (a hydrated aluminum silicate clay mineral) is a mixture consisting principally of the mineral kaolinite and containing varying amounts of other minerals such as muscovite, quartz, feldspar, and anatase [50]. It is prepared for pharmaceutical and medicinal purposes by levigating with water to remove sand and other impurities. The name is derived from Kao-ling (Chinese: "high ridge", a hill in China from where this clay was first obtained or mined). In general, clay minerals naturally possess various morphologies, including fiber, sheets, scrolls, rods, and tubes [51]. The morphological diversity is created in the process of the formation of clay minerals in nature.

Kaolinite is one of the most common clay minerals in the earth's crust and the most widespread phase among the other kaolin polymorphs (halloysite, dickite and nacrite) [52]. The most important functionalities of kaolin used as excipient are reported as diluent, binder, disintegrant, pelletizing and granulating, amorphizing, particle film coating, emulsifying and suspending agent [53]. Because of its uninjured bioactivity, kaolinite has been also used as active agent for treatment of some common diseases. It can be topically administered as hemostatic agent, dermatological protector, anti-inflammatory agent and in pelotherapy, or orally as gastrointestinal protector, and antibacterial, antiviral, detoxification or antidiarrheal agent [54,55]. Red kaolin is considerably more absorbent than other kaolin clays and is thus better suited to acne-prone or oily skin [56]. Even though Kaolin clay is not a great absorbent like other clays, especially bentonite clay, it can remove excess sebum from face. Kaolin clay is white and has a very soft texture. Although it is usually white, it may also come in different colors (mainly pinkish and greenish), depending on the type of other minerals present in that clay. The whiter the clay, the purer and better it is, suited for people with dry, sensitive, and mature skin. It is a natural detoxifier and exfoliator, tones skin and used with green tea, avocado, honey, witch hazel and apple cider vinegar as face mask [57]. Kaolin pneumoconiosis is generally regarded as an inhalational pneumoconiosis. However, on rare occasions kaolin may incite lung damage by the mechanism described above [58].

E. Bentonite

For a long time, bentonite has been used externally on skin. It could act as a barrier for toxic organo-phosphorous compound transfer across the skin, which suggests its physical protective action on skin [59]. Bentonite was effective on the improvement of diaper rash, and also had faster effects compared with *Calendula* [60]. There are different types of bentonite clay; each one is named after the dominant element in the clay, such as potassium, sodium, calcium, magnesium or aluminum. It is a powerful healing clay, is composed of volcanic ash, with a high percentage of montmorillonite, a group of soft minerals. The presence of iron and magnesium ions give Bentonite Clay a subtle greenish-grey color. When mixed with water, bentonite swells up like a sponge and becomes very slippery and almost gel-like [61]. Bentonite is a highly absorbent clay that pulls oils and toxins from the skin. Using a clay face mask can help remove impurities from the skin to treat acne or reduce the risk of pimples and skin infections [62]. Long-term occupational exposures to bentonite dust may cause structural and functional damage to the lungs [63] and systemic exposure may be detrimental to bones because aluminum competes with calcium for absorption [64]. Although, quaternium-18 bentonite presented no evidence of systemic toxicity [65]. Effectiveness of iron-rich clays for healing severe skin infections has recently been documented, drawing attention from the medical community [66]. Once the clay combines with water (perspiration) it gets to work, purifying and removing toxins [67]. Applying a lotion or cream with bentonite clay in it creates a barrier between skin and possible irritants. Bentonite clay also helps skincare products adhere to your skin and be more water resistant [68]. Colloidal clays, either natural processed bentonites or synthetic clays, have been used as binding agents because of their thixotropic properties. Most often, bentonite suspensions are also thixotropic, although rare cases of rheopectic behavior have also been reported [69]. The stabilization of emulsions using powders is not particularly common in cosmetic products, although powders such as veegum and bentonite are sometimes used [70-72].

6.3.7 ABSORBENCY

Powders should have ability to eliminate shiny skin in certain facial areas by absorbing sebaceous secretions and perspiration. Materials for this purpose should have a high absorptive capacity, but at the same time should not change the appearance of the powder on the skin [73]. There are several components of face powder which have this absorptive property such as kaolin, starch, microcrystalline cellulose, magnesium and calcium carbonate. ZnO and TiO2 are better in masking skin greasiness but chalk powder, kaolin and starch have better moisture absorption capacity.

A. Starch

Among all-natural available biopolymers, starch is the most commonly applied in the biomaterial fields due to its beneficial advantages such as low-cost, low-toxicity, biodegradability, and renewability. Despite these properties of starch materials, the industrial applications of starch are often limited because of its poor rheological properties and limited surface areas [74,75]. Soybean oil, corn flour, and potato starch are common ingredients in moisturizers, masks, and makeup. Corn starch is used as a thickener in cosmetic products, and more recently as a replacement for talc in natural baby powders [76]. Corn meal, or corn flour, is a cheap facial exfoliator that can be safely used in homemade cosmetic preparations. These are often used in face powders. In particular rice starch was very common as a basic ingredient in formulations. It was considered to give a 'peach-like' bloom to the face [77,78]. Because the particles are spherical it gives a very smooth feel when applied to the skin. It has excellent absorptive properties and in addition has good covering power. In the presence of water, it tends to cake, and cling to facial hair, giving an unpleasant appearance. It can also become sticky. Starch is synthesized in amyloplasts or chloroplasts, consists of amylose and amylopectin, and exists as semi-crystalline granules in plants [79]. Corn starch exists in two forms, amylose and amylopectin, containing glucose units connected linearly in chains of different lengths and, in amylopectin, with substantial branching. Wheat starch granules have a bimodal size distribution due to initiation of granule growth at different times. Rice starch granules, on average, are the smallest of the commercial starches (2–9 μm) [80,81]. Starch can be used as thickener, an adhesive, binder, encapsulating agent, film former, gelling agent, water binder, texturizer and fat-sparing agent and with numerous other applications. Starch can be modified by acid hydrolysis, oxidation, etherification, esterification and cross-linking. Various methods such as acid, phosphate and H_2O_2 treatments can be employed to modify starch [82]. Modified starches are now available which can be very beneficial in powder products. Modification of starch led to new products with new desirable properties. Corn starch samples modified by acid hydrolysis combined with heat moisture treatment were made by changing pH, moisture content and treated temperature. After modification, swelling power at temperature higher than 75°C of corn starches decreased while solubility of the starches increased [83]. They can be used as talc replacements in some products. Unfortunately, both starches and modified starches are ideal media for microbiological growth; it is therefore important that the grades used are sterilized prior to use, that the manufacturing environment is as clean as possible to prevent contamination and that sufficient preservatives are used in the formulation. Silver-starch nanocomposite material [AgNPs (<10 nm)] can be successfully employed to prevent the viability and growth of the common pathogens *Staphylococcus aureus*, *Escherichia coli* and *Candida albicans* [84].

B. Calcium carbonate (Chalk Powder)

Calcium carbonate occurs as an odorless and tasteless white powder or crystals. Calcium carbonates are one of the most abundant minerals in the earth's crust. It is obtained from the naturally occurring minerals aragonite, calcite, and vaterite. They occur in the form of limestone and chalk, formed from fossils, and marble, formed from the metamorphosis of sedimentary rock. They consist mostly (>98%) of $CaCO_3$, with trace amounts of magnesium carbonate, iron oxide, and aluminum silicates [78], [85]. It is mainly used in oral pharmaceutical formulations and is generally regarded as a nontoxic material. Calcium carbonate may be irritant to the eyes and on inhalation. Particle size is important and, for some applications requiring good weathering and impact performance (window profile), the ultrafine milled, high whiteness, natural version is normally used. Ground and precipitated calcium carbonate is used as an ingredient in the formulation of personal care products, cosmetics and toiletries. In make-up products, it is taken into use as a pigment extender, prolonger, whitener and oil absorber. Because calcium carbonate absorbs moisture it is frequently used as an ingredient in face powders to upsurge the capacity of the makeup to engross moisture and it makes a good absorber in primers, foundations, and finishing powders. It is known in the cosmetic-industry for its absorbent power, translucency, opacity, skin protecting properties, adhesion power that makes make-up to stay for long on the body, and light scattering properties [86]. The brightness and opacity of the calcium carbonates make them suitable for use in white and color cosmetics. They can even be considered as an extender of titanium dioxide and act as a natural source of calcium.To meet the brightness, polishing and opacifying requirements of the cosmetic industry, the calcium carbonates are available as limestone and marble-based products. While marble-based calcium carbonate exhibits high brightness, low oil absorption, and low yellow index, limestone calcium carbonate exhibits homogenous deposit, high brightness, higher yellow index and improved opacity [87]. A grit- free precipitate chalk or calcium carbonate is mildly alkaline, white, odorless, microcrystalline powder and it reduces the shine of talc and has a good covering power, it helps to absorb the perfume and is also grease resistant and perspiration absorbent. If this raw material is used in excess, the powder may acquire a dry feel, but moderate usage is most helpful to face powder formulas. In face powder formulations, chalk powder preserves certain balance between slip and adhesion, coverage power and transparency and develops "bloom effect" when face powder is applied [88]. Given that a variety of bacterial species may occur in the calcium carbonate powder used for cosmetic formulations, an understanding of their diversity and abundance is necessary to accurately assess the contamination of the finished product [89].

C. Magnesium Carbonate

Basic magnesium carbonate comprising a tubular aggregated particle of flaky fine crystals, having characteristics that a bulk density is as low as 0.2 to 0.3 g/mL, and a specific surface area is comparatively high and is 10 to 40 m2/g. There are two main branches of sedimentary petrology. One branch deal with carbonate rocks, namely limestones and dolomites, composed principally of calcium carbonate (calcite) and calcium magnesium carbonate (dolomite) [90]. $MgCO_3$ is used as an absorbent, opacifying agent, coloring agent, or to adjust the pH of cosmetic products. It is white, tasteless, odorless, amorphous, fine powder. It is used as an anticaking agent in free flow table salts due to its high hygroscopicity [91]. It is used in cosmetic industries especially in talcum powder, face powder, body powder, etc. Due to its marked absorptive powder it is incorporated in special soaps. The white powder is used in pharmaceutical preparations, hair bleach, powdered shampoo, cosmetic powder formulations, foot care and skin care. Among others, it is ideal as an absorbent/binder, bulking agent, and opacifier [92]. In the presence of dry skin, oil-absorbing products such as powders should be avoided. If a powder is desired, it should be low in magnesium carbonate and zinc oxide, since these two substances have an astringent or drying effect on the face [88]. It decreases the static friction coefficient and imparts fluffiness to the powder [78]. Magnesium protects the skin from free radical damage, inflammation, and it's necessary for the enzymes that regulate cell turnover and repair. A lot of people end up using it topically for the treatment of acne and acne rosacea. Magnesium carbonate cosmetic grade is packed with the utmost care in order to prevent moisture absorption by the material due to its hygroscopic property. It has a tremendous capacity to absorb oil from skin, prevents formulations from lump formation and acts as a fragrance enhancer. For this reason—often fragrance is added to magnesium carbonate as a separate step during formulation [93].

D. Avicel®/ Microcrystalline cellulose (MCC)

Because of its convenience of use, excellent toxicity profile and wide compatibility, Avicel® can be readily incorporated into a wide range of cosmetic formulations. It has use in cosmetics as an abrasive, absorbent, anti-caking agent, aqueous viscosity increasing agent, binder, bulking agent, emulsion stabilizer, slip modifier, and texturizer, which can be found in various hair and skin care products as well as makeup. It was discovered in 1955 by Battista and Smith and was first commercialized under the brand name Avicel® [94]. A purified, partially depolymerized alpha-cellulose made by acid hydrolysis of specialty wood pulp [95]. The physical network of insoluble particles formed by Avicel® is pseudoplastic, highly shear-thinning and thixotropic, making it ideal for suspensions, sprayable products, and emulsions. These microcrystals, which are insoluble, rod-shaped particles of less than 1 micron in length, can be dried to form commercial products known collectively as non-colloidal grades. During the drying process, hydrogen bonding causes the cellulose microcrystals to form larger, tightly-bound particles that cannot be redisposed later to recover the individual microcrystals [96]. It can be obtained from other sources like from other sources such as newsprint waste, corncobs, bagasse, rice straw as well as fast-growing plants including *Sesbania sesban*, *Pinus roxburghii* and *Crotalaria juncea* [97]. It is generally considered as the diluent having the best binding properties. It is a white fine crystalline powder, odorless and tasteless, made from free-flowing non-fibrous particles and compressed by its self-adhesion effects [98]. MCC produced from rice husk and cotton are the densest and least porous materials having the fastest flow and lowest compressibility. In contrast, MCC, as obtained from bagasse was the least dense and the most porous material and it was as compressible as Avicel® products rendering compacts of good strength [99]. It can be rapidly dispersed in water into the formulation, but insoluble in water, dilute acid or alkali solution, solution, and most organic solvents, and can absorb water to swell [100-102]. The large particle size grades of MCC-Avicel® PH 102, PH 302 and Pharmacel 102 were found to possess smaller quantities of structured water [103].

(a) **Slip:** Easy powder flowability and spreadability are two important parameters that are always considered at the time of manufacturing and evaluation of topical powder. Slip is the property that enables a powder to be easily and smoothly applied without any feeling of drag. As a property slip is hard to define in any quantifiable fashion but like powder grittiness it can be felt with the fingers or on the face. While several ingredients can contribute to giving a powder slip – such as the kaolin, the stearates and starch – by far the most important substance is talc (magnesium silicate) which is why it made up to 50% or more of some face powders. Talc is produced by different countries but Italian, French and some Indian varieties are of very good quality and most suitable for powders specifically face powders. It combines high spreadability (slip) with low translucency and covering power and feels smooth on the skin. kaolin improves homogeneity during spreading, imparts good coverage and bring consistency to the formulation. Alurninium hydrosilicate is a valuable basic material for powders It is smooth and fatty. It should be prepared properly by treating with acid, washing with water and then dried. It also has certain cooling effect. It absorbs fatty secretions and small amounts of water. It is completely non-toxic. Other substances used for softness and slip are zinc stearate, magnesium stearate, zinc undecanate, magnesium undecanate. The undecanates, in particular, are soft and have excellent slip but are expensive. properly purified stearates are extensively used [36]. Tapioca starch is particularly useful as it gives a very smooth feel to the product. Due to the chemically inert nature of talc and kaolin, they are the most commonly used ingredients in the formulation of dusting powder [104]. The presence of powders formed by spherical particles in the formula allows an excellent spreadability increasing the duration and decreasing the transferability of the make-up. The particle size of the talc can significantly affect the appearance and feel of the finished formulation; the smaller the particle sizes the smoother it will feel. However, very fine talc can start to feel gritty. It is also important to note that the finer the talc the opaquer it becomes, and it therefore becomes a question of balance to give the desired feel and opacity. In terms of extrinsic properties, it is well accepted that spherical powder particles positively contribute towards powder flowability and higher particle packing densities in the powder bed. Spherical morphologies are also typically associated with low levels of particle-particle friction which results in enhanced powder flow [105]. Micronized plastics such as polythene, polystyrene and nylon, not only exhibit good powder but also excellent thermal properties. They can impart a very smooth feel to formulas [106]. These particles are usually spherical and the ball-bearing effect comes into play. Typically, these can be used at between 5% and 10% but they are expensive so their use is somewhat limited. Spherical powders such as nylon, silica or polymethyl methacrylate contribute to two-way foundations by giving a silky-smooth feel, enhanced pay-off, and smoother skin application. Some, such as silica, act to absorb sebum and perspiration, therefore giving a uniform finish throughout the day. They can also act as light diffusers, minimizing the appearance of pores. The ideal level of spherical powders in two-way foundations generally ranges from 10% to 13%. However, if the formulation also contains microfine titanium dioxide or zinc oxide, for their sunscreen properties, the level of the spherical powders is usually increased to between 16% and 18%, to compensate for the coarse feel of the microfine pigments. Increasing the level of spherical powders used results in a greater slip, but at the expense of creaminess. Excessive amounts of spherical powders can lead to unstable pressed cakes and to break-up of the cake during use. The silicas, in addition to the silicates, are useful in maintaining the free-flowing properties of powders in high humidity [12].

(b) **Adhesion:** Adhesive improves the consistency of face powders, ensuring a smooth application. The staying power of a face powder, its ability to stick to the skin, is referred to by cosmetic chemists as its adhesiveness. Lack of adhesion was a common problem with early face powders and many women resorted to using a vanishing or cold cream before powdering to help their face powder stay in place. Known for its smoothing effects and adhesive texture, dimethicone is used in powders to enhance makeup wear and give the skin an airbrushed finish. Also, talc inclusion in a face powder increases its adhesiveness to the skin and avoids the powder dissipating in a short period.. Cocoa seed butter imparts silky texture on the skin, delivering superior adhesion whether worn on a bare face or with a full beat. Zinc oxide possesses moderate adhesive properties and is comparatively inert [39]. The materials primarily used for imparting adhesive characters are metal soaps primarily zinc stearate and magnesium stearate talc, magnesium and calcium salts of myristic acid. Magnesium stearate has better adhesive property than zinc stearate and is more preferred in face powders. But zinc stearate is more predominantly used in talcum powders. Super quality magnesium and zinc stearates are available with excellent color, texture and minimum of odor. They also give a velvety softness to the product. As they are waterproof, they maintain the complexion intact in inclement weather. Magnesium stearate is used 3-10% in face powders and any other pharmaceutical powders. Magnesium stearate is permitted for use in the European Union and other countries including China, Japan, Australia and New Zealand, and was granted generally recognized as safe (GRAS) status in the US [107]. Stearates of lithium and calcium are also available for use for the same purpose. Lithium stearate in particular, has also got good covering properties and fluffy texture. Magnesium and calcium salts of myristic acid are also used for their adhesion properties. Magnesium myristate has better adhesion character and a better texture. Cosmetic quality talc, which is a purified hydrated magnesium silicate has adhesion properties. Though it is available in various countries, Italian product is the best and used for face powders. Titanium dioxide is three to four times better as a covering agent than zinc oxide, but it has less adhesion and does not blend quite as well. For a face powder in which an appreciable quantity of covering power is desirable, the judicious use of TiO_2 or ZnO or a blend of the two is necessary [16]. The adhesion character of the powders can be increased by incorporating 1-2% of cetyl alcohol, stearyl alcohol, glyceryl monostearate, petrolatum, lanolin or similar fats.

(c) **Bloom:** Opalescent, or pearly finish, products contain ingredients such as bismuth oxychloride that give them a shimmery glow. The materials chiefly used to impart bloom are chalk, rice starch and prepared starch. Silk Powder is produced from high quality silk using sophisticated technology in order to retain its chemical properties, and is made up of 100% fibroin, which contains 18 kinds of amino acids and trace elements essential to the human body. It serves as an ideal protein enricher for high quality cosmetics. It is in the form of a yellow powder of 200 mesh diameter that can be applied to a wide range of cosmetics. Users can expect it to help maintain moisture levels in the skin and prevent dryness. Superfine Silk Powder is valued as a filler in mineral makeup formulations to help soften the appearance of fine lines, provide moisture balance, absorb excess oil and provide a silky slip [108]. In addition to being a great filler base for mineral makeup, Superfine Silk Powder can also be used in any type of powdered formulations where oil absorption and a silky slip are desired. It is an exceptional alternative to talc in body and face powders. It helps decrease reflective light from the surface of the skin and creates a soft glow. The fine particle size makes it easy to incorporate into cosmetic formulations. Sericin, which is a protein synthesized by the domestic silkworm, *Bombyx mori, is on*e of these substances. Sericin becomes gel by itself, and forms a film when combined with some polymers by cross-linking and therefore can be used in manufacturing cosmetics and pharmaceuticals [109]. Also known as synthetic pearl, it's the primary ingredient included in most powders that are referred to as "mineral makeup." Some cosmetic companies claim that bismuth oxychloride is natural and better for skin than talc. The truth is that in many ways' talc is a more natural, unadulterated, pure ingredient than bismuth oxychloride. Bismuth oxychloride, an insoluble inorganic pigment which seldom occurs in nature, is used in cosmetics because it has a distinct shimmery, pearlescent appearance and a fine white powder texture that adheres well to skin. However, it is heavier than talc. Far from natural, it was designed to be a replacement for talc. Among its boasted beneficial properties are its great slip and its sheen that offers the wearer a dewy look. It was permanently listed by the FDA as a coloring agent in 1977 and for use as a synthetic ingredient. Women have been advised to scan makeup labels for bismuth oxychloride, the ingredient that gives makeup its pearly finish. It can cause skin irritation and acne flare-ups [110]. Because of its molecular crystalline shape, many individuals experience itching from bismuth oxychloride, which worsens when they sweat.

(d) **Colors:** The colors used in face powders came mainly from two sources: inorganic pigments like iron oxides (ochres, sienna and umbers) and organic lakes and toners; both types being increasingly controlled by legislation. Inorganic pigments were originally sourced from nature but synthetic forms were later preferred. Synthetics were less likely to have contaminants, were free from grit, more uniform in color from batch to batch and, being purer, had a greater strength of color than their natural counterparts. Inorganic pigments were very stable and had an indefinite shelf life but lacked a certain brilliance so, despite being less stable when exposed to light, organic lakes were often included into face powders as well. Any lake color selected needed to be tested for stability and checked to ensure that it did not readily dissolve in water or oil, otherwise the color would bleed in areas where perspiration or sebum was present. Even if no bleeding occurred, sebum could still have an adverse effect on a powder. Many face powders turned darker and yellower, or darker and redder after they had been on the skin for a while, a problem exacerbated by the fact that color changes were greater where more sebum was produced making an evenly applied face powder look blotchy after a while. Various synthetic or natural inorganic pigments used are iron oxides for yellows, reds, and browns and ultramarine for green and blue [112]. Toxic lead and arsenic compounds are not used. Organic lakes and pigments produce better brilliance but should be selected from certified dyes. The organic pigments must not bleed in oil or water and should be light-fast. The choice of color is mainly users' taste. Various colors with various shades are used to fulfil the satisfaction of the users. The color of the thin film of the pigment may be different from the color effect given by the powder viewed in bulk [113]. Since the ingredients in the base were white or off-white, they would also affect the powder shade. Consequently, if a manufacturer was making up powders in light, medium and heavy grades, the colors used in each would need to be adjusted to compensate for the varying levels of titanium dioxide and/or zinc oxide used in the different grades to ensure that all were the same shade. As well as the inorganic pigments and lakes other coloring agents have been added to face powders over the years. These include metallic powders (mica, aluminum, bronze) to give gold, silver and other metal effects; synthetic bismuth oxychloride and synthetic pearl pigments to give the powder a pearlescent sheen; and various forms of resins and plastics [114]. Women expected their powder shades to remain the same batch after batch and would change brands if they found too much fluctuation from one purchase to another. In the past, the colors were checked by eye using samples taken during the milling process which were compared to a reference powder kept on file. The introduction of color measurement by colorimeter greatly improved the accuracy of this procedure. The secret to producing powders of a consistent color was standardization. Standardization of raw materials, proportions, moisture content manufacturing, storage and packaging was the only way to produce consistent results.

(e) **Perfumes:** From the Renaissance into the nineteenth century, perfume wearing and perfume type were ungendered, and men and women adorned them equally. Sweet floral blends were deemed exclusively feminine, while sharper, woodsy, pine, and cedar notes were characterized as masculine [115]. However, perfume is an essential component of powders. Users put more importance to perfume. But it should not be overemphasized at the time of manufacturing. Normally the products are perfumed lightly, particularly face powders and compacts. The odor must be fragrant and pleasant. An attractive scent was essential if a powder was to enjoy good sales. This enabled the scent in the powder to work with the woman's perfume rather than against it. Care had to be taken when selecting a perfume as the powder base could modify the perfume's odor, making it smell musty. In addition, the scent could also discolor the powder and darken the shade. Various perfumes or fragrance which are used, either flowery fragrance or synthetic odor. The selection of proper fragrance is very vital for the products. Sometime combination of fragrances gives a better appeal [116]. Compatibility of perfume with other constituents of the formulation is to be checked properly before use. Constituents of powder preparation may change the character of fragrance. The addition of a perfume to a powder generally required the powder to be matured or aged for up to a month before it was packaged and sold. Depending on the manufacturing process, ageing could be done before or after the powder was made. If the perfume was mixed into a portion of the powder, e.g. the kaolin, it would be stored and matured before being incorporated into the rest of the powder mix; if it was sprayed on to the powder during the mixing process then the entire powder mixture would be aged before it was packaged.

6.3.8 EVALUATION OF POWDERS

There are various methods available to measure the powder flow. The compendial methods include measurement of angle of repose, bulk density, tapped density, Carr's compressibility index or Hausner ratio. With technological advances, innovative methods of characterization of powder flow such as cohesivity determination, avalanching determination, shear cell, dielectric imaging, atomic force microscopy, penetrometry. These methods suffer from various limitations including reproducibility, performance conditions, and predictability [117]. General tests include determination of contents in the formulation along with the stability test. This is carried out to know whether the product remains stable for prolongedtime (i.e. shelf life). Other tests are also carried out. They are:

(a) *Shade Test*: In this test, the variations of color shade are determined and controlled. It is carried out by spreading the powder sample on a white paper and appearance is observed which is compared with the standard one. Another method involves, applying powder sample and standard one with the help of puff on the skin and then comparing it. The puff used to perform this test is also used for the final product. Evaluation of color is carried out by using artificial light.

(b) *Color Dispersion Test*: in this test, a sample of powder is spread on a white paper and with the help of magnifying glass., segregation or bleeding of the color is observed. the color should be properly distributed in the powder base of the formulation.

(c) *Pay-off Test*: This test is carried out to check the adhesive property of powders with the puff. This test is mainly carried out on compact powders.

(d) *Pressure Test*: For compaction purposes in compact powders, pressure required. Uniform pressure should be applied to avoid formation of air pockets, which will lead to either breaking or cracking of compact powders. This is because low pressure will make the compact powder soft, whereas high pressure will lead to formation of hard cake. With the help of penetrometer, uniformity of hardness of the cake is checked. This is done by taking the reading at different points on compact powder and then comparing them.

(e) *Breakage Test*: In this test, compact powders are allowed to fall on a wooden surface from a height of about 8-10 inches. This is carried out several times and then checking is done to see whether any breakage has occurred on compact powder. If the compact powder remains unbroken, then it shows the resistance to travel and normal handling by the users.

(f) *Flow Property Test*: This test is carried out maim} on body powders to determine their flow property (from the container upon usage). This intern helps in easy application of powder to skin. In this method, angle of repose of powder is measured by allowing the powder product to fall on a plate through a funnel. Then the height and the radius of heap formed is measured, and even the time taken for the powder to fall is noted.

(g) *Particle Size Determination*: With the help of microscope, sieve analysis or by utilizing other techniques and instrument, particle size of powder product is determined.

(h) *Abrasive Character*: Abrasive character of powder can be determined by, rubbing, the powder on a smooth surface of the skin. Then with the help of a microscope, the effects of powder are studied.

(i) *Moisture Content*: Moisture content present in the powder can be determined by using following formula. This is usually carried out by using various suitable analytical methods. These methods are also suitable for determining limits for color.

$$\text{Moisture Content \%} = \frac{\text{Weight of Water in Sample}}{\text{Weight of Dry Sample}} \times 5$$

6.3.9 REGULATORY REQUIREMENTS

A. REACH/MSDS

All cosmetic ingredients, including those which are specifically used in cosmetic powders, have to fulfill REACH requirements as individual chemicals. REACH governs the registration, evaluation, authorization and restriction of chemicals in the European Union. Its purpose is to ensure a high level of protection of human health and the environment, the promotion of alternative methods for the assessment of hazards of substances and the free circulation of substances in the internal market while enhancing competitiveness and innovation. Data of such tests and any classification according to GHS/CLP (Globally Harmonized System) which has been implemented in the EU in form of the Regulation (EC) No 1272/2008 on the classification, labeling and packaging of substances and mixtures - CLP Regulation) will be available via the material safety data sheet (MSDS). Each individual hazard classification needs to be considered in the safety assessment of the cosmetic ingredients [119,120].

(a) **Occupational Exposure Limits: Apart from chemical substance-**specific regulations via REACH or product type specific regulations like the Cosmetics Regulation, occupational exposure limits (OEL) are defined for certain ingredients. As the above introduced occupational exposure scenario for solid particles (dust) is quite different and conservative compared to the typical consumer exposure during the typical use of cosmetic products like loose powders, OELs may serve as a first rough estimate for consumer exposure or professional use in a hairdresser salon in safety assessments of powder products [121].

(b) **Cosmetic Use: In contrast to** the occupational scenario, the intentional application of cosmetic products is quite different as both the exposure duration as well as the typical quantities of airborne particles is less prominent. Furthermore, the toxic potential of the ingredients used is significantly lower compared to general industrial chemicals, as all of them have to be approved as safe for the use in such consumer products.

However, there are special restrictions for the UV filters titanium dioxide and zinc oxide if the materials contain particles in the nano-size range; as listed in Annex VI entry 27a and 30a (list of UV filters allowed in cosmetic products) as usage restriction of: "Not to be used in applications that may lead to exposure of the end-user's lungs by inhalation". As in the EU, the US FDA requires cosmetic products to be safe without setting specific requirements as to how such safety, specifically of powders, has to be assessed. Cosmetic products and ingredients are not subject to the US FDA pre-market approval authority, except for color additives. The US FDA lays the responsibility on the cosmetic firms for checking the safety of their products and ingredients before introducing them into the market. Regarding Cu, Zn and Fe, there is no regulation of the levels in lipsticks or powders. There is only consideration about the metals' uses and restrictions. US Regulations such as Proposition 65 in California have ingredient specific restrictions similar to those of the EU Cosmetic Regulation. Ingredients deemed to be of concern due to inhalation, e.g. titanium dioxide commonly used as a colorant or pearl in powdered cosmetics, have considerations, which must be met to ensure their safety when typically used in consumer products. The ingredient is assessed as 'of concern' if meets three criteria: being unbound, airborne and of respirable size. These criteria were used in several safety evaluations applying the particle size of 10 μm as the cut-off for the respirable fraction of airborne particles [122-126].

EPILOGUE

Face powder is an indispensable article of a lady's cosmetic range. From the mask-like covering in ancient times to the natural look which is the choice of the present day, face powders have been and still remain one of the basics of the cosmetic industry. A great deal of changes has taken place in face powder fashion during the last couple of decades. Tinted, shiny, enhanced by our modern cosmetics, the woman of today is able, with only modest effort, to be more attractive than she has ever been in the past. A face powder is a cosmetic product which has as its prime function the ability to complement skin color by imparting a velvet finish to it. A good fair powder should produce a smooth furnish to the facial skin, masking visible imperfections of the face and shine due to moisture or grease from perspiration or secretion of sebaceous and sweat glands or from preparations used on the skin. The powder must produce a lasting effect, so that frequent application is unnecessary. The preparation should make the face pleasant to look and touch. The degree of opacity can vary from opaque, in case of clown make-up, to almost transparent. It must adhere to the skin and be reasonably resistant to the mixed secretions of the skin. Pressed powders nowadays are usually talc-free and pressure-blasted into compacts without the need for caking agents. They're infinitely finer, softer and more natural-looking. With brands offering up options that promise to smooth, set and even hydrate, powders are undergoing an essential overhaul. Powder-encapsulated spheres of hyaluronic acid dispense a seamless sweep of cashmere-soft, oil-balancing powder on skin, while the hydrating microspheres settle into lines to plump them out and prevent creasing. Now, it's the turn of powder as next generation technology is pushing it forward and into the future problem - solving issues that have turned many into powder refuseniks.

SUMMARY

Face powder is a cosmetic product used to provide a special touch on the skin, to control oil and combat shines, or, in addition to provide a matt finishing effect on the skin. This matt effect, combined with the high transparency of the powder can develop a special soft-focus effect on the skin, blurring the appearance of wrinkles and lines as well as reducing the visibility of discoloration to enhance skin appearance. Certain types of pigmented facial powders are meant tobe worn alone with no base foundation. Powder tones the face and gives an even appearance. Besides toning the face, some powders with sunscreen can also reduce skin damage from sunlight and environmental stress. It comes packaged either as a compact or as loose powder. It can be applied with a sponge, brush, or powder puff. Uniform distribution over the face is achieved more easily when a loose powder is applied. In recent years, the so-called mineral-based foundation products have become increasingly popular in the cosmetic consumer market and can demand a premium price from the consumer.

ABBREVIATIONS

Microcrystalline cellulose (MCC); Generally Recognized as Safe (GRAS); Reactive Oxygen Species (ROS); Registration, Evaluation and Authorization of Chemicals (REACH); CLP (Classification, Labelling and Packaging); Globally Harmonized System (GHS); Material Safety Data Sheet (MSDS); Acetylcholinesterase (AChE)

BIBLIOGRAPHY AND WEBLIOGRAPHY

1. Loose Face Powders. Cosmetics and Skin, 28th April 2017.
2. M. S. Balsam, Edward Sagarin. Cosmetics: Science and Technology Volume 1 of Cosmetics, Science and Technology, M. S. Balsam, Edition 2 (illustrated), published by John Wiley & Sons Canada, Limited, 1972, ISBN 0471046469, 9780471046462
3. Make-up tips. How to Choose and Use Face Powder? Expert-Advice, Paula's Choice (LLC) Skincare. Available From: https://www.paulaschoice.com/expert-advice/makeup-tips/face/how-choose-apply-face-powder.html

4. Make-up. How to Choose The Right Face Powder For You? Available From: https://www.beautifulwithbrains.com/how-to-choose-the-right-face-powder-for-you/
5. Peter Elsner, Howard I. Maibach. Cosmeceuticals: Drugs vs. Cosmetics Volume 23 of Cosmetic science and technology series, published by CRC Press, 2000 ISBN 0824703057, 9780824703059
6. John Toedt, Darrell Koza, Kathleen Van Cleef-Toedt. Chemical Composition of Everyday Products ABC-Clio e-book Gale virtual reference library, published by Greenwood Publishing Group, 2005 ISBN 0313325790, 9780313325793
7. Arcano N. 5 Interesting Uses for Face Powder You Probably Didn't Know About. Preview, Oct 10, 2017.
8. Intantya. Types of Face Powder and Its Functions. The Carousel by Avoskin, 2 January 2017.
9. Finishing Powder vs Setting Powder: What's The Difference? Available From: https://camerareadycosmetics.com/blogs/news/finishing-powder-vs-setting-powder-what-is-the-difference
10. Paula Begoun. The Complete Beauty Bible: The Ultimate Guide to Smart Beauty, published by Rodale, 2004 ISBN 1579549993, 9781579549992
11. Stan Place, Bobbi Ray Madry. The Art and Science of Professional Makeup Skin Series, published by Cengage Learning, 1989. ISBN 0873503619, 9780873503617
12. H. Butler. Poucher's Perfumes, Cosmetics and Soaps Edition 10, illustrated, published by Springer Science & Business Media, 2013 ISBN 9401727341, 9789401727341
13. Blumenthal D. Beauty: A Dusting Of Powder. The New York Times, OCT. 28, 1984
14. Ralph Gordon Harry. Harry's Cosmeticology 7th edition, edited by Meyer R. Rosen, published by Chemical Publishing Company, 2015 ISBN 0820601764, 9780820601762
15. Talc. Available From: https://www.fda.gov/cosmetics/cosmetic-ingredients/talc
16. S.K. Singh. Handbook on Cosmetics (Processes, Formulae with Testing Methods), published by Asia Pacific Business Press Inc., 2010 ISBN 8178331292, 9788178331294, pp 336
17. Gordon RE, Fitzgerald S, Millette J. Asbestos in commercial cosmetic talcum powder as a cause of mesothelioma in women. Int J Occup Environ Health. 2014 Oct;20(4):318-32. doi: 10.1179/2049396714Y.0000000081. Epub 2014 Sep 3. Erratum in: Int J Occup Environ Health. 2015;21(4):347-8. PubMed PMID: 25185462; PubMed Central PMCID: PMC4164883.
18. Talc (without asbestos fibres) (respirable fraction) [MAK Value Documentation, 2006] (respirable fraction) 2006. Documentations and Methods First published: 31 January 2012 https://doi.org/10.1002/3527600418.mb1480796nfae0022
19. Ashour MS, Abdelaziz AA, Hefni H, el-Tayeb OM. Microbial contamination of cosmetics and personal care items in Egypt--body lotions and talcum powders. J Clin Pharm Ther. 1989 Jun;14(3):207-12. PubMed PMID: 2760119.

20. Muscat JE, Huncharek MS. Perineal talc use and ovarian cancer: a critical review. Eur J Cancer Prev. 2008 Apr;17(2):139-46. doi: 10.1097/CEJ.0b013e32811080ef.
21. Cramer DW, Vitonis AF, Terry KL, Welch WR, Titus LJ. The Association Between Talc Use and Ovarian Cancer: A Retrospective Case-Control Study in Two US States. Epidemiology. 2016 May;27(3):334-46. doi: 10.1097/EDE.0000 000000000434.
22. TrabertB. Body Powder and Ovarian Cancer Risk-What Is the Role of Recall Bias? Cancer Epidemiol Biomarkers Prev. 2016 Oct;25(10):1369-1370.
23. Penninkilampi R, Eslick GD. Perineal Talc Use and Ovarian Cancer: A Systematic Review and Meta-Analysis. Epidemiology. 2018 Jan;29(1):41-49. doi: 10.1097/EDE.0000000000000745.
24. Casey R, Larkin TP. Ovarian Cancer and "Tainted Talc": What Treating Physicians Need to Know. Mo Med. 2019 Mar-Apr;116(2):83-86.
25. Fletcher NM, Harper AK, Memaj I, Fan R, Morris RT, Saed GM. Molecular Basis Supporting the Association of Talcum Powder Use With Increased Risk of Ovarian Cancer. Reprod Sci. 2019 Feb 28:1933719119831773. doi: 10.1177/1933719119831773
26. Talc Overview. Available From: https://www.flexicon.com/Materials-Handled/Talc.html
27. Levy SB. Chapter 29. UV Filters. In: André O. Barel, Marc Paye, Howard I. Maibach. Handbook of Cosmetic Science and Technology, 3rd Edition, published by CRC Press, 2014. ISBN 9781842145647, pp-318
28. Titanium Dioxide. Available From: http://www.safecosmetics.org/get-the-facts/chemicals-of-concern/titanium-dioxide-2/
29. Smijs, Threes G, and Stanislav Pavel. “Titanium dioxide and zinc oxide nanoparticles in sunscreens: focus on their safety and effectiveness.” Nanotechnology, science and applications vol. 4 95-112. 13 Oct. 2011, doi:10.2147/NSA.S19419
30. Skocaj M, Filipic M, Petkovic J, Novak S. Titanium dioxide in our everyday life; is it safe? Radiol Oncol. 2011 Dec;45(4):227-47. doi: 10.2478/v10019-011-0037-0. Epub 2011 Nov 16.
31. Weir A, Westerhoff P, Fabricius L, Hristovski K, von Goetz N. Titanium dioxide nanoparticles in food and personal care products. Environ Sci Technol. 2012 Feb 21;46(4):2242-50. doi: 10.1021/es204168d.
32. IARC Working Group on the Evaluation of Carcinogenic Risk to Humans. Carbon Black, Titanium Dioxide, and Talc. Lyon (FR): International Agency for Research on Cancer; 2010. (IARC Monographs on the Evaluation of Carcinogenic Risks to Humans, No. 93.) 1, Exposure Data. Available from: https://www.ncbi.nlm.nih.gov/books/NBK326523/
33. Carmo TLL, Siqueira PR, Azevedo VC, Tavares D, Pesenti EC, Cestari MM, Martinez CBR, Fernandes MN. Overview of the toxic effects of titanium dioxide nanoparticles in blood, liver, muscles, and brain of a Neotropical detritivorous fish. Environ Toxicol. 2019 Apr;34(4):457-468. doi: 10.1002/tox.22699.

34. Sagawa Y, Futakuchi M, Xu J, Fukamachi K, Sakai Y, Ikarashi Y, Nishimura T, Suzui M, Tsuda H, Morita A. Lack of promoting effect of titanium dioxide particles on chemically-induced skin carcinogenesis in rats and mice. J Toxicol Sci. 2012;37(2):317-27.
35. Xu J, Sagawa Y, Futakuchi M, Fukamachi K, Alexander DB, Furukawa F, Ikarashi Y, Uchino T, Nishimura T, Morita A, Suzui M, Tsuda H. Lack of promoting effect of titanium dioxide particles on ultraviolet B-initiated skin carcinogenesis in rats. Food Chem Toxicol. 2011 Jun;49(6):1298-302. doi: 10.1016/j.fct.2011.03.011. Epub 2011 Mar 23.
36. Chapter 3. Powders and Compacts. In. B.M. Mithal, R.N. Saha. A Handbook Of Cosmetics. Vallabh Prakashan, 2006 ISBN 9788185731223, 8185731225. Page 23.
37. Winkler, Hans Christian et al. "Critical review of the safety assessment of titanium dioxide additives in food." Journal of nanobiotechnology vol. 16,1 51. 1 Jun. 2018, doi:10.1186/s12951-018-0376-8
38. Leone, Federica et al. "Nanostructured ZnO as Multifunctional Carrier for a Green Antibacterial Drug Delivery System-A Feasibility Study." Nanomaterials (Basel, Switzerland) vol. 9,3 407. 11 Mar. 2019, doi:10.3390/nano9030407
39. Kołodziejczak-Radzimska, Agnieszka, and Teofil Jesionowski. "Zinc Oxide-From Synthesis to Application: A Review." Materials (Basel, Switzerland) vol. 7,4 2833-2881. 9 Apr. 2014, doi:10.3390/ma7042833
40. Gupta, Mrinal et al. "Zinc therapy in dermatology: a review." Dermatology research and practice vol. 2014 (2014): 709152. doi:10.1155/2014/709152
41. Pasquet J, Chevalier Y, Couval E, Bouvier D, Bolzinger MA. Zinc oxide as a new antimicrobial preservative of topical products: interactions with common formulation ingredients. Int J Pharm. 2015 Feb 1;479(1):88-95. doi: 10.1016/j.ijpharm.2014.12.031.
42. Sirelkhatim A, Mahmud S, Seeni A, Kaus NHM, Ann LC, Bakhori SKM, Hasan H, Mohamad D. Review on Zinc Oxide Nanoparticles: Antibacterial Activity and Toxicity Mechanism. Nanomicro Lett. 2015;7(3):219-242. doi: 10.1007/s40820-015-0040-x.
43. The Science & Safety Behind Your Favorite Products (Zinc Oxide). Available From: https://cosmeticsinfo.org/ingredient/zinc-oxide-0
44. Ma, Jinxia et al. "Preparation of Zinc Oxide-Starch Nanocomposite and Its Application on Coating." Nanoscale research letters vol. 11,1 (2016): 200. doi:10.1186/s11671-016-1404-y
45. Lin, Pei-Hui et al. "Zinc in Wound Healing Modulation." Nutrients vol. 10,1 16. 24 Dec. 2017, doi:10.3390/nu10010016
46. The Ultimate Guide to Zinc oxide. Available From: https://www.alyaka.com/magazine/ultimate-guide-zinc-oxide/
47. Jiang J, Pi J, Cai J. The Advancing of Zinc Oxide Nanoparticles for Biomedical Applications. Bioinorg Chem Appl. 2018 Jul 5;2018:1062562. doi: 10.1155/2018/1062562.

48. Siddiqi KS, Ur Rahman A, Tajuddin, Husen A. Properties of Zinc Oxide Nanoparticles and Their Activity Against Microbes. Nanoscale Res Lett. 2018 May 8;13(1):141. doi: 10.1186/s11671-018-2532-3.
49. Williams, Lynda B, and Shelley E Haydel. "Evaluation of the medicinal use of clay minerals as antibacterial agents." International geology review vol. 52,7/8 (2010): 745-770. doi:10.1080/00206811003679737
50. Ngole-Jeme, Veronica M, and Georges-Ivo E Ekosse. "A Comparative Analyses of Granulometry, Mineral Composition and Major and Trace Element Concentrations in Soils Commonly Ingested by Humans." International journal of environmental research and public health vol. 12,8 8933-55. 31 Jul. 2015, doi:10.3390/ijerph120808933
51. Zhou Y, Liu Q, Xu P, Cheng H, Liu Q. Molecular Structure and Decomposition Kinetics of Kaolinite/Alkylamine Intercalation Compounds. Front Chem. 2018 Jul 27;6:310. doi: 10.3389/fchem.2018.00310.
52. Li X, Ouyang J, Zhou Y, Yang H. Assembling strategy to synthesize palladium modified kaolin nanocomposites with different morphologies. Sci Rep. 2015 Sep 3;5:13763. doi: 10.1038/srep13763.
53. Massaro M, Colletti CG, Lazzara G, Riela S. The Use of Some Clay Minerals as Natural Resources for Drug Carrier Applications. J FunctBiomater. 2018 Oct 19;9(4). pii: E58. doi: 10.3390/jfb9040058.
54. Glick JB, Kaur RR, Siegel D. Achieving hemostasis in dermatology-Part II: Topical hemostatic agents. Indian Dermatol Online J. 2013 Jul;4(3):172-6. doi: 10.4103/2229-5178.115509.
55. COOP COCO (Blog). How to choose clay? Tips and tricks, Tutorials and recipes, 26 June 2015.
56. Awad ME, López-Galindo A, Setti M, El-Rahmany MM, Iborra CV. Kaolinite in pharmaceutics and biomedicine. Int J Pharm. 2017 Nov 25;533(1):34-48. doi: 10.1016/j.ijpharm.2017.09.056.
57. Sinha R. Kaolin Clay For Skin: What Is It, Benefits, And How To Use It. STYLECRAZE (Skin Care Ideas), June 27, 2019.
58. Herman SJ, Olscamp GC, Weisbrod GL. Pulmonary kaolin granulomas. J Can Assoc Radiol. 1982 Dec;33(4):279-80.
59. Moosavi, Maryam. "Bentonite Clay as a Natural Remedy: A Brief Review." Iranian journal of public health vol. 46,9 (2017): 1176-1183.
60. Adib-Hajbaghery, Mohsen et al. "The effects of Bentonite and Calendula on the improvement of infantile diaper dermatitis." Journal of research in medical sciences: the official journal of Isfahan University of Medical Sciences vol. 19,4 (2014): 314-8.
61. Cosmetic Clays in Skin Care. Chagrin Valley Soap & Salve Co, June 25, 2019.
62. Berry J. Bentonite clay: 11 benefits and uses. Medical News Today, 22 May 2019.
63. Maxim LD, Niebo R, McConnell EE. Bentonite toxicology and epidemiology - a review. InhalToxicol. 2016 Nov;28(13):591-617.

64. Chapter 5. Do it yourself. In: Julie Gabriel. The Green Beauty Guide, Health Communications, Inc. Deerfield Beach, Florida 2008, Page 87. eISBN-13: 978-0-7573-9788-2, eISBN-10: 0-7573-9788-3
65. Safety Assessment of Alkonium Clays as Used in Cosmetics. Cosmetics Ingredient Review, January 6, 2016, Page 12. Available From: https://www.cir-safety.org/sites/default/files/alkcly122015Rev%20Tent.pdf
66. Williams LB, Haydel SE, Ferrell RE. Bentonite, Bandaids, and Borborygmi. Elements (Que). 2009 Apr 1;5(2):99-104.
67. Web Sojourner Williams LLC. DIY All Natural, Oil Absorbing Translucent Facial Powder. Face, September 9, 2014.
68. What Is Calcium Bentonite Clay? Available From: https://www.healthline.com/health/calcium-bentonite-clay#1
69. Ghica MV, Hîrjău M, Lupuleasa D, Dinu-Pîrvu CE. Flow and Thixotropic Parameters for Rheological Characterization of Hydrogels. Molecules. 2016 Jun 16;21(6). pii: E786. doi: 10.3390/molecules21060786.
70. Binks BP, Clint JH, Whitby CP. Rheological behavior of water-in-oil emulsions stabilized by hydrophobic bentonite particles. Langmuir. 2005 Jun 7;21(12):5307-16.
71. Cho YJ, Kim DM, Song IH, Choi JY, Jin SW, Kim BJ, Jeong JW, Jang CE, Chu K, Chung CM. An Oligoimide Particle as a Pickering Emulsion Stabilizer. Polymers (Basel). 2018 Sep 27;10(10). pii: E1071. doi: 10.3390/polym10101071.
72. Fernández L, Scher H, Jeoh T, VanderGheynst JS. Room-temperature storage of microalgae in water-in-oil emulsions: influence of solid particle type and concentration in the oil phase. Bioprocess Biosyst Eng. 2015 Dec;38(12):2451-60.
73. Chapter 2. Corundum and Emery Supply-Demand Relationships. In: John J. McKetta Jr. Encyclopedia of Chemical Processing and Design: Volume 12 - Corrosion to Cottonseed. CRC Press, 1981, Page 87. ISBN 0824724623, 9780824724627
74. Zhang B, Cui D, Liu M, Gong H, Huang Y, Han F. Corn porous starch: preparation, characterization and adsorption property. Int J Biol Macromol. 2012 Jan 1;50(1):250-6. doi: 10.1016/j.ijbiomac.2011.11.002.
75. Dura A, Błaszczak W, Rosell CM. Functionality of porous starch obtained by amylase or amyloglucosidase treatments. CarbohydrPolym. 2014 Jan 30;101:837-45. doi: 10.1016/j.carbpol.2013.10.013.
76. Kirschner C. 5 alternatives to talc powder. Mother Nature Network, June 13, 2019.
77. Schlossman ML. Chapter 43. Decorative Products. In. André Barel, Marc Paye, Howard I. Maibach. Handbook of Cosmetic Science and Technology Edition 2, CRC Press, 2005, Page 568. ISBN 0849354838, 9780849354830
78. Schlossman ML. Chapter 19. Decorative Products. In. Peter Elsner, Howard I. Maibach. Cosmeceuticals: Drugs vs. Cosmetics Volume 23 of Cosmetic science and technology series EBSCO ebook academic collection, CRC Press, 2000, Page 291, ISBN 0824742397, 9780824742393

79. García N.L., Famá L., Dufresne A., Aranguren M., Goyanes S. A comparison between the physic-chemical properties of tuber and cereal starches. Food Res. Int. 2009;42:976–982. doi: 10.1016/j.foodres.2009.05.004
80. Wang, Kai, Henry RJ, Gilvert RG. "Causal Relations Among Starch Biosynthesis, Structure, and Properties." Springer Science Reviews, vol. 2, no. 1-2, May 2014, pp. 15–33., doi:10.1007/s40362-014-0016-0.
81. Peng M, Gao M, Båga M, Hucl P, Chibbar RN. Starch-branching enzymes preferentially associated with A-type starch granules in wheat endosperm. Plant Physiol. 2000 Sep;124(1):265-72.
82. Sun Q, Zhu X, Si F, Xiong L. Effect of acid hydrolysis combined with heat moisture treatment on structure and physicochemical properties of corn starch. J Food Sci Technol. 2015 Jan;52(1):375-82. doi: 10.1007/s13197-013-0998-7. Epub 2013 Apr 28.
83. Kaur M, Oberoi DP, Sogi DS, Gill BS. Physicochemical, morphological and pasting properties of acid treated starches from different botanical sources. J Food Sci Technol. 2011 Aug;48(4):460-5. doi: 10.1007/s13197-010-0126-x. Epub 2010 Oct 29.
84. Božanić DK, Djoković V, Dimitrijević-Branković S, Krsmanović R, McPherson M, Nair PS, Georges MK, Radhakrishnan T. Inhibition of microbial growth by silver-starch nanocomposite thin films. J Biomater Sci Polym Ed. 2011;22(17):2343-55. doi: 10.1163/092050610X539532. PubMed PMID: 25593372; PubMed Central PMCID: PMC4288800.
85. Chapter 4 Fillers and reinforcements. In. Clive Maier, Theresa Calafut. Polypropylene: The Definitive User's Guide and Databook Plastics Design Library, Page 50. William Andrew, 1998 ISBN 0815518714, 9780815518716
86. Schaefer K. Natural Calcium Carbonates for Oral Care and Color Cosmetics. Cosmetics & Toiletries® Magazine, June 11, 2010.
87. Anstead DF. Chapter 7. Miscellaneous Raw Materials. In. H. W. Hibbott. Handbook of Cosmetic Science: An Introduction to Principles and Applications, page 121. Elsevier, 2016 ISBN 1483186474, 9781483186474.
88. Chapter 13. Facial Adornment. In. Zoe Diana Draelos. Cosmetics and Dermatologic Problems and Solutions, Third Edition (revised). Taylor & Francis, 2011, Page 95-99. ISBN 1841847402, 9781841847405
89. Di Maiuta N, Schwarzentruber P. Molecular detection of bacteria in calcium carbonate powder used in cosmetic formulations. Int J Cosmet Sci. 2011 Oct;33(5):426-31. doi: 10.1111/j.1468-2494.2011.00648.x.
90. Chapter 5 Group 14 C Si Ge Sn and Pb Alkaline Earth Compounds. In. Richard C. Ropp. Encyclopedia of the Alkaline Earth Compounds, Page 360. Newnes, 2012 ISBN 0444595538, 9780444595539.
91. Magnesium carbonate. Available From: https://www.revolvy.com/page/Magnesium-carbonate
92. Select Minerals for the North America Personal Care. Available From: http://www.dpl-us.com/wp-content/uploads/2015/08/personalcare.pdf

93. Chapter 7. Color cosmetics. In. S.D. Williams, W.H. Schmitt. Chemistry and Technology of the Cosmetics and Toiletries Industry, Page 164. Springer Science & Business Media, 2012 ISBN 9400915551, 9789400915558.
94. Sherif S. Z. Hindi, "Microcrystalline Cellulose: The Inexhaustible Treasure for Pharmaceutical Industry." Nanoscience and Nanotechnology Research, vol. 4, no. 1 (2017): 17-24. doi: 10.12691/nnr-4-1-3.
95. Qin Y, Qiu X, Zhu JY. Understanding Longitudinal Wood Fiber Ultra-structure for Producing Cellulose Nanofibrils Using Disk Milling with Diluted Acid Prehydrolysis. Sci Rep. 2016 Oct 31;6:35602. doi: 10.1038/srep35602.
96. Lynch G. Rheology Modification with Avicel® in Personal Care Applications. Available From: http://www.cosmeticsciencetechnology.com/articles/samples/181.pdf
97. Setu, Md Nurul Islam, et al. "Preparation of Microcrystalline Cellulose from Cotton and Its Evaluation as Direct Compressible Excipient in the Formulation of Naproxen Tablets." Dhaka University Journal of Pharmaceutical Sciences, vol. 13, no. 2, May 2015, pp. 187–192., doi:10.3329/dujps.v13i2.21899.
98. Chaerunisaa, Anis Yohana, et al. "Microcrystalline Cellulose as Pharmaceutical Excipient." Pharmaceutical Formulation Design - Recent Practices [Working Title], 2019, doi:10.5772/intechopen.88092.
99. Rojas J, Lopez A, Guisao S, Ortiz C. Evaluation of several microcrystalline celluloses obtained from agricultural by-products. J Adv Pharm Technol Res. 2011 Jul;2(3):144-50. doi: 10.4103/2231-4040.85527.
100. Kamel, S., et al. "Pharmaceutical Significance of Cellulose: A Review." Express Polymer Letters, vol. 2, no. 11, 2008, pp. 758–778., doi:10.3144/express polymlett.2008.90.
101. FMC, 2013. Fun facts about Avicel® microcrystalline cellulose also known as cellulose gel. Available From: http://www.fmcbiopolymer.com/ Food/Home /News/FiftyYearsofAvicel.aspx
102. Microcrystalline Cellulose powder. SIDLEY CHEMICAL, 7 March, 2014.
103. Heng PW, Liew CV, Soh JL. Pre-formulation studies on moisture absorption in microcrystalline cellulose using differential thermo-gravimetric analysis. Chem Pharm Bull (Tokyo). 2004 Apr;52(4):384-90.
104. Garg T, Rath G, Goyal AK. Comprehensive review on additives of topical dosage forms for drug delivery. Drug Deliv. 2015 Dec;22(8):969-987.
105. Muñiz-Lerma JA, Nommeots-Nomm A, Waters KE, Brochu M. A Comprehensive Approach to Powder Feedstock Characterization for Powder Bed Fusion Additive Manufacturing: A Case Study on AlSi7Mg. Materials (Basel). 2018 Nov 27;11(12). pii: E2386. doi: 10.3390/ma11122386.
106. Hesse N, Dechet MA, Bonilla JSG, Lübbert C, Roth S, Bück A, Schmidt J, Peukert W. Analysis of Tribo-Charging during Powder Spreading in Selective Laser Sintering: Assessment of Polyamide 12 Powder Ageing Effects on Charging Behavior. Polymers (Basel). 2019 Apr 3;11(4). pii: E609, doi: 10.3390/polym11040609.

107. Hobbs CA, Saigo K, Koyanagi M, Hayashi SM. Magnesium stearate, a widely-used food additive, exhibits a lack of in vitro and in vivo genotoxic potential. Toxicol Rep. 2017 Oct 16;4:554-559. doi: 10.1016/j.toxrep.2017.10.003.
108. Silk Powder (200 Mesh) Raw Material. Available from: https://www.newdirectionsaromatics.com/products/raw-materials/silk-powder-200-mesh.html
109. Shi L, Yang N, Zhang H, Chen L, Tao L, Wei Y, Liu H, Luo Y. A novel poly(γ-glutamic acid)/silk-sericin hydrogel for wound dressing: Synthesis, characterization and biological evaluation. Mater Sci Eng C Mater Biol Appl. 2015 Mar;48:533-40. doi: 10.1016/j.msec.2014.12.047.
110. Material Safety Data Sheet Bismuth Oxychloride MSDS," Sciencelab.com, May 21, 2013. Available From: http://www.sciencelab.com/msds.php?msdsId=9923103.
111. van Lotringen I. Cream or powder makeup - which is better? Cosmopolitan (UK), May 5, 2015.
112. Bale S. Chapter 20. Natural Finishes. In. Jacob Deva Racusin, Ace McArleton. The Natural Building Companion: A Comprehensive Guide to Integrative Design and Construction (Yestermorrow Design/Build library), Published by Chelsea Green Publishing, 2012, Page 363. ISBN 1603583394, 9781603583398
113. Yusuf M, Shabbir M, Mohammad F. Natural Colorants: Historical, Processing and Sustainable Prospects. Nat Prod Bioprospect. 2017 Feb;7(1):123-145. doi: 10.1007/s13659-017-0119-9.
114. Marzec A, Szadkowski B, Rogowski J, Maniukiewicz W, Szynkowska MI, Zaborski M. Characteristics of Hybrid Pigments Made from Alizarin Dye on a Mixed Oxide Host. Materials (Basel). 2019 Jan 24;12(3). pii: E360. doi: 10.3390/ma12030360.
115. Herz RS. Perfume. In: Gottfried JA, editor. Neurobiology of Sensation and Reward. Boca Raton (FL): CRC Press/Taylor & Francis; 2011. Chapter 17. Available from: https://www.ncbi.nlm.nih.gov/books/NBK92802/
116. Lenochová P, Vohnoutová P, Roberts SC, Oberzaucher E, Grammer K, Havlíček J. Psychology of fragrance use: perception of individual odor and perfume blends reveals a mechanism for idiosyncratic effects on fragrance choice. PLoS One. 2012;7(3):e33810. doi: 10.1371/journal.pone.0033810.
117. Shah RB, Tawakkul MA, Khan MA. Comparative evaluation of flow for pharmaceutical powders and granules. AAPS PharmSciTech. 2008;9(1):250-8. doi: 10.1208/s12249-008-9046-8. Epub 2008 Feb 15. PubMed PMID: 18446489; PubMed Central PMCID: PMC2976911.
118. Amparo Salvador, Alberto Chisvert. Analysis of Cosmetic Products, Edition 2, published by Elsevier Science, 2017 ISBN 0444635165, 9780444635167
119. Globally Harmonized System of Classification and Labelling of Chemicals, ST/SG/AC. 10/30/Rev.6 (sixth revised edition), United Nations, New York and Geneva (2015)
120. EU Regulation (EC) No 1272/2008 of the European Parliament and of the Council of 16 December 2008 on Classification, Labelling and Packaging of Substances and Mixtures, Amending and Repealing Directives 67/548/EEC and 1999/45/EC,

and Amending Regulation (EC) No 1907/2006. Official Journal of the European Union, L 353/1, 31/12/2008.

121. Steiling W, Almeida JF, Assaf Vandecasteele H, Gilpin S, Kawamoto T, O'Keeffe L, Pappa G, Rettinger K, Rothe H, Bowden AM. Principles for the safety evaluation of cosmetic powders. Toxicol Lett. 2018 Nov;297:8-18. doi: 10.1016/j.toxlet.2018.08.011.

122. OEHHA (Office of Environmental Health Hazard Assessment), 2011. https://oehha.ca.gov/proposition-65/chemicals/titanium-dioxide-airborne-unbound-particles-respirable-size. Office of Environmental Health Hazard Assessment (OEHHA) of the California Environmental Protection Agency, 2011.

123. Monographs on the Evaluation of Carcinogenic Risks to Human, vol. 65 (1996), pp. 171-172.

124. Łodyga-Chruścińska, E.; Sykuła, A.; Więdłocha, M. Hidden Metals in Several Brands of Lipstick and Face Powder Present on Polish Market. Cosmetics 2018, 5(4), 57 DOI: https://doi.org/10.3390/cosmetics5040057.

125. Abdul Kader Mohiuddin. Heavy Metals in Cosmetics: The Notorious Daredevils and Burning Health Issues. Am J Biomed Sci & Res. 2019 - 4(5). AJBSR.MS.ID.000829. DOI: 10.34297/AJBSR.2019.04.000829

126. Mohiuddin AK. Cosmetics Safety: Gray Areas with Darker Inside. Journal of Medical Research and Health Sciences Volume 2 issue 8, Page 688-693 August, 2019. DOI https://doi.org/10.15520/jmrhs.v2i8.97

CHAPTER 7

ACNE PROTECTION

7.1 BACKGROUND

Historic Panorama of Acne Protection - The word 'acne' appears to evolve from Greek word 'acme' which means 'point or spot'. Although acne is described in very ancient writings dating back to Eber's Papyrus, its clear description is found after Fuch's coined the term 'Acne Vulgaris' and Erasmus Wilson separated it from acne rosacea. The roots of acne have been traced to three well known ancient civilizations viz, Egyptians, Greeks and Romans.

- Some Egyptian writings have mentioned that Pharaohs suffered from acne and had also made efforts to resolve it. In Ebers Papyrus the word 'aku-t' is cited that was later translated as 'boils, blains, sores, pustules or any inflammatory swelling' and is described to be treated with some animal origin preparations and honey. Ancient Egyptians around 3rd century was of the opinion that acne is caused by telling lies. Tutankhamun, Egyptian Pharaoh of the 18th dynasty had acne as evident from the anti-acne remedies in his tomb. From the historical records, both Hippocrates and Aristotle were aware of this ailment. Aristotle also explained this condition in detail.
- The ancient Greeks knew acne as 'tovoot'- 'the first growth of the beard' hence it was associated with puberty. Ancient Romans has guided initial treatment of acne.
- In ancient Rome, acne was treated with baths as people there believed that the pores of the skin may be lifted and cleaned with a mixture of sulfur in the mineral baths. Cassius in 3 AD interpreted that since this disorder is related to puberty, it is known by the name of 'akmas'. In the 4th century AD, the court physician of Theodosius advised acne victims to wipe their "pimples" with a cloth while watching a falling star and the pimples would then 'fall from the body.
- Ibn Sina (980-1037) in his legendary text 'Al Qanoon Fil Tib' (The Cannon of Medicine) has depicted the etiopathogenesis and clinical presentation of Busoore labaniya (acne).

- In the Elizabethan era (1558–1603), the appearance of women was given primordial importance. Acne at that time was also contributed to witchcraft. For the management of these pimples, different type of mercury makeup was also in use. The caustic mercury erodes the flesh. Hence forth, people restored to the sulfur treatments of antique times.
- Riolanus and Jonston associated acne with disorders of menstruation in 1638 and 1648 respectively. Jonston (1648) also linked acne with heterosexual behavior pattern in a manner very close to present day psychosomatic ideas on the subject.
- In 1920, Jack Breitbart of the Revlon Corporation invented benzoyl peroxide for the treatment of acne which was more effective and smelled better than the sulfur treatments of the past.
- Around 1930, laxatives were in common use for the treatment of acne.
- In 1950s Tetracycline was for the first time prescribed for acne as it was noticed that acne was caused by bacteria.
- In 1960s, the topical treatment Retin-A was developed to alleviate acne. Retin-A has produced great results and is still in use.
- In 1980s, a novel medication Accutane (Isotretinoin) for acne appeared in the markets of America. It was found extremely effective but severe side effects were also noted viz., stroke, seizure, heart attack, and hair loss.
- In 1990, laser therapy made its evolvement in treating acne and is now widely used remedy as it clears the recent as well as old scars left by acne besides active lesions.
- In 2000, the blue/red therapy was developed along with laser therapy for easy treatment of acne. Microneedling with dermaroller emerged as a novel treatment modality for the treatment of acne scars.
- Fernandes, in 2006, developed percutaneous collagen induction therapy with the derma-roller.
- Vaccine against inflammatory acne has been tested successfully in mice in 2007 and many such studies and trials are detailed in several journals till then.

7.2 ABSTRACT

Acne, also known as acne vulgaris (AV), is a long-term skin disease that occurs when hair follicles are clogged with dead skin cells and oil from the skin. It is characterized by blackheads or whiteheads, pimples, oily skin, and possible scarring. An intact stratum corneum and barrier, normal natural moisturizing factor and hyaluronic acid levels, normal Aquaporin-3 (AQP3) expression (localized at the basal lateral membranes of collecting duct cells in the kidney), and balanced sebum secretion are qualities of the skin that fall in the middle of the oily–dry spectrum. Patients rarely, if ever, complain about reduced sebum production, but elevated sebum production, yielding oily skin that can be a precursor to acne, is a common complaint. Several factors are known to influence sebum production. AV is mostly triggered by *Propionibacterium acnes* in adolescence, under the influence of normal circulating dehydroepiandrosterone (DHEA). It is a very common skin disorder which can present with inflammatory and non-inflammatory lesions chiefly on the face but can also occur on the upper arms, trunk, and back. Age, in particular, has a significant and well-known impact, as sebum levels are usually low in childhood, rise in the middle-to-late teen years, and remain stable into the seventh and eighth decades until endogenous androgen synthesis dwindles. Sebum, the oily secretion of the sebaceous glands containing wax esters, sterol esters, cholesterol, di- and triglycerides, and squalene, imparts an oily quality to the skin and is well known to play an important role in acne development. Acne can't be prevented or cured, but it can be treated effectively. The pimples and bumps heal slowly, and when one begins to go away, others seem to crop up. Depending on its severity, acne can cause emotional distress and scar the skin. Acne may cause scarring of the skin, but generally causes no long-term health problems. In self-body image, some parts of the body including face play an important role. The existence of even a minor lesion in this part may be unpleasant for the patient and seems large. This image can cause mental disorders including depression and anxiety, low self-esteem, and a decrease in social relationships. However, high levels of anxiety and depression in patients with facial acne are not related to oxidative stress, according to a study published online in the Journal of Cosmetic Dermatology.

Keywords: acne, skin care, comedones, pustules, acne scars, sebum, *Propionibacterium acnes*

Exhibit 1. Important terminology
1. Whiteheads -closed plugged pores
2. Blackheads -open plugged pores
3. Papules-Small red, tender bumps
4. Pimples-pustules, which are papules with pus at their tips
5. Nodules-Large, solid, painful lumps beneath the surface of the skin
6. Cystic lesions-Painful, pus-filled lumps beneath the surface of the skin
7. Hirsutism- abnormal growth of hair on a woman's face and body.
8. Alopecia-the partial or complete absence of hair from areas of the body where it normally grows; baldness.

7.3 INTRODUCTION

AV is a multifaceted skin disorder, affecting more than 85% of young individuals worldwide. It is the most common skin disease, and although it usually manifests during puberty and worsens throughout adolescence, epidemiological studies suggest that it can arise at any age. Apart from the classic belief that acne results from sebaceous gland hyperplasia, abnormal follicular differentiation with increased keratinization, microbial hyper-colonization of the follicular canal, and increased inflammation primarily through activation of the adaptive immune system may also be contributors. There are various types of acne, such as acne vulgaris, acne rosacea, acne cosmetica, acne fulminans, and acne mechanica. In 2011, around 20% of the population in the US was affected with acne. According to the lesion type, acne can be classified into four main categories: non-inflammatory (purely comedone acne), mild papular, scarring papular, and nodular; the latter three are inflammatory acne lesions. Acne treatment aims to lessen the inflammatory or non-inflammatory acne lesions, improve appearance, prevent or minimize potential adverse effects, and minimize any scarring. Pharmacological therapy is not always desirable because of the development of antibiotic resistance or the potential risk of adverse effects. Non-pharmacological therapies can be viable alternatives for conventional therapies. Acne severity is classified according to different scales. It is widely agreed, however, that the mild and moderate forms of acne display primary lesions only, while severe acne also includes nodules, cysts, and eventually open lesions. It is noteworthy that acne severity and scarring have been related to P. acnes inflammatory factors, bacterial growth metabolites such as allergens, toxins, or porphyrins, and enzymes. Acne is always accompanied by a variety of other signs and symptoms such as erythema, desquamation, burning, itching, dyschromia, and pain. Furthermore, acne causes significant psychological morbidity in affected patients. Currently available systemic products include the retinoid isotretinoin, antibiotics, or oral contraceptives, all of which are indicated for more severe acne, acne resistant to other therapies, and nodulocystic, scarring acne. Although acne is widespread with numerous treatment options available, the condition is still not considered curable, prompting further investigation by the pharmaceutical industry. Commonly used treatments aim to reduce the number of inflammatory lesions, inhibit comedones, suppress the growth of *Propionibacterium acne* or reduce sebaceous gland size and secretory activity. People with acne often turn to complementary and alternative medicine (CAM), such as herbal medicine, acupuncture, and dietary modifications, because of their concerns about the adverse effects of conventional medicines. Some researchers have concluded that genetic predisposition and hormonal influences play a more important role in acne than diet. Chinese herbal medicine, manual healing therapies (such as acupuncture and massage), and other traditional and folk remedies may follow similar mechanisms in the treatment of acne.

Methodological and reporting quality limitations in the included studies weakened any evidence. All mainstream products can cause severe side effects including, paradoxically, the typical signs and symptoms of acne, and there is therefore a demand for new innovative treatments.

7.3.1 ETIOLOGY

The pathogenesis is multifactorial with four primary pathogenic factors including: (a) abnormal hyperkeratinization of the pilosebaceous duct with comedo formation caused by increased androgens; (b) an increase in sebum production from the enlarged sebaceous gland caused by increased androgens; (c) colonization and proliferation of the duct with bacteria, most commonly P. acnes, although clear evidence of a causal relationship between P. acnes and AV is lacking; and (d) an inflammatory response caused by the immunological activity of P. acnes [74].The adequate control of the four pathogenic mechanisms involved in the appearance of acne lesions is key to treatment success [1-7]. Several exacerbating factors have been suggested including diet, menstruation, sweating, personal stress, ultraviolet radiation, application of pomades and occupation [8]. Use of medications like lithium, steroids, and anticonvulsants, exposure to excess sunlight, use of occlusive wear like shoulder pads, headbands backpacks, and underwire brassieres, endocrine disorders like polycystic ovarian syndrome and even pregnancy have also reported [26]. The association between diet and acne can no longer be dismissed. Compelling evidence shows that high glycemic load diets may exacerbate acne (also, LGL diet that resulted in the improvement of acne lesions) [9-12]. Food with a high glycemic index is rapidly absorbed, increases serum glucose levels and stimulates increased glucose-dependent insulin signaling [13]. Elevated insulin levels stimulate the secretion of androgens and cause an increased production of sebum, growth of the sebaceous glands and hyperkeratinization, which plays a fundamental role in pathogenesis of AV [9], [14-17]. High plasma levels of Insulin-Like Growth Factor 1 (IGF 1) which are caused by consumption of milk, stimulates proliferation of sebocytes, resulting in the development and progression of acne lesions. Skim milk contains less estrogen than whole milk. Estrogen is a hormone that may reduce acne [9], [18-25]. There is a common medical and lay belief that women experience perimenstrual acne flares [27-31]. Summer aggravation of acne reported by 80% of patient in a study due to sweating and increased humidity [32]. Acne has also been associated with impaired health-related quality of life (HRQoL), at times with negative impacts as great as that of severe and even life-threatening diseases [33]. However, Zari et.al, 2017 and Bagatin et. al, 2019 revealed a positive association with menstruation, heat and humidity, sweating, use of makeup and cosmetic products, oily hair products, use of topical steroids, sleep disorders, excessive skin washing, possible resistance to P. acnes and squeezing pimples [34,35]. Bondade et.al, 2019 found undesirable stressful life events and psychiatric comorbidity were more in acne patients than in controls [36]. Stress and depression positively correlate with acne severity [34], [37]. Acne can also develop in neonates but in most cases resolves spontaneously [38]. Acne neonatorum, which presents within the first four weeks of life, occurs in up to 20% of newborns. Additionally, childhood acne is strongly correlated with the development of persistent acne later in life.

Exhibit 2. Sebaceous Gland and Acne [88], [101-115]
• The sebaceous gland (SG) is integral to the structure and function of the skin, providing 90% of its surface lipids. While much of the focus relating to the sebaceous gland comes from its central role in AV. • If sebum interferes with the process of follicular keratinization in the pilosebaceous unit, pore blockage may occur, contributing to lesion formation and acne. • Low levels of linoleic acid have been observed in skin surface lipids of acne patients. Depletion of linoleic acid in sphingolipids has been hypothesized to be involved in the follicular hyperkeratosis, which is a crucial event involved in the comedones formation. After 10 weeks of omega-3 fatty acid or γ-linoleic acid supplementation, inflammatory and non-inflammatory acne lesions decreased significantly. • Typical western diet, comprised of milk and hyperglycaemic foods, may have potentiating effects on serum insulin and insulin-like growth factor-I (IGF-I) levels. Several studies have shown that elevated levels of serum IGF-I correlate with overproduction of sebum and acne. Also, there is a relationship between female acne and insulin resistance (IR). This association is independent of hyperandrogenemia. Anti-insulin drugs may an adjunctive treatment of female acne. • Another hallmark of sebum in acne patients is the presence of lipoperoxides, mainly due to the peroxidation of squalene and a decrease in the level of vitamin E, the major sebum antioxidant. • The researchers found that the levels of serum vitamins A and E and zinc were significantly lower in the people with acne. • When sebocytes were incubated with an H-1 receptor antagonist, diphenhydramine (DPH), at non-cytotoxic doses, a significant decrease in squalene levels, a biomarker for sebum, was observed. Acne sebum presents a higher level of squalene peroxide. • Retinoids are also suggested to influence the biological function of sebocytes. Retinoic acid receptors and retinoid X receptors are expressed in human sebocytes. • Acne patients produced higher rates of testosterone and 5α-dihydrotestosterone (5α-DHT) in their skin than healthy individuals.

Contd...

- Androgens are important hormones that influence sebum production from the sebaceous glands. Highest density of these has been demonstrated in sebaceous glands. Androgens are not directly correlated with acne severity, but affect acne severity as seen in difference between their levels in different grades of acne.
- Dehydroepiandrosterone (DHEA) has been also shown to regulate sebum production especially in postmenopausal women.
- In AV, increased sebum production peaks in mid-adolescence at a time that GH and IGF-I reach their highest serum levels.
- At puberty, sebum production is increased by the multiple factors including androgens, corticotropin-releasing hormone, vitamin D and insulin-like growth factor-1 (IGF-1).
- In acne-involved skin the complete CRH system [Neuropeptides (NPs)] is abundant especially in the sebaceous glands.
- Inflammation is being regarded as a key component of the pathogenesis of acne. The main factors associated with acneiform lesion development are follicular hyperkeratinization, sebum production by sebaceous glands, and inflammation.
- Cytokines are present in normal sebaceous glands, and they are affected by many factors. In a stressed environment, the amounts of released cytokines increase significantly.
- The sebum excretion rate exerts a profound influence on the rate of growth of P. acnes and may determine, along with availability of water, whether a particular follicle is capable of being colonized. Certain P. acnes strains to be responsible for opportunistic infections worsening acne lesions.

7.3.2 EPIDEMIOLOGY

Acne is a very common skin disease with the prevalence among adolescent is 80% or more [13, [29], [39-45]. Among them, 80% are teenagers [46-49]. Although this inquisitive nature is considered a normal aspect of the maturation process, approximately 80% to 90% of teenagers in the Western world experience behavioral/emotional and physical/psychological effects caused by acne [50]. About 60% of affected adolescents have mild acne for which they use non-prescription preparations without consulting a physician. The remaining 40% constitute the population of acne patients seen in medical practice [4]. It is less common in African-Americans and Asians than in the Caucasian population [9]. About 20% of the affected individuals develop severe acne which results in scarring [26]. In youths, overweight and obesity are inversely associated with acne in a dose-dependent manner [51]. Overweight and obesity are associated with acne in girls aged 18 and 19, but the same association was not observed in boys [52]. However, Stewart et.al 2019 found no significant association between increased BMI and AV [53]. Western nutrition is characterized by high calorie uptake, high glycemic load, high fat, and meat intake, as well as increased consumption of insulin- and IGF-1-level elevating dairy proteins. Intake of instant noodles, junk food, carbonated drinks, snacks, processed cheeses, pork, chicken, nuts and seaweed were significantly higher in acne patients than in the controls. Moreover, positive associations between acne and the consumption of other dairy products like instant breakfast drink, sherbet, cream cheese and cottage cheese have been reported [54]. Wang et. al, 2019 reviewed that a nearly 50% of normal women with acne did not have clinical or biochemical evidence of hyperandrogenism [55]. More than 60% of women had an increase in the number of inflammatory acne lesions in the late luteal phase of the menstrual cycle [27-31]. Acne is common during pregnancy. In fact, more than one out of every two pregnant women can expect to develop acne [56]. Girls must be made aware that cosmetic usage may be a potential aggravating factor for their facial acne [57]. Because certain chemicals in personal care products are suspected endocrine disrupters (e.g, phthalates, parabens, triclosan) [58]. There are many causes for acneiform eruptions including exposure to halogenated aromatic hydrocarbons and use of antibiotics like macrolides and penicillin. Other drugs that can also induce acneiform eruptions include nystatin, isoniazid, corticotropin, naproxen, and hydroxychloroquine. Many organisms can also induce acneiform eruptions like infections by *Proteus, Klebsiella, Escherichia coli*, and *Enterobacter*. Pityrosporum folliculitis caused by *Malassezia furfur* may also present on the trunk and upper extremities with pruritic eruptions [59]. Black individuals are more prone to post-inflammatory hyperpigmentation and specific subtypes such as 'pomade acne'. The heritability of acne is almost 80% in first-degree relatives [60]. George et.al, 2018 revealed Food items and cosmetics were attributed to exacerbation by 47.3% and 40% of patients respectively. About 48% patients had first degree relatives with present or past history of acne [61]. Daily soft drink consumption significantly increases the risk of moderate-to-severe acne in adolescents, especially when the sugar intake from any type of soft drink exceeds 100 g per day [84].

Exhibit 3. Acne Myths/Misconception Vs Study Result

Myth/Misconception	Study Result
In particular, no effect has been established between chocolate, dairy products, shellfish, or fatty foods [116].	Dark chocolate consumption appears to affect the facial skin of young men by enhancing corneocyte desquamation and promoting bacterial colonization of the residual skin surface components [117].
	Any dairy, such as milk, yogurt, and cheese, was associated with an increased OR for acne in individuals aged 7–30 years [20].
	Four ounces of shrimp provides about 325 -375 milligrams of omega-3 fatty acids [118]. After 10 weeks of omega-3 fatty acid supplementation,

Contd...

	inflammatory and non-inflammatory acne lesions decreased significantly [105].
	Isotretinoin, Retinol (Vitamin A), carotenoids (provitamin A) and retinoids (Vitamin A metabolites) are absorbed better with parallel intake of vegetable oils [11].
Weight loss and the use of metformin are both associated with lower plasma insulin levels and decreased androgen levels and therefore for acne patients, a weight loss diet may be indicated [119,120].	Low glycemic loads, with or without metformin, has been associated with greater reduction in acne lesion counts compared with high loads [53].
There were no significant correlations between IGF-1and acne severity [120].	Plasma IGF-1 levels positively correlate with severity of acne [18].
Too much sex or masturbation may worsen acne. when females begin having a regular sex life their acne will be improved [116], [121]. Masturbation results in general debility, unnatural pale eyes and forehead acne [122].	Despite popular myth, diet, lack of exercise, lack of hygiene, greasy hair hanging over the face, and masturbation do not have any effect [123]. After adjustment for sex and age, the presence of acne remained highly associated with less sexual activity [124].
open comedones or blackheads are full of dirt [125].	The dark color of blackheads has nothing to do with dirt: They look dark because this kind of blackhead is "open" and the skin pigment melanin reacts with oxygen in the air [83].
One should pop pimples at first sight.	Although squeezing pimples may make skin look better in the short term, it might force the pus even deeper into skin, which can make it become even more inflamed and the chance that the area will become dark as it tries to heal [83].
Sitting in the Sun to Clear Pimples	AV is aggravated by sunlight. Acne solaris a form of acne that appears and relapses after sun exposure. However, clinicians should not be didactic in their recommendations regarding diet, hygiene and face-washing, and sunlight to patients with acne. Advice should be individualized [126-128].

(a) **Pathophysiology:** Acne is proposed to be an IGF-1-mediated disease, modified by diets and smoking increasing insulin/IGF1-signalling [62]. The main hormones responsible for the development of AV include androgens, insulin and insulin-like growth factor-1. Other factors involved in this process are corticotropin-releasing hormone, α-melanocyte-stimulating hormone and substance P [63]. During puberty, alteration of the sebaceous lipid profile, called dysmenorrhea, stress, irritation, cosmetics and potential dietary factors lead to inflammation and formation of different types of acne lesions [64,65]. Distended follicles rupture and release proinflammatory chemicals into the dermis, stimulating inflammation. P. acnes, *Staphylococcus epidermis*, and Malassezia furfur induce inflammation and induce follicular epidermal proliferation [65]. Androgens also affect the barrier function of the skin, and disturbances of barrier function may stimulate epidermal DNA synthesis. This leads to epidermal hyperplasia, which may also contribute to follicular hyperkeratosis in acne [66]. Foam cells are lipid-loaded macrophages and neutrophils that are generated from a massive uptake of oxidized lipid. Foam cells are a pathological hallmark of atherosclerosis, and have also been found in acne lesions [67]. Sphingolipids are a class of lipids composed of a backbone of spingoid bases that are modified to produce ceramide (Cer) and more complex compounds, such as sphingomyelin (SM) and glycosphingolipids [68], have both structural and biological functions in human epidermis. Ceramide is the central molecule in the sphingolipid pathway [69]. They are among the most important epidermal sphingolipids and compose about 50 % of intercellular stratum corneum lipids by mass and are involved in the prevention of transepidermal water loss [70]. Kaya et.al, 2019 reported AV patients had increased circulating levels of C16 SM, ceramide-1-phosphate (C1P) and lower circulating levels of C24 CER compared to healthy controls, which may provide prognostic value for the disease [71]. Sebum is particularly abundant at anatomic sites with high concentration of P. acnes, and the sebum component oleic acid has been reported to promote the growth of P. acnes in culture. Increased sebum production and follicular hyperkeratosis result in the development of microcomedones, and changes in follicular milieu in intensive growth of P. acnes. With proliferation, P acnes secretes various several proinflammatory products. These include lipases, proteases, hyaluronidases, and chemotactic factors. Immune response to P. acnes includes humoral and cell-mediated immunity as well as complement activation (**Figure 7.1**) [72,73].

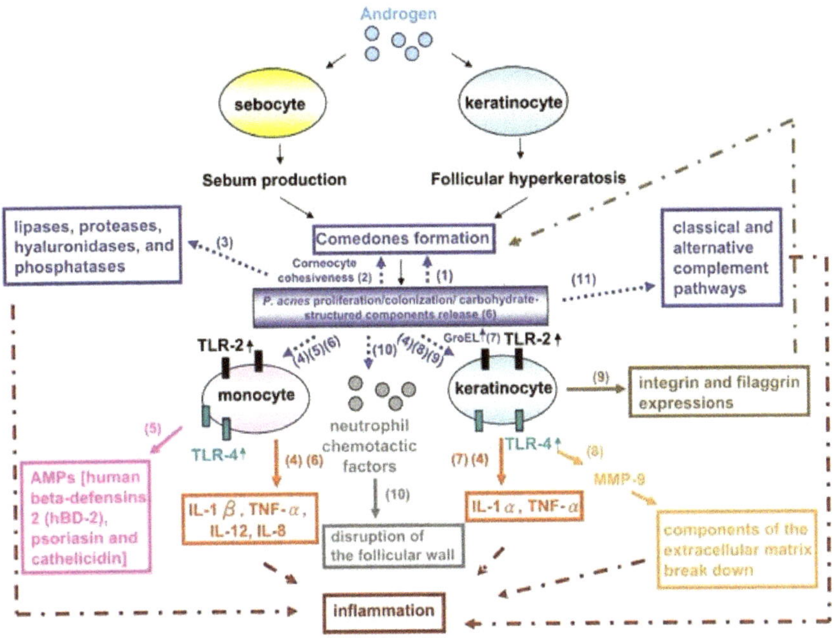

Figure 7.1 Molecular mechanisms by which P. acnes may contribute to the pathogenesis of AV [74]. (1) P. acnes is involved in the formation of microcomedones. (2) P. acnes colonization leads to an increase in the cohesiveness of corneocytes during the formation of comedones; (3) *in vitro* studies have suggested that P. acnes produces lipases, proteases, hyaluronidases, and phosphatases that may cause tissue injury; (4) P. acnes induces the expression of the proinflammatory cytokines IL-8, IL-12, IL-1α, IL-1β, and tumor necrosis factor alpha by innate cells, such as keratinocytes and monocytes, through the TLR2-dependent pathway; (5) host cells have developed a protective antimicrobial response to P. acnes such as antimicrobial lipids, AMPs (human beta-defensin 2, psoriasin and cathelicidin, exhibiting synergistic activities and inducing proinflammatory cytokines/ chemokines via TLR4- and CD14-dependent mechanisms; (6) the peptidoglycan-polysaccharide complexes and lipoteichoic acids of P. acnes stimulate proinflammatory cytokines released from monocytes, demonstrating their high antigenicity in severe acne patients. Increased expression of TLR2 and TLR4 *in vivo* was found in the epidermal layers of acne lesions for the sensing of peptidoglycans and lipopolysaccharides (LPSs), respectively; (7) P. acnes induces the growth of keratinocytes *in vitro* and upregulates the production of proinflammatory cytokines via a heat-shock GroEL protein; (8) MMPs, produced by different types of cells, including keratinocytes and sebocytes, play important roles in acne inflammation, dermal matrix destruction and hyperproliferative skin disorders. MMPs also cause rupture of the pilosebaceous follicle to exacerbate inflammation. For example, P. acnes induces the expression of MMP-9 in keratinocytes for the inflammatory process; (9) P. acnes lysates can directly modulate the differentiation of keratinocytes by inducing the expression of b1, a3, a6s, and aVb6 integrins and filaggrin during the formation of comedones; (10) P. acnes produces additional neutrophil chemotactic factors and is ingested by neutrophils within the sebaceous follicle, resulting in the release of hydrolases from neutrophils to disrupt the follicular wall; and (11) P. acnes results in the formation of C5a in inflammatory acne lesions by activating both the classical and alternative complement pathways.

(b) **Economic Burden of AV:** The economic burden of acne is substantial. This disorder is generally considered mild but represents a high economical and psychological burden for the society. Approximately 50 million individuals within the United States are affected by acne, making it one of the most common dermatological complaints in patients presenting to a general dermatology office [85]. Patients experience high levels of anxiety, depression, and low self-esteem which leads to impaired quality of life. Therefore, treatment should focus on early intervention to decrease the physical and esthetic burden of the disease, and improvement of quality of life [81]. The cost is estimated to exceed $1 billion per year in the USA for direct acne therapy, with $100 million spent on various acne products, as stated by Changqiang et.al, 2019 [75]. According to Bhate et. al, 2013, it was over 3 billion dollars per year in terms of treatment and loss of productivity [79]. With the rapid economic growth and concomitant changes in lifestyle in China, the demand for facial beauty has been surprisingly increased. In the general esthetic pursuit of fairer skin in East Asia, Chinese people increasingly pay attention to post-acne outcomes such as scars and PIH, in addition to the disease per se [76]. Zhang et.al, 2017 revealed that higher brand-name usage and a broader range of topical steroids prescribed by specialists than primary care, which were associated with increased costs. The most common drug class utilized was topical antibiotics, accounting for 63% of all prescriptions [77]. Acne affects a large proportion of the Canadian population and has psychosocial and financial consequences. A 2016 study shows Oral isotretinoin 3-month costs ranged from $400to $500 (approx.) [78]. Many methods have been performed to achieve a satisfying outcome in acne scars but some of them were high cost and also were associated with low results and some complications [80].

7.3.3 CLINICAL DIAGNOSIS

The diagnosis of AV is primarily clinical. The common differential diagnosis of acne includes folliculitis, keratosis pilaris, perioral dermatitis, seborrheic dermatitis and rosacea. History and physical examination can help determine if there is an underlying cause of the acne, such as an exacerbating medication or endocrinologic abnormality causing hyperandrogenism (e.g., polycystic ovarian syndrome). Other dermatologic manifestations of androgen excess include seborrhea, hirsutism and androgenetic alopecia. Endocrinologic testing is not ordered routinely for women with regular menstrual cycles. Older women, especially those with new-onset acne and other signs of androgen excess (e.g., hirsutism, androgenic alopecia, menstrual irregularities, infertility), should be tested for androgen excess with measurements of total and free serum testosterone, dihydroepiandrosterone, and luteinizing and follicle-stimulating hormone levels. Pelvic ultrasonography may show the presence of polycystic ovaries. In prepubertal children with acne, signs of hyperandrogenism include early-onset accelerated growth, pubic or axillary hair, body odor, genital maturation and advanced bone age [82].

Exhibit 4. Grading severity of acne [26], [82,83]

Grade	Severity	Clinical findings
I	**Mild**	Open and closed comedones (blackheads or whiteheads) with few inflammatory papules and pustules. Open comedones are due to plugging of the pilosebaceous orifice by sebum on the skin surface. Closed comedones are due to keratin and sebum plugging the pilosebaceous orifice below the skin surface. The more oil builds up, the more likely it is that bacteria will multiply and lead to inflammatory acne. Acne is also considered to be "mild acne" if someone only has a few pimples, or only has small ones.
II	**Moderate**	Inflammatory lesions present as a small papule with erythema. Inflamed pimples are called "papules" (small bumps) or "pustules" (filled with yellow pus), mainly on face.
III	**Moderately severe**	Numerous papules and pustules, and occasional inflamed nodules, also on chest and back
IV	**Severe**	People who have severe forms of acne have a lot of papules and pustules, as well as nodules on their skin. These nodules are often reddish and painful. The acne may lead to scarring.

Exhibit 5. Clinical Diagnosis of Acne [86], [89-100]

Diagnosis	Differentiating characteristics
Bacterial folliculitis	Abrupt eruption; spreads with scratching or shaving; variable distribution. Because both AV and folliculitis can present as inflammatory erythematous papules, pustules or nodules, they are often hard to distinguish.
Acne keloidalis nuchae	Often seen in black patients; lesions localized to the posterior neck; initially papules and pustules that may progress to confluent keloids
Acneiform eruptions	Secondary to systemic medications, topical corticosteroid medications, contrast dye, and cosmetic products; may be abrupt in onset and correlation with exposure; improvement with cessation of exposure.

Contd...

Chloracne	Comedones, pustules, and cysts that localize to the post-auricular area, axillae, and groin; history of exposure to halogenated aromatic hydrocarbons; patient may have other systemic manifestations
Favre-Racouchot	Open and closed comedones on periorbital and malar areas; no inflammatory lesions; patients are usually older with a history of significant sun exposure
Periorificial dermatitis	Papules and pustules in the periorificial distribution; often exacerbated by topical corticosteroid use
Pyoderma faciale	Rapid onset of erythema, abscesses, cysts, and possible sinus tracts, no comedones
Syringoma	Noninflammatory papules that typically localize to the eyelids and malar cheeks; skin biopsy test results show dilated cysts with tadpole appearance
Drug-induced acne	There are many causes for acneiform eruptions including exposure to halogenated aromatic hydrocarbons and use of antibiotics like macrolides and penicillin. Other drugs that can also induce acneiform eruptions include nystatin, isoniazid, corticotropin, naproxen, hydroxychloroquine, cyclosporin A, antimycotics, gold salts, isotretinoin, clofazimine, epidermal growth factor receptor inhibitors (cetuximab, gefitinib, and erlotinib), and interferon-beta.
Hidradenitis suppurativa (HS), also called acne inversus.	Double comedo; starts as a painful boil; sinus tracts. A nearly 40% of individuals with HS report an affected first-degree relative, suggesting a hereditary component with an autosomal dominant transmission pattern. It is a chronic inflammatory skin condition with lesions including deep-seated nodules and abscesses, draining tracts, and fibrotic scars. These lesions most commonly occur in intertriginous areas and areas rich in apocrine glands. Among the most common are axillary, groin, perianal, perineal, and inframammary locations.
Miliaria	"Heat rash" in response to exertion or heat exposure; non-follicular papules, pustules, and vesicles. Miliaria is a clinical diagnosis. Laboratory tests are often inconclusive and not helpful. Dermoscopy has been found to be a useful tool, particularly in people with darker skin, revealing large white globules with surrounding darker halos (white bullseye). When in doubt, a skin punch biopsy would be useful to help with diagnosis.
Perioral dermatitis	Papules and pustules confined to the chin and nasolabial folds; clear zone around the vermilion border.

Contd...

Adenoma sebaceum	Small waxy papules over the medial cheeks, nose, and forehead; multiple lesions associated with tuberous sclerosis; skin biopsy test results show dermal fibrosis and vascular proliferation and dilatation (angiofibromas). Facial angiofibromas are also a feature of multiple endocrine neoplasia type I and, rarely, Birt-Hogg-Dubé syndrome.
Pseudofolliculitis barbae	Affects curly-haired persons who regularly shave closely, with a high prevalence in men of subequatorial African ancestry and, to a much lesser extent, Indo-Europeans. But it can affect both men and women of all ethnicities. Invariably reported as being associated with shaving, also evidence suggests a strong genetic component in patients with persistent PFB.
Rosacea	Erythema and telangiectasias; no comedones. Rosacea can also involve the eyes and even a bulbous nose. Acne is seen most commonly in teens, while rosacea occurs most often much later. Also, unlike in patients with rosacea, blackheads are generally present, and bumps and pimples on the trunk and arms are common.
Seborrheic dermatitis	Greasy scales and yellow-red coalescing macules or papules. Seborrheic dermatitis presents as ill-defined erythematous patches with greasy scale distributed on the eyebrows, glabella, paranasal skin, nasolabial folds, beard, scalp, and chest. Azelaic acid may be especially valuable in this application because of its efficacy in treating concomitant rosacea and acne.

Exhibit 6. Laboratory tests in patients with suspected hormonal acne [29]	
Testosterone	Minimal to modest elevations of <200 ng/dL are suggestive of a benign cause of ovarian or adrenal cause while above this level; neoplasia of ovarian or adrenal origin should be suspected.
Androstenedione	Secreted equally by ovaries and adrenals and follows a circadian rhythm making early morning samples, the best to analyze.
DHEA	High levels of DHEA >8,000 ng/dL and dehydroepiandrosterone sulfate (DHEAS) should raise concern of adrenal tumors, while levels of DHEAS (4,000–8,000 ng/dL) indicate benign adrenal hyperplasia.
SHBG	Decreased levels of SHBG lead to free unbound testosterone in excess, resulting in more manifested signs.
Prolactin	Elevated prolactin could point out to hypothalamic or pituitary causes for further assessment and investigation.

Contd...

17-Hydroxy progesterone	Elevated (>200 ng/dl) in congenital adrenal hyperplasia or non-classic congenital adrenal hyperplasia due to deficiency or absence of 21α-hydroxylase.
Luteinizing hormone	Follicle-stimulating hormone (FSH) ratio: a ratio of >2 is indicative of possible PCOS.
Fasting and postprandial insulin	Overweight and obese patients should be checked for insulin levels.
Serum cortisol	High levels are an indication of adrenal neoplasia.

7.3.4 ACNE SCARS

Acne affects the face in a majority of cases, with many patients experiencing some degree of scarring, the severity of which correlates to acne grade. Acne scars result from an altered wound healing response to cutaneous inflammation, with inflammatory cell infiltrates found in nearly 80% of atrophic scars. Almost all scars (99%) originate from papules and pustules (inflammatory lesions) and post-inflammatory lesions [175]. Different P. acnes phylotypes differentially activate epidermal innate immunity, contributing to variations in acne severity. In patients not prone to scarring, early lesions have a large, nonspecific immune response that subsides in resolving lesions. In contrast, in patients prone to scarring, early lesions are characterized by a smaller number of skin-homing CD4+ T-cells compared to non-scarring patients, a response that becomes more active in resolving lesions [141]. Studies report the incidence of acne scarring in the general population to be 1 to 11%. Having acne scars can be emotionally and psychologically distressing to patients. Rather than fading with time, the appearance of scars often worsens with normal aging or photodamage [137].

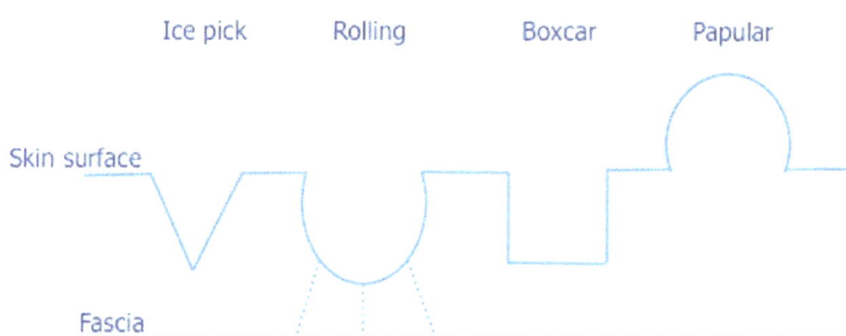

Figure 7.2 Acne Scar Types [139]. Ice pick scars are narrow, deep, and extend vertically to the deep dermis or subcutaneous tissue. Rolling scars occur from fibrous anchoring of the dermis to the subcutis, leading to superficial shadowing and an undulating appearance to the overlying skin. Boxcar scars are round-to-oval depressions with sharply demarcated vertical edges. Papular scars, unlike the depressed morphology of ice pick, rolling, and boxcar scars, are exophytic in nature and produce a cobblestone-like appearance.

Exhibit 7. Acne Effects [83], [136-140]	
Atrophic scars	Atrophic acne scarring is an unfortunate, permanent complication of AV, which may be associated with significant psychological distress. It is most likely related to inflammatory mediators and enzymatic degradation of collagen fibers and subcutaneous fat. The most basic, practical, system divides atrophic acne scars into the following three main types: a) icepick, b) rolling, and c) boxcar scars
(a) Icepack	Icepick scars are narrow (<2 mm), deep, sharply margined epithelial tracts that extend vertically to the deep dermis or subcutaneous tissue.
(b) Rolling	Rolling scars occur from dermal tethering of otherwise relatively normal-appearing skin and are usually wider than 4 to 5 mm. Abnormal fibrous anchoring of the dermis to the subcutis leads to superficial shadowing and a rolling or undulating appearance to the overlying skin.
(c) Boxcar	Boxcar scars are round to oval depressions with sharply demarcated vertical edges, similar to varicella scars. They are clinically wider at the surface than icepick scars and do not taper to a point at the base.
Hypertrophic scars	These raised scars can form on chest, back or shoulders, particularly in people who have severe acne. They develop if too much connective tissue is produced while the wound is healing. This type of acne scar is less common.
Papular Scars	Papular scars can clinically mimic closed comedones, acne, and granulomas, leading to an unnecessary delay in appropriate treatment. Active acneiform lesions causing any type of scars should be treated aggressively with systemic therapy to prevent further progression of scarring. Papular scars are 3 to 4mm skin-colored cobblestone-like papules distributed anywhere on the body but, in our clinical experience, most commonly on the chin, nose, and back. Also known as white papular acne scars, these flesh-colored papules are often incorrectly diagnosed as acne and do not respond to traditional acne treatments.
Keloid Scars	Keloids result from abnormal wound healing in response to skin trauma or inflammation. Keloid development rests on genetic and environmental factors. Higher incidences are seen in darker skinned individuals of African, Asian, and Hispanic descent. Keloid scars also form when too much connective tissue is made. Unlike hypertrophic scars, though, they are bigger than the original inflamed area. This is a very rare type of acne scarring. In keloids, the fibroblastic phase continues, unchecked, resulting in the clinical and histopathological findings.

7.3.5 PSYCHOLOGICAL IMPACT OF AV

Along with acne, having acne scars is a risk factor for suicide and also may be linked to poor self-esteem, depression, anxiety, altered social interactions, body image alterations, embarrassment, anger, lowered academic performance, and unemployment [137]. Studies have also shown that the psychological impact of acne appears to affect more females than males [35]. Facial appearance has an important role in self-perception, as well as in the interaction with others; face lesions cause a significant impact on women's quality of life [147]. The psychological impact of acne is generally significant and largely underestimated; stress during professional and private life, anxiety and sleep quality, in particular, have a reciprocal relationship with disease susceptibility and severity [145]. Suicidal ideation was found in 6–7% of acne patients. Psychological issues such as social dysfunction such as reduced/avoidance of social interactions with peers and opposite gender also reported. Acne can negatively influence the intension to participate in sports [142]. Psychiatric symptoms such as somatization, obsession, sensitivity, hostility, phobia, paranoid ideation, and psychoticism were associated with this skin disorder [143]. The degree of impairment in QOL significantly increased with increase of clinical severity of acne, with presence of post acne hyper pigmentation and scarring. In a study in Middle East, 23% of acne female students reported that they had difficulty in sports because of acne; while, a study among Scottish students found that 10% of acne sufferers avoided swimming and other sports because of embarrassment [144]. The management of adult female acne should encompass not just medical treatment of the symptoms, but also a comprehensive, holistic approach to the patient as a whole, her lifestyle factors and the impact of acne on her quality of life [145]. Compared with heterosexuals, sexual minorities report higher rates of depression, suicidal ideation, and body image issues. Consequentially, sexual minorities with acne may be a group at high risk for development of mental health problems [146]. Sexual distress was particularly higher in female than in male patients with Acne Inversa. Surprisingly, the severity of cutaneous alterations correlated neither with sexual dysfunctions nor with sexual distress [148]. The relationship between isotretinoin and depression is the most debated aspect of isotretinoin therapy [149]. It is prudent for the practitioner to continue to use isotretinoin to treat severe acne, while at the same time informing patients and their relatives that depressive symptoms should be actively assessed at each visit and, if necessary, referral to a psychiatrist and a discontinuation of isotretinoin should be considered [150].

7.3.6 ACNE MANAGEMENT

In recent years, due to better understanding of the pathogenesis of acne, new therapeutic modalities and various permutation and combinations have been designed. In topical agents; benzoyl peroxide, antibiotics, retinoids, etc are the mainstay of treatment; can be given in combinations. While systemic therapy includes oral antibiotics, hormonal therapy, and isotretinoin, depending upon the need of patients it has to be selected. Physical treatment in the form of lesion removal, photo-therapy is also helpful in a few of them. Due to convenience, lower cost, and difficulty getting an appointment with a dermatologist, the use of over-the-counter acne treatments is on the rise. Commonly referred to as "cosmeceuticals," OTC acne treatments come in lotions, creams, washes, kits, scrubs, brushes, and devices. Due to the sheer number of different OTC brands, plus newer products constantly being developed, it is hard for both physicians and patients to keep abreast of the numerous products. However, all treatments for AV are theoretically designed to target one or more of the pathogenic pathways involved in the development of AV lesions. In moderate acne, combination therapy has shown the most favorable results and typically consists of a regimen including benzoyl peroxide, topical antibiotics, and a topical retinoid (tretinoin, adapalene, or tazorotene). Tretinoin, adapalene, and tazorotene demonstrate similar effectiveness in the reduction of inflammatory, noninflammatory, and total lesion counts after 12 weeks of treatment. Oral antibiotics may be tried for patients with a predominance of inflammatory lesions who have not responded favorably to the above topical treatments.

Exhibit 8. Different treatment options for acne [305]

Treatment Methods	Examples
Topical	Retinoids: adapalene, isotretinoin, motretinide, retinoyl-β-glucuronide, tazarotene, tretinoin
	Antibiotics: clindamycin, erythromycin
	Diverse: azelaic acid, benzoyl peroxide, chemical peels, corticosteroids, dapsone, hydrogen peroxide, niacinamide, salicylic acid, sodium sulfacetamide, sulfur, triclosan
Systemic	Retinoids: isotretinoin
	Antibiotics: azithromycin, clindamycin, co-trimoxazole, doxycycline, erythromycin, levofloxacin, lymecycline, minocycline, roxithromycin
	Hormonal: contraceptives
	Diverse: clofazimine, corticosteroids, ibuprofen, zinc sulfate
Complementary and Alternative Medicines (CAM)	*Achillea millefolium*, amaranth, antimicrobial peptides, arnica, asparagus, basil oil, bay, benzoin, birch, bittersweet nightshade, black cumin, black walnut, borage, Brewer's yeast, burdock root, calendula, celandine, chamomile, chaste tree, *Commiphora mukul*, copaiba oil, coriander, cucumber, duckweed, Du Zhong extract, English walnut, *Eucalyptus dives*,

Contd...

	fresh lemon, garlic, geranium, grapefruit seeds, green tea, jojoba oil, juniper twig, labrador tea, lemon grass, lemon, minerals, neem, oak bark, onion, orange peel, orange, Oregon grape root, patchouli, pea, petitgrain, pine, pomegranate rind extract, poplar, probiotics, pumpkin, resveratrol, rose myrtle, rhubarb, *Rosa damascena*, rosemary, rue, safflower oil, sandalwood, seaweed, soapwort, *Sophora flavescens*, specific antibodies, stinging nettle, sunflower oil, *Taraxacum officinale*, taurine bromamine, tea tree oil, thyme, turmeric, vinegar, vitex, witch hazel, *Withania somnifera* and yerba mate extract
Physical Treatment	Comedone extraction, cryoslush therapy, cryotherapy, electrocauterization, intralesional corticosteroids and optical treatments

7.3.7 ACNE PREVENTION

The relationship between diet and acne is highly controversial. Several studies during the last decade have led dermatologists to reflect on a potential link between diet and acne. Selected dietary factors on the course of AV are milk and dairy products, chocolate, glycemic load of the diet, dietary fiber, fatty acids, antioxidants, zinc, vitamin A and iodine.

(a) *Milk and dairy products*: High intakes (≥2 glasses per day) of full-fat dairy products were associated with moderate to severe acne. No significant associations were found between acne and intake of semi-skimmed or skimmed dairy products, and not with moderate intakes of any fat variety of dairy products [151]. Also, no significant association between yogurt/cheese and acne development was observed by Aghasi et.al, 2018 [152]. However, a person can reduce or prevent acne breakouts by consuming fewer dairy products, and fewer foods with a high glycemic index. Acne that occurs after ingestion of foods rich in iodine appears suddenly and is characterized by many papules. The association between acne and milk may also be a result of the iodine content of milk [9].

(b) *Chocolate Restriction*: Chocolate consumption primed human blood mononuclear cells to release more proinflammatory cytokines, interleukin-1β, and TNFα, upon stimulation with Propionibacterium acnes. Because over-inflammation is an important contributor to acne pathogenesis and the anti-inflammatory dose effect of antibiotics has been demonstrated to be most effective in treating acne, it is plausible that altered cytokine profiles can contribute to worsening acne [154]. Dark chocolate contains more antioxidants than milk chocolate, which would lead to the conclusion that it may have much smaller comedogenic effects [9]. Some say that avoiding things like meat, milk or chocolate improved their complexion.

(c) *Glycemic Load*: The improvement in acne and insulin sensitivity after a low-glycemic-load diet suggests that nutrition-related lifestyle factors may play a role in the pathogenesis of acne [155]. A high glycemic index (GI) and glycemic load (GL) diet may stimulate acne proliferative pathways by influencing biochemical factors associated with acne. A low GI and GL diet decreased IGF-1 concentrations, a well-established factor in acne pathogenesis [156]. Having fast food like fries/chips and soda can dramatically increase the calories, carbohydrate, fat, and GL of the nutritionally promoted fast-food meal [157]. Cordain et.al, 2002 suggested that a low-fat intake and low glycemic load diet may be the cause of acne absence in both populations [158]. Processed foods, especially those with a high glycemic index, have been known to exacerbate acne. One study found that a control group consuming more fish and vegetables had a lower incidence rate of acne. Therefore, adopting a whole foods diet and reducing the intake of dairy products may help significantly reduce acne [159].

(d) *Dietary Fiber*: Patients with AV consumed daily 30 g of high fiber breakfast cereal (13 g fiber/serving), a significant improvement in the skin condition was shown [159]. Fiber aids elimination of toxins and used hormones from the body. Fruits, vegetables, oats, other whole grains, beans and lentils are good sources. Some soluble dietary fiber components, such as oat bran, pectin, and guar gum, stimulate fecal excretion of bile acids. High fiber intakes promote increased bacterial mass but do not alter the microflora composition [160]. Gastrointestinal dysfunction is an important risk factor for diseases of the sebaceous glands and is correlated with their occurrence and development [161], conversely proper digestion improves acne conditions. One study involving over 13,000 adolescents showed that those with acne were more likely to experience gastrointestinal symptoms such as constipation, halitosis, and gastric reflux. In particular, abdominal bloating was 37% more likely to be associated with acne and other seborrheic diseases [162].

(e) *Anti-oxidants*: Al-Shobaili, 2014 revealed that plasma levels of malondialdehyde in acne patients were significantly higher as compared with that of the controls, whereas activities of the antioxidant enzymes superoxide dismutase and catalase were lower. Moreover, total antioxidant capacity was also low in acne patients as compared with that of the controls [39]. Polyphenols are antioxidant molecules found in many foods including nuts, fruits, vegetables, chocolate, wine, and tea. Polyphenols have antimicrobial, anti-inflammatory, and antineoplastic properties. Recent studies suggest that tea polyphenols may be used for reducing sebum production in the skin and for treatment of AV. Again, green tea and green tea-lotus combination topicals could be used to treat skin diseases that are associated with increased sebum secretion, such as AV [163-165]. Apple polyphenols (APP) inhibited Dexamethasone-induced lipid production and expression of sterol response element-binding protein-1 and its target enzymes, acetyl-CoA carboxylase and fatty acid synthase, in the sebocytes. Thus, APP may be useful to regulate sebum production and may alleviate sebum-involved skin disease [166]. Low vitamin A, E and zinc plasma levels have an important role in the pathogenesis of acne and in the aggravation of this condition. Supportive treatment with these vitamins and zinc in severe acne may lead to satisfactory results [167], [114].

(f) *Frequent Cleansing and Sun Protection*: Washing and over-the-counter cleansers are common interventions in AV, but the clinical evidence for their benefit is poorly understood [168]. Cleansers reduced both inflammatory and non-inflammatory acne lesion counts, and might be helpful for acne treatment [169]. In addition to containing dyes and perfumes that can irritate and exacerbate acne, these cleansers often are too harsh and can result in excessive drying of the skin, which leads to overcompensation by the oil glands and ultimately to more oil on the surface of the skin [170]. However, cleansing the acne patient involves several considerations, including matching skin type to the right type of cleanser, optimal times and methods of cleansing, treating parts of the body other than the face, and patient perceptions of the cause and treatment of acne. Soap-free cleansing products that have a similar pH to skin (5.5) are more suitable for people with acne. A reference pH range of 4.5 to 5.5 was considered normal for women, and 4 to 5.5 was considered normal for men. Studies have shown that lowering the pH reduces the inflammatory TH2 response (CD4+ cells, orchestrate protective type 2 immune responses) and quickens barrier function recovery, thereby preventing epidermal hyperproliferation [171]. While sunscreens are often irritants, the best options for young, oily, acne-prone skin tend to have a water or light liquid base. Moisturizing sunscreens are appropriate for patients with dry, sun-damaged skin, as well as those who wear makeup, have other skin diseases, or are easily irritated by products [44].

(g) *Avoid Stress/Tobacco*: Stress is a well-attested contributor to AV pathogenesis. The basis for the association between emotional stress and the onset or exacerbation of acne is in several cutaneous neurogenic factors which interact with a pathogenic cascade in acne. Stress stimulates the release of pro-inflammatory cytokines and CRH, leading to increased levels of cortisol. Sleep deprivation associated with modern lifestyle and stress have an important impact on the hypothalamic-pituitary-adrenal axis and in increased secretion of stress-related hormones, and may also be an aggravating factor for acne. Pythagorean Self-Awareness Intervention is a feasible and possibly effective stress management method for AV [258-260]. Clinical evidence and experimental data showed a straight correlation between smoking habit and post-pubertal acne in which the clinically non-inflammatory (atypical) post-adolescent acne is the most frequent [131].The comedonal form predominates in smokers and is characterized by the presence of micro and macro-comedones and few inflammatory lesions, which led the authors to describe this clinical form as "smoker's face." The sebaceous gland is sensitive to acetylcholine that is stimulated by nicotine. Acetylcholine leads to cellular modulation and differentiation, inducing hyper-keratinization and influencing sebum production and composition, as well as reducing antioxidant agents and increasing peroxidation of sebum components, such as squalene [261]. Among patients with adolescent acne, the probability to be affected by current acne in smokers was between 2.6–6.3 times higher than in non-smokers [131]. However, it is worth bearing in mind that many successful quitters have found it motivational to watch their skin regain its tone and elasticity just weeks after smoking cessation [262].

7.3.8 TOPICAL DRUGS

Topical treatment is the mainstay of acne therapy. The most commonly prescribed topical medications for acne include benzoyl peroxide, clindamycin, and retinoids. Despite their effectiveness in treating mild to moderate acne vulgaris, these topical medications are found to be irritating, and are historically associated with poor tolerability and diminished patient adherence. Thus, choosing the right formulation that will be effective and well tolerated is essential. Antibiotics targeting P. acnes have been the mainstay in acne treatment for the past four decades. Among them, macrolides, clindamycin, and tetracyclines are the most widely prescribed. Novel formulations that optimize drug concentration and utilize improved delivery vehicles have helped to enhance the tolerability and efficacy, and allow for less frequent application or co-application of drugs that were previously considered incompatible. In the near future, more effective treatments with less side effects are expected. The use of topical anti-androgens, coenzyme-A carboxylase inhibitors, and insulin growth factor-1inhibitors to control sebum production seem promising. Selective RAR-agonists have the potential of becoming an alternative to the currently available retinoid therapy in the management of infundibular dyskeratosis with a better safety profile. Antibiotic use will probably decline as more effective options for controlling *Cutinebacterium acnes* colonization and the inflammation cascade emerge.

A. Benzoyl Peroxide

Benzoyl peroxide (BP) has been an important component of topical therapy for acne vulgaris for more than five decades due to its ability to markedly reduce *Propionibacterium acnes* and inflammatory acne lesions and its ability to moderately reduce noninflammatory acne lesions [180]. It has mild sebostatic and keratolytic effects without a concern for the development of drug-resistant bacteria. Studies suggested that AEs at the application site occurred more often in Japanese patients than Western patients, most of the AEs were mild [172], [177]. It is most effective when used in combination with other acne vulgaris therapies [35]. BP is a bactericidal agent. Combining BP with a topical antibiotic in a stable formulation has been proven in clinical trials to reduce total P acnes count by 99.7% after 1 week of therapy, eliminating both susceptible and resistant strains of P acnes [179]. However, we have recently noticed BP's benefits as monotherapy in the treatment of acne. Topical BP also has mild sebostatic effects contributing to its keratolytic activity and efficacy in treating comedonal acne. BP is available as both over-the-counter and prescription formulations in concentrations of 2.5%, 5%, and 10% [82]. Available preparations include lotions, creams, gels, foams, solutions, cleansing bars, cleansing lotions, cloths, pads, masks, and shaving creams. Each application vehicle has specific instructions for the frequency of use. Combination products with BP and topical antibiotics or adapalene are more effective than either medication used alone [173]. Concentrations of BP above 5% are not recommended for use in adult women. It can also cause photosensitivity and bleaching of clothing [35]. It is used as 2.5%, 4% and 5% concentration in gel base [26]. BP in concentrations of 2.5%, 5% and 10% are equally effective at treating inflammatory acne. However, higher concentrations are associated with more adverse effects. It useful as monotherapy for mild acne or as an adjunct in the treatment of moderate to severe acne vulgaris [178]. Comedonal acne is more typical in young adolescents, but can occur in combination with inflammatory papules and pustules at any time. Topical retinoids have long been advocated for the treatment of comedonal acne. Adapalene 0.3%- BP 2.5% was found to be effective in patients with severe acne. Clindamycin-BP 1.2%/3.75% gel and clindamycin-BP 1.2%/2.5% gel was both found to be effective in severe acne with an apparent BP-dose response [181]. Clindamycin 1.2%-BP 3.75% gel may afford similar benefits to adapalene 0.3%-BP 2.5% gel in this sometimes difficult to treat patient population [174]. When acupuncture was combined with BP, serum excretion rate in women was reduced compared to BP alone [176]. In addition to use for facial acne vulgaris, cleanser formulations of BP are commonly used for truncal AV due to ease of use on a large body-surface area and to avoid bleaching of fabric. Short contact therapy utilizing a 2-minute skin contact time with BP 9.8% emollient foam used once daily over a 2-week duration was highly effective in reducing the quantity of P acnes organisms on the back and provided comparable colony count reduction to "leave on" therapy using BP 5.3% emollient foam [182]. The FDA classifies benzoyl peroxide as pregnancy risk category C [186].

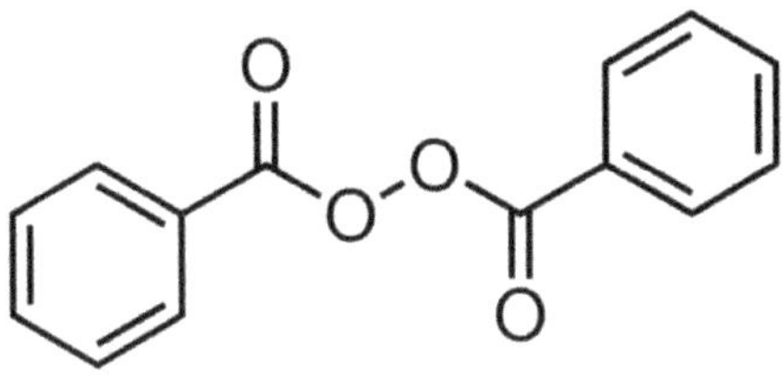

Figure 7.3 Benzoyl peroxide

B. Clindamycin

Due to the significant increase of P. acnes strains resistant to clindamycin and erythromycin, the use of these substances alone is contra-indicated [185]. *Cutibacterium acnes* (C. acnes) can become an exacerbating factor in acne vulgaris, where clindamycin was found to be resistant, as reported by Aoki et.al, 2019 [187]. Clindamycin can be administered into the body by multiple routes. It is available topically as a foam, gel, lotion, or solution for treatment of acne vulgaris. The most common side effects experienced with topical use include pruritis, xeroderma, erythema, burning, exfoliation, or oily skin [183]. Treatment with clindamycin phosphate 1.2% and tretinoin 0.025% resulted in continuous improvement of facial acne over 12 weeks, along with improved QOL and a tolerable safety profile, supporting the use of this combination in clinical practice [184]. Tolerability profile of ClinP/Tret gel is beneficial when combining different topical therapies and formulations in a given patient, as cutaneous irritation is an adverse factor that can reduce adherence and prevent a successful therapeutic outcome [189]. It is also easy for patients to handle and apply, and has the advantage of not containing BP which can bleach hair and fabrics [190]. ClinP/Tret gel has a favorable safety profile following UV/visible irradiation and a low potential for phototoxicity and photo-allergy, currently available for the once-daily topical treatment of acne [191]. Patients with Fitzpatrick Skin Type V and VI treated with clindamycin phosphate 1.2%/ BP 3.75% gel experienced significant reductions in facial acne severity, lesion counts and PIH severity/distribution. Tolerability was excellent [188]. A triple-combination regimen incorporating oral minocycline (dosed by patient weight), BP foaming cloths 6% QD, and clindamycin phosphate 1.2%/ tretinoin 0.025% gel QD can substantially improve moderate to severe acne vulgaris [192]. Zeichner et.al, 2013 reported similar cutaneous S/Es with a fixed-dose tretinoin 0.025%/clindamycin phosphate 1.2% gel in combination with a benzoyl peroxide 6% foaming cloth compared with ClinP/Tret gel alone for facial acne [193]. Clindamycin often discussed along with the macrolides but are not chemically related, it belongs to a group of medicines known as lincosamide or lincomycin antibiotics. Clindamycin is pregnancy category B.

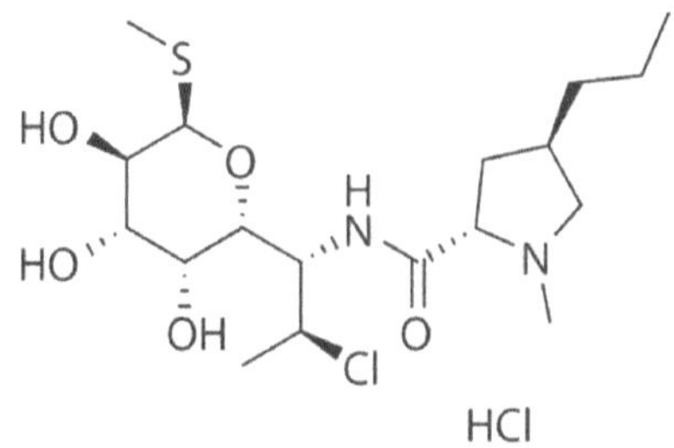

Figure 7.4 Clindamycin Hydrochloride

C. Retinoids

Topical retinoids are creams, lotions and gels containing medicine derived from Vitamin A. These compounds result in proliferation and reduced keratinization of skin cells independent of their functions as a vitamin and devoid of bacterial resistance. American Academy of Dermatology (AAD) states "retinoids are the core of topical therapy for acne because they are comedolytic, resolve the precursor microcomedone lesion, and are anti-inflammatory;" further, they "allow for maintenance of clearance" [194]. Local adverse effects, including erythema, dryness, itching, and stinging, occur frequently during the early treatment phase. Their impact varies with the vehicle formation, skin type, frequency and mode of application, use of moisturizers, and environmental factors such as sun exposure or temperature [195]. Retinoids act to normalize desquamation by reducing keratinocyte proliferation and promoting differentiation. Isotretinoin, tretinoin, and tazarotene also suppress Toll-like receptor expression. Blocking these pathways reduces the release of inflammatory cytokines and nitric oxide and inhibits cellular inflammation [194]. Topical retinoids are safe and efficacious for the treatment of AV. They should be used in combination with benzoyl peroxide to optimize results in patients. Adapalene has a superior tolerability profile amongst topical retinoids [199]. Developed in response to concerns about the instability of tretinoin, the naphthoic acid derivative adapalene was found in vitro to be photostable and not degraded in the presence of BP. Again, adapalene/BP was rated as more successful with a significantly greater reduction in all lesions counts compared to any other therapy after the trial [204]. Higher concentrations of retinoids such as adapalene 0.3%/BP 2.5% have shown increased efficacy, particularly among patients with moderately severe and severe acne – a population at high risk for scarring [196]. Adapalene supplied as a 0.1% cream, gel, and lotion and 0.3% gel are prescription only products. It is less irritating compared to other topical retinoids, applied once daily, either in the morning or at bedtime to a clean face. The patient should be advised to wash the face with a gentle cleanser and allow the face to dry thoroughly [197]. Tretinoin 0.05% gel exhibits a greater anti-acne efficacy than adapalene 0.1% gel, but has higher skin irritation potential [198]. Chandrashekhar et.al, 2015 stated tretinoin 0.025% nanogel formulation is more efficacious and better tolerated than its conventional 0.05% gel formulation [200]. Harper et.al, 2019 detailed a similar polymeric formulation of tretinoin 0.05% lotion with an incidence of erythema, dryness, and skin burning [201]. Combination of tretinoin 0.05% cream and Aloe vera topical gel (50%) with was well tolerated and significantly more effective than tretinoin 0.05% cream alone for the treatment of mild to moderate acne vulgaris [202]. Deshmukh et. al, 2019 found that topical combination of 1% Nadifloxacin and 0.025% Tretinoin was caused greater reduction in facial acne lesions than 1% Clindamycin and 0.025% Tretinoin in patients of mild to moderate AV. This could be due to the fact that Nadifloxacin is reported to have potent action against P. acnes, *Staphylococcus epidermidis*, and methicillin-resistant *Staphylococcus aureus* (MRSA), with no cross-resistance [203].

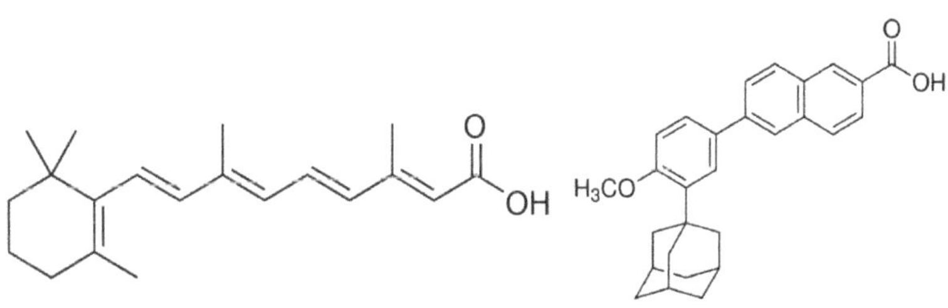

Tretinoin Adapalene

Figure 7.5 Retinoids

Exhibit 9. News of celebrities who got rid of their acne	
News	**Comment**
Natalie Portman says going vegan changed everything [129].	The frequency of vegetables and fish intake was significantly higher in the control group than in the acne group [54].
Victoria Beckham eats a lot of salmon [129].	Salmon is rich omega-3 fatty acids. There is some evidence that fish oil supplementation is associated with an improvement in overall acne severity, especially for individuals with moderate to severe acne [130].
Rihanna cuts back on booze. I cut out all alcohol and overdo the water," she said [129].	Among patients with adolescent acne, the probability to be affected by current acne in smokers was between 2.6–6.3 times higher than in non-smokers.

Contd...

Scarlett Johansson always washes her face and makeup brushes [129]	Antibacterial face washes can have a positive effect in mild acne, but might also irritate more sensitive skin. There is no clear evidence that acne vulgaris is related to poor hygiene or that frequent face washing lessens acne [82]. Acne is unavoidable but can be controlled by regular washing of the face by a pH balancing wash which is available as benzoyl peroxide and salicylic acid face wash [26].
Cameron Diaz wrote that fast food was plaguing her skin. In "The Body Book," Diaz wrote "My acne wasn't totally gone, but it was significantly better." [129]	Plenty of fast-food items are high on the glycemic index, elicit a rapid shift in blood glucose and insulin levels. Insulin also stimulates the synthesis of androgens leading to high sebum production, a recognized correlate of acne severity [10]. On the contrary, low-glycemic-index foods increased SHBG and reduced androgen levels; this is important since higher SHBG levels were associated with lower acne severity [11].
"Whenever it's been really bad, I've gone to the dermatologist to get those cortisone shots. Those are amazing....." Emma Stone [132].	Low doses of corticosteroids, such as prednisone (2.5 or 5mg), can suppress adrenal androgen production and are recommended in late congenital adrenal hyperplasia, acute inflammatory lesions in AFA, and short-term treatment of very severe acne [35]. While short-term use of corticosteroids is associated with mild side effects, long-term use can result in hypertension, peptic ulcer disease, ocular damage, neuropsychiatric effects, hematologic and musculoskeletal effects. Patients need close monitoring and follow up and should also be advised not to exceed the prescribed treatment and to only discontinue use under medical supervision [133,134].
After years of struggling with breakouts, Bella Thorne turned to the powerful anti-acne drug Accutane [132].	Isotretinoin is a vitamin A-derivative 13-cis-retinoic acid, which is the most effective therapy for acne to date. It targets all four processes during acne development, including normalization of follicular desquamation, reduction of sebaceous gland activity, inhibition of the proliferation of *Propionibacterium acnes* and anti-inflammatory effects. It cured around 85% of patients after an average treatment course of 4 months. However, the risk of depression associated with the use of isotretinoin has been a major concern for a long time [75].

Contd...

"I never used to understand the importance of washing my brushes, but it's so important" Miley Cyrus [132]	With each use, your makeup brushes become coated with more than just residue. They pick up sebum, dead skin and airborne dust and dirt. They need to be cleaned regularly AND properly. If not, all of this debris will build up and negatively affect future makeup applications and decrease the life expectancy of brushes. The most dangerous consequence of dirty brushes – they become a playground for bacteria that can cause skin problems and possible infection [135].

(a) **Azelaic Acid:** Azelaic acid is a naturally occurring saturated C9-dicarboxylic acid which is shown to be effective in the treatment of comedonal acne and inflammatory acne, as well as hiperpigmentary skin disorders [210]. It is an antiacne drug by inhibiting thioredoxin reductase enzyme of *Propionibacterium acnes* that affects the inhibition of bacterial DNA synthesis which occurs in the cytoplasm. Azelaic acid (20% cream or 15% gel) is recommended as the first line of treatment in monotherapy for non-inflammatory and inflammatory acne, applied twice a day [35]. Azelaic acid 15% foam is effective and safe in the treatment of facial acne vulgaris [205]. Treatment with azelaic acid 20 % cream significantly improves acne severity and disease-related QoL in adult women [209]. Azelaic acid must penetrate through the stratum corneum to the sebaceous tissue and into cytoplasm by passing through thick peptidoglycan of P. acnes. Thus, it is necessary to increase the penetration of azelaic acid that formulated based ethosome. Azelaic acid ethosome-based cream showed better activity to against P. acnes than marketed azelaic acid preparation (Zelface® cream) [206]. Combined azelaic acid 20% and salicylic acid 20% are recommended at early stage of treatment if patients have more inflammatory lesions, while trichloroacetic acid 25% chemical peel is recommended if patients have more non-inflammatory lesions. Chemical peeling is effective in controlling mild-moderate acne in SPT III-IV (Fitzpatrick skin type) [207]. Again, a hormonal blockade conducted by ethinylestradiol plus a new generation of progesterone derived of spironolactone with anti-androgenic activity was compared to topical treatment with azelaic acid, it showed better statistical improvement in women with mild to moderate acne [208].

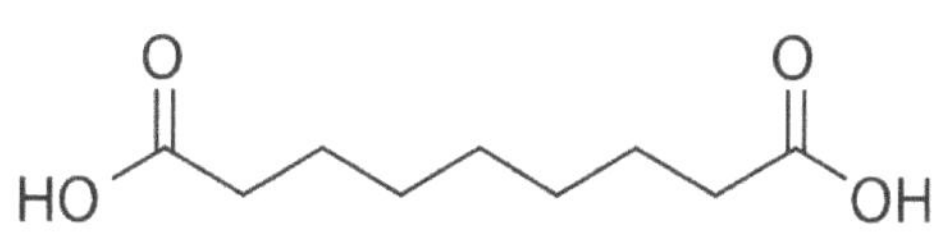

Figure 7.6 Azelaic Acid

(b) **Dapsone:** Topical dapsone is used for both comedonal and papular acne, though there are some concerns with G6PD deficient individuals [26]. Treatment of AV with dapsone gel, 5% requires twice-daily dosing, and some patients may not adhere to this regimen. Dapsone gel, 7.5% applied topically once daily is an effective, safe, and well-tolerated treatment for acne over 12 weeks and offers similar local tolerability compared with vehicle and had a safety and tolerability profile similar to that of twice-daily dapsone gel, 5% in patients aged ≥12 years [218,219], [221], [223,224]. However, Monotherapy with dapsone gel, 5% administered twice daily was safe and effective for treatment of facial acne in women with and well tolerated in patients with all skin phototypes who were treated for moderate acne [220], [222]. Dapsone 7.5% gel is a viable option to add to the armamentarium for treatment of truncal AV [216]. Draelos et.al, 2017 found that Treatment response with dapsone gel, 7.5% in racial subgroups was similar [225]. Tanghetti et.al, 2018 revealed that once-daily dapsone gel, 7.5% was efficacious for acne regardless of baseline total lesion count, with superior efficacy in females and similar tolerability in males and females [226]. It has been shown to be useful when combined with doxycycline and then alone as maintenance for long periods, with the advantage of having no risk for bacterial resistance in patients with AV [35]. The combination oral doxycycline hyclate 100 mg with topical dapsone 5% gel twice daily is an effective and well-tolerated regimen to treat moderate to severe acne vulgaris. After discontinuation of doxycycline, topical dapsone 5% gel is effective at maintaining a therapeutic response. Topical dapsone 5% gel can be used effectively for long-term acne maintenance treatment without the risk of developing antibiotic resistance [217]. Incorporation of dapsone in methylprednisolone aceponate 0.1 % ointment broaden the therapeutic options for topical treatment, in particular for patients with chronic inflammatory dermatoses associated with a neutrophilic pathogenesis [212]. Drugs which inhibit cytochrome P-450 should be used with caution in patients receiving dapsone [213]. Careful patient selection and close monitoring during treatment are mandatory to provide safe and effective use of dapsone [215]. Bilosomes as novel vesicular carrier for the cutaneous delivery of the sulfone compound, Dapsone, for topical treatment of acne represented about 1.5-fold higher drug retained in the bilosomes treated skin, compared to dapsone alcoholic solution. [214].

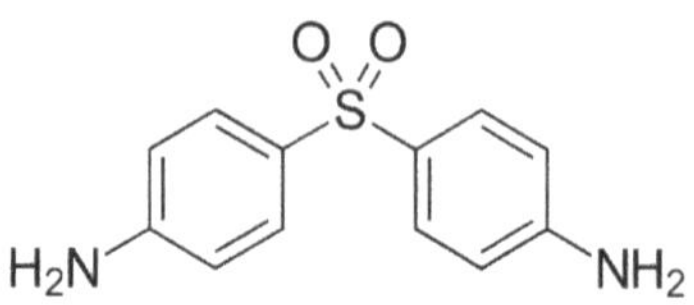

Figure 7.7 Dapsone

(c) **Acetyl Coenzyme A Carboxylase Inhibitor:** The increasing emergence of microbial resistance associated with antibiotics, teratogenicity, particularly associated with systemic isotretinoin, and the need for an adverse drug profile, which can be tolerated by the patient, make the need of new pathogenesis relevant anti-acne agents an emerging issue. The compounds under investigation include olumacostat glasaretil, cortexolone 17α-propionate, stearoyl-CoA desaturase 1 inhibitors, agents affecting the melanocortin system, omiganan, and minocycline [229]. Olumacostat glasaretil (OG) is a small molecule inhibitor of acetyl coenzyme A (CoA) carboxylase (ACC), the enzyme that controls the first rate-limiting step in fatty acid biosynthesis. Inhibition of ACC activity in the sebaceous glands is designed to substantially affect sebum production, because over 80% of human sebum components contain fatty acids. OG inhibits de novo lipid synthesis in primary and transformed human sebocytes, including the synthesis of triglycerides, diglycerides, cholesteryl esters, wax esters, and phospholipids [226]. OG was well tolerated and showed evidence of efficacy [227]. It reduces both saturated and monounsaturated fatty acyl chains in sebaceous lipids. Topical OG application decreases hamster ear sebaceous gland size and shows efficacy in treating patients with acne vulgaris [228]. Triglycerides and fatty acids together make up the largest portion of sebum content; therefore, OG has the potential to decrease sebum output. Further, when evaluated in animal models, topical OG consistently reduced sebaceous gland size. Dermira, a biopharmaceutical company, released data from a Phase 2b trial conducted for a topical sebum production inhibitor, OG (formerly DRM01) [229].

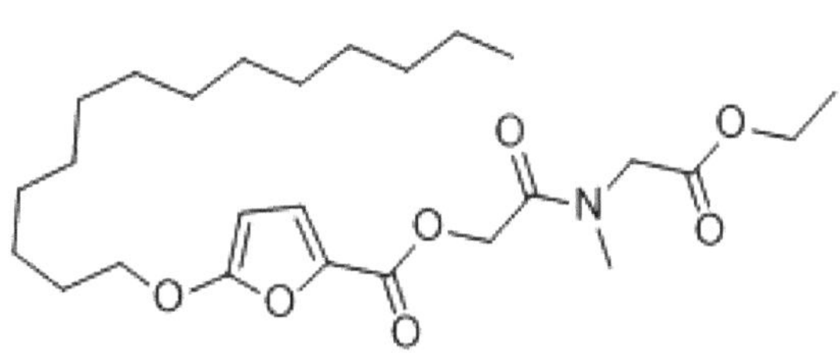

Figure 7.8 Olumacostat glasaretil

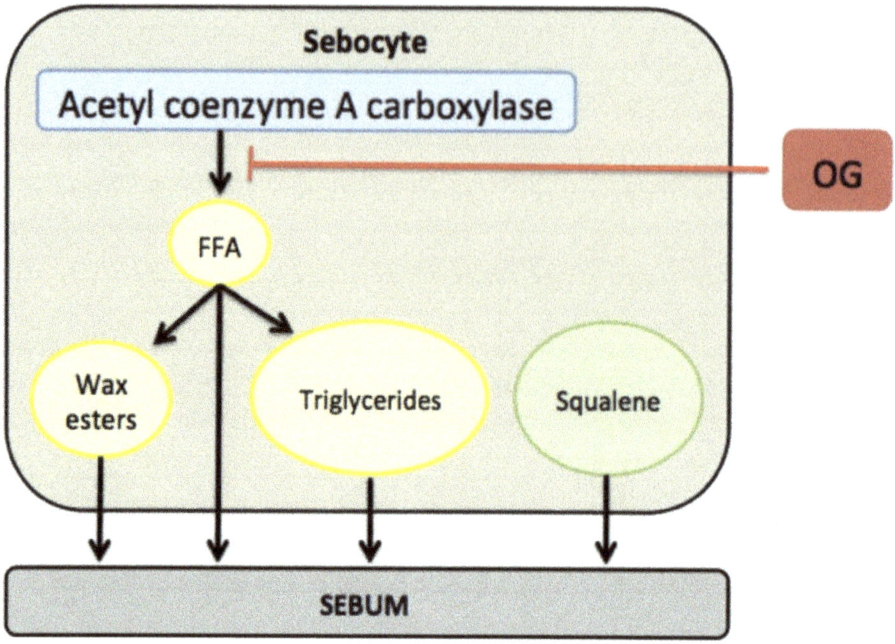

Figure 7.9 Olumacostat glasaretil (OG) blocks acetyl coenzyme-A carboxylase in sebocytes to inhibit the production of free fatty acids (FFA) [229]

(d) **Topical Anti-androgens:** Topical spironolactone may be effective for the treatment of acne patients with increased sebum secretion. The 5% spironolactone topical gel resulted in a decrease in the total acne lesions (TLC) in acne vulgaris, while it had no significant efficacy in the acne severity index [230]. RCTs have shown mixed results in the improvement of acne, which indicates that topical spironolactone gel is not an effective alternative for systemic spironolactone [231]. Cortexolone 17α-propionate 1% cream was very well tolerated, and was significantly better than placebo regarding TLC [232]. Cortexolone 17α-propionate competitively inhibits endogenous androgen binding at the human androgen receptor level without inhibiting the skin 5α-reductase. Cortexolone 17α-propionate 1% cream was also clinically more effective than tretinoin 0.05% cream but this difference was not statistically significant [98]. Stearoyl-CoA desaturase-1 (SCD-1) catalyzes the formation of delta9-monounsaturated fatty acids from saturated precursors. Upon topical application to the skin of mice as a 1% solution, XEN103 induces pronounced sebaceous gland atrophy with a rapid onset after a few days of dosing, both sebaceous gland numbers and size is reduced by 50 to 75%, and without any signs of skin irritation [233]. Omiganan pentahydrochloride is a synthetic, cationic, antimicrobial peptide that is being developed for the prevention of catheter-related infections and the treatment of acne and rosacea. It has been demonstrated to be rapidly bactericidal and fungicidal, with significant dose-dependent activity against a broad spectrum of infectious organisms. These results further confirm that the drug has the potential as a topical antimicrobial agent [234].

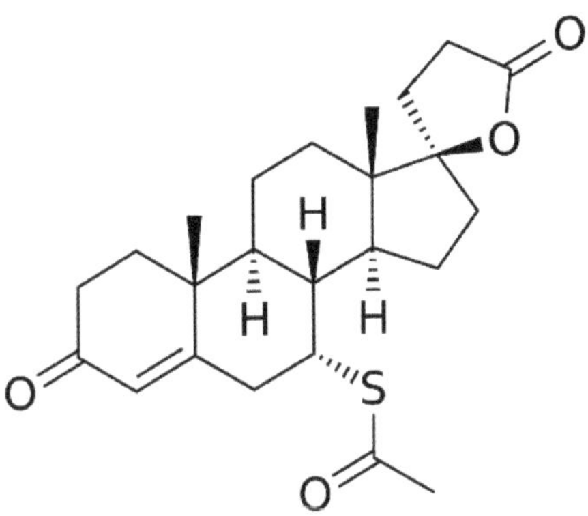

Spironolactone

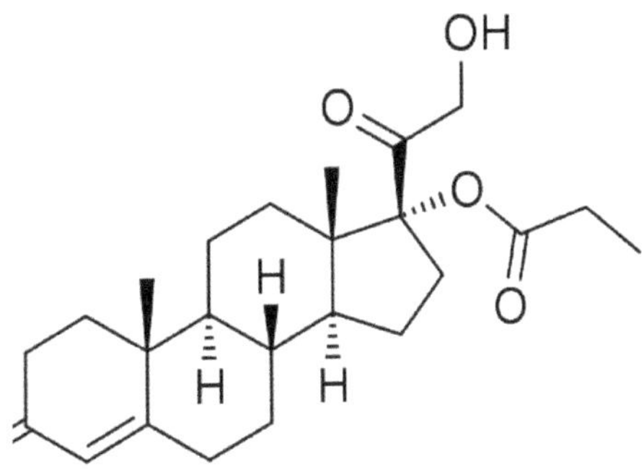

Cortexolone 17α-propionate

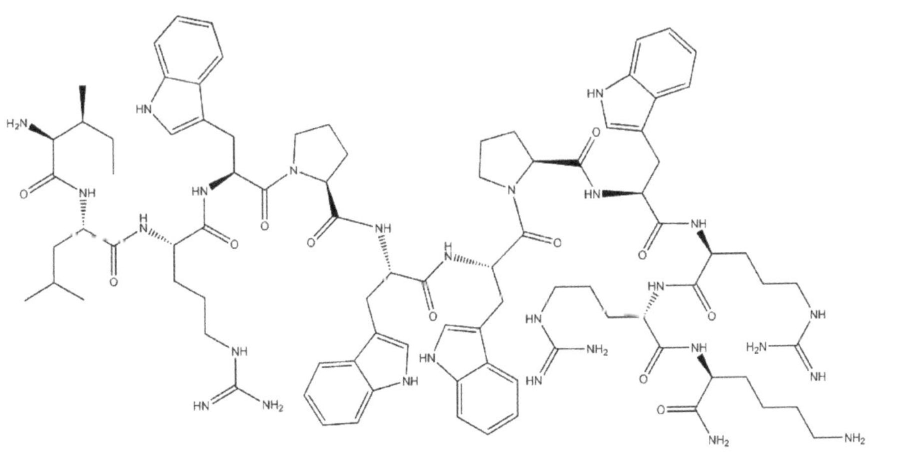

Omiganan pentahydrochloride

Figure 7.10 Topical Anti-androgens

(e) **Minocycline:** Oral tetracyclines-especially doxycycline and minocycline-are frequently prescribed for the treatment of moderate-to-severe acne, given their anti-inflammatory properties and their effect on P. acnes reduction. Minocycline is an effective treatment for moderate to moderately-severe inflammatory acne vulgaris. It is an oral antibiotic, use has lessened due to safety concerns (including potentially irreversible pigmentation), a relatively high cost, and no evidence of any greater benefit than other acne treatments [235]. FMX101 4% is a topical minocycline foam is a new class of topical minocycline products has been developed for the treatment of acne and rosacea that decreases the risk for antibiotic resistance while maintaining safety and efficacy, hydrophilic gel studies reported greater treatment efficacy than the lipophilic foam studies. reduced both inflammatory and noninflammatory lesions and improved Investigator's Global Assessment scores in patients with moderate-to-severe acne [236,237]. Once-daily topical application of minocycline foam 4% did not lead to significant systemic exposure to minocycline. It appears to be a well-tolerated treatment option for individuals with moderate-to-severe acne [238]. BPX-01) was developed to directly deliver minocycline through the epidermis and into the pilosebaceous unit to achieve localized treatment with lower doses of the drug [239]. However, because BPX-01 (another topical minocycline in trial) is topical and exhibits negligible systemic exposure, the likelihood of adverse events associated with oral minocycline use is much lower. BPX-01 2% formulation is a promising treatment for moderate-to-severe nonnodular, inflammatory acne vulgaris in both reduction of inflammatory lesions and also an overall improvement in facial acne according to IGA [240].

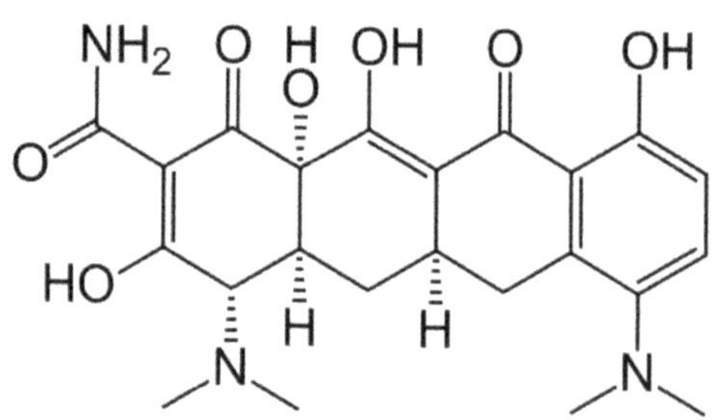

Figure 7.11 Minocycline

(f) **Oral Drugs for Acne Management:** Not all acne clears up with topical medications. Oral medications, also called systemic medications, work internally to improve the skin. Persistent or severe cases of acne are difficult to control, and in the majority of cases require oral medications. A hot, humid climate with an increased risk of sweating can also make it worse. Severe acne (sometimes called cystic acne or nodular acne) creates large, deep, inflamed breakouts. Topical medications can't get deep enough to effectively treat these types of blemishes. All oral acne medications are prescription only. There are no over-the-counter alternatives. People who shave should use safety razors with a sharp blade or an electric shaver. Most patients on oral antibiotics should notice improvements after about 6 weeks. A course may last from 4 to 6 months. Pregnant or breastfeeding mothers should take an erythromycin instead of tetracycline. Long-term oral antibiotic use in acne may be associated with a variety of adverse effects including antibiotic resistance, pharyngitis, inflammatory bowel disease, and breast and colon cancer.

A. Isotretinoin

Isotretinoin is a retinoic acid derivative mostly used in the treatment of cystic acne vulgaris [254]. Oral isotretinoin is FDA-approved for the treatment of severe recalcitrant AV but can also be used to treat patients with moderate acne that is either treatment-resistant or relapses quickly after discontinuation of oral antibiotic therapy. Several studies have shown that isotretinoin effectively decreases sebum production, the number of acne lesions, and acne scarring [98]. The treatment for the average patient is carried out during two to ten months [248]. Isotretinoin is the most effective treatment available, but serious adverse effects, including a possible association with depression and suicide, limit its use, further studies are needed to identify those patients who would benefit from an early referral to a mental health professional when Isotretinoin is initiated [241]. However, Huang et.al, 2017 revealed that Isotretinoin treatment for acne does not appear to be associated with an increased risk for depression. Moreover, the treatment of acne appears to ameliorate depressive symptoms [242]. Botsali et.al, 2019 further ensured an improvement for neurocognitive functions in isotretinoin patients and none of them was evaluated as depressive by the psychiatric examination [243]. iPLEDGE is the mandatory regulatory program for isotretinoin in the United States, aimed to prevent isotretinoin-related teratogenicity [244]. Isotretinoin is still the best treatment for severe nodulocystic acne. However, it must be taken into consideration its teratogenic effect on pregnant women and its association with inflammatory bowel disease, depression and suicidal ideas [245]. Soyuduru et.al., 2019 found that five months of isotretinoin therapy in AV patients causes insulin resistance and the increase in insulin resistance is not dependent on age, BMI, BFM, and lipid levels of these patients [246]. Isotretinoin can induce hyperhomocysteinemia and decreased serum folic acid level, which may be a risk for cardiovascular disease and thrombosis, as well as psychoses. Van et.al, 2019 revealed a study in Vietnam where a low dose isotretinoin treatment had effectiveness in decrease the severity of disease without significant changes in the plasma homocysteine level as well as the serum folic acid level [247]. Fouladgar et.al, 2018 stated that corneal sensitivity decreases after three months of treatment with isotretinoin. This decrease is more pronounced at higher ages and in women [249]. Approximately 80% of pregnant women are exposed to isotretinoin within the recommended 30 days of contraception or during pregnancy. North America and the European Union, implemented the pregnancy prevention program [250]. Tasli et.al, 2018 stated complaint of nasal obstruction [251]. Conventional and low dose isotretinoin regimens are associated with increased dermcidin (an antimicrobial peptide secreted by sweat glands that attacks any bacteria on our skin) expression [252]. Reduced dermcidin concentration in sweat in patients with inflammatory acne may permit proliferation of P. acnes in pilosebaceous units, resulting in progression of inflammatory acne [253]. Isotretinoin was the main component found in milk 10 to 12 hours after a dose while the metabolite was the primary component in milk 22 to 24 hours after the previous dose [255]. A review of adverse reaction reports on retinoids causing a breast reaction submitted to a French pharmacovigilance center found 22 cases of gynecomastia was associated with isotretinoin use. Fourteen of the cases were gynecomastia, 6 were galactorrhea and 2 were of both gynecomastia and galactorrhea. Gynecomastia and/or galactorrhea was unilateral for almost half of the reported retinoid cases [256]. Exposing to isotretinoin among pregnant women has still occurred due to detrimental adherence to risk reduction programs which resulted in live-born infants with different kinds of abnormalities. Despite the known serious adverse effect of isotretinoin, the use of drug was not based on the guidelines in some cases, which needs more attention to prevent the severe drug related problems [257].

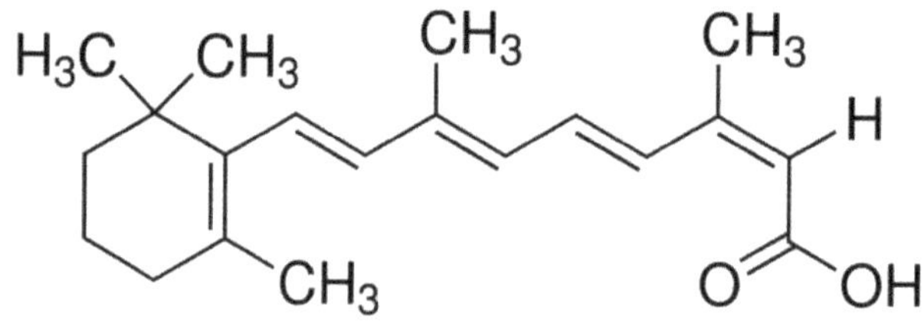

Figure 7.12 Isotretinoin

B. Spironolactone

Spironolactone, a synthetic 17-lactone steroid, acts as a non-selective mineralocorticoid receptor antagonist with moderate affinity for both progesterone and androgen receptors [266]. It is an effective second-line treatment option for post-adolescent acne, with a low risk of short-term adverse effects such as hyperkalemia [268]. A reduction in sebum may be achieved by blocking dihydrotestosterone binding to the androgen receptor within sebocytes and inhibiting androgen-induced sebocyte proliferation. The systemic effects of spironolactone on adrenal synthesis of androgen precursors may also contribute to clinical efficacy, although at therapeutic doses this may be unlikely. The diuretic effect of spironolactone may benefit women who experience a premenstrual acne flare associated with fluid retention [267]. The safety of long-term spironolactone use is well established given that it has been approved by the U.S. FDA since 1960. Because androgens mediate increased sebum production, they have been implicated in the pathophysiology of acne which led to the current acceptance of spironolactone as a non-antibiotic alternative to traditional systemic treatments for women with acne [231]. Spironolactone regulates sebaceous gland activity by blocking androgen receptor. It is a valuable alternative in women with acne in whom oral isotretinoin has failed. Combined oral contraceptives and spironolactone are good options [265]. First and second-generation oral contraceptives decrease the efficacy of spironolactone, confirming the interest of using two third or fourth-generation oral contraceptives [263]. In monotherapy, 80% of the patients present menstrual irregularity. The combined use of spironolactone with topical retinoid seems to provide a superior response to the retinoid treatment isolated in adult female acne. It can be used to promote androgen blockade in patients using levonorgestrel intrauterine devices or to increase androgen blockade in those who opt for combined oral contraceptive pills. A retrospective study of spironolactone found that there is no need for periodic control of potassium levels in young women, who do not have nephropathies, and are not users of other medications that may increase potassium levels [35]. Spironolactone (25 mg per day) can also be used in males. It decreases the production of androgens and blocks the actions of testosterone. If given to females, then pregnancy should be avoided because the drug can cause feminization of the fetus [26]. For this, spironolactone is classified as a Pregnancy Category C. Without the need for regular blood testing or the risk of severe teratogenicity, spironolactone is an attractive alternative to treatment with isotretinoin [231]. Spironolactone may have similar clinical effectiveness to that of oral tetracycline-class antibiotics [264]. A study shows the effectiveness of spironolactone to treat acne in Asian women, with a 47% good response using an initial dose of 200 mg per day, then reducing the dose every 4 weeks. Spironolactone's side effects are dose-dependent, and the most frequent are increase of diuresis, headache, dizziness, menstrual irregularity, breast pain, fatigue, and hyperpotassemia [265].

C. Oral Antibiotics

Oral antibiotic medications are commonly prescribed as second-line therapy for patients with mild-to-moderate acne that is not adequately controlled with topical agents alone and oral antibiotics have been a mainstay in the treatment of acne for decades and function by exerting an antibacterial effect by reducing the follicular colonization of *Propionibacterium acnes*. Systemic antibiotics also have anti-inflammatory and immunomodulatory properties. Tetracyclines, including sub-antimicrobial dose doxycycline, macrolides (notably azithromycin), trimethoprim-sulfamethoxazole, cephalosporins, and fluoroquinolones as treatment options for acne vulgaris. Antibiotic use for acne not only promotes resistance in Propionibacterium acnes, but also affects other host bacteria with pathogenic potential. [269,270]. Limiting systemic antibiotic use may also reduce the risk of inflammatory bowel disease (for tetracyclines), pharyngitis (for tetracyclines), C. difficile infection, and candida vulvovaginitis; however, studies have shown that these associations are limited. Penicillin, erythromycin, and cephalosporin are thought to have the best safety profile during pregnancy. There are three categories of antibiotic agents that range from those that are likely to reduce the effectiveness of OCPs (rifampin), those that are associated with OCP failure in three or more reported cases (ampicillin, amoxicillin, metronidazole, and tetracycline), and those that were associated with OCP failure in at least one case report (cephalexin, clindamycin, dapsone, erythromycin, griseofulvin, isoniazid, phenoxymethylpenicillin, talampicillin, and trimethoprim) [98].

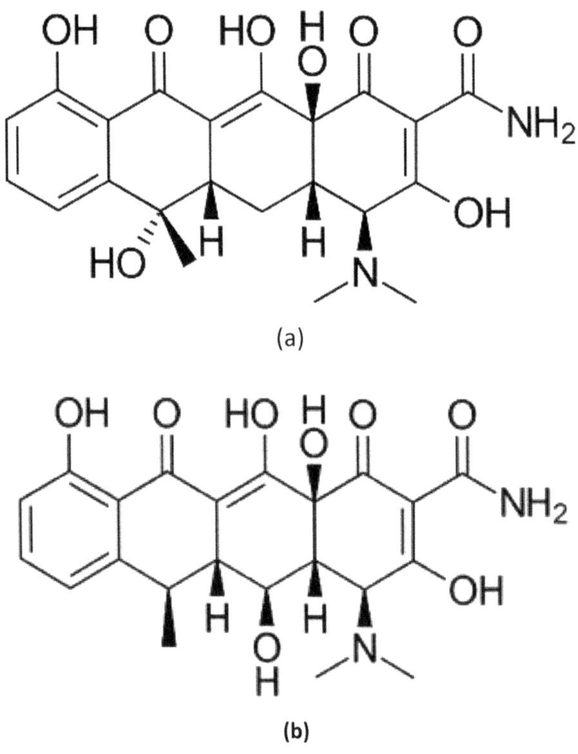

Figure 7.13 (a) Tetracycline and (b) Doxycycline

Tetracycline treatments, which include minocycline, doxycycline, and tetracycline, are considered first-line therapy in patients with moderate-to-severe inflammatory acne except in certain circumstances including pregnancy, age < 8 years, or known allergy [271]. Tetracycline medications including minocycline and doxycycline are classified as FDA pregnancy category D. Tetracycline agents should not be used during pregnancy because use during the second and third trimester is known to cause discoloration of the teeth and bones [272, 273]. GI side effects, including "pill esophagitis," are perhaps the most common concerning side effect associated with the use of oral doxycycline [274]. Oral azithromycin pulse therapy may be a good alternative to doxycycline in the management of acne for those unable to tolerate doxycycline [275].

Exhibit 10. Factors Differentiate Doxycycline and Minocycline for the Treatment of Acne Vulgaris [274]

Point of Comparison	Study Results
Phototoxicity	Minocycline exhibits negligible photosensitivity while doxycycline exhibits dose-related phototoxicity.
Vestibular side effects	Vestibular side effects, such as vertigo and dizziness, are not characteristic side effects associated with doxycycline use. Minocycline-associated vertigo usually becomes evident after the first dose or within the first few doses, which allows discontinuation of therapy should this side effect occur.
Efficacy comparisons	Although both minocycline and doxycycline have a long overall track record of widespread use with well-recognized efficacy, and safety when used to treat AV, prescription tracking data as depicted above has more recently shown that doxycycline is most commonly prescribed by dermatologists, followed by immediate-release minocycline formulations and extended-release minocycline tablets.
Other adverse reactions	potentially serious adverse effects that have been reported with minocycline and are very unlikely or nonexistent with doxycycline. These include drug-associated lupus-like syndrome, autoimmune hepatitis, and drug hypersensitivity syndrome with associated systemic manifestations (i.e., hepatitis, pneumonitis), in addition to other minocycline-specific side effects, such as vertigo/dizziness and patterns of cutaneous and/or mucosal hyperpigmentation.

Azithromycin, 500 mg thrice weekly for 12 weeks, is a safe and effective treatment of acne vulgaris with excellent patient compliance with few S/Es [276,277]. Oral desloratadine had antiacne properties, and when combined with azithromycin plus isotretinoin protocol, it significantly improves severe acne lesions and minimizes the ADEs [278]. Nakase et.al, 2016 reported low-level fluoroquinolone-resistant mutants with the Ser101Leu or Asp105Gly substitution in GyrA could be obtained from selection with *ciprofloxacin* and *levofloxacin* during in vitro mutation experiments [279]. Other antibiotics such as amoxicillin, erythromycin and bactrim are sometimes used, and if bacterial overgrowth or infection is masquerading as acne, other antibiotics such as ciprofloxacin may be used in pseudomonas related 'acne' [26]. *Metronidazole* gel (2%) is an effective, safe, and well-tolerated topical medication for moderate AV. Its mechanism of action is thought to be associated with its anti-inflammatory, immunosuppressive, and/or antimicrobial properties [280]. Metronidazole has an excellent record of safety during pregnancy and is frequently used as the treatment of choice for several common non-dermatologic infections during pregnancy [281].

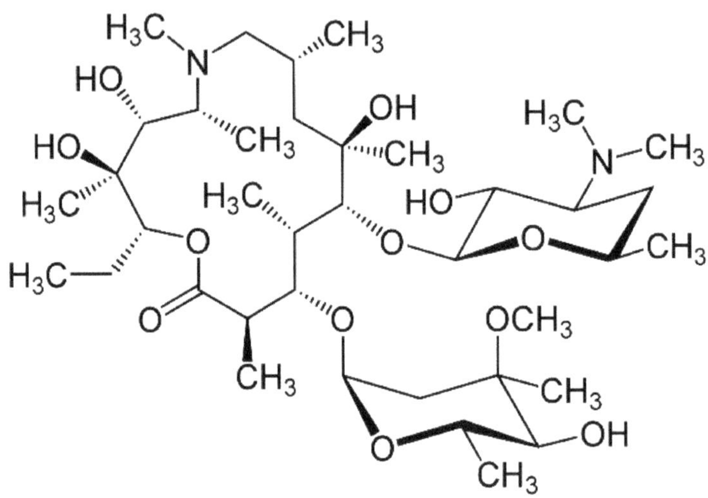

(a)

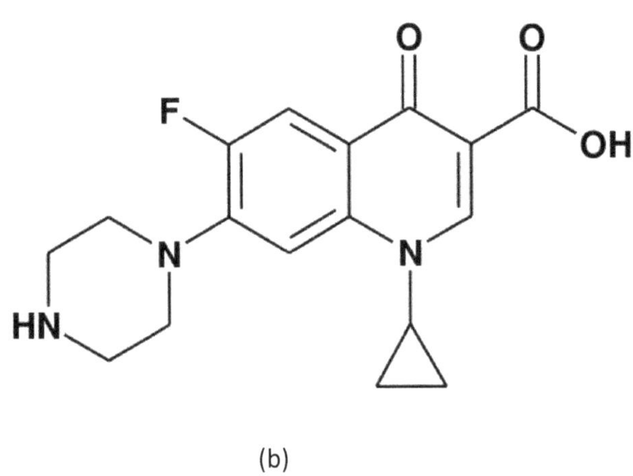

(b)

Figure 7.14 (a) Azithromycin and (b) Ciprofloxacin

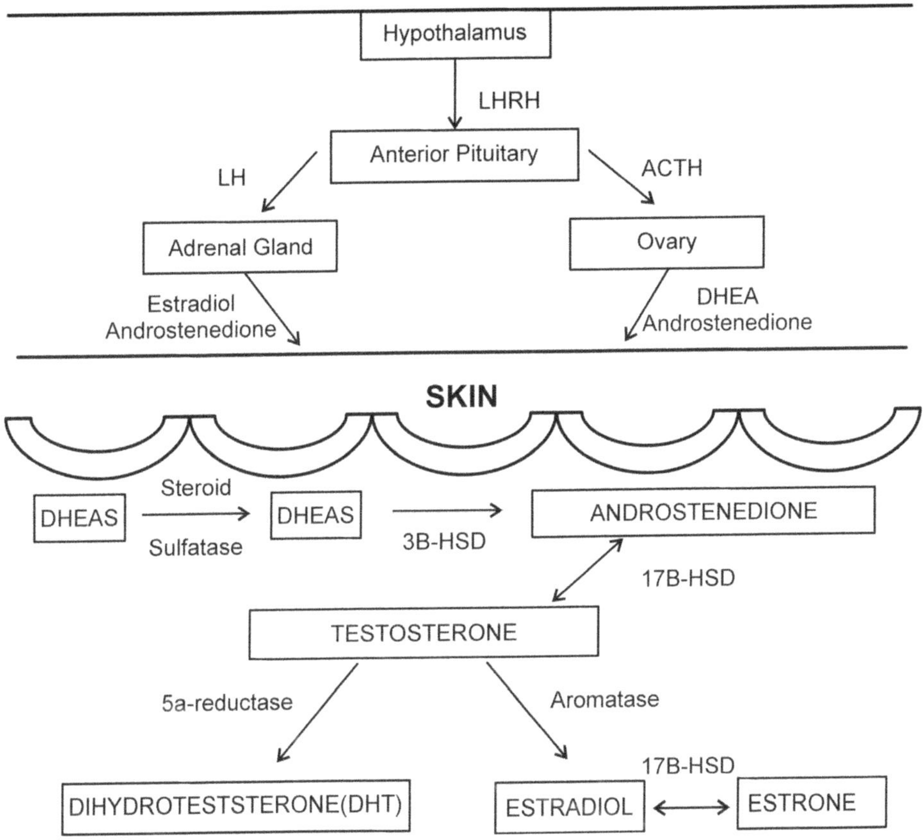

Figure 7.15 Hormonal regulation of skin pathogenesis [211]. Intracrine secretion involves the synthesis of active androgens in peripheral organs, such as the skin, where the androgens exert their action in the same cells where synthesis takes place without release into the general circulation. A large portion of androgens are also synthesized in the skin from inactive adrenal precursors including, dehydroepiandrosterone (DHEA), DHEA-sulfate (DHEA-S), and androstenedione. Besides sebaceous glands, other androgen-sensitive components of skin are hair follicles, sweat glands, epidermis, and dermis, containing enzymes responsible for converting DHEA, DHEA-S, and androstendione into the potent androgens dihydrotestosterone (DHT) and testosterone. DHT and testosterone are the major androgens that interact with the androgen receptors on sebaceous glands with DHT being 5 to 10 times more potent than testosterone. This conversion of inactive adrenal precursors to potent androgen occurs in sebaceous glands in the presence of several key steroidogenic enzymes: 3-Beta-hydroxysteroid dehydrogenase (3B-HSD), 17-Beta-hydroxysteroid dehydrogenase (17B-HSD), and 5α-reductase. Estrogen is known to suppress sebum production when given in sufficient amounts. Other mechanisms for estrogen's effect include direct opposition effect on testosterone and inhibition of testosterone secretion. In addition, through the metabolization of estrogen in the liver, estrogen increases sex hormone-binding globulin (SHBG). SHBG has a high affinity for testosterone and will bind to it preferentially over estrogen. Since testosterone and its conversion to DHT are the primary androgens in acne, increased SHBG leads to improvement in acne.

D. Oral Contraceptive Pills (OCPs)

Currently, there are three types of oral contraceptive pills: combined estrogen-progesterone, progesterone only and the continuous or extended use pill. The use of combined pills for acne has been formally approved by the FDA for specific brands. The majority of women take OCP's to prevent pregnancy, but 14% used them for non-contraceptive reasons [282]. The beneficial effect of OCPs is related to a decrease in ovarian and adrenal androgen precursors; to an increase in SHBG, which limits free testosterone; and to a decrease in 3a-androstenediol glucuronide conjugate, the catabolite of DHT formed in peripheral tissues (**Figure 7.15**) [306]. There are now four different combined oral contraceptive pills that are FDA approved for the treatment of acne since its first introduction in 1960. Hormonal therapies are effective and well tolerated options for the treatment of acne vulgaris in adolescents with and without endocrine disorders. They can be used as monotherapy or in conjunction with benzoyl peroxide, topical retinoic acid, or antibiotics [291]. In the case of hormonal disturbances, the use of hormonal contraception not only improves the cosmetic situation of the patient but is also necessary to decrease the risks related to hyperandrogenemia [286]. According to WHO recommendations, the contraindications to oral contraception are as follows: pregnancy, breast feeding, history of deep venous thrombosis and thromboembolic event, active liver disease, smoking after the age of 35 years, migraine, breast cancer, hypertension, diabetes mellitus with vascular changes, and long-term immobilization [287]. There was a significant reduction in the expression of TLR-2 (Toll-like receptor expression) in the skin of adult females with facial acne who used azelaic acid 15% gel or combined oral contraceptive (drospirenone + ethinylestradiol). Rocha et.al, 2017 suggested a possible anti-inflammatory effect of oral contraceptive and azelaic acid in AFA via modulation of this receptor [283]. Contraceptive pills can have side effects such as headaches, breast tenderness and nausea. The pills that reduced acne had ethinyl estradiol in them, combined with one of the following drugs: levonorgestrel, norethindrone, norgestimate, drospirenone, cyproterone acetate, chlormadinone acetate, dienogest or desogestrel. Cyproterone acetate has not been approved for contraceptive use in Germany, but it can be prescribed for the treatment of acne [284]. Cyproterone acetate (2 mg of cyproterone acetate and 0.35 of ethinyl estradiol) after 3 months of treatment caused visible improvement in acne in 40%. More than 85% of patient finished the study, which suggests very good compliance and tolerability [285]. Animal studies showed that cyproterone acetate in high doses only is associated with congenital malformations. There is a possibility of abnormal sexual differentiation of the fetus or other teratogenic effects [288]. Chlormadinone acetate was more effective in the treatment of acne than levonorgestrel and was more antiandrogenic than dienogest [289]. ethinyl estradiol/chlormadinone acetate 30 mcg/2 mg once daily is more effective for the treatment of acne and dysmenorrhea in women with mild to moderate AV and dysmenorrhea than ethinyl estradiol/ drospirenone 30 mcg/3 mg [289].

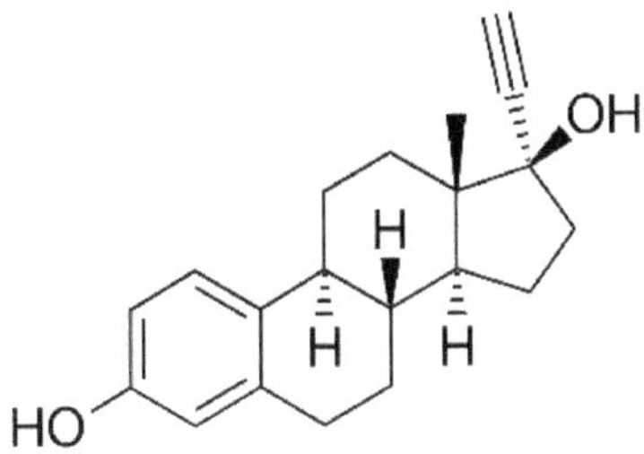

(a) Ethinyl estradiol

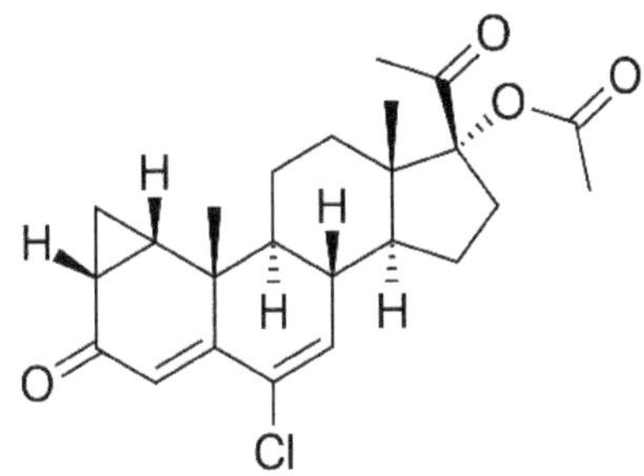

(b) Cyproterone acetate

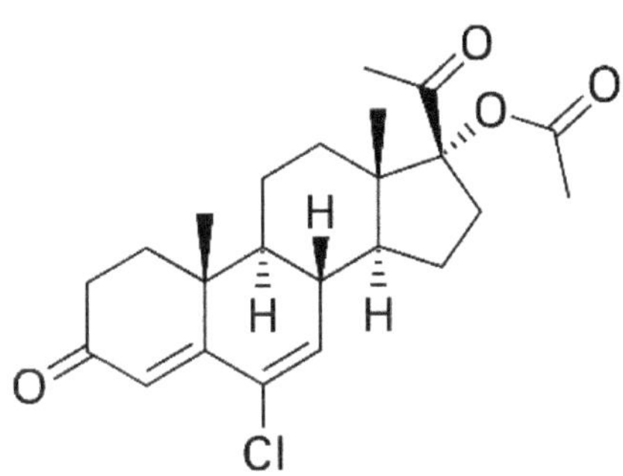

(c) Chlormadinone acetate

Figure 7.16 Hormonal contraceptives

7.3.9 LASER THERAPY

Laser therapies are increasingly becoming part of or an adjunct to the medical treatment of active acne and are a useful treatment modality. Studies of lasers in the treatment of acne, including erbium glass, Nd:YAG, pulse dye laser (PDL), potassium titanyl phosphate (KTP) laser, and laser-based photodynamic therapy, have been published [292,293]. Lasers including infrared wavelengths and pulsed dye lasers; light devices including blue light, red light, and broadband light; and photodynamic therapy with aminolevulinic acid and methylaminolevulinic acid have been shown to be effective in the treatment of acne vulgaris. The optimal outcomes are achieved with photodynamic therapy combined with medical therapy. Acne scarring has been best treated with lasers, including nonablative infrared lasers, fractional nonablative and ablative laser resurfacing, and most recently needle-based radiofrequency devices. Unique combination of lasers appears to be safe in patients with Fitzpatrick Skin Type IV, and might be useful in treating moderate-to-severe acne vulgaris. Kang et.al, 2019 stated that approximately 80% of the patients reported overall satisfaction.

Laser therapy is advantageous because it is an in-office treatment, which ensures patient adherence to therapy. In addition, it offers no systemic side effects that might complicate treatment when using oral acne medications. Although many different lasers have been studied for the treatment of acne, only a few studies to date have have evaluated a combination of lasers, which include PDL with either a 1,064-nm Nd:YAG or a 1,450-nm diode laser. Lasers studied include the 1,540-nm erbium:glass laser, 1,550-nm fractionated erbium: glass laser, pulsed-dye laser (PDL), q-switched 1,064-nm neodymium-doped yttrium aluminium garnet (Nd:YAG) laser, fractional 1,320-nm Nd:YAG laser, 1,450-nm diode laser, and 532-nm potassium titanyl phosphate laser. In addition, the 1,450-nm diode laser has been shown to reduce sebum production [295]. The novel IPL filter at wavelength of 400-600 nm and 800-1,200 nm provides an effective option to treatment of inflammatory acne lesions, especially for Pillsbury I-II acne patients, with minimal reversible side effects, such as transient post-inflammatory pigmentation. Intense pulsed light (IPL) has become a well-recognized method in the treatment of acne vulgaris [296]. Various types of lasers have been utilized in the treatment of scars since the 1980s, beginning with continuous wave argon, CO_2, and Nd:YAG 1064 lasers, followed by the application of PDL and Er:YAG lasers for scar revision [297] Most recently, fractional photothermolysis with ablative and non-ablative fractionated lasers have found use as effective treatments for scars. For hypertrophic scars and keloids, the most common non-ablative laser has been the pulsed dye laser (PDL: 585 to 595 nm). For atrophic facial scars, the most commonly used non-ablative lasers are Nd:YAG and 1450-nm diode laser. One study reported an improvement of 40 to 45% with 1320-nm Nd:YAG or 1450-nm diode laser treatment after an average of three consecutive monthly treatment sessions, as assessed by patient satisfaction surveys, histologic evaluations, and skin texture measurements. Non-ablative lasers have minimal downtime and produce gradual results, with the most significant improvement noted between 3 and 6 months following the final laser treatment [298]. PDL is effective in improving the vascularity, pliability, color, and height of hypertrophic scars and keloids. Previous studies have reported a 57% to 83% improvement in clinical appearance and texture of hypertrophic scars after one to two PDL treatments [299,300]. Non-ablative fractional lasers (NAFL) have been shown to significantly improve the pigmentation and thickness of surgical scars, atrophic scars, hypertrophic scars, and hypopigmented scars. A study by Tierney et al. comparing 1550-nm NAFL to 595-nm PDL for the treatment of surgical scars showed that NAFL outperformed PDL and 83% of patients preferred the half of the scar treated with a non-ablative fractional laser [301,302]. A study by Niwa et al. examined NAFL in the treatment of hypertrophic scars and found 26% to 75% clinical improvement after two to three treatment sessions done at 4-week intervals [297]. Ablative laser resurfacing, with CO_2 or Er:YAG lasers, has been shown to be effective for traumatic and surgical scars, especially when resurfaced within 6 to 10 weeks after trauma or surgery or even immediately after surgery. CO_2 and Er:YAG lasers are also effective for atrophic scars due to their ability to smooth scar texture and stimulate collagen production within facial atrophic scars, although patients must consider the potential for significant downtime as re-epithelialization typically takes 4 to 7 days with Er:YAG and 7 to 10 days with the CO_2 laser. While requiring more downtime, ablative lasers usually produce a higher degree of clinical improvement [303,304]. For acne scars, previous head-to-head studies have suggested that CO_2 laser produces superior results while Er:YAG is better tolerated with less downtime. Raised scars and shallow boxcar scars improve the most with laser resurfacing, while icepick scars are more challenging to treat and may necessitate secondary resurfacing. Non-ablative lasers are also useful for acne scars [294,303].

EPILOGUE

A better understanding of the pathophysiological mechanisms driving acne has allowed for the development of more effective topical and systemic therapies. These can be prescribed in logical combinations to target each relevant pathological factor and thus ensure optimal acne management. Each patient should receive education regarding acne and the available treatment options. A realistic explanation of the benefits, risks and expected outcomes of each therapy must be provided to promote autonomy. Patients also need to understand that, although most cases of acne can be cleared with available treatments, therapy requires time, and in the early weeks of treatment their acne may worsen. However, with frequent reassurance and follow-up, many patients will comply with treatment and achieve an acceptable outcome. Maintenance therapy is an important consideration as acne represents a chronic disease and frequently recurs without an ongoing treatment regimen. Among all pathogenetic factors of acne, inflammation seems to be rediscovered and anti-inflammatory concepts seem to become the new trend of systemic and topical acne treatment. Acne scars may have a damaging effect on a person's physical, mental, and social well-being. Although a wide range of treatments are used, there is a lack of high-quality evidence on which are the most effective for acne scars. Despite the interest on the development of topical treatments for acne in the last decades, systemic treatment is still a milestone, especially in the treatment of moderate-to-severe scarring types of the disease. The establishment of new systemic drugs for acne is based on the consideration of successes and pitfalls of the past and the emerging knowledge of the future.

SUMMARY

Acne is estimated to affect approximately 10% of the global population, making it the eighth most prevalent disease worldwide. Several studies have confirmed that acne can affect a person's quality of life, self-esteem, and mood in an adverse manner. Acne treatments take a considerable share of dermatology OTC product market. Also, increasingly various prescription acne treatments are becoming qualified as OTC products due to their history of long-term safety and efficacy. The issue of antibiotic resistance also impacts the prescribing patterns and treatment algorithms. The standard of care for the treatment of mild-to-moderate acne still lies with topical therapies. Poor adherence is one of the critical and negatively impacting factors affecting acne treatment outcomes. Moreover, limited patient education and awareness about acne treatment is also a roadblock to successful treatment. The acne therapy market is moving from mono therapy towards combination therapy options. The most likely reason is higher efficacy of combinations that consider the multifactorial pathogenesis of acne, reduced resistance levels, and the ease of single product use versus two separate mono therapies. Laser and light modalities, although not sufficiently studied for first-line use, show promise for the future.

ABBREVIATIONS

Acne Vulgaris (AV); Aquaporin-3 (AQP3); Dehydroepiandrosterone (DHEA); complementary and alternative medicine (CAM); Insulin-Like Growth Factor 1 (IGF-1); Health-Related Quality of Life (HRQoL); Dehydroepiandrosterone (DHEA); Sex Hormone-Binding Globulin (SHBG); Ceramide (Cer); Sphingomyelin (SM); Follicle-Stimulating Hormone (FSH); 5α-dihydrotestosterone (5α-DHT); Polycystic ovary syndrome (PCOS); sebaceous gland (SG); eicosapentaenoic acid (EPA); docosahexaenoic acid (DHA); Adult Female Acne (AFA); Benzoyl peroxide (BP); post inflammatory hyperpigmentation (PIH); American Academy of Dermatology (AAD); methicillin-resistant Staphylococcus aureus (MRSA); combined oral contraceptive (COC); randomized controlled trials (RCTs); Investigator's Global Assessment (IGA); Intense pulsed light (IPL); Non-ablative fractional lasers (NAFL)

BIBLIOGRAPHY AND WEBLIOGRAPHY

1. Valente Duarte De Sousa IC. New and emerging drugs for the treatment of acne vulgaris in adolescents. Expert OpinPharmacother. 2019 Mar 8:1-16. doi: 10.1080/14656566.2019.1584182. [Epub ahead of print] PubMed PMID: 30848961.
2. Bellew S, Thiboutot D, Del Rosso JQ. Pathogenesis of acne vulgaris: what's new, what's interesting and what may be clinically relevant. J Drugs Dermatol. 2011 Jun;10(6):582-5. PubMed PMID: 21637898.

3. Aydemir EH. Acne vulgaris. Turk Pediatri Ars. 2014 Mar 1;49(1):13-6. doi: 10.5152/tpa.2014.1943. eCollection 2014 Mar. Review. PubMed PMID: 26078626; PubMed Central PMCID: PMC4462260.
4. Gollnick HP. From new findings in acne pathogenesis to new approaches in treatment. J Eur Acad Dermatol Venereol. 2015 Jun;29 Suppl 5:1-7. doi: 10.1111/jdv.13186. Review. PubMed PMID: 26059819.
5. Cong TX, Hao D, Wen X, Li XH, He G, Jiang X. From pathogenesis of acne vulgaris to anti-acne agents. Arch Dermatol Res. 2019 Mar 11. doi: 10.1007/s00403-019-01908-x. [Epub ahead of print] Review. PubMed PMID: 30859308.
6. Yang JH, Yoon JY, Kwon HH, Min S, Moon J, Suh DH. Seeking new acne treatment from natural products, devices and synthetic drug discovery. Dermatoendocrinol. 2017 Oct 4;9(1):e1356520. doi: 10.1080/19381980.2017.1356520. eCollection 2017. Review. PubMed PMID: 29484092; PubMed Central PMCID: PMC5821150.
7. Beylot C. [Mechanisms and causes of acne]. Rev Prat. 2002 Apr 15;52(8):828-30. Review. French. PubMed PMID: 12053788.
8. Eichenfield LF, Del Rosso JQ, Mancini AJ, Cook-Bolden F, Stein Gold L, Desai S, Weiss J, Pariser D, Zeichner J, Bhatia N, Kircik L. Evolving perspectives on the etiology and pathogenesis of acne vulgaris. J Drugs Dermatol. 2015 Mar;14(3):263-72. Review. PubMed PMID: 25738848.
9. Kucharska A, Szmurło A, Sińska B. Significance of diet in treated and untreated acne vulgaris. Postepy Dermatol Alergol. 2016 Apr;33(2):81-6. doi: 10.5114/ada.2016.59146. Epub 2016 May 16. Review. PubMed PMID: 27279815; PubMed Central PMCID: PMC4884775.
10. Reynolds RC, Lee S, Choi JY, Atkinson FS, Stockmann KS, Petocz P, Brand-Miller JC. Effect of the glycemic index of carbohydrates on Acne vulgaris. Nutrients. 2010 Oct;2(10):1060-72. doi: 10.3390/nu2101060. Epub 2010 Oct 18. PubMed PMID: 22253996; PubMed Central PMCID: PMC3257617.
11. Pappas A. The relationship of diet and acne: A review. Dermatoendocrinol. 2009 Sep;1(5):262-7. PubMed PMID: 20808513; PubMed Central PMCID: PMC2836431.
12. Nguyen QG, Markus R, Katta R. Diet and acne: an exploratory survey study of patient beliefs. Dermatol Pract Concept. 2016 Apr 30;6(2):21-7. doi: 10.5826/dpc.0602a05. eCollection 2016 Apr. PubMed PMID: 27222768; PubMed Central PMCID: PMC4866623.
13. Romańska-Gocka K, Woźniak M, Kaczmarek-Skamira E, Zegarska B. The possible role of diet in the pathogenesis of adult female acne. Postepy Dermatol Alergol. 2016 Dec;33(6):416-420. doi: 10.5114/ada.2016.63880. Epub 2016 Dec 2. Review. PubMed PMID: 28035217; PubMed Central PMCID: PMC5183780.
14. Emiroğlu N, Cengiz FP, Kemeriz F. Insulin resistance in severe acne vulgaris. Postepy Dermatol Alergol. 2015 Aug;32(4):281-5. doi: 10.5114/pdia.2015.53047. Epub 2015 Aug 12. PubMed PMID: 26366152; PubMed Central PMCID: PMC4565837.

15. Mishra JS, More AS, Kumar S. Elevated androgen levels induce hyperinsulinemia through increase in Ins1 transcription in pancreatic beta cells in female rats. Biol Reprod. 2018 Apr 1;98(4):520-531. doi: 10.1093/biolre/ioy017. PubMed PMID: 29365042; PubMed Central PMCID: PMC6279097.
16. Assaf HA, Abdel-Maged WM, Elsadek BE, Hassan MH, Adly MA, Ali SA. Survivinas a Novel Biomarker in the Pathogenesis of Acne Vulgaris and Its Correlation to Insulin-Like Growth Factor-I. Dis Markers. 2016;2016:7040312. Epub 2016 Oct 10. PubMed PMID: 27803511; PubMed Central PMCID: PMC5075610.
17. Çerman AA, Aktaş E, Altunay İK, Arıcı JE, Tulunay A, Ozturk FY. Dietary glycemic factors, insulin resistance, and adiponectin levels in acne vulgaris. J AmAcad Dermatol. 2016 Jul;75(1):155-62. doi: 10.1016/j.jaad.2016.02.1220. Epub 2016 Apr 6. PubMed PMID: 27061046.
18. Rahaman SMA, De D, Handa S, Pal A, Sachdeva N, Ghosh T, Kamboj P. Association of insulin-like growth factor (IGF)-1 gene polymorphisms with plasma levels of IGF-1 and acne severity. J Am Acad Dermatol. 2016 Oct;75(4):768-773. doi: 10.1016/j.jaad.2016.05.019. Epub 2016 Jul 27. PubMed PMID: 27476104.
19. Melnik BC. Linking diet to acne metabolomics, inflammation, and comedogenesis: an update. Clin CosmetInvestig Dermatol. 2015 Jul 15;8:371-88. doi: 10.2147/CCID.S69135. eCollection 2015. Review. PubMed PMID: 26203267; PubMed Central PMCID: PMC4507494.
20. Juhl CR, Bergholdt HKM, Miller IM, Jemec GBE, Kanters JK, Ellervik C. Dairy Intake and Acne Vulgaris: A Systematic Review and Meta-Analysis of 78,529 Children, Adolescents, and Young Adults. Nutrients. 2018 Aug 9;10(8). pii: E1049. doi: 10.3390/nu10081049. Review. PubMed PMID: 30096883; PubMed Central PMCID: PMC6115795.
21. Danby FW. Acne: Diet and acnegenesis. Indian Dermatol Online J. 2011 Jan;2(1):2-5. doi: 10.4103/2229-5178.79851. PubMed PMID: 23130204; PubMed Central PMCID: PMC3481796.
22. Kim H, Moon SY, Sohn MY, Lee WJ. Insulin-Like Growth Factor-1 Increases the Expression of Inflammatory Biomarkers and Sebum Production in Cultured Sebocytes. Ann Dermatol. 2017 Feb;29(1):20-25. doi: 10.5021/ad.2017.29.1.20. Epub 2017 Feb 3. PubMed PMID: 28223742; PubMed Central PMCID: PMC5318522.
23. Cappel M, Mauger D, Thiboutot D. Correlation between serum levels of insulin-like growth factor 1, dehydroepiandrosterone sulfate, and dihydrotestosterone and acne lesion counts in adult women. Arch Dermatol. 2005 Mar;141(3):333-8. PubMed PMID: 15781674.
24. Adebamowo CA, Spiegelman D, Berkey CS, Danby FW, Rockett HH, Colditz GA, Willett WC, Holmes MD. Milk consumption and acne in teenaged boys. J Am Acad Dermatol. 2008 May;58(5):787-93. doi: 10.1016/j.jaad.2007.08.049. Epub 2008 Jan 14. PubMed PMID: 18194824; PubMed Central PMCID: PMC4391699.
25. Keri JE, Rosenblatt AE. [In Process Citation]. J Clin Aesthet Dermatol. 2008 Sep;1(3):22-6. PubMed PMID: 21203358; PubMed Central PMCID: PMC3013591.

26. Sutaria AH, Schlessinger J. Acne Vulgaris. [Updated 2018 Nov 14]. In: StatPearls [Internet]. Treasure Island (FL): StatPearls Publishing; 2019 Jan-. Available from: https://www.ncbi.nlm.nih.gov/books/NBK459173/
27. Stoll S, Shalita AR, Webster GF, Kaplan R, Danesh S, Penstein A. The effect of the menstrual cycle on acne. J Am Acad Dermatol. 2001 Dec;45(6):957-60. PubMed PMID: 11712049.
28. Geller L, Rosen J, Frankel A, Goldenberg G. Perimenstrual flare of adult acne. J Clin Aesthet Dermatol. 2014 Aug;7(8):30-4. PubMed PMID: 25161758; PubMed Central PMCID: PMC4142818.
29. Elsaie ML. Hormonal treatment of acne vulgaris: an update. Clin CosmetInvestig Dermatol. 2016 Sep 2;9:241-8. doi: 10.2147/CCID.S114830. eCollection 2016. Review. PubMed PMID: 27621661; PubMed Central PMCID: PMC5015761.
30. Zeichner JA, Baldwin HE, Cook-Bolden FE, Eichenfield LF, Fallon-Friedlander S, Rodriguez DA. Emerging Issues in Adult Female Acne. J Clin Aesthet Dermatol. 2017 Jan;10(1):37-46. Epub 2017 Jan 1. Review. PubMed PMID: 28210380; PubMed Central PMCID: PMC5300732.
31. Raghunath RS, Venables ZC, Millington GW. The menstrual cycle and the skin. Clin Exp Dermatol. 2015 Mar;40(2):111-5. doi: 10.1111/ced.12588. Epub 2015 Feb 11. Review. PubMed PMID: 25683236.
32. Sardana K, Sharma RC, Sarkar R. Seasonal variation in acne vulgaris--myth or reality. J Dermatol. 2002 Aug;29(8):484-8. PubMed PMID: 12227481.
33. Tanghetti EA, Kawata AK, Daniels SR, Yeomans K, Burk CT, Callender VD. Understanding the burden of adult female acne. J Clin Aesthet Dermatol. 2014 Feb;7(2):22-30. PubMed PMID: 24578779; PubMed Central PMCID: PMC3935648.
34. Zari S, Alrahmani D. The association between stress and acne among female medical students in Jeddah, Saudi Arabia. Clin CosmetInvestig Dermatol. 2017 Dec 5;10:503-506. doi: 10.2147/CCID.S148499. eCollection 2017. PubMed PMID: 29255370; PubMed Central PMCID: PMC5722010.
35. Bagatin E, Freitas THP, Machado MCR, Ribeiro BM, Nunes S, Rocha MADD. Adult female acne: a guide to clinical practico. An Bras Dermatol. 2019 Jan-Feb;94(1):62-75. doi: 10.1590/abd1806-4841.20198203. Review. PubMed PMID: 30726466; PubMed Central PMCID: PMC6360964.
36. Bondade S, Hosthota A, Basavaraju V. Stressful life events and psychiatric comorbidity in acne-a case control study. Asia Pac Psychiatry. 2019 Mar;11(1):e12340. doi: 10.1111/appy.12340. Epub 2018 Nov 8. PubMed PMID: 30406964.
37. Uhlenhake E, Yentzer BA, Feldman SR. Acne vulgaris and depression: a retrospective examination. J Cosmet Dermatol. 2010 Mar;9(1):59-63. doi: 10.1111/j.1473-2165.2010.00478.x. PubMed PMID: 20367674.
38. Özçelik S, Kulaç İ, Yazıcı M, Öcal E. Distribution of childhood skin diseases according to age and gender, a single institution experience. Turk Pediatri Ars. 2018 Jun 1;53(2):105-112. doi: 10.5152/TurkPediatriArs.2018.6431. eCollection 2018 Jun. PubMed PMID: 30116131; PubMed Central PMCID: PMC6089785.

39. Minh PPT, Bich DD, Hai VNT, Van TN, Cam VT, Khang TH, Gandolfi M, Satolli F, Feliciani C, Tirant M, Vojvodic A, Lotti T. Microneedling Therapy for Atrophic Acne Scar: Effectiveness and Safety in Vietnamese Patients. Open Access Maced J Med Sci. 2019 Jan 29;7(2):293-297. doi: 10.3889/oamjms.2019.098. eCollection 2019 Jan 30. PubMed PMID: 30745984; PubMed Central PMCID: PMC6364723.
40. Tasoula E, Gregoriou S, Chalikias J, Lazarou D, Danopoulou I, Katsambas A, Rigopoulos D. The impact of acne vulgaris on quality of life and psychic health in young adolescents in Greece. Results of a population survey. An Bras Dermatol. 2012 Nov-Dec;87(6):862-9. PubMed PMID: 23197205; PubMed Central PMCID: PMC3699905.
41. Gollnick HP, Zouboulis CC. Not all acne is acne vulgaris. DtschArztebl Int. 2014 Apr 25;111(17):301-12. doi: 10.3238/arztebl.2014.0301. Review. PubMed PMID: 24828100; PubMed Central PMCID: PMC4098044.
42. Taylor M, Gonzalez M, Porter R. Pathways to inflammation: acne pathophysiology. Eur J Dermatol. 2011 May-Jun;21(3):323-33. doi: 10.1684/ejd.2011.1357. Review. PubMed PMID: 21609898.
43. Purdy S, de Berker D. Acne. BMJ. 2006 Nov 4;333(7575):949-53. Review. PubMed PMID: 17082546; PubMed Central PMCID: PMC1633755.
44. Goodman G. Cleansing and moisturizing in acne patients. Am J Clin Dermatol. 2009;10 Suppl 1:1-6. doi: 10.2165/0128071-200910001-00001. Review. PubMed PMID: 19209947.
45. Tasoula E, Gregoriou S, Chalikias J, Lazarou D, Danopoulou I, Katsambas A, Rigopoulos D. The impact of acne vulgaris on quality of life and psychic health in young adolescents in Greece. Results of a population survey. An Bras Dermatol. 2012 Nov-Dec;87(6):862-9. PubMed PMID: 23197205; PubMed Central PMCID: PMC3699905.
46. Sparavigna A, Tenconi B, De Ponti I, La Penna L. An innovative approach to the topical treatment of acne. Clin CosmetInvestig Dermatol. 2015 Apr 9;8:179-85. doi: 10.2147/CCID.S82859. eCollection 2015. Review. PubMed PMID: 25914552; PubMed Central PMCID: PMC4399783.
47. Purdy S, de Berker D. Acne vulgaris. BMJ Clin Evid. 2011 Jan 5;2011. pii: 1714. Review. PubMed PMID: 21477388; PubMed Central PMCID: PMC3275168.
48. Purdy S, Langston J, Tait L. Presentation and management of acne in primary care: a retrospective cohort study. Br J Gen Pract. 2003 Jul;53(492):525-9. PubMed PMID: 14694664; PubMed Central PMCID: PMC1314642.
49. Costa CS, Bagatin E, Martimbianco ALC, da Silva EM, Lúcio MM, Magin P, Riera R. Oral isotretinoin for acne. Cochrane Database Syst Rev. 2018 Nov 24;11:CD009435. doi: 10.1002/14651858.CD009435.pub2. PubMed PMID: 30484286; PubMed Central PMCID: PMC6383843.
50. Ettel DL, Lamanno LR, Neyra SA, Ettel WJ, Ettel GL III, Mitchell MK. Teens and Technology Transforming Acne Treatment. Perm J. 2017;21:16-192. doi: 10.7812/TPP/16-192. PubMed PMID: 28898196; PubMed Central PMCID: PMC5593518.
51. Snast I, Dalal A, Twig G, Astman N, Kedem R, Levin D, Erlich Y, Leshem YA, Lapidoth M, Hodak E, Levi A. Acne and Obesity: A Nationwide Study of 600,404

Adolescents. J Am Acad Dermatol. 2019 Apr 9. pii: S0190-9622(19)30589-4. doi: 10.1016/j.jaad.2019.04.009. [Epub ahead of print] PubMed PMID: 30978426.

52. Halvorsen JA, Vleugels RA, Bjertness E, Lien L. A population-based study of acne and body mass index in adolescents. Arch Dermatol. 2012 Jan;148(1):131-2. doi: 10.1001/archderm.148.1.131. PubMed PMID: 22250253.

53. Stewart TJ, Bazergy C. Hormonal and dietary factors in acne vulgaris versus controls. Dermatoendocrinol. 2018 Feb 22;10(1):e1442160. doi: 10.1080/19381980.2018.1442160. eCollection 2018. PubMed PMID: 29904568; PubMed Central PMCID: PMC5997051.

54. Melnik B. Dietary intervention in acne: Attenuation of increased mTORC1 signaling promoted by Western diet. Dermatoendocrinol. 2012 Jan 1;4(1):20-32. doi: 10.4161/derm.19828. PubMed PMID: 22870349; PubMed Central PMCID: PMC3408989.

55. Wang YY, Li SW, Luo S, Qin L, Zeng X, Li L, Li XH. How to Evaluate Acne in Reproductive-Age Women: An Epidemiological Study in Chinese Communities. Biomed Res Int. 2019 Feb 3;2019:6126808. doi: 10.1155/2019/6126808. eCollection 2019. PubMed PMID: 30854398; PubMed Central PMCID: PMC6378077.

56. Acne During Pregnancy. Available From: https://www.webmd.com/skin-problems-and-treatments/acne/acne-during-pregnancy-treatments-causes#1

57. Perera MPN, Peiris WMDM, Pathmanathan D, Mallawaarachchi S, Karunathilake IM. Relationship between acne vulgaris and cosmetic usage in Sri Lankan urban adolescent females. J Cosmet Dermatol. 2018 Jun;17(3):431-436. doi: 10.1111/jocd.12431. Epub 2017 Sep 22. PubMed PMID: 28941014.

58. Taylor KW, Baird DD, Herring AH, Engel LS, Nichols HB, Sandler DP, Troester MA. Associations among personal care product use patterns and exogenous hormone use in the NIEHS Sister Study. J Expo Sci Environ Epidemiol. 2017 Sep;27(5):458-464. doi: 10.1038/jes.2016.82. Epub 2017 Jan 25. PubMed PMID: 28120835; PubMed Central PMCID: PMC5526738.

59. Nair PA, Salazar FJ. Acneiform Eruptions. [Updated 2018 Dec 2]. In: StatPearls [Internet]. Treasure Island (FL): StatPearls Publishing; 2019 Jan-. Available from: https://www.ncbi.nlm.nih.gov/books/NBK459207/

60. Bhate K, Williams HC. Epidemiology of acne vulgaris. Br J Dermatol. 2013 Mar;168(3):474-85. doi: 10.1111/bjd.12149. Review. PubMed PMID: 23210645.

61. George RM, Sridharan R. Factors Aggravating or Precipitating Acne in Indian Adults: A Hospital-Based Study of 110 Cases. Indian J Dermatol. 2018 Jul-Aug;63(4):328-331. doi: 10.4103/ijd.IJD_565_17. PubMed PMID: 30078878; PubMed Central PMCID: PMC6052742.

62. Melnik BC, Schmitz G. Role of insulin, insulin-like growth factor-1, hyperglycaemic food and milk consumption in the pathogenesis of acne vulgaris. Exp Dermatol. 2009 Oct;18(10):833-41. doi: 10.1111/j.1600-0625.2009.00924.x.Epub 2009 Aug 25. Review. PubMed PMID: 19709092.

63. Cong TX, Hao D, Wen X, Li XH, He G, Jiang X. From pathogenesis of acne vulgaris to anti-acne agents. Arch Dermatol Res. 2019 Mar 11. doi:

10.1007/s00403-019-01908-x. [Epub ahead of print] Review. PubMed PMID: 30859308.

64. Dréno B. What is new in the pathophysiology of acne, an overview. J Eur Acad Dermatol Venereol. 2017 Sep;31 Suppl 5:8-12. doi: 10.1111/jdv.14374. Review. PubMed PMID: 28805938.
65. Alexeyev OA, Dekio I, Layton AM, Li H, Hughes H, Morris T, Zouboulis CC, Patrick S. Why we continue to use the name Propionibacterium acnes. Br J Dermatol. 2018 Nov;179(5):1227. doi: 10.1111/bjd.17085. Epub 2018 Sep 19. PubMed PMID: 30101491.
66. Bergfeld WF. The pathophysiology of acne vulgaris in children and adolescents, Part 1. Cutis. 2004 Aug;74(2):92-7. Review. PubMed PMID: 15379361.
67. Jiang H, Li C. Common Pathogenesis of Acne Vulgaris and Atherosclerosis. Inflammation. 2019 Feb;42(1):1-5. doi: 10.1007/s10753-018-0863-y. Review. PubMed PMID: 30073565.
68. Hanamatsu H, Ohnishi S, Sakai S, Yuyama K, Mitsutake S, Takeda H, Hashino S, Igarashi Y. Altered levels of serum sphingomyelin and ceramide containing distinct acyl chains in young obese adults. Nutr Diabetes. 2014 Oct 20;4:e141. doi: 10.1038/nutd.2014.38. PubMed PMID: 25329603; PubMed Central PMCID: PMC4217001.
69. Futerman AH, Hannun YA. The complex life of simple sphingolipids. EMBO Rep. 2004 Aug;5(8):777-82. Review. PubMed PMID: 15289826; PubMed Central PMCID: PMC1299119.
70. Borodzicz S, Rudnicka L, Mirowska-Guzel D, Cudnoch-Jedrzejewska A. The role of epidermal sphingolipids in dermatologic diseases. Lipids Health Dis. 2016 Jan 19;15:13. doi: 10.1186/s12944-016-0178-7. Review. PubMed PMID: 26786937; PubMed Central PMCID: PMC4717587.
71. Kaya S, Aslan İ, Kıraç E, Karaarslan T, Aslan M. Serum Sphingolipidomic Analysis in Acne Vulgaris P Kolar SL, Tsai CM, Torres J, Fan X, Li H, Liu GY. Propionibacterium acnes-induced immunopathology correlates with health and disease association. JCI Insight. 2019 Mar 7;4(5). pii: 124687. doi: 10.1172/jci.insight.124687. eCollection 2019 Mar 7. PubMed PMID: 30843879.atients. Ann Clin Lab Sci. 2019 Mar;49(2):242-248. PubMed PMID: 31028071.
72. Webster GF. The pathophysiology of acne. Cutis. 2005 Aug;76(2 Suppl):4-7. PubMed PMID: 16164150.
73. Knor T. The pathogenesis of acne. Acta Dermatovenerol Croat. 2005;13(1):44-9. PubMed PMID: 15788147.
74. Liu PF, Hsieh YD, Lin YC, Two A, Shu CW, Huang CM. Propionibacterium acnes in the pathogenesis and immunotherapy of acne vulgaris. Curr Drug Metab. 2015;16(4):245-54. Review. PubMed PMID: 26264195.
75. Li C, Chen J, Wang W, Ai M, Zhang Q, Kuang L. Use of isotretinoin and risk of depression in patients with acne: a systematic review and meta-analysis. BMJ Open. 2019 Jan 21;9(1):e021549. doi: 10.1136/bmjopen-2018-021549. Erratum in: BMJ Open. 2019 Mar 15;9(3):e021549corr1. PubMed PMID: 30670500; PubMed Central PMCID: PMC6347928.

76. Xiao Y, Chen L, Jing D, Deng Y, Chen X, Su J, Shen M. Willingness-to-pay and benefit-cost analysis of chemical peels for acne treatment in China. Patient Prefer Adherence. 2019 Feb 22;13:363-370. doi: 10.2147/PPA.S194615. eCollection 2019. PubMed PMID: 30863024; PubMed Central PMCID: PMC6391120.
77. Zhang M, Silverberg JI, Kaffenberger BH. Prescription patterns and costs of acne/rosacea medications in Medicare patients vary by prescriber specialty. J Am Acad Dermatol. 2017 Sep;77(3):448-455.e2. doi: 10.1016/j.jaad.2017.04.1127. Epub 2017 Jun 23. PubMed PMID: 28651825; PubMed Central PMCID: PMC5557700.
78. Czilli T, Tan J, Knezevic S, Peters C. Cost of Medications Recommended by Canadian Acne Clinical Practice Guidelines. J Cutan Med Surg. 2016 Nov;20(6):542-545. Epub 2016 Jun 8. PubMed PMID: 27281440.
79. Tassavor M, Payette MJ. Estimated cost efficacy of U.S. Food and Drug Administration-approved treatments for acne. Dermatol Ther. 2019 Jan;32(1):e12765. doi: 10.1111/dth.12765. Epub 2018 Nov 19. PubMed PMID: 30288869.
80. Saadawi AN, Esawy AM, Kandeel AH, El-Sayed W. Microneedling by dermapen and glycolic acid peel for the treatment of acne scars: Comparative study. J Cosmet Dermatol. 2019 Feb;18(1):107-114. doi: 10.1111/jocd.12827. Epub 2018 Dec 9. PubMed PMID: 30548170.
81. Castillo DE, Keri JE. Chemical peels in the treatment of acne: patient selection and perspectives. Clin CosmetInvestig Dermatol. 2018 Jul 16;11:365-372. doi: 10.2147/CCID.S137788. eCollection 2018. Review. PubMed PMID: 30038512; PubMed Central PMCID: PMC6053170.
82. Kraft J, Freiman A. Management of acne. CMAJ. 2011 Apr 19;183(7):E430-5. doi: 10.1503/cmaj.090374. Epub 2011 Feb 28. Review. PubMed PMID: 21398228; PubMed Central PMCID: PMC3080563.
83. InformedHealth.org [Internet]. Cologne, Germany: Institute for Quality and Efficiency in Health Care (IQWiG); 2006-. Acne: Overview. 2013 Jan 16 [Updated 2016 Jul 28]. Available from: https://www.ncbi.nlm.nih.gov/books/NBK279211/
84. Huang X, Zhang J, Li J, Zhao S, Xiao Y, Huang Y, Jing D, Chen L, Zhang X, Su J, Kuang Y, Zhu W, Chen M, Chen X, Shen M. Daily Intake of Soft Drinks and Moderate-to-Severe Acne Vulgaris in Chinese Adolescents. J Pediatr. 2019 Jan;204:256-262.e3. doi: 10.1016/j.jpeds.2018.08.034. Epub 2018 Sep 28. PubMed PMID: 30274928.
85. Coyner T. Insights Into the Management of Acne Vulgaris: Clinical Considerations for Acne Treatment. Journal of the Dermatology Nurses' Association: January/February 2018 - Volume 10 - Issue 1S - p S1. doi: 10.1097/JDN.0000000000000375.
86. Titus S, Hodge J. Diagnosis and treatment of acne. Am Fam Physician. 2012 Oct 15;86(8):734-40. Review. PubMed PMID: 23062156.
87. Freiman A, Barankin B. Five things to know about...: acne. CMAJ. 2012 Sep 18;184(13):1497. doi: 10.1503/cmaj.090639. Epub 2012 Feb 21. Review. PubMed PMID: 22353591; PubMed Central PMCID: PMC3447019.

88. Makrantonaki E, Ganceviciene R, Zouboulis C. An update on the role of the sebaceous gland in the pathogenesis of acne. Dermatoendocrinol. 2011 Jan;3(1):41-9. doi: 10.4161/derm.3.1.13900. PubMed PMID: 21519409; PubMed Central PMCID: PMC3051853.
89. Sun KL, Chang JM. Special types of folliculitis which should be differentiated from acne. Dermatoendocrinol. 2017 Sep 27;9(1):e1356519. doi: 10.1080/19381980.2017.1356519. eCollection 2017. Review. PubMed PMID: 29484091; PubMed Central PMCID: PMC5821164.
90. Nair PA, Salazar FJ. Acneiform Eruptions. [Updated 2018 Dec 2]. In: StatPearls [Internet]. Treasure Island (FL): StatPearls Publishing; 2019 Jan-. Available from: https://www.ncbi.nlm.nih.gov/books/NBK459207/
91. Du-Thanh A, Kluger N, Bensalleh H, Guillot B. Drug-induced acneiform eruption. Am J Clin Dermatol. 2011 Aug 1;12(4):233-45. doi: 10.2165/11588900-000000000-00000. Review. PubMed PMID: 21668032.
92. Kazandjieva J, Tsankov N. Drug-induced acne. Clin Dermatol. 2017 Mar - Apr;35(2):156-162. doi: 10.1016/j.clindermatol.2016.10.007. Epub 2016 Oct 27. PubMed PMID: 28274352.
93. Pontello R Jr, Kondo RN. Drug-induced acne and rose pearl: similarities. An Bras Dermatol. 2013 Nov-Dec;88(6):1039-40. doi: 10.1590/abd1806-4841.20132586. PubMed PMID: 24474128; PubMed Central PMCID: PMC3900370.
94. Ballard K, Shuman VL. Hidradenitis Suppurativa. [Updated 2019 Feb 28]. In: StatPearls [Internet]. Treasure Island (FL): StatPearls Publishing; 2019 Jan-. Available from: https://www.ncbi.nlm.nih.gov/books/NBK534867/
95. Pink A, Anzengruber F, Navarini AA. Acne and hidradenitis suppurativa. Br J Dermatol. 2018 Mar;178(3):619-631. doi: 10.1111/bjd.16231. Epub 2018 Jan 30. Review. PubMed PMID: 29380349.
96. Guerra KC, Krishnamurthy K. Miliaria. [Updated 2018 Dec 26]. In: StatPearls [Internet]. Treasure Island (FL): StatPearls Publishing; 2019 Jan-. Available from: https://www.ncbi.nlm.nih.gov/books/NBK537176/
97. Adotama P, Tinker D, Mitchell K, Glass DA 2nd, Allen P. Barber Knowledge and Recommendations Regarding Pseudofolliculitis Barbae and Acne Keloidalis Nuchae in an Urban Setting. JAMA Dermatol. 2017 Dec 1;153(12):1325-1326. doi: 10.1001/jamadermatol.2017.3668. PubMed PMID: 29049485; PubMed Central PMCID: PMC5817432.
98. Tan AU, Schlosser BJ, Paller AS. A review of diagnosis and treatment of acne in adult female patients. Int J Womens Dermatol. 2017 Dec 23;4(2):56-71. doi: 10.1016/j.ijwd.2017.10.006. eCollection 2018 Jun. Review. PubMed PMID: 29872679; PubMed Central PMCID: PMC5986265.
99. Tolaymat L, Hall MR. Dermatitis, Perioral. [Updated 2018 Oct 27]. In: StatPearls [Internet]. Treasure Island (FL): StatPearls Publishing; 2019 Jan-. Available from: https://www.ncbi.nlm.nih.gov/books/NBK525968/
100. Bikowski J. Facial seborrheic dermatitis: a report on current status and therapeutic horizons. J Drugs Dermatol. 2009 Feb;8(2):125-33. Review. PubMed PMID: 19213227.

101. Iftikhar U, Choudhry N. Serum levels of androgens in acne & their role in acne severity. Pak J Med Sci. 2019 Jan-Feb;35(1):146-150. doi: 10.12669/pjms.35.1.131. PubMed PMID: 30881413; PubMed Central PMCID: PMC6408631.

102. Hoover E, Krishnamurthy K. Physiology, Sebaceous Glands. [Updated 2018 Oct 27]. In: StatPearls [Internet]. Treasure Island (FL): StatPearls Publishing; 2019 Jan-. Available from: https://www.ncbi.nlm.nih.gov/books/NBK499819/

103. Ottaviani M, Camera E, Picardo M. Lipid mediators in acne. Mediators Inflamm. 2010;2010. pii: 858176. doi: 10.1155/2010/858176. Epub 2010 Aug 25. Review. PubMed PMID: 20871834; PubMed Central PMCID: PMC2943135.

104. Downing DT, Stewart ME, Wertz PW, Strauss JS. Essential fatty acids and acne. J Am Acad Dermatol. 1986 Feb;14(2 Pt 1):221-5. PubMed PMID: 2936775.

105. Jung JY, Kwon HH, Hong JS, Yoon JY, Park MS, Jang MY, Suh DH. Effect of dietary supplementation with omega-3 fatty acid and gamma-linolenic acid on acne vulgaris: a randomised, double-blind, controlled trial. Acta DermVenereol. 2014 Sep;94(5):521-5. doi: 10.2340/00015555-1802. PubMed PMID: 24553997.

106. Silva JR, Burger B, Kühl CMC, Candreva T, Dos Anjos MBP, Rodrigues HG. Wound Healing and Omega-6 Fatty Acids: From Inflammation to Repair. Mediators Inflamm. 2018 Apr 12;2018:2503950. doi: 10.1155/2018/2503950. eCollection 2018. Review. PubMed PMID: 29849484; PubMed Central PMCID: PMC5925018.

107. Kartal D, Yildiz H, Ertas R, Borlu M, Utas S. Association between isolated female acne and insulin resistance: a prospective study. G Ital Dermatol Venereol. 2016 Aug;151(4):353-7. Epub 2015 Sep 15. PubMed PMID: 26373866.

108. Hwang YL, Lee MH, Oh HI, Kim HJ, Lim CA, Lee JH, Kim CD. Isoginkgetin Inhibits Insulin-Like Growth Factor-1-Induced Sebum Production in Cultured Human Sebocytes. Ann Dermatol. 2018 Jun;30(3):394-396. doi: 10.5021/ad.2018.30.3.394. Epub 2018 Apr 23. PubMed PMID: 29853769; PubMed Central PMCID: PMC5929972.

109. Picardo M, Ottaviani M, Camera E, Mastrofrancesco A. Sebaceous gland lipids. Dermatoendocrinol. 2009 Mar;1(2):68-71. PubMed PMID: 20224686; PubMed Central PMCID: PMC2835893.

110. Tolaymat L, Zito PM. Adapalene. [Updated 2019 Feb 2]. In: StatPearls [Internet]. Treasure Island (FL): StatPearls Publishing; 2019 Jan-. Available from: https://www.ncbi.nlm.nih.gov/books/NBK482509/.

111. Eady EA, Layton AM, Cove JH. A honey trap for the treatment of acne: manipulating the follicular microenvironment to control Propionibacterium acnes. Biomed Res Int. 2013;2013:679680. doi: 10.1155/2013/679680. Epub 2013 May 14. PubMed PMID: 23762853; PubMed Central PMCID: PMC3666392.

112. Pelle E, McCarthy J, Seltmann H, Huang X, Mammone T, Zouboulis CC, Maes D. Identification of histamine receptors and reduction of squalene levels by an antihistamine in sebocytes. J Invest Dermatol. 2008 May;128(5):1280-5. Epub2007 Nov 15. PubMed PMID: 18007585.

113. Seo YJ, Li ZJ, Choi DK, Sohn KC, Kim HR, Lee Y, Kim CD, Lee YH, Shi G, Lee JH, Im M. Regional difference in sebum production by androgen susceptibility in

human facial skin. Exp Dermatol. 2014 Jan;23(1):70-2. doi: 10.1111/exd.12291. PubMed PMID: 24289322.

114. Ozuguz P, DogrukKacar S, Ekiz O, Takci Z, Balta I, Kalkan G. Evaluation of serum vitamins A and E and zinc levels according to the severity of acne vulgaris. CutanOculToxicol. 2014 Jun;33(2):99-102. doi: 10.3109/15569527.2013.808656. Epub 2013 Jul 5. PubMed PMID: 23826827.

115. Vongraviopap S, Asawanonda P. Dark chocolate exacerbates acne. Int J Dermatol. 2016 May;55(5):587-91. doi: 10.1111/ijd.13188. Epub 2015 Dec 29. PubMed PMID: 26711092.

116. Goodman G. Acne--natural history, facts and myths. Aust Fam Physician. 2006 Aug;35(8):613-6. Review. PubMed PMID: 16894437.

117. Chalyk N, Klochkov V, Sommereux L, Bandaletova T, Kyle N, Petyaev I. Continuous Dark Chocolate Consumption Affects Human Facial Skin Surface by Stimulating Corneocyte Desquamation and Promoting Bacterial Colonization. J Clin Aesthet Dermatol. 2018 Sep;11(9):37-41. Epub 2018 Sep 1. PubMed PMID: 30319730; PubMed Central PMCID: PMC6169599.

118. Web George Mateljan Foundation. Shrimp What's New and Beneficial About Shrimp. Available From: http://www.whfoods.com/genpage.php?pfriendly=1&tname=foodspice&dbid=107

119. Kidson W. Polycystic ovary syndrome: a new direction in treatment. Med J Aust. 1998 Nov 16;169(10):537-40. Review. PubMed PMID: 9861912.

120. Aizawa H, Niimura M. Elevated serum insulin-like growth factor-1 (IGF-1) levels in women with postadolescent acne. J Dermatol. 1995 Apr;22(4):249-52. PubMed PMID: 7608381.

121. Mahmood NF, Shipman AR. The age-old problem of acne. Int J Womens Dermatol. 2016 Dec 2;3(2):71-76. doi: 10.1016/j.ijwd.2016.11.002. eCollection 2017 Jun. PubMed PMID: 28560299; PubMed Central PMCID: PMC5440448.

122. Rössner S. John Harvey Kellogg (1852-1943): "Masturbation results in general debility, unnatural pale eyes and forehead acne". Obes Rev. 2006 May;7(2):227-8. PubMed PMID: 16629878.

123. Ayer J, Burrows N. Acne: more than skin deep. Postgrad Med J. 2006 Aug;82(970):500-6. Review. PubMed PMID: 16891439; PubMed Central PMCID: PMC2585707.

124. Misery L, Wolkenstein P, Amici JM, Maghia R, Brenaut E, Cazeau C, VoisardJJ, Taïeb C. Consequences of acne on stress, fatigue, sleep disorders and sexual activity: a population-based study. Acta DermVenereol. 2015 Apr;95(4):485-8. doi: 10.2340/00015555-1998. PubMed PMID: 25365961.

125. Zelickson AS, Strauss JS, Mottaz J. Ultrastructural changes in open comedones following treatment of cystic acne with isotretinoin. Am J Dermatopathol. 1985 Jun;7(3):241-4. PubMed PMID: 2413783.

126. Allen HB, LoPresti PJ. Acne vulgaris aggravated by sunlight. Cutis. 1980 Sep;26(3):254-6. PubMed PMID: 6448731.

127. Padilha-Gonçalves A, Alvimar Ferreira J. [Solar acne]. Med CutanIbero Lat Am. 1977;5(4):271-4. Portuguese. PubMed PMID: 152828.

128. Magin P, Pond D, Smith W, Watson A. A systematic review of the evidence for 'myths and misconceptions' in acne management: diet, face-washing and sunlight. Fam Pract. 2005 Feb;22(1):62-70. Epub 2005 Jan 11. Review. PubMed PMID: 15644386.
129. Praderio C. Here's how 13 celebrities got rid of their acne. INSIDER (Health), September 15, 2017.
130. Khayef G, Young J, Burns-Whitmore B, Spalding T. Effects of fish oil supplementation on inflammatory acne. Lipids Health Dis. 2012 Dec 3;11:165. doi: 10.1186/1476-511X-11-165. PubMed PMID: 23206895; PubMed Central PMCID: PMC3543297.
131. Capitanio B, Sinagra JL, Ottaviani M, Bordignon V, Amantea A, Picardo M. Acne and smoking. Dermatoendocrinol. 2009 May;1(3):129-35. PubMed PMID: 20436880; PubMed Central PMCID: PMC2835905.
132. Orenstein H. How 32 Celebrities With Acne Handle Blemishes and Breakouts. SEVENTEEN, November 8, 2018.
133. Gabros S, Zito PM. Topical Corticosteroids. [Updated 2019 Jan 10]. In: StatPearls [Internet]. Treasure Island (FL): StatPearls Publishing; 2019 Jan-. Available from: https://www.ncbi.nlm.nih.gov/books/NBK532940/
134. Yasir M, Sonthalia S. Corticosteroid Adverse Effects. [Updated 2019 Mar 24]. In: StatPearls [Internet]. Treasure Island (FL): StatPearls Publishing; 2019 Jan-. Available from: https://www.ncbi.nlm.nih.gov/books/NBK531462/
135. Cleaning Makeup Brushes Like A Pro. Available From: https://kjbennett.com/category/beauty-tutorial/
136. Fife D. Practical evaluation and management of atrophic acne scars: tips for the general dermatologist. J Clin Aesthet Dermatol. 2011 Aug;4(8):50-7. PubMed PMID: 21909457; PubMed Central PMCID: PMC3168245.
137. Fabbrocini G, Annunziata MC, D'Arco V, De Vita V, Lodi G, Mauriello MC, Pastore F, Monfrecola G. Acne scars: pathogenesis, classification and treatment. Dermatol Res Pract. 2010;2010:893080. doi: 10.1155/2010/893080. Epub 2010 Oct 14. PubMed PMID: 20981308, PubMed Central PMCID: PMC2958495.
138. Kravvas G, Al-Niaimi F. A systematic review of treatments for acne scarring. Part 1: Non-energy-based techniques. Scars Burn Heal. 2017 Mar 30;3:2059513117695312. doi: 10.1177/2059513117695312. eCollection 2017 Jan-Dec. Review. PubMed PMID: 29799567; PubMed Central PMCID: PMC5965325.
139. Gan SD, Graber EM. Papular scars: an addition to the acne scar classification scheme. J Clin Aesthet Dermatol. 2015 Jan;8(1):19-20. PubMed PMID: 25610520; PubMed Central PMCID: PMC4295854.
140. McGinty S, Siddiqui WJ. Keloid. [Updated 2019 Mar 19]. In: StatPearls [Internet]. Treasure Island (FL): StatPearls Publishing; 2019 Jan-. Available from: https://www.ncbi.nlm.nih.gov/books/NBK507899/
141. Connolly D, Vu HL, Mariwalla K, Saedi N. Acne Scarring-Pathogenesis, Evaluation, and Treatment Options. J Clin Aesthet Dermatol. 2017 Sep;10(9):12-23. Epub 2017 Sep 1. Review. PubMed PMID: 29344322; PubMed Central PMCID: PMC5749614.

142. Hazarika N, Archana M. The Psychosocial Impact of Acne Vulgaris. Indian J Dermatol. 2016 Sep-Oct;61(5):515-20. doi: 10.4103/0019-5154.190102. PubMed PMID: 27688440; PubMed Central PMCID: PMC5029236.
143. Behnam B, Taheri R, Ghorbani R, Allameh P. Psychological impairments in the patients with acne. Indian J Dermatol. 2013 Jan;58(1):26-9. doi: 10.4103/0019-5154.105281. PubMed PMID: 23372208; PubMed Central PMCID: PMC3555368.
144. Alanazi MS, Hammad SM, Mohamed AE. Prevalence and psychological impact of Acne vulgaris among female secondary school students in Arar city, Saudi Arabia, in 2018. Electron Physician. 2018 Aug 25;10(8):7224-7229. doi: 10.19082/7224. eCollection 2018 Aug. PubMed PMID: 30214705; PubMed Central PMCID: PMC6122864.
145. Dreno B, Bagatin E, Blume-Peytavi U, Rocha M, Gollnick H. Female type of adult acne: Physiological and psychological considerations and management. J Dtsch Dermatol Ges. 2018 Oct;16(10):1185-1194. doi: 10.1111/ddg.13664. Epub 2018 Sep 24. Review. PubMed PMID: 30248242.
146. Gao Y, Wei EK, Arron ST, Linos E, Margolis DJ, Mansh MD. Acne, sexual orientation, and mental health among young adults in the United States: A population-based, cross-sectional study. J Am Acad Dermatol. 2017 Nov;77(5):971-973. doi: 10.1016/j.jaad.2017.06.004. PubMed PMID: 29029907; PubMed Central PMCID: PMC6181754.
147. Vilar GN, Santos LA, Sobral Filho JF. Quality of life, self-esteem and psychosocial factors in adolescents with acne vulgaris. An Bras Dermatol. 2015 Sep-Oct;90(5):622-9. doi: 10.1590/abd1806-4841.201533726. PubMed PMID: 26560206; PubMed Central PMCID: PMC4631226.
148. Kurek A, Peters EM, Chanwangpong A, Sabat R, Sterry W, Schneider-Burrus S. Profound disturbances of sexual health in patients with acne inversa. J Am Acad Dermatol. 2012 Sep;67(3):422-8, 428.e1. doi: 10.1016/j.jaad.2011.10.024. Epub 2011 Dec 17. PubMed PMID: 22182915.
149. Bray AP, Kravvas G, Skevington SM, Lovell CR. Is there an association between isotretinoin therapy and adverse mood changes? A prospective study in a cohort of acne patients. J Dermatolog Treat. 2019 Feb 18:1-6. doi: 10.1080/09546634.2019.1577545. [Epub ahead of print] PubMed PMID: 30717601.
150. Hull PR, D'Arcy C. Acne, depression, and suicide. Dermatol Clin. 2005 Oct;23(4):665-74. Review. PubMed PMID: 16112443.
151. Ulvestad M, Bjertness E, Dalgard F, Halvorsen JA. Acne and dairy products in adolescence: results from a Norwegian longitudinal study. J Eur Acad Dermatol Venereol. 2017 Mar;31(3):530-535. doi: 10.1111/jdv.13835. Epub 2016 Jul 16. PubMed PMID: 27422392.
152. Aghasi M, Golzarand M, Shab-Bidar S, Aminianfar A, Omidian M, Taheri F. Dairy intake and acne development: A meta-analysis of observational studies. Clin Nutr. 2018 May 8. pii: S0261-5614(18)30166-3. doi: 10.1016/j.clnu.2018.04.015. [Epub ahead of print] PubMed PMID: 29778512.
153. Harris S. Can dietary changes help acne? MedicalNewsToday, 31 July 2018.

154. Delost GR, Delost ME, Lloyd J. The impact of chocolate consumption on acne vulgaris in college students: A randomized crossover study. J Am Acad Dermatol. 2016 Jul;75(1):220-2. doi: 10.1016/j.jaad.2016.02.1159. PubMed PMID: 27317522.

155. Smith RN, Mann NJ, Braue A, Mäkeläinen H, Varigos GA. A low-glycemic-load diet improves symptoms in acne vulgaris patients: a randomized controlled trial. Am J ClinNutr. 2007 Jul;86(1):107-15. PubMed PMID: 17616769.

156. Burris J, Shikany JM, Rietkerk W, Woolf K. A Low Glycemic Index and Glycemic Load Diet Decreases Insulin-like Growth Factor-1 among Adults with Moderate and Severe Acne: A Short-Duration, 2-Week Randomized Controlled Trial. J AcadNutr Diet. 2018 Oct;118(10):1874-1885. doi: 10.1016/j.jand.2018.02.009. Epub 2018 Apr 22. PubMed PMID: 29691143.

157. Bove A, Hebreo J, Wylie-Rosett J, Isasi CR. Burger King and Subway: key nutrients, glycemic index, and glycemic load of nutritionally promoted items. Diabetes Educ. 2006 Sep-Oct;32(5):675-90. PubMed PMID: 16971703.

158. CordainL, Lindeberg S, Hurtado M, Hill K, Eaton SB, Brand-Miller J. Acne vulgaris: a disease of Western civilization. Arch Dermatol. 2002 Dec;138(12):1584-90. PubMed PMID: 12472346.

159. Klepchukova A. Acne: Everything You Need to Know. Flo Health, Inc., March 18, 2019.

160. National Research Council (US) Committee on Diet and Health. Diet and Health: Implications for Reducing Chronic Disease Risk. Washington (DC): National Academies Press (US); 1989. 10, Dietary Fiber. Available from: https://www.ncbi.nlm.nih.gov/books/NBK218764/

161. Bowe WP, Logan AC. Acne vulgaris, probiotics and the gut-brain-skin axis - back to the future? Gut Pathog. 2011 Jan 31;3(1):1. doi: 10.1186/1757-4749-3-1. PubMed PMID: 21281494; PubMed Central PMCID: PMC3038963.

162. Zhang H, Liao W, Chao W, Chen Q, Zeng H, Wu C, Wu S, Ho HI. Risk factors for sebaceous gland diseases and their relationship to gastrointestinal dysfunction in Han adolescents. J Dermatol. 2008 Sep;35(9):555-61. doi: 10.1111/j.1346-8138.2008.00523.x. PubMed PMID: 18837699.

163. Saric S, Notay M, Sivamani RK. Green Tea and Other Tea Polyphenols: Effects on Sebum Production and Acne Vulgaris. Antioxidants (Basel). 2016 Dec 29;6(1). pii: E2. doi: 10.3390/antiox6010002. Review. PubMed PMID: 28036057; PubMed Central PMCID: PMC5384166.

164. Database of Abstracts of Reviews of Effects (DARE): Quality-assessed Reviews [Internet]. York (UK): Centre for Reviews and Dissemination (UK); 1995-. Polyphenols as novel treatment options for dermatological diseases: a systematic review of clinical trials. 2014. Available from: https://www.ncbi.nlm.nih.gov/books/NBK291682/

165. Mahmood T, Akhtar N, Moldovan C. A comparison of the effects of topical green tea and lotus on facial sebum control in healthy humans. Hippokratia. 2013 Jan;17(1):64-7. PubMed PMID: 23935347; PubMed Central PMCID: PMC3738281.

166. Lee KE, Youm JK, Lee WJ, Kang S, Kim YJ. Polyphenol-rich apple extract inhibits dexamethasone-induced sebaceous lipids production by regulating SREBP1 expression. Exp Dermatol. 2017 Oct;26(10):958-960. doi: 10.1111/exd.13319. Epub 2017 Apr 21. PubMed PMID: 28191675.
167. El-Akawi Z, Abdel-Latif N, Abdul-Razzak K. Does the plasma level of vitamins A and E affect acne condition? Clin Exp Dermatol. 2006 May;31(3):430-4. PubMed PMID: 16681594.
168. Stringer T, Nagler A, Orlow SJ, Oza VS. Clinical evidence for washing and cleansers in acne vulgaris: a systematic review. J Dermatolog Treat. 2018 Nov;29(7):688-693. doi: 10.1080/09546634.2018.1442552. Epub 2018 Feb 25. Review. PubMed PMID: 29460655.
169. Choi YS, Suh HS, Yoon MY, Min SU, Kim JS, Jung JY, Lee DH, Suh DH. A study of the efficacy of cleansers for acne vulgaris. J Dermatolog Treat. 2010 May;21(3):201-5. doi: 10.3109/09546630903401454. PubMed PMID: 20394494.
170. Draelos ZD. The effect of a daily facial cleanser for normal to oily skin on the skin barrier of subjects with acne. Cutis. 2006 Jul;78(1 Suppl):34-40. PubMed PMID: 16910029.
171. Prakash C, Bhargava P, Tiwari S, Majumdar B, Bhargava RK. Skin Surface pH in Acne Vulgaris: Insights from an Observational Study and Review of the Literature. J Clin Aesthet Dermatol. 2017 Jul;10(7):33-39. Epub 2017 Jul 1. PubMed PMID: 29104722; PubMed Central PMCID: PMC5605222.
172. Kawashima M, Nagare T, Doi M. Clinical efficacy and safety of benzoyl peroxide for acne vulgaris: Comparison between Japanese and Western patients. J Dermatol. 2017 Nov;44(11):1212-1218. doi: 10.1111/1346-8138.13996. Epub 2017 Aug 9. Review. PubMed PMID: 28791735; PubMed Central PMCID: PMC5697687.
173. Matin T, Goodman MB. Benzoyl Peroxide. [Updated 2019 Jan 2]. In: StatPearls [Internet]. Treasure Island (FL): StatPearls Publishing; 2019 Jan-. Available from: https://www.ncbi.nlm.nih.gov/books/NBK537220/
174. Gold MH, Baldwin H, Lin T. Management of comedonal acne vulgaris with fixed-combination topical therapy. J Cosmet Dermatol. 2018 Apr;17(2):227-231. doi: 10.1111/jocd.12497. Epub 2018 Jan 30. Review. PubMed PMID: 29380941.
175. Dréno B, Bissonnette R, Gagné-Henley A, Barankin B, Lynde C, Kerrouche N, Tan J. Prevention and Reduction of Atrophic Acne Scars with Adapalene 0.3%/Benzoyl Peroxide 2.5% Gel in Subjects with Moderate or Severe Facial Acne: Results of a 6-Month Randomized, Vehicle-Controlled Trial Using Intra-Individual Comparison. Am J Clin Dermatol. 2018 Apr;19(2):275-286. doi: 10.1007/s40257-018-0352-y. PubMed PMID: 29549588; PubMed Central PMCID: PMC5978908.
176. Mansu SSY, Liang H, Parker S, Coyle ME, Wang K, Zhang AL, Guo X, Lu C, Xue CCL. Acupuncture for Acne Vulgaris: A Systematic Review and Meta-Analysis. Evid Based Complement Alternat Med. 2018 Mar 12;2018:4806734. doi: 10.1155/2018/4806734. eCollection 2018. Review. PubMed PMID: 29721027; PubMed Central PMCID: PMC5867647.

177. Sagransky M, Yentzer BA, Feldman SR. Benzoyl peroxide: a review of its current use in the treatment of acne vulgaris. Expert OpinPharmacother. 2009 Oct;10(15):2555-62. doi: 10.1517/14656560903277228. Review. PubMed PMID: 19761357.
178. Fakhouri T, Yentzer BA, Feldman SR. Advancement in benzoyl peroxide-based acne treatment: methods to increase both efficacy and tolerability. J Drugs Dermatol. 2009 Jul;8(7):657-61. Review. PubMed PMID: 19588642.
179. Kircik LH. The role of benzoyl peroxide in the new treatment paradigm for acne. J Drugs Dermatol. 2013 Jun 1;12(6):s73-6. PubMed PMID: 23839205.
180. What is the Role of Benzoyl Peroxide Cleansers in Acne Management?: Do they Decrease Propionibacterium acnes Counts? Do they Reduce Acne Lesions? J Clin Aesthet Dermatol. 2008 Nov;1(4):48-51. PubMed PMID: 21218192; PubMed Central PMCID: PMC3016935.
181. Stein Gold L, Baldwin HE, Lin T. Management of Severe Acne Vulgaris With Topical Therapy. J Drugs Dermatol. 2017 Nov 1;16(11):1134-1138. Review. PubMed PMID: 29141062.
182. Leyden JJ, Del Rosso JQ. The effect of benzoyl peroxide 9.8% emollient foam on reduction of Propionibacterium acnes on the back using a short contact therapy approach. J Drugs Dermatol. 2012 Jul;11(7):830-3. PubMed PMID: 22777224.
183. Murphy PB, Le JK. Clindamycin. [Updated 2019 Feb 17]. In: StatPearls [Internet]. Treasure Island (FL): StatPearls Publishing; 2019 Jan-. Available from: https://www.ncbi.nlm.nih.gov/books/NBK519574/
184. Ohlson J, Dakovic R, Berg M. Observational Study of Clindamycin Phosphate and Tretinoin Gel for the Treatment of Acne. J Drugs Dermatol. 2019 Apr 1;18(4):328-334. PubMed PMID: 31012560.
185. Dréno B, Layton A, Zouboulis CC, López-Estebaranz JL, Zalewska-Janowska A, Bagatin E, Zampeli VA, Yutskovskaya Y, Harper JC. Adult female acne: a new paradigm. J Eur Acad Dermatol Venereol. 2013 Sep;27(9):1063-70. doi: 10.1111/jdv.12061. Epub 2013 Jan 10. Review. PubMed PMID: 23302006.
186. Kong YL, Tey HL. Treatment of acne vulgaris during pregnancy and lactation. Drugs. 2013 Jun;73(8):779-87. doi: 10.1007/s40265-013-0060-0. Review. PubMed PMID: 23657872.
187. Aoki S, Nakase K, Hayashi N, Noguchi N. Transconjugation of erm(X) conferring high-level resistance of clindamycin for Cutibacterium acnes. J Med Microbiol. 2019 Jan;68(1):26-30. doi: 10.1099/jmm.0.000875. Epub 2018 Nov 15. PubMed PMID: 30431414.
188. Amar L, Kircik LH. Treatment of Moderate Acne Vulgaris in Fitzpatrick Skin Type V or VI: Efficacy and Tolerability of Fixed Combination Clindamycin Phosphate 1.2%/Benzoyl Peroxide 3.75% Gel. J Drugs Dermatol. 2018 Oct 1;17(10):1107-1112. PubMed PMID: 30365592.
189. Del Rosso JQ. Clindamycin Phosphate 1.2%/Tretinoin 0.025% Gel for the Treatment of Acne Vulgaris: Which Patients are Most Likely to Benefit the Most? J Clin Aesthet Dermatol. 2015 Jun;8(6):19-23. PubMed PMID: 26155323; PubMed Central PMCID: PMC4479365.

190. Ochsendorf F. Clindamycin phosphate 1.2% / tretinoin 0.025%: a novel fixed-dose combination treatment for acne vulgaris. J Eur Acad Dermatol Venereol. 2015 Jun;29 Suppl 5:8-13. doi: 10.1111/jdv.13185. Review. PubMed PMID: 26059820.

191. Murray J, Potts A. The phototoxic and photoallergy potential of clindamycin phosphate 1.2%/ tretinoin 0.025% gel for facial acne: results of two single-center, evaluator-blinded, randomized, vehicle-controlled phase 1 studies in healthy volunteers. J Drugs Dermatol. 2014 Jan;13(1):16-22. PubMed PMID: 24385115.

192. Zaenglein AL, Shamban A, Webster G, Del Rosso J, Dover JS, Swinyer L, Stein L, Lin X, Draelos Z, Gold M, Thiboutot D. A phase IV, open-label study evaluating the use of triple-combination therapy with minocycline HCl extended-release tablets, a topical antibiotic/retinoid preparation and benzoyl peroxide in patients with moderate to severe acne vulgaris. J Drugs Dermatol. 2013 Jun 1;12(6):619-25. PubMed PMID: 23839176.

193. ZeichnerJA, Wong V, Linkner RV, Haddican M. Efficacy and safety of tretinoin 0.025%/clindamycin phosphate 1.2% gel in combination with benzoyl peroxide 6% cleansing cloths for the treatment of facial acne vulgaris. J Drugs Dermatol. 2013 Mar;12(3):277-82. PubMed PMID: 23545909.

194. Leyden J, Stein-Gold L, Weiss J. Why Topical Retinoids Are Mainstay of Therapy for Acne. Dermatol Ther (Heidelb). 2017 Sep;7(3):293-304. doi: 10.1007/s13555-017-0185-2. Epub 2017 Jun 5. Review. PubMed PMID: 28585191; PubMed Central PMCID: PMC5574737.

195. Thielitz A, Gollnick H. Topical retinoids in acne vulgaris: update on efficacy and safety. Am J Clin Dermatol. 2008;9(6):369-81. doi: 10.2165/0128071-200809060-00003. Review. PubMed PMID: 18973403.

196. Tan J, Tanghetti E, Baldwin H, Stein Gold L, Lain E. The Role of Topical Retinoids in Prevention and Treatment of Atrophic Acne Scarring: Understanding the Importance of Early Effective Treatment. J Drugs Dermatol. 2019 Mar 1;18(3):255-260. PubMed PMID: 30909329.

197. Tolaymat L, Zito PM. Adapalene. [Updated 2019 Feb 2]. In: StatPearls [Internet]. Treasure Island (FL): StatPearls Publishing; 2019 Jan-. Available from: https://www.ncbi.nlm.nih.gov/books/NBK482509/

198. Jain S. Topical tretinoin or adapalene in acne vulgaris: an overview. J Dermatolog Treat. 2004 Jul;15(4):200-7. Review. PubMed PMID: 15764031.

199. Kolli SS, Pecone D, Pona A, Cline A, Feldman SR. Topical Retinoids in Acne Vulgaris: A Systematic Review. Am J Clin Dermatol. 2019 Jan 23. doi: 10.1007/s40257-019-00423-z. [Epub ahead of print] Review. PubMed PMID: 30674002.

200. Chandrashekhar BS, Anitha M, Ruparelia M, Vaidya P, Aamir R, Shah S, Thilak S, Aurangabadkar S, Pal S, Saraswat A, Sanmukhani JJ. Tretinoin Nanogel 0.025% Versus Conventional Gel 0.025% in Patients with Acne Vulgaris: A Randomized, Active Controlled, Multicentre, Parallel Group, Phase IV Clinical Trial. J Clin Diagn Res. 2015 Jan;9(1):WC04-9. doi: 10.7860/JCDR/2015/10663.5469. Epub 2015 Jan 1. PubMed PMID: 25738069; PubMed Central PMCID: PMC4347160.

201. Harper JC, Roberts WE, Zeichner JA, Guenin E, Bhatt V, Pillai R. Novel tretinoin 0.05% lotion for the once-daily treatment of moderate-to-severe acne vulgaris: assessment of safety and tolerability in subgroups. J Dermatolog Treat. 2019 Apr 2:1-8. doi: 10.1080/09546634.2019.1587884. [Epub ahead of print] PubMed PMID: 30935257.

202. Hajheydari Z, Saeedi M, Morteza-Semnani K, Soltani A. Effect of Aloe vera topical gel combined with tretinoin in treatment of mild and moderate acne vulgaris: a randomized, double-blind, prospective trial. J Dermatolog Treat. 2014 Apr;25(2):123-9. doi: 10.3109/09546634.2013.768328. Epub 2013 May 6. PubMed PMID: 23336746.

203. Deshmukh SN, Badar VA, Mahajan MM, Dudhgaonkar DS, Mishra D. Comparison of efficacy and safety of topical 1% nadifloxacin and tretinoin 0.025% combination therapy with 1% clindamycin and tretinoin 0.025% combination therapy in patients of mild-to-moderate acne. Perspect Clin Res. 2018 Oct-Dec;9(4):161-164. doi: 10.4103/picr.PICR_109_17. PubMed PMID: 30319945; PubMed Central PMCID: PMC6176694.

204. Kircik LH. Synergy and its clinical relevance in topical acne therapy. J Clin Aesthet Dermatol. 2011 Nov;4(11):30-3. PubMed PMID: 22125656; PubMed Central PMCID: PMC3225138.

205. Hashim PW, Chen T, Harper JC, Kircik LH. The Efficacy and Safety of Azelaic Acid 15% Foam in the Treatment of Facial Acne Vulgaris. J Drugs Dermatol. 2018 Jun 1;17(6):641-645. PubMed PMID: 29879251.

206. Apriani EF, Rosana Y, Iskandarsyah I. Formulation, characterization, and in vitro testing of azelaic acid ethosome-based cream against Propionibacterium acnes for the treatment of acne. J Adv Pharm Technol Res. 2019 Apr-Jun;10(2):75-80. doi: 10.4103/japtr.JAPTR_289_18. PubMed PMID: 31041186; PubMed Central PMCID: PMC6474161.

207. Abdel Hay R, Hegazy R, Abdel Hady M, Saleh N. Clinical and dermoscopic evaluation of combined (salicylic acid 20% and azelaic acid 20%) versus trichloroacetic acid 25% chemical peel in acne: an RCT. J Dermatolog Treat. 2019 Mar 1:1-6. doi: 10.1080/09546634.2018.1484876. [Epub ahead of print] PubMed PMID: 29862871.

208. Rocha M, Sanudo A, Bagatin E. The effect on acne quality of life of topical azelaic acid 15% gel versus a combined oral contraceptive in adult female acne: A randomized trial. Dermatoendocrinol. 2017 Oct 13;9(1):e1361572. doi: 10.1080/19381980.2017.1361572. eCollection 2017. PubMed PMID: 29484094; PubMed Central PMCID: PMC5821159.

209. Kainz JT, Berghammer G, Auer-Grumbach P, Lackner V, Perl-Convalexius S, Popa R, Wolfesberger B. Azelaic acid 20 % cream: effects on quality of life and disease severity in adult female acne patients. J Dtsch Dermatol Ges. 2016 Dec;14(12):1249-1259. doi: 10.1111/ddg.12889. Epub 2016 Nov 29. PubMed PMID: 27897372.

210. Burchacka E, Potaczek P, Paduszyński P, Karłowicz-Bodalska K, Han T, Han S. New effective azelaic acid liposomal gel formulation of enhanced pharmaceutical

bioavailability. Biomed Pharmacother. 2016 Oct;83:771-775. doi: 10.1016/j.biopha.2016.07.014. Epub 2016 Jul 30. PubMed PMID: 27484346.

211. Ebede TL, Arch EL, Berson D. Hormonal treatment of acne in women. J Clin Aesthet Dermatol. 2009 Dec;2(12):16-22. PubMed PMID: 20725580; PubMed Central PMCID: PMC2923944.

212. Wohlrab J, Michael J. Dapsone for topical use in extemporaneous preparations. J Dtsch Dermatol Ges. 2018 Jan;16(1):34-40. doi: 10.1111/ddg.13409. Epub 2017 Dec 27. PubMed PMID: 29280553.

213. Subramaniam A, Corallo C, Nagappan R. Dapsone-associated methaemoglobinaemia in patients with a haematologic malignancy. Anaesth Intensive Care. 2010 Nov;38(6):1070-6. PubMed PMID: 21226440.

214. El-Nabarawi MA, Shamma RN, Farouk F, Nasralla SM. Bilosomes as a novel carrier for the cutaneous delivery for dapsone as a potential treatment of acne: Preparation, characterization and in-vivo skin deposition assay. J Liposome Res. 2019 Apr 22:1-26. doi: 10.1080/08982104.2019.1577256. [Epub ahead of print] PubMed PMID: 31010357.

215. Molinelli E, Paolinelli M, Campanati A, Brisigotti V, Offidani A. Metabolic, pharmacokinetic, and toxicological issues surrounding dapsone. Expert Opin Drug MetabToxicol. 2019 May;15(5):367-379. doi: 10.1080/17425255.2019.1600670. Epub 2019 Apr 19. PubMed PMID: 30943794.

216. Del Rosso JQ, Kircik L, Tanghetti E. Management of Truncal Acne Vulgaris with Topical Dapsone 7.5% Gel. J Clin Aesthet Dermatol. 2018 Aug;11(8):45-50. Epub 2018 Aug 1. PubMed PMID: 30214667; PubMed Central PMCID: PMC6122512.

217. Kircik LH. Use of Dapsone 5% Gel as Maintenance Treatment of Acne Vulgaris Following Completion of Oral Doxycycline and Dapsone 5% Gel Combination Treatment. J Drugs Dermatol. 2016 Feb;15(2):191-5. PubMed PMID: 26885787.

218. Stein Gold LF, Jarratt MT, Bucko AD, Grekin SK, Berlin JM, Bukhalo M, Weiss JS, Berk DR, Chang-Lin JE, Lin V, Kaoukhov A. Efficacy and Safety of Once-Daily Dapsone Gel, 7.5% for Treatment of Adolescents and Adults With Acne Vulgaris: First of Two Identically Designed, Large, Multicenter, Randomized, Vehicle-controlled Trials. J Drugs Dermatol. 2016 May 1;15(5):553-61. PubMed PMID: 27168264.

219. Thiboutot DM, Kircik L, McMichael A, Cook-Bolden FE, Tyring SK, Berk DR, Chang-Lin JE, Lin V, Kaoukhov A. Efficacy, Safety, and Dermal Tolerability of Dapsone Gel, 7.5% in Patients with Moderate Acne Vulgaris: A Pooled Analysis of Two Phase 3 Trials. J Clin Aesthet Dermatol. 2016 Oct;9(10):18-27. Epub 2016 Oct 1. PubMed PMID: 27847545; PubMed Central PMCID: PMC5104308.

220. Alexis AF, Burgess C, Callender VD, Herzog JL, Roberts WE, Schweiger ES, Stockton TC, Gallagher CJ. The Efficacy and Safety of Topical Dapsone Gel, 5% for the Treatment of Acne Vulgaris in Adult Females With Skin of Color. J Drugs Dermatol. 2016 Feb;15(2):197-204. PubMed PMID: 26885788.

221. Eichenfield LF, Lain T, Frankel EH, Jones TM, Chang-Lin JE, Berk DR, Ruan S, Kaoukhov A. Efficacy and Safety of Once-Daily Dapsone Gel, 7.5% for Treatment of Adolescents and Adults With Acne Vulgaris: Second of Two Identically

Designed, Large, Multicenter, Randomized, Vehicle-Controlled Trials. J Drugs Dermatol. 2016 Aug 1;15(8):962-9. PubMed PMID: 27537997.

222. Taylor SC, Cook-Bolden FE, McMichael A, Downie JB, Rodriguez DA, Alexis AF, Callender VD, Alvandi N. Efficacy, Safety, and Tolerability of Topical Dapsone Gel, 7.5% for Treatment of Acne Vulgaris by Fitzpatrick Skin Phototype. J Drugs Dermatol. 2018 Feb 1;17(2):160-167. PubMed PMID: 29462223.

223. Jarratt MT, Jones TM, Chang-Lin JE, Tong W, Berk DR, Lin V, Kaoukhov A. Safety and Pharmacokinetics of Once-Daily Dapsone Gel, 7.5% in Patients With Moderate Acne Vulgaris. J Drugs Dermatol. 2016 Oct 1;15(10):1250-1259. PubMed PMID: 27741344.

224. Al-Salama ZT, Deeks ED. Dapsone 7.5% Gel: A Review in Acne Vulgaris. Am J Clin Dermatol. 2017 Feb;18(1):139-145. doi: 10.1007/s40257-016-0242-0. Review. PubMed PMID: 28005194.

225. DraelosZD, Rodriguez DA, Kempers SE, Bruce S, Peredo MI, Downie J, Chang-Lin JE, Berk DR, Ruan S, Kaoukhov A. Treatment Response With Once-Daily Topical Dapsone Gel, 7.5% for Acne Vulgaris: Subgroup Analysis of Pooled Data from Two Randomized, Double-Blind Stu. J Drugs Dermatol. 2017 Jun 1;16(6):591-598. PubMed PMID: 28686777.

226. TanghettiE, Harper J, Baldwin H, Kircik L, Bai Z, Alvandi N. Once-Daily Topical Dapsone Gel, 7.5%: Effective for Acne Vulgaris Regardless of Baseline Lesion Count, With Superior Efficacy in Females. J Drugs Dermatol. 2018 Nov 1;17(11):1192-1198. PubMed PMID: 30500139.

227. Bissonnette R, Poulin Y, Drew J, Hofland H, Tan J. Olumacostatglasaretil, a novel topical sebum inhibitor, in the treatment of acne vulgaris: A phase IIa, multicenter, randomized, vehicle-controlled study. J Am Acad Dermatol. 2017 Jan;76(1):33-39. doi: 10.1016/j.jaad.2016.08.053. Epub 2016 Oct 28. PubMed PMID: 28029390.

228. Melnik BC. OlumacostatGlasaretil, a Promising Topical Sebum-Suppressing Agent that Affects All Major Pathogenic Factors of Acne Vulgaris. J Invest Dermatol. 2017 Jul;137(7):1405-1408. doi: 10.1016/j.jid.2017.01.026. Review. PubMed PMID: 28647025.

229. Endly DC, Miller RA. Oily Skin: A review of Treatment Options. J Clin Aesthet Dermatol. 2017 Aug;10(8):49-55. Epub 2017 Aug 1. Review. PubMed PMID: 28979664; PubMed Central PMCID: PMC5605215.

230. Afzali BM, Yaghoobi E, Yaghoobi R, Bagherani N, Dabbagh MA. Comparison of the efficacy of 5% topical spironolactone gel and placebo in the treatment of mild and moderate acne vulgaris: a randomized controlled trial. J Dermatolog Treat. 2012 Feb;23(1):21-5. doi: 10.3109/09546634.2010.488260. Epub 2010 Oct 22. PubMed PMID: 20964565.

231. Charny JW, Choi JK, James WD. Spironolactone for the treatment of acne in women, a retrospective study of 110 patients. Int J Womens Dermatol. 2017 Mar 13;3(2):111-115. doi: 10.1016/j.ijwd.2016.12.002. eCollection 2017 Jun. PubMed PMID: 28560306; PubMed Central PMCID: PMC5440451.

232. Trifu V, Tiplica GS, Naumescu E, Zalupca L, Moro L, Celasco G. Cortexolone 17α-propionate 1% cream, a new potent antiandrogen for topical treatment of

acne vulgaris. A pilot randomized, double-blind comparative study vs. placebo and tretinoin 0·05% cream. Br J Dermatol. 2011 Jul;165(1):177-83. doi: 10.1111/j.1365-2133.2011.10332.x.Epub 2011 Jun 2. PubMed PMID: 21428978.

233. Meingassner JG, Aschauer H, Winiski AP, Dales N, Yowe D, Winther MD, Zhang Z, Stütz A, Billich A. Pharmacological inhibition of stearoyl CoA desaturase in the skin induces atrophy of the sebaceous glands. J Invest Dermatol. 2013 Aug;133(8):2091-4. doi: 10.1038/jid.2013.89. Epub 2013 Feb 27. PubMed PMID: 23446987.

234. Rubinchik E, Dugourd D, Algara T, Pasetka C, Friedland HD. Antimicrobial and antifungal activities of a novel cationic antimicrobial peptide, omiganan, in experimental skin colonisation models. Int J Antimicrob Agents. 2009 Nov;34(5):457-61. doi: 10.1016/j.ijantimicag.2009.05.003. Epub 2009 Jun 12. PubMed PMID: 19524411.

235. Garner SE, Eady A, Bennett C, Newton JN, Thomas K, Popescu CM. Minocycline for acne vulgaris: efficacy and safety. Cochrane Database Syst Rev. 2012 Aug 15;(8):CD002086. doi: 10.1002/14651858.CD002086.pub2. Review. PubMed PMID: 22895927.

236. Gold LS, Dhawan S, Weiss J, Draelos ZD, Ellman H, Stuart IA. A novel topical minocycline foam for the treatment of moderate-to-severe acne vulgaris: Results of 2 randomized, double-blind, phase 3 studies. J Am Acad Dermatol. 2019 Jan;80(1):168-177. doi: 10.1016/j.jaad.2018.08.020. Epub 2018 Aug 27. PubMed PMID: 30165171.

237. Bonati LM, Dover JS. Treating Acne With Topical Antibiotics: Current Obstacles and the Introduction of Topical Minocycline as a New Treatment Option. J Drugs Dermatol. 2019 Mar 1;18(3):240-244. PubMed PMID: 30909327.

238. Jones TM, Ellman H, deVries T. Pharmacokinetic Comparison of Once-Daily Topical Minocycline Foam 4% vs Oral Minocycline for Moderate-to-Severe Acne. J Drugs Dermatol. 2017 Oct 1;16(10):1022-1028. PubMed PMID: 29036256.

239. Alexis A, Del Rosso JQ, Desai SR, Downie JB, Draelos ZD, Feser C, Forconi R, Fowler JF Jr, Gold M, Kaufman-Janette J, Lain E, Lee M, Ling M, Shamban AT, Werschler WP, Daniels A. BPX-01 Minocycline Topical Gel Shows Promise for the Treatment of Moderate-to-severe Inflammatory Acne Vulgaris. J Clin Aesthet Dermatol. 2018 Nov;11(11):25-35. Epub 2018 Nov 1. PubMed PMID: 30588271; PubMed Central PMCID: PMC6303111.

240. Jeong S, Hermsmeier M, Osseiran S, Yamamoto A, Nagavarapu U, Chan KF, Evans CL. Visualization of drug distribution of a topical minocycline gel in human facial skin. Biomed Opt Express. 2018 Jun 27;9(7):3434-3448. doi: 10.1364/BOE.9.003434. eCollection 2018 Jul 1. PubMed PMID: 29984108; PubMed Central PMCID: PMC6033575.

241. Oliveira JM, Sobreira G, Velosa J, Telles Correia D, Filipe P. Association of Isotretinoin With Depression and Suicide: A Review of Current Literature. J Cutan Med Surg. 2018 Jan/Feb;22(1):58-64. doi: 10.1177/1203475417719052. Epub 2017 Jul 14. Review. PubMed PMID: 28705050.

242. Huang YC, Cheng YC. Isotretinoin treatment for acne and risk of depression: A systematic review and meta-analysis. J Am Acad Dermatol. 2017 Jun;76(6):1068-

1076.e9. doi: 10.1016/j.jaad.2016.12.028. Epub 2017 Mar 11. Review. Erratum in: J Am Acad Dermatol. 2017 Nov 14;:. PubMed PMID: 28291553.

243. BotsaliA, Kocyigit P, Uran P. The Effects of Isotretinoin on Affective and Cognitive Functions are Disparate in Adolescent Acne Vulgaris Patients. J Dermatolog Treat. 2019 Apr 15:1-17. doi: 10.1080/09546634.2019.1606396. [Epub ahead of print] PubMed PMID: 30985218.

244. Charrow A, Xia FD, Lu J, Waul M, Joyce C, Mostaghimi A. Differences in isotretinoin start, interruption, and early termination across race and sex in the iPLEDGE era. PLoS One. 2019 Mar 26;14(3):e0210445. doi: 10.1371/journal.pone.0210445. eCollection 2019. PubMed PMID: 30913210; PubMed Central PMCID: PMC6435230.

245. Gómez-Flores M, Poletti-Vázquez DE, García-Hidalgo L, Fierro-Arias L, Herz-Ruelas M, Garza-Gómez J, Rosas-Ortiz JF. Second joint position paper: Use of isotretinoin in severe acne. Rev Med Inst Mex Seguro Soc. 2019 Jan 28;56(5):441-446. Spanish. PubMed PMID: 30777411.

246. SoyuduruG, ÖsoyAdışen E, KadıoğluÖzer İ, Aksakal AB. The effect of isotretinoin on insulin resistance and adipocytokine levels in acne vulgaris patients. Turk J Med Sci. 2019 Feb 11;49(1):238-244. doi: 10.3906/sag-1806-44. PubMed PMID: 30761880.

247. Van TLT, Minh PN, Thuy PTT, Gandolfi M, Satolli F, Feliciani C, Tirant M, Vojvodic A, Lotti T. Efficacy of Oral Low-Dose Isotretinoin in the Treatment of Acne Vulgaris in Vietnam. Open Access Maced J Med Sci. 2019 Jan 20;7(2):279-282. doi: 10.3889/oamjms.2019.094. eCollection 2019 Jan 30. PubMed PMID: 30745980; PubMed Central PMCID: PMC6364726.

248. Thomazini BF, Lamas CA, Dolder MAH. Safety of isotretinoin treatment as measured by liver parameters. HistolHistopathol. 2018 Dec 17:18075. doi: 10.14670/HH-18-075. [Epub ahead of print] PubMed PMID: 30556579.

249. FouladgarN, Khabazkhoob M, Hanifnia AR, Yekta A, Mirzajani A. Evaluation of the effects of isotretinoin for treatment of acne on corneal sensitivity. J CurrOphthalmol. 2018 Sep 6;30(4):326-329. doi: 10.1016/j.joco.2018.06.005. eCollection 2018 Dec. PubMed PMID: 30555965; PubMed Central PMCID: PMC6276732.

250. Kim NR, Yoon SR, Choi JS, Ahn HK, Lee SY, Hong DS, Yun JS, Hong SY, Kim YH, Han JY. Isotretinoin exposure in pregnant women in Korea. ObstetGynecol Sci. 2018 Nov;61(6):649-654. doi: 10.5468/ogs.2018.61.6.649. Epub 2018 Oct 12. PubMed PMID: 30474010; PubMed Central PMCID: PMC6236094.

251. TasliH, Yurekli A, Gokgoz MC, Karakoc O. Effects of oral isotretinoin therapy on the nasal cavities. Braz J Otorhinolaryngol. 2018 Nov 12. pii: S1808-8694(18)30253-2. doi: 10.1016/j.bjorl.2018.10.004. [Epub ahead of print] PubMed PMID: 30472003.

252. El Aziz Ragab MA, Omar SS, Collier A, El-Wafa RAHA, Gomaa N. The effect of continuous high versus low dose oral isotretinoin regimens on dermcidin expression in patients with moderate to severe acne vulgaris. Dermatol Ther. 2018 Nov;31(6):e12715. doi: 10.1111/dth.12715. Epub 2018 Nov 5. PubMed PMID: 30397984.

253. Nakano T, Yoshino T, Fujimura T, Arai S, Mukuno A, Sato N, Katsuoka K. Reduced expression of dermcidin, a peptide active against propionibacterium acnes, in sweat of patients with acne vulgaris. Acta DermVenereol. 2015 Sep;95(7):783-6. doi: 10.2340/00015555-2068. PubMed PMID: 25673161.
254. Ustun I, Rifaioglu EN, Sen BB, Inam MU, Gokce C. Gynecomastia: a rare complication of isoretinoin? CutanOculToxicol. 2013 Mar;32(1):93-4. doi: 10.3109/15569527.2012.705406. Epub 2012 Jul 20. PubMed PMID: 22813063.
255. Drugs and Lactation Database (LactMed) [Internet]. Bethesda (MD): National Library of Medicine (US); 2006-. Acitretin. [Updated 2019 Apr 1]. Available from: https://www.ncbi.nlm.nih.gov/books/NBK501367/
256. Drugs and Lactation Database (LactMed) [Internet]. Bethesda (MD): National Library of Medicine (US); 2006-. Isotretinoin. [Updated 2018 Dec 3]. Available from: https://www.ncbi.nlm.nih.gov/books/NBK501634/
257. Khiali S, Gharekhani A, Entezari-Maleki T. Isotretinoin; A review on the Utilization Pattern in Pregnancy. Adv Pharm Bull. 2018 Aug;8(3):377-382. doi: 10.15171/apb.2018.044. Epub 2018 Aug 29. Review. PubMed PMID: 30276133; PubMed Central PMCID: PMC6156490.
258. Albuquerque RG, Rocha MA, Bagatin E, Tufik S, Andersen ML. Could adult female acne be associated with modern life? Arch Dermatol Res. 2014 Oct;306(8):683-8. doi: 10.1007/s00403-014-1482-6. Epub 2014 Jun 21. Review. PubMed PMID: 24952024.
259. Chatzikonstantinou F, Miskedaki A, Antoniou C, Chatzikonstantinou M, Chrousos G, Darviri C. A novel cognitive stress management technique for acne vulgaris: a short report of a pilot experimental study. Int J Dermatol. 2019 Feb;58(2):218-220. doi: 10.1111/ijd.14227. Epub 2018 Sep 19. PubMed PMID: 30229883.
260. Jović A, Marinović B, Kostović K, Čeović R, Basta-Juzbašić A, BukvićMokos Z. The Impact of Pyschological Stress on Acne. Acta Dermatovenerol Croat. 2017 Jul;25(2):1133-141. Review. PubMed PMID: 28871928.
261. Yang YS, Lim HK, Hong KK, Shin MK, Lee JW, Lee SW, Kim NI. Cigarette smoke-induced interleukin-1 alpha may be involved in the pathogenesis of adult acne. Ann Dermatol. 2014 Feb;26(1):11-6. doi: 10.5021/ad.2014.26.1.11. Epub2014 Feb 17. PubMed PMID: 24648681; PubMed Central PMCID: PMC3956775.
262. Mohtady O. How Your Skin Changes When Your Smoke. Digital Therapeutics, Inc, SEPTEMBER 26, 2018.
263. Isvy-Joubert A, Nguyen JM, Gaultier A, Saint-Jean M, Le Moigne M, Boisrobert E, Khammari A, Dreno B. Adult female acne treated with spironolactone: a retrospective data review of 70 cases. Eur J Dermatol. 2017 Aug 1;27(4):393-398. doi: 10.1684/ejd.2017.3062. PubMed PMID: 28862134.
264. Barbieri JS, Choi JK, Mitra N, Margolis DJ. Frequency of Treatment Switching for Spironolactone Compared to Oral Tetracycline-Class Antibiotics for Women With Acne: A Retrospective Cohort Study 2010-2016. J Drugs Dermatol. 2018 Jun 1;17(6):632-638. PubMed PMID: 29879250.
265. Rocha MA, Bagatin E. Adult-onset acne: prevalence, impact, and management challenges. Clin CosmetInvestig Dermatol. 2018 Feb 1;11:59-69. doi:

10.2147/CCID.S137794. eCollection 2018. Review. PubMed PMID: 29440921; PubMed Central PMCID: PMC5798558.

266. Garthwaite SM, McMahon EG. The evolution of aldosterone antagonists. Mol Cell Endocrinol. 2004 Mar 31;217(1-2):27-31. PubMed PMID: 15134797.

267. Layton AM, Eady EA, Whitehouse H, Del Rosso JQ, Fedorowicz Z, van Zuuren EJ. Oral Spironolactone for Acne Vulgaris in Adult Females: A Hybrid Systematic Review. Am J Clin Dermatol. 2017 Apr;18(2):169-191. doi: 10.1007/s40257-016-0245-x. Review. PubMed PMID: 28155090; PubMed Central PMCID: PMC5360829.

268. Grandhi R, Alikhan A. Spironolactone for the Treatment of Acne: A 4-Year Retrospective Study. Dermatology. 2017;233(2-3):141-144. doi: 10.1159/000471799. Epub 2017 May 5. PubMed PMID: 28472793.

269. Amin K, Riddle CC, Aires DJ, Schweiger ES. Common and alternate oral antibiotic therapies for acne vulgaris: a review. J Drugs Dermatol. 2007 Sep;6(9):873-80. Review. PubMed PMID: 17941358.

270. Farrah G, Tan E. The use of oral antibiotics in treating acne vulgaris: a new approach. Dermatol Ther. 2016 Sep;29(5):377-384. doi: 10.1111/dth.12370. Epub 2016 Jun 16. Review. PubMed PMID: 27306750.

271. Zaenglein AL, Pathy AL, Schlosser BJ, Alikhan A, Baldwin HE, Berson DS, Bowe WP, Graber EM, Harper JC, Kang S, Keri JE, Leyden JJ, Reynolds RV, Silverberg NB, Stein Gold LF, Tollefson MM, Weiss JS, Dolan NC, Sagan AA, Stern M, Boyer KM, Bhushan R. Guidelines of care for the management of acne vulgaris. J Am Acad Dermatol. 2016 May;74(5):945-73.e33. doi: 10.1016/j.jaad.2015.12.037. Epub 2016 Feb 17. Review. PubMed PMID: 26897386.

272. Cross R, Ling C, Day NP, McGready R, Paris DH. Revisiting doxycycline in pregnancy and early childhood--time to rebuild its reputation? Expert Opin Drug Saf. 2016;15(3):367-82. doi: 10.1517/14740338.2016.1133584. Epub 2016 Jan 25. Review. PubMed PMID: 26680308; PubMed Central PMCID: PMC4898140.

273. Muanda FT, Sheehy O, Bérard A. Use of antibiotics during pregnancy and risk of spontaneous abortion. CMAJ. 2017 May 1;189(17):E625-E633. doi: 10.1503/cmaj.161020. PubMed PMID: 28461374; PubMed Central PMCID: PMC5415390.

274. Del Rosso JQ. Oral Doxycycline in the Management of Acne Vulgaris: Current Perspectives on Clinical Use and Recent Findings with a New Double-scored Small Tablet Formulation. J Clin Aesthet Dermatol. 2015 May;8(5):19-26. Review. PubMed PMID: 26029331; PubMed Central PMCID: PMC4445892.

275. Kim JE, Park AY, Lee SY, Park YL, Whang KU, Kim HJ. Comparison of the Efficacy of Azithromycin Versus Doxycycline in Acne Vulgaris: A Meta-Analysis of Randomized Controlled Trials. Ann Dermatol. 2018 Aug;30(4):417-426. doi: 10.5021/ad.2018.30.4.417. Epub 2018 Jun 28. PubMed PMID: 30065581; PubMed Central PMCID: PMC6029975.

276. Kapadia N, Talib A. Acne treated successfully with azithromycin. Int J Dermatol. 2004 Oct;43(10):766-7. PubMed PMID: 15485538.

Erythematous Surgical Scars: A Randomized, Controlled, Open-Label Study. Dermatol Surg. 2016 Jan;42(1):70-6. doi: 10.1097/DSS.0000000000000582. PubMed PMID: 26673432.

301. Tierney E, Mahmoud BH, Srivastava D, Ozog D, Kouba DJ. Treatment of surgical scars with nonablative fractional laser versus pulsed dye laser: a randomized controlled trial. Dermatol Surg. 2009 Aug;35(8):1172-80. doi: 10.1111/j.1524-4725.2009.01085.x.Epub 2009 Feb 23. PubMed PMID: 19250300.

302. Tierney EP, Eisen RF, Hanke CW. Fractionated CO2 laser skin rejuvenation. Dermatol Ther. 2011 Jan-Feb;24(1):41-53. doi: 10.1111/j.1529-8019.2010.01377.x. Review. PubMed PMID: 21276157.

303. Alexiades-Armenakas MR, Dover JS, Arndt KA. The spectrum of laser skin resurfacing: nonablative, fractional, and ablative laser resurfacing. J Am Acad Dermatol. 2008 May;58(5):719-37; quiz 738-40. doi: 10.1016/j.jaad.2008.01.003. PubMed PMID: 18423256.

304. You HJ, Kim DW, Yoon ES, Park SH. Comparison of four different lasers for acne scars: Resurfacing and fractional lasers. J PlastReconstrAesthet Surg. 2016 Apr;69(4):e87-95. doi: 10.1016/j.bjps.2015.12.012. Epub 2016 Jan 7. PubMed PMID: 26880620.

305. Fox L, Csongradi C, Aucamp M, du Plessis J, Gerber M. Treatment Modalities for Acne. Molecules. 2016 Aug 13;21(8). pii: E1063. doi: 10.3390/molecules 21081063. Review. PubMed PMID: 27529209; PubMed Central PMCID: PMC6273829.

306. Lemay A, Poulin Y. Oral contraceptives as anti-androgenic treatment of acne. J ObstetGynaecol Can. 2002 Jul;24(7):559-67. Review. PubMed PMID: 12196847.

www.ingramcontent.com/pod-product-compliance
Ingram Content Group UK Ltd.
Pitfield, Milton Keynes, MK11 3LW, UK
UKHW062155030826
14089UKWH00025B/28

9 789390 211340